Medical Radiology

Radiation Oncology

Series editors

Luther W. Brady
Hans-Peter Heilmann
Michael Molls
Carsten Nieder

For further volumes:
http://www.springer.com/series/4353

Carsten Nieder • Laurie E. Gaspar
Editors

Decision Tools for Radiation Oncology

Prognosis, Treatment Response and Toxicity

Springer

Editors
Carsten Nieder
Department of Oncology
Nordland Hospital Trust Bodø
University of Tromsø
Bodø
Norway

Laurie E. Gaspar
Department of Radiation Oncology
School of Medicine
University of Colorado
Aurora, CO
USA

ISSN 0942-5373 ISSN 2197-4187 (electronic)
ISBN 978-3-642-37101-1 ISBN 978-3-642-37102-8 (eBook)
DOI 10.1007/978-3-642-37102-8
Springer Heidelberg New York Dordrecht London

Library of Congress Control Number: 2014933277

Printed on acid-free paper

Springer is part of Springer Science+Business Media (www.springer.com)

Foreword

"Decision Tools for Radiation Oncology: Prognosis, Treatment Response, and Toxicity," edited by Carsten Nieder and Laurie E. Gaspar, searches the literature for common databases, reviewing the steadily increasing number of nomograms along with prognostic models. It represents a logical addition to the prior publications in this series—"Radiation Oncology: An Evidence-Based Approach" edited by Jiade J. Lu and Luther W. Brady and the subsequent two volumes, "Decision Making in Radiation Oncology," also edited by Jiade J. Lu and Luther W. Brady.

The volume by Nieder and Gaspar expands on the risk of relapse and the biology of the various cancer sites with an emphasis on lymphatic, vascular, and perineural spread of each cancer site, as well as the toxicities from treatment and their relationship to survival. It also examines pathology and gene signatures, as well as clinical data useful in computing the models.

The book explores trends toward individualized treatment concepts and underscores the importance of a balance between treatment effectiveness and side effects. It highlights the use of underlying prognostic expertise to ensure the effective utilization of resources, helping to avoid lengthy treatment for patients with potential short-term survival expectation. Therefore, it is mandatory that a firm understanding of limits in prognostic and predictive models precedes clinical implementation.

This volume represents a major contribution towards a comprehensive overview of key decision-making tools for Radiation Oncology. It will greatly help physicians to make informed choices in daily clinical practice and follow-up. In combination with the Lu/Brady volumes, it establishes critical foundations for future new tools in oncology. All volumes should be in the library of the practicing oncologist.

Luther W. Brady
Hans-Peter Heilmann
Michael Molls

Preface

Practicing radiation oncologists have to make several important decisions during treatment planning and realization, one patient at a time. Questions such as "is radiotherapy indicated, what is the optimal dose/fractionation regimen, what is the optimal technique and dose distribution, what are the risks and side effects" have to be addressed. This is often done in larger multidisciplinary teams, and ideally based on solid scientific evidence. Compared to earlier decades, we have now an incredibly large tool box, allowing for assessment of tumor biology and its surrogates, imaging biomarkers, host genetics, and dynamic tumor changes during treatment, to name a few. New research adding to these fields is being presented at each of the major international oncology meetings, including but not limited to prognostic scores and nomograms. It is critical to appraise the methodological strengths and weaknesses of such research and to put into context established decision tools.

The purpose of this book is to provide practicing radiation oncologists, as well as those in training, with a concise overview of the most important and up-to-date information pertaining to general and diagnosis-specific decision tools including staging systems. We strongly recommend starting with the introductory chapters, which provide necessary background information on statistical methods, principles of biomarker development, gene expression analyses, and other topics that are crucial for those who want to fully understand the applicability and limitations of prediction tools. Going towards increasingly individualized cancer therapy, we still need to rely on systematic evidence and sound treatment algorithms.

We are most grateful for the enthusiasm and courtesy all chapter authors showed during preparation of this truly international volume and for the fruitful discussion with many colleagues. We also appreciate the excellent support from the publisher. We hope that the reader will find this book to be a useful summary of new or refined decision tools and how they contribute to state-of-the-art radiation therapy. Only continued basic and clinical research will provide a better basis for tolerable and efficacious treatment regimens, exploiting the promises put forward by the emerging concepts of personalized medicine and adaptive radiation therapy.

Carsten Nieder
Laurie E. Gaspar

Contents

Contributors

Thomas B. Brunner Department of Radiation Oncology, University Hospital Freiburg, Freiburg, Germany

Hale Basak Caglar Department of Radiation Oncology, Acibadem University, Istanbul, Turkey

Francesc Casas Department of Radiation Oncology, University Clinic, Barcelona, Spain

Lynn Chang Department of Radiation Oncology, Fox Chase Cancer Center, Philadelphia, PA, USA

Joanna Y. Chin Harvard Radiation Oncology Program, Boston, MA, USA

Edward Chow Rapid Response Radiotherapy Program, Department of Radiation Oncology, University of Toronto, Odette Cancer Centre, Sunnybrook Health Sciences Centre, Toronto, ON, Canada

Andrea Damiani External consultant, Catholic University of Sacred Heart, Rome, Italy

Andre Dekker Department of Radiation Oncology (MAASTRO), GROW–School for Oncology and Developmental Biology, Maastricht University Medical Center (MUMC+), Maastricht, The Netherlands

Thomas F. DeLaney Connective Tissue Oncology Center, Francis H. Burr Proton Therapy Center, Radiation Oncology, Massachusetts General Hospital, Boston, MA, USA

Nicola Dinapoli Department of Radiotherapy, Pol. A. Gemelli, Catholic University of Sacred Heart, Rome, Italy

Juergen Dunst Department of Radiation Oncology, University Clinic Schleswig-Holstein, Kiel, Germany

Robert L. Eil Department of Surgery, Oregon Health & Science University, Portland, OR, USA

Nenad Filipovic BioIRC Centre for Bioengineering, Kragujevac, Serbia

Christine M. Fisher University of Colorado Cancer Center, Aurora, CO, USA

Anthony Fyles Department of Radiation Oncology, Princess Margaret Cancer Centre, University of Toronto, Toronto, ON, Canada

Laurie E. Gaspar University of Colorado, Denver, CO, USA

Meredith Elana Giuliani Department of Radiation Oncology, Princess Margaret Cancer Centre, University of Toronto, Toronto, Ontario, Canada

Susan A. Higgins Department of Therapeutic Radiology, Yale University School of Medicine, New Haven, CT, USA

Andrew J. Hope Department of Radiation Oncology, Princess Margaret Cancer Centre, University of Toronto, Toronto, Ontario, Canada

Branislav Jeremic Division of Radiation and Clinical Oncology, Stellenbosch University and Tygerberg Hospital, Cape Town, South Africa

Ping Jiang Department of Radiation Oncology, University Clinic Schleswig-Holstein, Kiel, Germany

Lisa A. Kachnic Department of Radiation Oncology, Boston Medical Center, Boston University School of Medicine, Boston, MA, USA

Chris R. Kelsey Duke Cancer Institute, Duke University Medical Center, Durham, NC, USA

Nataliya Kovalchuk Department of Radiation Oncology, Boston Medical Center, Boston University School of Medicine, Boston, MA, USA

Christine F. Lauro Department of Radiation Oncology, University of Colorado Denver, Aurora, CO, USA

Trevor Leong Division of Radiation Oncology, Peter MacCallum Cancer Centre, Melbourne, VIC, Australia

William P. Levin Department of Radiation Oncology, Abramson Cancer Center, Hospital of the University of Pennsylvania, Philadelphia, PA, USA

Kenneth Li Department of Clinical Oncology, Queen Elizabeth Hospital, Hong Kong SAR, China

Nina A. Mayr Department of Radiation Oncology, University of Washington School of Medicine, Seattle, WA, USA

Florence Mok Department of Clinical Oncology, Prince of Wales Hospital, Hong Kong SAR, China

Carsten Nieder Department of Oncology and Palliative Medicine, Nordland Hospital, Bodø, Norway; Faculty of Health Sciences, Institute of Clinical Medicine, University of Tromsø, Tromsø, Norway

Jacqueline Payton Department of Pathology and Immunology, Washington University School of Medicine in St. Louis, St. Louis, MO, USA

Cordula Petersen Department of Radiotherapy and Radiooncology, University Medical Center Hamburg-Eppendorf, Hamburg, Germany

Michael Poon Rapid Response Radiotherapy Program, Department of Radiation Oncology, University of Toronto, Odette Cancer Centre, Sunnybrook Health Sciences Centre, Toronto, ON, Canada

Marko Popovic Rapid Response Radiotherapy Program, Department of Radiation Oncology, University of Toronto, Odette Cancer Centre, Sunnybrook Health Sciences Centre, Toronto, ON, Canada

Rachel A. Rabinovitch University of Colorado Cancer Center, Aurora, CO, USA

Ramachandran Rashmi Department of Radiation Oncology, Washington University School of Medicine in St. Louis, St. Louis, MO, USA

Danielle Rodin Rapid Response Radiotherapy Program, Department of Radiation Oncology, University of Toronto, Odette Cancer Centre, Sunnybrook Health Sciences Centre, Toronto, ON, Canada

Tracey E. Schefter Department of Radiation Oncology, University of Colorado Denver, Aurora, CO, USA

Rudolf Schwarz Department of Radiotherapy and Radiooncology, University Medical Center Hamburg-Eppendorf, Hamburg, Germany

Julie K. Schwarz Department of Radiation Oncology, Washington University School of Medicine in St. Louis, St. Louis, MO, USA; Department of Cell Biology and Physiology, Washington University School of Medicine in St. Louis, St. Louis, MO, USA

Paul W. Sperduto Minneapolis Radiation Oncology, University of Minnesota, Gamma Knife Center, Minneapolis, MN, USA

Maria A. Thomas Department of Radiation Oncology, Washington University School of Medicine in St. Louis, St. Louis, MO, USA

Charles R. Thomas Jr. Department Radiation Medicine, Oregon Health & Science University, Portland, OR, USA

J. Torres-Roca Department of Radiation Oncology, H Lee Moffitt Cancer Center, Tampa, FL, USA

Vincenzo Valentini Department of Radiotherapy, Pol. A. Gemelli, Catholic University of Sacred Heart, Rome, Italy

F. E. M. Voncken Department of Radiotherapy, The Netherlands Cancer Institute-Antoni van Leeuwenhoek Hospital, Amsterdam, The Netherlands

Luhua Wang Department of Radiation Oncology, Chinese Medical Academy of Sciences, Beijing, China

Stephanie E. Weiss Department of Radiation Oncology Fox Chase Cancer Center, Chief of Adult Brain Tumors Radiotherapy and Radiosurgery, Philadelphia, PA, USA

Lynn D. Wilson Department of Therapeutic Radiology, Yale University School of Medicine, New Haven, CT, USA

Erin Wong Rapid Response Radiotherapy Program, Department of Radiation Oncology, University of Toronto, Odette Cancer Centre, Sunnybrook Health Sciences Centre, Toronto, ON, Canada

Melissa R. Young Department of Therapeutic Radiology, Yale University School of Medicine, New Haven, CT, USA

William Yuh Department of Diagnostic Radiology, University of Washington School of Medicine, Seattle, WA, USA

Imran Zoberi Department of Radiation Oncology, Washington University School of Medicine in St. Louis, St. Louis, MO, USA

Introduction to Decision Tools

Meredith Elana Giuliani, Andrew J. Hope, and Anthony Fyles

Contents

Abstract

Decision tools are becoming critical to medical decision-making, due to the complexity of available information that outstrips the capacity to synthesize it without assistance. Tools such as decision trees, algorithms and nomograms may be used to facilitate treatment decisions, evaluating endpoints such as survival and toxicity. Incorporation of biologic and molecular data is increasingly being used in decision-making in cancer, for example in selecting systemic therapies, and will soon be expanded to include decisions about radiotherapy and surgery. Health technology is an integral part of decision tools development, allowing rapid access to data and distributed access to users. However, the limitations in the development and use of decision tools must be recognized, and solutions developed to facilitate their widespread implementation and improve healthcare outcomes.

The practice of medicine, and oncology specifically, is increasingly complex (Lenfant 2003; Davenport and Glaser 2002). Modern decision making in medicine requires the synthesis of multiple sources of information to make evidence based treatment decisions (Alper et al. 2004). With advances in genomics and proteomics these decision processes will likely become more complicated. In the near future, the amount of information available on any individual case will likely outreach human capacity to comprehend and synthesize without assistance.

Decision analysis is a discipline which aims to give a person, in a formal manner, insight into all facets of a problem which should influence the final decision (Hunink and Glasziou 2011). Decision analysis uses tools to identify, represent and assess all aspects of a decision (Skanes et al. 2012). These tools (i.e. decision tools) come in many different formats. For example, a decision tree is a visual representation of all the options and consequences that

M. E. Giuliani · A. J. Hope · A. Fyles (✉)
Department of Radiation Oncology,
Princess Margaret Cancer Centre,
University of Toronto, 610 University Avenue,
Toronto, Ontario M5G 2M9, Canada
e-mail: Anthony.Fyles@rmp.uhn.on.ca

C. Nieder and L. E. Gaspar (eds.), *Decision Tools for Radiation Oncology*, Medical Radiology. Radiation Oncology,
DOI: 10.1007/174_2013_843, © Springer-Verlag Berlin Heidelberg 2013
Published Online: 30 June 2013

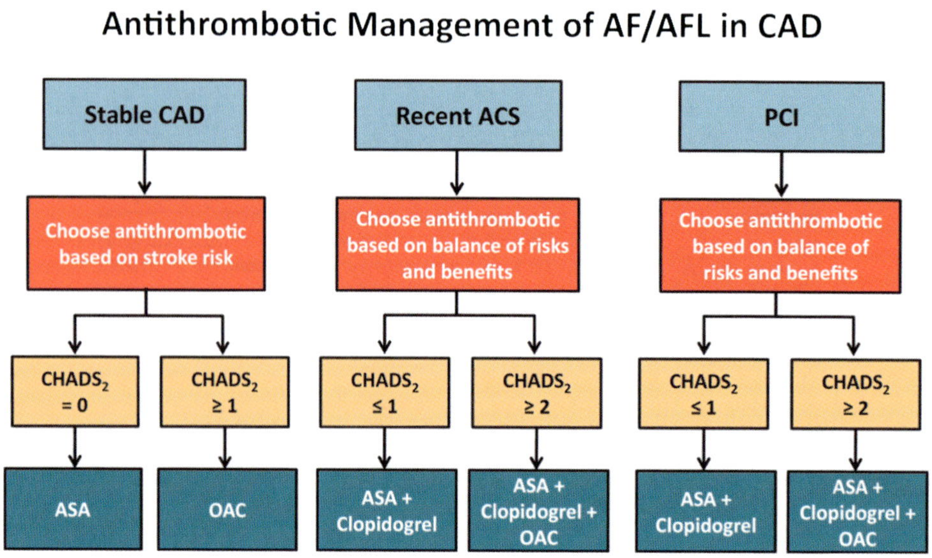

Fig. 1 An example of a clinical algorithm decision tool. Reprinted from Kanes et al. (2012), with permission from Elsevier

may follow each option (Hunink and Glasziou 2011). A clinical algorithm is a visual representation of a series of questions and subsequent actions which are based on answers to the questions (Hunink and Glasziou 2011). Figure 1 is an example of a clinical algorithm for anti-thrombotic therapy in patients with atrial fibrillation (Skanes et al. 2012). The aim of such decision tools is to keep all options for any given scenario in a broad perspective (Hunink and Glasziou 2011). Decision tools can also provide the health care professional with a consistent and reproducible process for estimating clinical outcomes, and provide the patient with definitive data on which to base a treatment decision. Nomograms are a graphical representation of a multivariable model that are often used in oncology for this purpose. In oncology it is not uncommon to use web-based nomograms as decision tools to give detailed information on risks of relapse and benefits of therapy to physicians and patients. More difficult is determining the patient's preference for treatment, and tolerance of side effects and/or preferences regarding quality-of-life vs. survival. Multi-criteria decision analysis techniques are one possible method to account for such diverse factors in decision making (Miot et al. 2012).

It is essential to understand the distinction between prognostic and predictive factors before one begins a discussion of the benefits and pitfalls of decisions tools. The distinction between these two terms is challenging for some individuals and can be misused (Italiano 2011). A prognostic factor is a "clinical or biologic characteristic that is objectively measurable and that provides information on the likely outcome of the cancer disease in an untreated individual" (Italiano 2011). In oncology prognostic factors such a tumor stage are used to identify patients at highest risk of relapse. Prognostic factors are used to determine the appropriate course of management.

In contrast, a predictive factor is a "clinical or biologic characteristic that provides information on the likely benefit from treatment (either in terms of tumor shrinkage or survival)" (Italiano 2011). In oncology predictive factors are used to identify sub-populations of patients who may benefit from a particular treatment such as hormone receptor status (ER/PR) in the use of adjuvant hormone therapy for breast cancer patients (Bast et al. 2001). In cardiology, hypertension and older age are predictive factors for stroke risk in patients with atrial fibrillation. A combination of predictive factors may be combined in a tool to determine the needs for anticoagulation therapy (Skanes et al. 2012).

Predictive and prognostic factors play a role in many diseases. For instance, there are established and validated decision support tools in management of atrial fibrillation. Mr. Smith is a 57 year-old man with newly diagnosed atrial fibrillation. Using a decision support model, $CHADS_2$ index (Gage et al. 2001), his risks of stroke can be assessed relative to known prognostic and predictive factors including congestive heart failure, hypertension, age >75, diabetes mellitus and prior stroke or transient ischemic attack (Gage et al. 2001). This score is used to guide clinician decision making around the need for a type of oral anticoagulants (Gage et al. 2004). See Fig. 1.

1 Decision Tools to Predict Survival

Survival is often the most important clinical endpoint for any disease. Disease, by its nature, limits health and longevity, and interventions designed to combat the disease should create a measurable improvement in survival. As such, survival is the gold standard endpoint for Phase III clinical trials.

Survival is measured from the 'start' of a disease until the time the subject expires. As the actual starting time of a disease is often unknown, the usual practice is to measure survival from either the time of diagnosis or the time of definitive intervention. If diagnosis date is used, the issue of lead time bias may be encountered when diagnostic tests shift the time point when disease is detected thereby 'extending' survival when in fact, only the duration of detectable disease increases, not the duration of survival at the same point in the disease process (Rothman 2002). This can lead to errors in the application of predictive tools, as described below.

As it is not usually possible or desired to wait until all patients have reached the end of their life before assessing the result of a treatment, a running estimate of survival for a group is necessary. Outcomes estimates for patient groups are often created using the Kaplan–Meier survival estimate (Kaplan and Meier 1958). This statistical approach tracks patients from the time of diagnosis or treatment until death, but for patients who remain alive, their survival information is incorporated in a 'censored' fashion. This allows groups of patients with surviving members to contribute to estimates of survival. More advanced methods to estimate survival include competing risk models, which attempt to account for other non-disease related events, in predicting survival or other endpoints. This is similar to a disease-specific-survival approach and helps interpret the effects of a treatment on a disease when other disease processes may influence survival. In a sufficiently large random sample, these non-treatment related factors are thought to be balanced in each arm of the study, but in smaller studies, non-treatment related factors may be distributed unevenly and may bias the results. These methods allow this issue to be addressed statistically.

It is critical to note that survival estimates are just that, estimates for a population group, and applying these estimates to individual patients has uncertainties. With sufficient power, factors that contribute to survival may allow more careful estimation of patient survival, but never an exact prediction. This distinction is of critical importance in any decision support tool, as the purported goal of such a tool is to provide predictive capacity to previously opaque outcomes. The relative uncertainties and assumptions in a model of survival are required elements of any discussion that uses information from a decision support tool.

Mr. Smith's stroke risk above was calculated to be approximately 4 %, but if only 5 patients in the whole study were included in his sub-group, there may be a very wide confidence interval on that estimate which could put the risk as low as 1 % or as high as 9 %. This range of uncertainty is almost as large as the difference between a low-risk group and a high risk group, but only applies to Mr. Smith's subgroup because of the relative rarity of those factors in combination.

2 Predicting Toxicity

Toxicity prediction is more complicated than survival, largely due to the inherent challenges of defining exactly what constitutes a toxicity. Most large clinical trials employ the Common Toxicity Criteria espoused by the NCI, but this system tends to lump multiple symptoms into larger classifications (Trotti et al. 2003). Predictions of toxicity are enhanced by use of specific symptoms as the endpoint (Heemsbergen et al. 2006). Beyond that, the toxicities associated with treatment can change over time or as treatments themselves change (Yom et al. 2007). As such, any decision support tool that evaluates toxicity must define carefully the toxicity endpoint, the treatment details, and outcomes. Furthermore, the potential for toxicity must be weighed against the natural history of the disease being treated and expected outcomes from that disease (in cancer, often death).

In our atrial fibrillation example, the main toxicity of anti-thrombotic management is that of unanticipated hemorrhagic events, which can be fatal. Hemorrhagic risks increase with the severity of anticoagulation (aspirin (ASA) vs. ASA+clopidogrel vs. low dose dabigatran vs. high dose dabigatran, rivaroxaban, or warfarin. The HAS-BLED score (Pisters et al. 2010) uses factors of hypertension, abnormal liver or renal function, history of stroke/bleeding, labile INR, age >65, excess alcohol, or concomitant use of bleed promoting drugs. A HAS-BLED score allows clinicians to estimate risks of bleeding from 1 % (score 0–1) to 12.5 % (score 5) and has been validated in a hospitalized elderly population. Patients at high risk of bleeding events on this scale warrant increased monitoring. The risks of non-treatment (i.e.: stroke with significant associated deficits) remain greater than the risk of toxicity (i.e.: bleeding, with less deficits than stroke) but each individual case requires a decision which balances both risks.

Toxicity prediction is also complicated by the duration of toxicity (Trotti et al. 2007). Long term low level toxicity may be less tolerable than short duration high toxicity that resolves. Toxicity metrics that attempt to integrate the effects on lifetime symptom burden will become more relevant as longer term toxicity information becomes available. Estimates of 'uncomplicated control' where a patient has the ideal outcome of cure and survival without toxicity may become the ideal endpoint for future decision support tools. Combinations of toxicity and survival including 'complicated control', 'complicated failure', and 'uncomplicated failure' will become more common in decision support tools as these predictions are included. A risk: benefit contour is one possible mechanism to assist in decision making between toxicity and control (Shakespeare et al. 2001) (see Fig. 2).

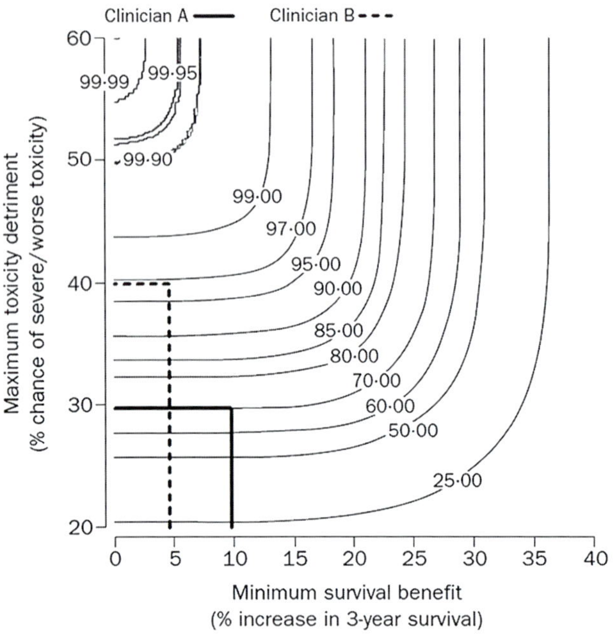

Fig. 2 A risk: benefit contour of toxicity versus survival. Confidence associated with absolute 3-year survival benefit and absolute toxicity detriment for chemoradiotherapy compared with radiotherapy alone. *Solid line* = clinician A; *dashed line* = clinician B. Reprinted from Shakespeare et al. (2001), with permission

3 Predicting Efficacy

Efficacy prediction focuses on the chance that a given treatment will prove effective in a given disease. Given the explosion of information regarding genotype and phenotypic response, nearly every treatment will soon have a myriad of factors which modulate or, in some cases, completely negate their effectiveness. Methods to incorporate biologic data into treatment choice are becoming standard for chemotherapy and targeted agents (Lau et al. 2007) and may soon apply to radiotherapy or surgical techniques as well. Again, the important endpoint when predicting efficacy is endpoint determination. For a cancer patient, efficacy can be defined as tumor shrinkage, increased survival, lack of progression, or even a change in patient reported outcomes of symptoms.

> Efficacy in patients with atrial fibrillation will be measured by multiple endpoints. First, the measure of anticoagulation (INR) which is associated with reduced risks of stroke or bleeding events. Other endpoints of interest may include 'rate of stroke' for a population or improvements in survival in patients with adequately adjusted INR.

An example for such a tool in oncology is Oncotype DxTM. OncotypeDxTM is a validated, complex genomic test which is used to predict breast-cancer recurrence in patients with early stage breast cancer (Cronin et al. 2007). The recurrence score generated by OncotypeDxTM is routinely used to guide clinician decision making around the use of adjuvant chemotherapy (Cronin et al. 2007).

4 Health Technology and Decision Tools

Health technology is an integral aspect in the use of decision tools. Health technology allows decision tools rapid access to data as well as facilitated distributed access to various tools.

One of the critical aspects of decision tool support is the integration with clinical records. Without the ability to access critical inputs, the decision support tools are limited. In addition, health technology can facilitie rapid and ubiquitous access to decision tools through the internet, such as the Memorial Sloan Kettering Prediction nomograms for prostate cancer recurrence risk (Memorial Sloan Kettering Cancer Centre 2013). Mobile health, or mHealth, technology can also place these decision tools at clinicians' fingertips through smart devices. Bioinformatics and health technology can allow multiple factors to be integrated into a decision tool beyond what could be accomplished in more simple decision tools. Such technology is essential to the development and clinical integration of genomic research but remains elusive due to logistical hurdles associated with gathering clinical information from many disparate clinical systems. Integrated health records systems with open standards to share relevant clinical information to decision support tools will be critical to implementing these tools in routine practice.

5 Drawbacks of Decision Tools

Decision support tools have risks and limitations, the most important of which is applicability. Each decision support tool is based on underlying data. If the tool's data does not apply to the situation the tool is used, then the decision support results may be incorrect. Worse, since the decision tool masks the underlying data, without careful understanding of the limitations of a given tool, there may not be a 'warning message'. For instance, changes in the time of disease detection can create a lead time bias which artificially inflates survival compared to survival estimates made from decision support tools that were generated in a previous diagnostic era. Another example would be changes in treatment methodology. If the type of intervention being applied has changes (surgical technique, medication, etc.), then the decision support tool may support an intervention that may cause harm, given the differences in underlying data.

Any decision support tool should describe the following limitations:

1. Describe the endpoints for the tool in detail.
2. Describe the population used to create the model.
3. Describe the intervention (in detail).
4. Describe the statistical uncertainty included in the prediction.

Validation of the decision tool is an important component of quality assurance for decision tools. External validation is ideal, although often not feasible. Kattan has argued that if the development dataset is large (over 1000 patients) internal validation using bootstrapping and other techniques may perform well (Kattan 2007). In the case of rare tumors with small datasets it may be difficult to find a validation cohort, therefore decisions about the benefits of the prediction model in the absence of validation must be made.

The widely used Adjuvant Online™ tool has been validated using a population-based cohort (Olivotto et al. 2005). However more recent validation efforts have highlighted the limitations as performance improved with the addition of biomarkers of proliferation and HER2 status. Thus the challenge in keeping decision tools up-to-date should not be underestimated, particularly in the era of rapidly expanding genetic and molecular prognostic and predictive factors.

6 Future Directions

Decision making in oncology involves sifting through a complicated mix of treatment uncertainties, patient preferences, risk of toxicities and costs. An optimal therapeutic ration balances these benefits and risks, modulated by the patient's preferences for therapeutic aggressiveness and tolerance for complications.

The widespread implementation of decision tools will result in the next wave of improved healthcare outcomes, akin to the improvements seen with adoption of treatments resulting from meta-analyses of large randomized trials in cancer. Development and implementation of validated online decision tools in medicine would be facilitated by one or more organizations that would allow providers and patients uniform evidence-based decisions about treatment and associated outcomes.

7 Organization of the Book

This chapter has served as an introduction to the concept of decision analysis and the tools used in this discipline. This volume will review the currently available decision tools, review their utility and pitfalls, and propose novel solutions incorporating upcoming genetic and other data that will be critical to optimal decision making in the future.

A site by site review of the existing clinical nomograms as well as the statistics which underpin the generation of survival data and the development of clinical nomograms, and prognostic and predictive factors for each cancer site will be presented. This book will provide a unique review of these important topics and pose pertinent questions which will underpin the future of oncology care.

References

Alper BS, Hand JA, Elliott SG et al (2004) How much effort is needed to keep up with the literature relevant for primary care? J Med Libr Assoc 92:429–437

Bast RC Jr, Ravdin P, Hayes DF et al (2001) 2000 update of recommendations for the use of tumor markers in breast and colorectal cancer: clinical practice guidelines of the American Society of Clinical Oncology. J Clin Oncol 19:1865–1878

Cronin M, Sangli C, Liu ML et al (2007) Analytical validation of the Oncotype DX genomic diagnostic test for recurrence prognosis and therapeutic response prediction in node-negative, estrogen receptor-positive breast cancer. Clin Chem 53:1084–1091

Davenport TH, Glaser J (2002) Just-in-time delivery comes to knowledge management. Harv Bus Rev 80:107–11

Gage BF, Waterman AD, Shannon W et al (2001) Validation of clinical classification schemes for predicting stroke: results from the National Registry of Atrial Fibrillation. JAMA 285: 2864–2870

Gage BF, van Walraven C, Pearce L et al (2004) Selecting patients with atrial fibrillation for anticoagulation: stroke risk stratification in patients taking aspirin. Circulation 110:2287–2292

Heemsbergen WD, Peeters ST, Koper PC et al (2006) Acute and late gastrointestinal toxicity after radiotherapy in prostate cancer patients: consequential late damage. Int J Radiat Oncol Biol Phys 66:3–10

Hunink M, Glasziou P (2011) Decision making in health and medicine. Cambridge University Press, New York

Italiano A (2011) Prognostic or predictive? It's time to get back to definitions! J Clin Oncol 29:4718 (author reply 4718–9)

Kanes AC, Healey JS, Cairns JA et al (2012) Focused 2012 update of the Canadian Cardiovascular Society atrial fibrillation guidelines: recommendations for stroke prevention and rate/rhythm control. Can J Cardiol 28:125–136

Kaplan EL, Meier P (1958) Nonparametric estimation from incomplete observations. J Am Stat Assoc 53:457–481

Kattan MW (2007) Outcome prediction in cancer. Elsevier, Oxford

Lau SK, Boutros PC, Pintilie M et al (2007) Three-gene prognostic classifier for early-stage non small-cell lung cancer. J Clin Oncol 25:5562–5569

Lenfant C (2003) Shattuck lecture—clinical research to clinical practice—lost in translation? N Engl J Med 349:868–874

Memorial Sloan Kettering Cancer Centre (2013) Prostate cancer nomograms. http://nomograms.mskcc.org/Prostate/PreTreatment.aspx. Accessed 1 Mar 2013

Miot J, Wagner M, Khoury H et al (2012) Field testing of a multicriteria decision analysis (MCDA) framework for coverage of a screening test for cervical cancer in South Africa. Cost Eff Resour Alloc 10:2

Olivotto IA, Bajdik CD, Ravdin PM et al (2005) Population-based validation of the prognostic model ADJUVANT! for early breast cancer. J Clin Oncol 23:2716–2725

Pisters R, Lane DA, Nieuwlaat R et al (2010) A novel user-friendly score (HAS-BLED) to assess 1-year risk of major bleeding in

patients with atrial fibrillation: the Euro Heart Survey. Chest 138:1093–1100
Rothman KJ (2002) Epidemiology: an introduction. Oxford University Press, New York
Shakespeare TP, Gebski VJ, Veness MJ et al (2001) Improving interpretation of clinical studies by use of confidence levels, clinical significance curves, and risk-benefit contours. Lancet 357:1349–1353
Skanes AC, Healey JS, Cairns JA et al (2012) Focused 2012 update of the Canadian cardiovascular society atrial fibrillation guidelines: recommendations for stroke prevention and rate/rhythm control. Can J Cardiol 28:125–136
Trotti A, Colevas AD, Setser A et al (2003) CTCAE v3.0: development of a comprehensive grading system for the adverse effects of cancer treatment. Semin Radiat Oncol 13:176–181
Trotti A, Pajak TF, Gwede CK et al (2007) TAME: development of a new method for summarising adverse events of cancer treatment by the Radiation Therapy Oncology Group. Lancet Oncol 8:613–624
Yom SS, Liao Z, Liu HH et al (2007) Initial evaluation of treatment-related pneumonitis in advanced-stage non-small-cell lung cancer patients treated with concurrent chemotherapy and intensity-modulated radiotherapy. Int J Radiat Oncol Biol Phys 68:94–102

Statistics of Survival Prediction and Nomogram Development

Vincenzo Valentini, Andrea Damiani, Andre Dekker, and Nicola Dinapoli

Contents

V. Valentini · N. Dinapoli (✉)
Department of Radiotherapy, Pol. A. Gemelli,
Catholic University of Sacred Heart, Rome, Italy
e-mail: nicola.dinapoli@rm.unicatt.it

A. Damiani
External consultant,
Catholic University of Sacred Heart,
Rome, Italy

A. Dekker
Department of Radiation Oncology (MAASTRO),
GROW–School for Oncology and Developmental Biology,
Maastricht University Medical Center (MUMC+),
Maastricht, The Netherlands

Abstract

Survival statistics are fundamental in outcome evaluation of clinical studies for modern cancer science. The use of survival statistics allows to compare results and to predict the effect of therapies, by using different statistical approaches that can be also combined together. Definition of survival statistics can be performed mainly in three different ways (Non-parametric-Kaplan-Meier, Parametric and Semi-parametric), each one having its own computational methods and being implemented in different ways. Modern cancer publications strengthen the value of diagnostic tools that can be used for predicting outcome of newly diagnosed patients. The nomograms are examples of these tools: they are usually drawn to facilitate physicians in manually solving complex equations required to calculate outcomes predicted by using Cox's proportional hazards models. The use of models to predict the outcome must follow adequate procedures for reliability evaluation and testing, in order to prevent the erroneous application on unsuitable patient populations.

1 Introduction: The Concept of "Survival"

The use of survival statisticsis a key topic for clinicians and oncologists, mainly because they are fundamental to evaluate the impact of treatments and therapies on patients. The measurements of 'survival' can be specified considering different endpoints, namely the outcome that a study tries to establish by using the survival statistics. The definition of 'survival' requires first of all to fix an observation starting point and finally a moment that is the 'survival time'. The most important difference between 'survival' data and other types of numerical continuous data (e.g. age, hemoglobin level, weight etc.) is that the event occurring (death, local recurrence, metastases onset etc.) is not necessarily

C. Nieder and L. E. Gaspar (eds.), *Decision Tools for Radiation Oncology*, Medical Radiology. Radiation Oncology,
DOI: 10.1007/174_2013_854, © Springer-Verlag Berlin Heidelberg 2013
Published Online: 6 July 2013

Table 1 Summary of the most common survival endpoints used in oncology

Survival endpoints				
Endpoint	Power	Initial event	Final event	Biases
Overall survival (OS)	Very high	Diagnosis time Clinical trial enrollment (for randomized controlled trials)	Death	Other than cancer death causes
Disease specific survival (DSS)	High	Diagnosis time Clinical trial enrollment (for randomized controlled trials)	Cancer death	The definition of 'cancer related death' in some cases could be questionable (e.g. suicide in cancer patient)
Disease free survival (DFS)	High	End of primary cancer treatment	Local relapse or metastases onset	Definition of 'complete response' and 'local relapse' or 'metastases' findings influenced by diagnostic times and imaging interpretation
Metastases free survival (MFS)	Average	Diagnosis time Clinical trial enrollment (for randomized controlled trials)	Distant metastasis finding	Definition of 'metastases' findings influenced by diagnostic times and imaging interpretation
Local control (LC)	Average	End of primary cancer treatment	Local relapse	Definition of 'complete response' and 'local relapse' findings influenced by diagnostic times and imaging interpretation
Progression free survival (PFS)	Poor	End of (primary) cancer treatment	Progression finding	Adequate diagnostic definition of 'progression' according to pre-defined criteria (RECIST 1.1), diagnostic times

observed in all subjects, while all subjects are followed for a time that can be lower or higher according to the start of the observation and the time of the last follow-up or event. The weight and the clinical impact of survival statistics strictly depend from the chosen outcome, because different survival endpoints may be affected by different confounding factors influencing the final observations of clinicians involved in the research data collection.

According to the type of the study and the observed population there are many different types of survival outcomes that can be analyzed. Not all outcomes have the same *power significance* from a clinical point of view: finding differences in the overall survival (OS) in a study population compared to another outcome is always considered the best way for finalizing the need to select patients for a given type of therapy, but it is not always possible to get significant differences in OS. In Table 1 the most common survival endpoints in oncology have been summarized. In many cases the use of another kind of 'response' to the treatment, defined by using shared and well defined *evaluation criteria* (Eisenhauer et al. 2009), could be used.

As previously stated the collection of survival data has to consider the possibility that patients can show the event at a given time after the start, but it is also possible that during the observation time a patient does not show the event, or in other cases the patients could be 'lost' during follow up. The survival statistics have the possibility to take into account all these situations: usually, when compiling survival tables in statistical software packages, observers indicate the presence of the event at a given time using the number '1', if the patient does not show the event at the time of last follow up this condition is indicated by the number '0'. These cases are usually indicated as '*censored*', because as in a census the survival data are updated by considering the condition of the whole observed population at a given moment. Patients lost on follow up should be excluded from the analysis, by assigning them a conventional value (e.g. '−1') that the statistical software simply will not consider for the survival analysis or they can be considered simply as censored at the time of last follow up. However, using this last method, the possibility to decrease the median follow up time for a whole patient cohort could be higher, because the follow up time of the lost patients will not be further updated moving far from the beginning of the accrual. For other kinds of statistical analysis (that do not consider the survival time) having these patients at one's disposal could be still useful, so they should not be deleted completely from the data collection tables.

The survival analyses can be performed mainly in three different ways that will be described in the three following sections:

1. Non parametric analysis —Kaplan-Meier: a model describing the observed survival outcome(s) (without underlying parameters).
2. Parametric analysis —Exponential, Weibull: models using *parameters* to describe and calculate the survival by a mathematical function that fits the survival data.
3. Semi-parametric analysis—Cox's Proportional Hazards Model (CPHM): a model that allows to *calculate* the

Table 2 Data for Kaplan Meier survival curve definition

Kaplan-Meier data table						
1	2	3	4	5	6	7
Rank i	Overall Survival time t	Status (observed events) d	FUP Status d_{fup}	No. Patient at risk n	Proportion of surviving patients at each step i: with $d_i = 1 \Rightarrow p_i = 1 - \frac{d_i}{n_i}$ with $d_i = 0 \Rightarrow p_i = p_{i-1}$	Overall surviving fraction at time t: with $d_i = 1 \Rightarrow S_i = p_i \cdot S_{i-1}$ with $d_i = 0 \Rightarrow S_i = S_{i-1}$
1	1	0	1	20	1.000000	1.000000
2	2	1	0	19	0.947368	0.947368
3	2	0	1	19	0.947368	0.947368
4	3	0	1	17	0.947368	0.947368
5	4	1	0	16	0.937500	0.888158
6	6	0	1	15	0.937500	0.888158
7	8	1	0	14	0.928571	0.824718
8	9	0	1	13	0.928571	0.824718
9	9	1	0	13	0.923077	0.761278
10	10	1	0	11	0.909091	0.692071
11	11	0	1	10	0.909091	0.692071
12	12	0	1	9	0.909091	0.692071
13	13	1	0	8	0.875000	0.605562
14	14	1	0	7	0.857143	0.519053
15	15	0	1	6	0.857143	0.519053
16	16	0	1	5	0.857143	0.519053
17	18	1	0	4	0.750000	0.389290
18	22	0	1	3	0.750000	0.389290
19	23	1	0	2	0.500000	0.194645
20	24	0	1	1	0.500000	0.194645

The height of the *steps* in the curve is given by the values calculated in the column 7. The mathematical procedure to achieve these values is given by the formulas in the header of the columns

expected survival for a single subject by using specific parameters *and* observational survival data (*baseline hazard*).

2 Non-Parametric Analysis: Kaplan-Meier

The Kaplan-Meier (KM) survival curves represent the visual description of the survival phenomenon in a given patient population. The creation of these curves requires first of all the collection of survival times and the status of the patients, split in *censored* (not checked endpoint) and patients with *checked endpoint*. In Table 2 an example of data collection is shown: the *censored* patients are shown in column 3 using the number 0, while the *checked* ones (patients showing the *event*) using the number 1. The related KM survival curve is shown in Fig. 1. In KM survival curves the proportion of surviving patients in a given population is shown, step by step, and the height of the steps is proportional to the number of patients showing the occurring event (death, local relapse, metastases finding etc.) during follow up time and inversely proportional to the number of subjects *at risk* at the moment of the event. In column 7 of Table 2 each step contributing to the graph appearance is calculated. A typical aspect of a KM survival curve is given by the height of the steps, which grows moving away from the beginning of the observation time. This is a consequence of the fact that each step represents a single patient for whom the event occurs at a definite time, while the small vertical lines along the horizontal segments of the curve represent the *censored* patients. The absolute number of remaining patients after a sequence of occurred events is increasingly smaller, so being the fraction of each patient showing the event over the number of remaining patients consistently larger ($1/n_i$), and finally being represented by a longer vertical segment in the curve.

When the patient with the highest follow up time shows the event '1' the KM curve falls to 0 in the value of Survival Probability, and generally events in the rightmost part of the curve seem more effective at influencing the outcome than

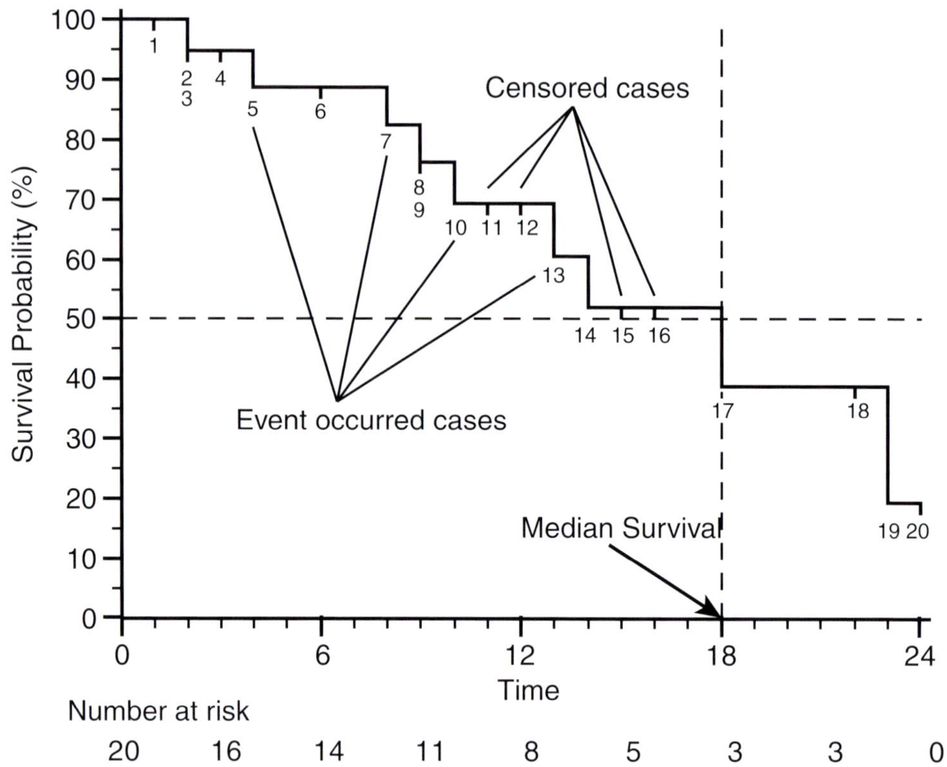

Fig. 1 Example of Kaplan-Meier survival curve: labels show the events and the censored cases, the *dashed lines* show how to calculate the median survival of the case series, by drawing a line that moves from the value of 50 % of survival probability to a vertical step in the curve, and drawing a second line that drops down to the timeline. In the line below the graph the value of the number at risk is shown every 3 months in the timeline

events in the leftmost part. Researchers have to be very careful in selecting adequate follow up times to be displayed and the number of patients in order to prevent unreliable behaviors shown by KM survival curves, which could lead readers to incorrect conclusions. Another feature that can be easily obtained by the KM survival curves is the *median survival*. In Fig. 1 it has been found by drawing a horizontal line starting from the 50 % of survival probability on the vertical axis and finding the intersection with a vertical segment of the curve, the value of the median survival is given by the intersection of a vertical line starting from this segment with the horizontal axis. Despite the value of the median survival, which is widely reported in literature, it is important to point out that it is not always a good indicator to compare different treatments administered to different patients cohorts. Furthermore the impact of median follow up time and the shape of the KM survival curve should always be considered together. A basic but good tool to achieve a summary is the possibility, provided by many statistical software packages, to add under the *x* axis of the graph the '*number at risk*' at regular intervals (also shown in Fig. 1). The 'number at risk' is defined as the number of patients who are known not to have experienced some *event* at that time-point nor having been censored before the time-point: as a rule of thumb the curve can be particularly unreliable when the number of patients remaining at risk is less than 15 (Machin et al. 2006).

Another critical topic in the evaluation of KM survival curves is the evaluation of follow up maturity, and this is usually reported by indicating the *median follow up time* (MFUP). Different ways for calculating the MFUP have been proposed but the most widely used is the one using the '*reverse Kaplan-Meier*' estimation of the OS (Schemper and Smith 1996): patients still alive (censored) are patients for whom the follow up time is known, while for patients that experienced death we cannot know if there would have been further follow up after the time of death. So the solution is to create a column in the statistical software that swaps the value of the overall survival endpoint, setting '1' for censored patients ('0' in the column of the overall survival status) and '0' for dead patients ('1' in the column of the overall survival status). The results should be similar to column 3 (OS status) and 4 (FUP status) of Table 2. Finally a new KM curve can be calculated by using this *follow up status* column as a series of events, and then the MFUP can be calculated in the same way as for calculating the median survival described before (Fig. 2, MFUP = 15 months). The value of MFUP should always be taken into account (and always mentioned in publications describing survival statistics) when reading statements about median OS. Figure 3 shows how the value of different MFUP compared with identical median OS can impact the reliability of the latter calculated by KM survival curves.

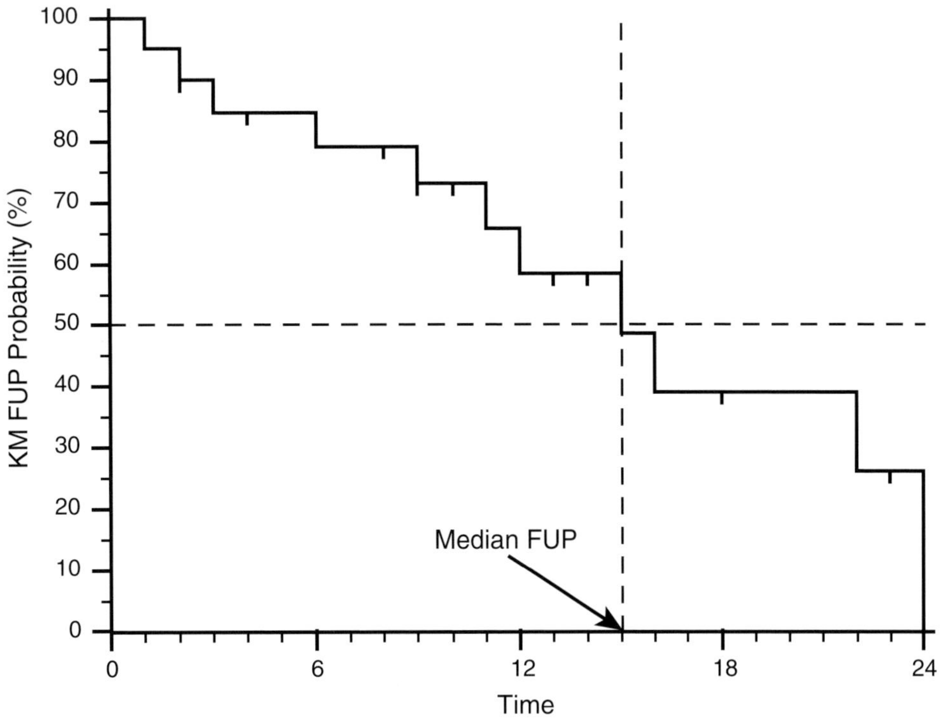

Fig. 2 Calculation of the median follow-up (MFUP) time for the case series in Table 2. Using as 'status' value the column d_{fup} in Table 2 a new KM survival curve has been drawn. The value of the MFUP is achieved by using the same method to get the median OS in Fig. 1, by drawing a horizontal line from the value of 50 % of survival (in this plot it corresponds to the 50 % of KM FUP probability) and then finding the intersection with a vertical segment of the KM curve. Starting from this segment a vertical line is drawn down to the horizontal axis (the FUP time) to get the value, in this case 15 months

A good evaluation of the reliability of the median overall (and other kinds of) survival can be achieved by comparing it to the value of the MFUP. No exact criteria are known to give a judgment about this comparison; but large differences in the two values are suspicious for unreliable median survival value. Finally much care has to be used in considering the MFUP as the only parameter to evaluate the maturity of the follow up of a patient series because it has been proven misleading in some cases (Shuster 1991).

2.1 Comparison Among Kaplan-Meier Survival Curves

The KM survival analysis is extensively used by researchers to compare the effect of a *factor* on different patients populations. When the hypothesis is that a *factor* can affect the outcome in terms of survival, typical statistical software packages allow us to compare populations and plot a graph with two (or more) overlapping curves, in order to show how it leads to differences in the survival outcome. The *factor* cannot be a continuous variable, rather it must be a categorical variable (e.g. sex, different chemotherapy regimens, experimental drug versus placebo etc.) or a classification of the patient population in two (or more) categories using a pre-defined cut-off on a continuous numerical variable (e.g. the level of a serum marker, the radiation dose, an age cut-off etc.). The analysis across different patients series is usually performed by using the *Logrank test*, also referred as the Mantel-Cox test (Mantel 1966). The Logrank test compares estimates of the hazard functions of the two groups at each observed event time. It is constructed by computing the observed and expected number of events in one of the groups at each observed event time and then adding these to obtain an overall summary across all time points where an event occurs. Finally, in order to get the value of *significance* of the Logrank test, a χ^2 statistics is calculated over this summation for the different populations and the value of the probability to reject the null hypothesis (that is: the *factor* doesn't affect the survival outcome) can be achieved by referring to $z = \sqrt{\chi^2_{Logrank}}$, and thus calculating the final *p value*.

Many variables can influence the final result of the *p value*. First of all the number of patients enrolled in the analysis, due to the fact that of course calculations of the observed and expected *events* are directly influenced by the total number of cases. So, when observing relatively small differences among different KM survival curves, the increase of the number of the observed patients can provide a strategy to support the hypothesis that the *factor* actually influences the outcome. Starting from the KM Logrank test calculation, when a protocol is planned, it is useful to calculate in advance the population needed to discriminate a significant difference in survival rates, by using as hypothesis the rates observed on smaller populations not yet giving significant results. Many software packages offer the possibility to perform such a power calculation very easily. An example of similar curves calculated over different population sizes is given in Fig. 4. It shows two graphs: plot 'a'

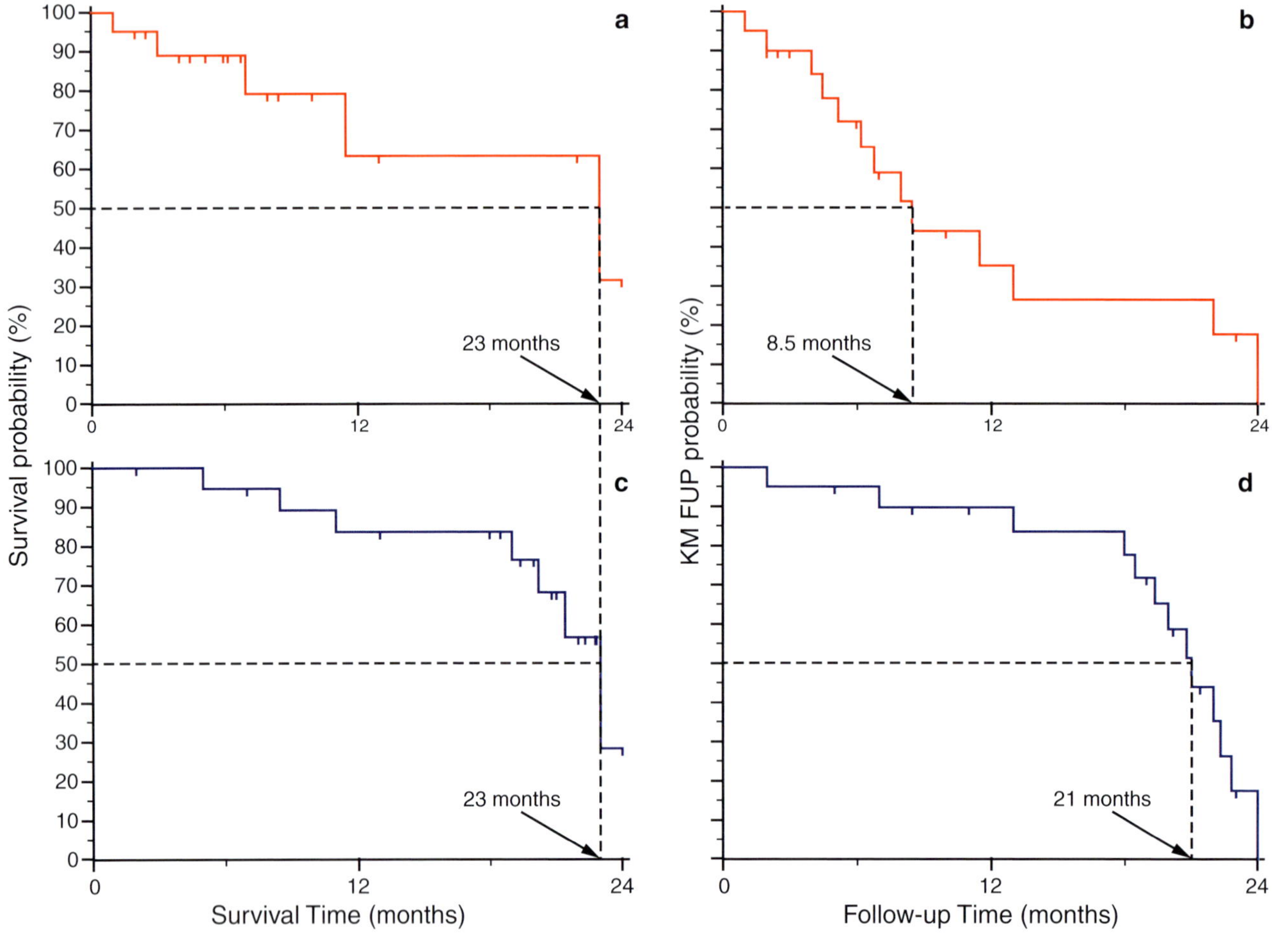

Fig. 3 Example of use of median follow-up (MFUP) times to evaluate the consistence of observed overall (OS) survival. The two series have the same median OS time (23 months: **a**, **c**), but different values of MFUP times can be calculated using a KM approach. The *red series* shows many censored cases in the left part of the curve 'a', giving a median follow-up time that is 8.5 months (**b**). However it is very low if compared with the median overall survival found in the fig. '*a*', and so the latter value could be definitely not reliable. Using the KM computation approach the blue series shows a more adequate median follow-up time of 21 months (**d**), that gives consistence to related OS value

represents two KM survival curves for two populations of patients, each one counting 30 patients. The 'blue' population seems to have a better survival than the 'red' one. But the Logrank test gives a $p = 0.10$ and so, it is not significant; in the plot 'b' we have simply doubled the number of cases, each patients group counting 60 cases, and kept the position of the events in the timeline similar to the case series in the plot 'a': the final shape of the curves in 'a' and 'b' seems very similar, but now the Logrank test provides a statistically significant value of $p = 0.02$. Another feature that can be shown in the KM survival curves by many statistical software packages is the width of the *confidence intervals* (CI) for the survival curves (the dashed lines in Fig. 4). The overlap between the CI areas is larger in plot 'a' than in plot 'b', furthermore the CI of the survival probability at 36 months has been drawn by using arrowheads lines on the survival axis and the level of uncertainty of the calculation of this value is apparently larger for the case series in plot 'a' than in plot 'b'. These features of the graphs represent the visual appearance of the significance in the difference between the two populations, and can be added to plots by researchers, if needed, to enhance the characteristics of the case series.

Another parameter usually calculated by statistical tools is the *hazard ratio* (HR). The HR is the ratio of the hazard rates corresponding to the conditions described by two levels of an explanatory variable. For example, in a study comparing a population undergoing an experimental therapy regimen versus a control population, the population treated with the experimental regimen may show the event at half the rate per unit time as the control population. The hazard ratio would be 0.5, indicating higher hazard of

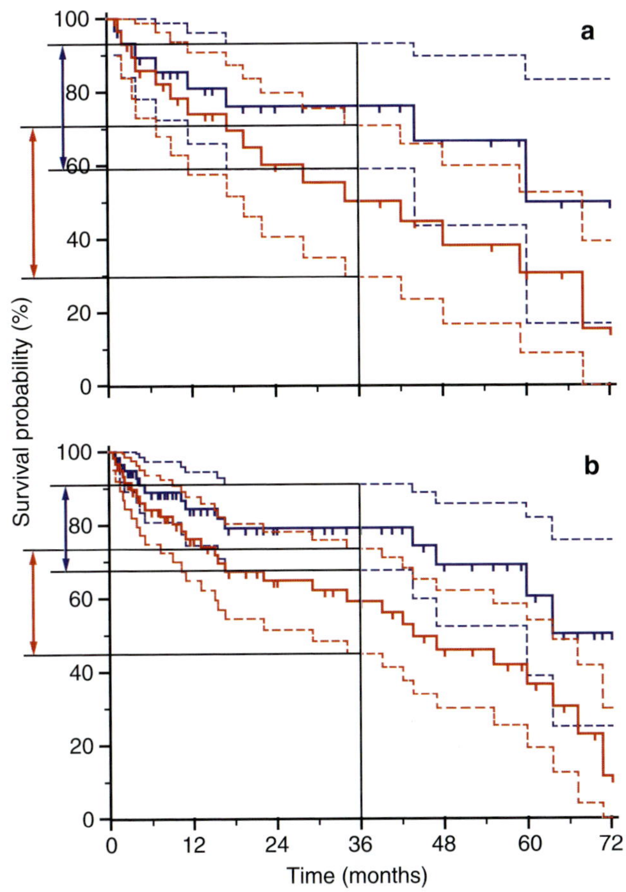

Fig. 4 Comparison of Kaplan-Meier survival curves for different populations. In the graph '**a**' each series counts 30 patients, the Logrank test p value is not significant (0.10). In the graph '**b**' each series counts 60 patients and the p value is 0.02 (significant). The confidence intervals are plotted as *dashed lines*, the values of the survival confidence intervals at 36 months are shown as *arrowheads lines* on the survival axis, being the width of the confidence intervals smaller in the plot '**b**' than in the plot '**a**' because of the difference in the number of patients per series

showing an event from the untreated population. The HR can be calculated by the Eq. (1):

$$HR = \frac{O_A/E_A}{O_B/E_B} \tag{1}$$

In this equation O_X is the summation of the *observed events* (death, local recurrence etc.) while E_X is the summation of the *expected events* in two different populations (A and B). It is possible to calculate the CI for the HR too, giving an idea of the reliability of the results. When the $HR = 1$ there is no difference between the two examined populations. An $HR < 1$ means that the hazard is lower for population on numerator while a $HR > 1$ means that it is higher. The HRs calculated for the two populations (each one divided in two groups, red and blue) in Fig. 4 are summarized in Table 3.

Another important concept in studying survival, slightly different from the *HR*, is the *odds ratio* (OR). The OR is calculated from Eq. (2):

$$OR = \frac{(O_{Ex}/Ex)/[1 - (O_{Ex}/Ex)]}{(O_{Nex}/Nex)/[1 - (O_{Nex}/Nex)]} \tag{2}$$

where *O* is the number of *observed events* (death, recurrence etc.) in the *exposed* (O_{Ex}) *or not exposed* (O_{Nex}) patients, *Ex* is the total number of patients *exposed* to a given factor, *Nex* is the total number of the patients *not exposed* to the factor (controls). OR's are very important in meta-analyses because they can be primarily used to compute the comparison among different studies related to similar outcome and inclusion criteria. In this context the final objective is to get the results of different source studies in order to identify patterns among study results, sources of disagreement among those results, or other interesting relationships that may come to light in the context of multiple studies (Greenland and O' Rourke 2008).

3 Parametric Analysis

It is possible to refer the *hazard* to an instantaneous value, defining it as *hazard rate*. It shows the risk in a specific time interval related to a given observed population and it can be calculated using Eq. (3):

$$\lambda_t = \frac{d_t}{f_t + F_t} \tag{3}$$

where *d* is the number of events observed in the given time interval *t*, while the denominator is the cumulated time-to event since the beginning of the interval. For example, if during our chosen time interval of 30 days among the 10 patients under observation one exhibits an event at day 5 and another one shows an event at day 15, we have $\lambda_t = 2/(20 + 240) = 2/260 = 0.00769$ because 2, the numerator, is the number of events, 20 is the sum of 5 and 15 (cumulated time-to-event for patients who show the event) and we add the product of 8 patients who did not show the event by 30 days (interval duration), giving 240. This is the same as assigning 30 days as time-to-event for patients with no events. The method is perfectly consistent because the number of affected patients is well represented by the numerator of the fraction. In some clinical conditions it is possible to assume that the *hazard rate* doesn't change during a long observation time, thus remaining constant. In this case the *survival function* can be computed as an *exponential function* in which survival is given in the form of Eq. (4):

$$S(t) = e^{-\lambda t} \tag{4}$$

Table 3 Hazard ratios for the populations plotted in the Fig. 4

Hazard-ratio for data in Fig. 4			
Data origin	HR	95 % CI	P value
a	2.0000	0.8985–4.4518	0.1008
b	2.0714	1.1393–3.7661	0.0211

The absolute value of the HRs for the two populations 'a' and 'b' is almost identical, but CIs are largely different. For the population 'a' it goes from about 0.9 to 4.5, being too large if compared with the value of the HR. Moreover the lowest value of the CI is below 1, meaning that there is uncertainty on the possibility that the *factor* actually changes the hazard between the two subpopulations studied in the group 'a'

and the only parameter involved in the function is the constant λ, since time t is the independent variable of Eq. (4). In this particular condition it could be very easy to fit the *survival function* to a single parameter, and use it to predict the outcome in a given patients population. Unfortunately, analyzing the majority of clinical situations, the *hazard rate* is modified during time, being λ itself a value subject to change over time. For example the rate of local recurrence after the surgery, or the mortality due to post-operative complications, can be higher in the first months after surgery than after some years of follow up. In these conditions it is sometimes feasible to assess the variation of the *hazard rate* as a function of time t. A model that can describe this behavior is the *Weibull distribution* described by Eq. (5):

$$S(t) = e^{-(\lambda t)^{\kappa}} \tag{5}$$

In this equation the parameter κ can assume different values reflecting the trend in the *hazard rate* variation during time:

$\kappa < 1$: the *hazard rate* is highest in the first part of the curve, meaning that there is a factor that can increase proportionally the number of the events during the first part of the follow-up time;

$\kappa = 1$: the *hazard rate* is constant over time. It means that the trend of the Weibull distribution is identical to an exponential distribution with the same λ value: with $\kappa = 1 \Rightarrow S(t) = e^{-(\lambda t)^{\kappa}} = e^{-\lambda t}$;

$\kappa > 1$: the *hazard rate* is highest in the second part of the curve, while in the first part it seems to have slowed giving to the survival curve a two phases appearance with opposite convexity, upward in the first part, downward in the second part.

The appearance of three Weibull distribution curves according different values of κ is shown in Fig. 5. Figure 6 shows an example of non parametric distribution (Kaplan-Meier) with corresponding fitted exponential and Weibull distributions.

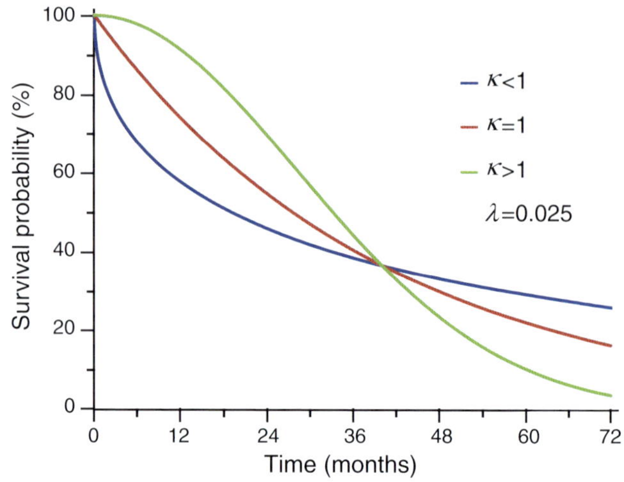

Fig. 5 Example of three *Weibull distribution* curves with different values of κ and equal λ. With $\kappa<1$ (*blue curve*) the *hazard rate* is higher in the first part of the curve, and the survival probability decreases faster in this tract than the curve with $\kappa = 1$, that is the *exponential distribution*. The *green curve* shows the trend of the *Weibull distribution* with $\kappa > 1$, with the classical 'two phases' convexity trend, oriented upwards in the first part of the curve and downwards in the second part

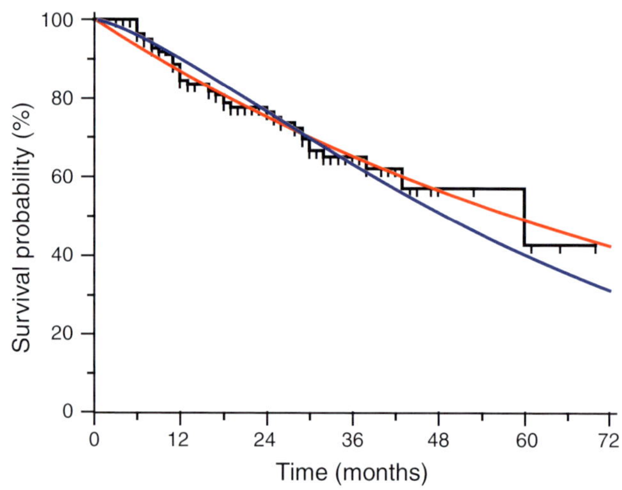

Fig. 6 Example of two parametric models (*red* exponential, *blue* Weibull) fitted to a given empirical Kaplan-Meier distribution (*black*). The value of the parameters change according the function used: *exponential*, $\lambda = 0.01186$; *Weibull*, $\lambda = 0.01551$, $\kappa = 1.33906$

4 Semi-parametric Analysis: Cox's Proportional Hazards Model

The value of the *hazard rate* can be a function of time and can be expressed as $\lambda(t)$. This variability in most real clinical situations cannot be expressed correctly using parametric survival functions. In order to assess this trend it is possible to find the relation between *hazard rate* and time by using the specific plot shown in Fig. 7, where two survival curves are plotted against the *complementary log transformation* (CLT), that is $\log\{-\log[S(t)]\}$ against $\log(t)$. This graph points out the correlation between survival rate and time, allowing to find if there is a constant rate rather than a variable rate of λ. When the CLT shows a good fit of the data points around a regression line (Fig. 7a2) it means that the *hazard rate* is roughly constant, and the *survival function* can be expressed in the exponential form shown in Eq. (4). In other cases (Fig. 7b2) there could not be a good fit of the data along the regression line function. In order to enhance these findings it is also possible to display the *difference* between the CLT points and the data points predicted by the regression function using the *plot of residuals* (Fig. 7a3, b3). This graph shows the *distance* between each point from the predicted one on the y axis, and gives a direct measure of the agreement of the *survival predicted function* with the observed data. In the ideal condition of a parametric fitting with exponential form the observed points should align on the horizontal line traced from the value of '0' in the y axis as in Fig. 7a3, but in all other cases the results are much more similar to the plot shown in Fig. 7b3, where there is no alignment in the plot of residuals. In this case λ has to be expressed as function of time in the form $\lambda(t)$. In Fig. 8 the plot of two survival curves is compared to the corresponding CLTs. The two series show a different survival rate and the CLT graph shows that the *hazard rate* is not constant, not having a linear-like appearance. But the two CLT lines show similar trends, seemingly 'parallel' because there is an approximately constant vertical distance between them at any given time. This typical appearance means that there is a *proportion* between the survival rates in the two populations. Starting from this kind of findings in the survival curves among populations differentiated by specific *factors* D. R. Cox published his fundamental paper where he described the *proportional hazards regression model* (PHRM, Cox 1972). In the main assumption of the model the hazard for a particular patient has to be related to the *average* underlying hazard of the whole examined population. We denote this average hazard as $\lambda_0(t)$, and the hazard for the specific patient can be specified as:

$$\lambda(t) = h(t) \cdot \lambda_0(t) \tag{6}$$

where $h(t)$ is a function of time t (Machin et al. 2006). In this condition it does not matter which is the function of distribution of the hazards allowing to model any survival data collection characterized by a time-dependent *hazard rate*. The only assumption to be satisfied in the PHRM is that *the hazards in the groups must remain proportional to each other over time*. In the PHRM usually the *factors* that can affect the outcome are named *covariates*. The *covariates* are variables that can be numerical and continuous (e.g. age, hemoglobin level, a serum-marker level etc.) or can be categorical (e.g. sex, tumor clinical stage, therapy protocol etc.). The relation that exists among survival and *covariates* can be calculated by using the following assumptions and equations:

1. Each *numerical covariate* affects the outcome by the product between its coefficient β and its own value x;
2. For *categorical covariates* each possible value has to be tested, during modeling procedures, as *dummy variable*, so the final results of the β coefficients can be different for each category of the covariate. If the category is not significant the value of the corresponding product $\beta \cdot x$ must be put to '0', if significant $\beta \cdot x =$ the value of coefficient found with regression;
3. Being $x_i\beta = \beta_1 x_{i1} + \beta_2 x_{i2} + \cdots + \beta_n x_{in}$ the sum of the products of each covariate x related to patient i with its own coefficient β, the survival probability $S_i(t)$ for patient i at a given time t can be calculated using the following expressions:

$$S_i(t) = e^{\{-H_i(t)\}} = e^{\left\{-H_0(t)\cdot e^{[x_i\beta]}\right\}} \tag{7}$$

$$S_i(t) = \left\{e^{[-H_0(t)]}\right\}^{e^{\{x_i\beta\}}} = S_0(t)^{e^{\{x_i\beta\}}} \tag{8}$$

where $H_0(t)$ is the *baseline hazard* at time t and $S_0(t)$ is the *baseline survival* at time t. They are the value of the *hazard function* and *survival function* achieved just with all the covariates values set to '0' at the time t. The statistical software packages usually provide either a table with the values of $H_0(t)$ or the values of $S_0(t)$ after the computation of the PHRM. Note that the *survival at mean of covariate* (further output usually calculated) *cannot* be used in place of $S_0(t)$ that is the survival with all covariates values set to '0', as previously stated. An example of application of PHRM is given in the following section, the dataset is shown in Appendix 1.

A population of 144 patients has been followed after the diagnosis of a kind of cancer for a maximum follow-up time of 70 months (MFUP = 29 months). The first problem to solve when defining a PHRM is the sample size. As a rule of thumb, the maximum number of covariates that can be analyzed in a binary outcome model (such as a PHRM) is given by the minimum value of the frequencies of the two response levels divided by 10 (Harrel 2001). So in this example we have 39 cases with *censor status* = 1 and 105 cases with *censor status* = 0. In this case being the minimum value of the frequencies = 39 we cannot analyze more than 4 (4×10 = 40) covariates in the model. So a set of 4 *factors* has been investigated: two *factors* (Factor 1 and Factor 2) are divided in two categories each; the last two factors are numerical and continuous: the age of the patients and a serum marker level. A series of Kaplan-Meier survival curves has been drawn: in Fig. 9 the appearance is

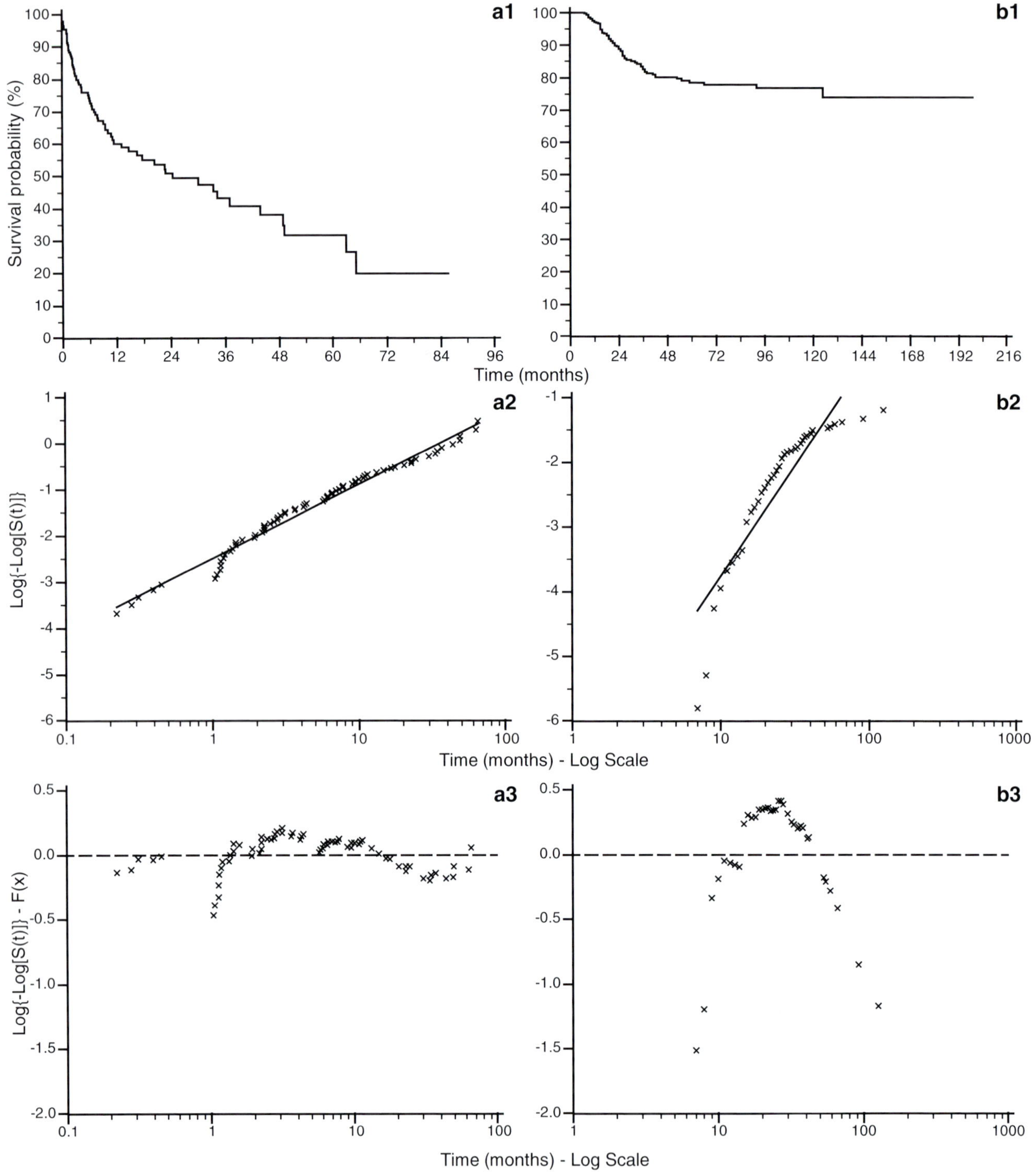

Fig. 7 Comparison between a case series described by exponential survival function (**a**) and a case series with different survival function (**b**). The graphs n. 1 show the survival functions. The graphs n. 2 show the *complementary log transformation*: the graph **a2** shows a better linear fit of survival values than graph **b2**. The graphs n. 3 show the value of residuals (difference between the *complementary log transformation value* and the *log-linear regression function value*): the absolute value of the residuals is larger for the b case series showing unacceptable fitting with the exponential survival function calculated over the data

shown of the subpopulations of patients categorized according to Factor 1 (categories '1' and '0'), Factor 2 (categories '1' and '0'), the two age classes (using a cut-off value of 37 years) and the two classes of serum marker level (generically defined 'low' and 'high' level). When analyzing continuous variables in order to detect

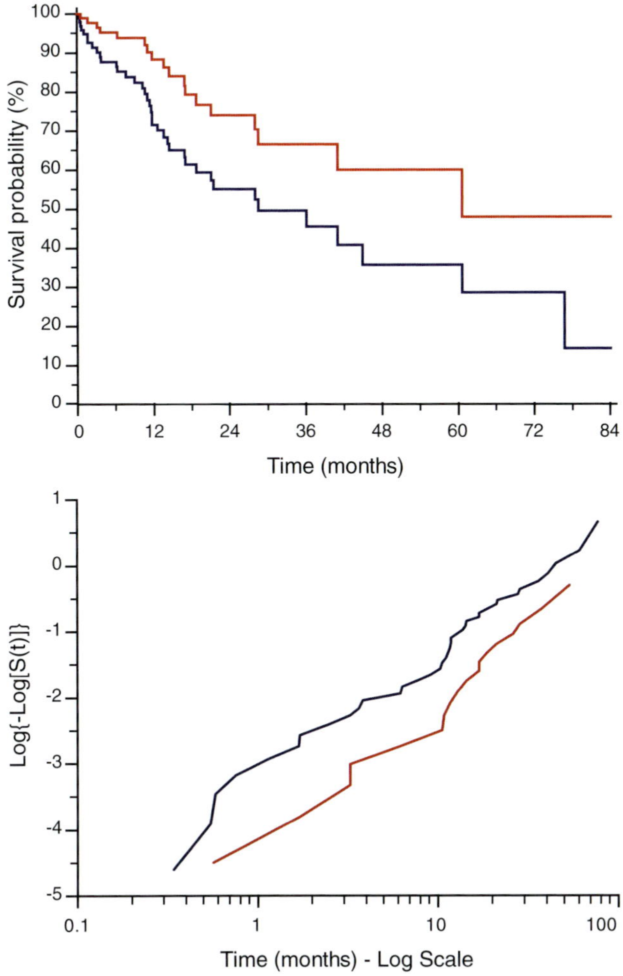

Fig. 8 Comparison between two survival curves and corresponding *complementary log transformation curves*. The two CLT lines are not exactly *linear* but they seem to have the same trend being fairly parallel, meaning that there is a *proportion* in the survival rate between the two populations

relationships between those values and survival it can be useful to distinguish *classes* by dividing the population according to a specific cut-off. The cut-off value can be identified by the researcher looking at the data for 'anomalous' correlations or by using simple statistical methods, such as dividing the population in classes found by using the mean or, better, the median value of the continuous variable. This is an effective method because the median value of a continuous variable bisects the overall population into two subgroups with (nearly) the same number of cases (if the population is even the two subpopulations are equivalent, if it is odd the number of cases for each subpopulation is different for one case). Looking at the example for all the analyses the distinction between the curves is statistically significant according to the Logrank test (Fig. 9). But when one wants to analyze the impact of *combined factors* on the survival probability of a single case the approach based on the Kaplan-Meier survival function cannot be used, e.g. trying to combine all the covariates for a single patient showing Factor 1 = 0 (worse survival), Factor 2 = 0 (better survival), age <37 years (better survival) and marker level = high (worse survival). The best way to analyze the effect of all these combined covariates on survival is through the PHRM. In this example the analysis (performed by MedCalc Software, © 1993–2013 MedCalc Software, Acacialaan 22, B-8400 Ostend, Belgium) using the PHRM, gave the results shown in Table 4. The overall model significance is very high ($p < 0.0001$) but among the covariates, age, Factor 1 = 0 and Factor 2 = 0 are significant, while the marker level, Factor 1 = 1 and Factor 2 = 1 are not. Please note that, looking at the Kaplan-Meier Logrank test analyses in Fig. 9, the marker level seemed to have a slightly better significance than age ($p_{marker\ level} = 0.0214 < p_{age} = 0.0234$), but this finding has not been confirmed by the PHRM analysis. The use of a preliminary Kaplan-Meier analysis on single covariates is not trivial, because it can help the researcher in detecting covariates that are likely to affect the outcome and simplifying the multivariate analysis performed by the PHRM.

The assessment of a PHRM needs of course some kind of validation. It is very important to verify whether the impact of an independent variable meets the proportional hazard assumption: this verification can be performed using many tests of proportional hazards that are related to time-weighted score tests of the proportional hazards hypothesis, and can be visualized as a weighted least-squares line fitted to the residual plot (Grambsch and Therneau 1994; Schoenfeld 1982). An example of this verification is given in Fig. 10 where the scaled Schoenfeld residuals for the significant covariates are shown: the lack of some kind of regular trend (linear or with some other kind of regular shape) in the positions of scaled residuals for the three plots means that the null hypothesis (presence of proportional hazards over time) can be accepted. In Table 5 the results of proportional hazards test are shown. None of the covariates or the global model behavior show lack of proportionality as confirmed by the p values >0.05 in all cases.

Once a PHRM has been calculated the objective of a researcher could be trying to use it to determine a prediction of survival for new patients with similar characteristics in order to address them to a better tailored care pathway. This is one of the most interesting applications of predictive models realized by using these statistical techniques. But getting a good result in a Cox regression analysis is only the first step, because the achieved *results* that fit the data of the analyzed population must be *verified* on different patients populations in order to achieve a *predictive* model. In fact, a PHRM is only the snapshot describing a single study population, and the prediction based only on this kind of findings could be lacking in reliability and, on the other hand,

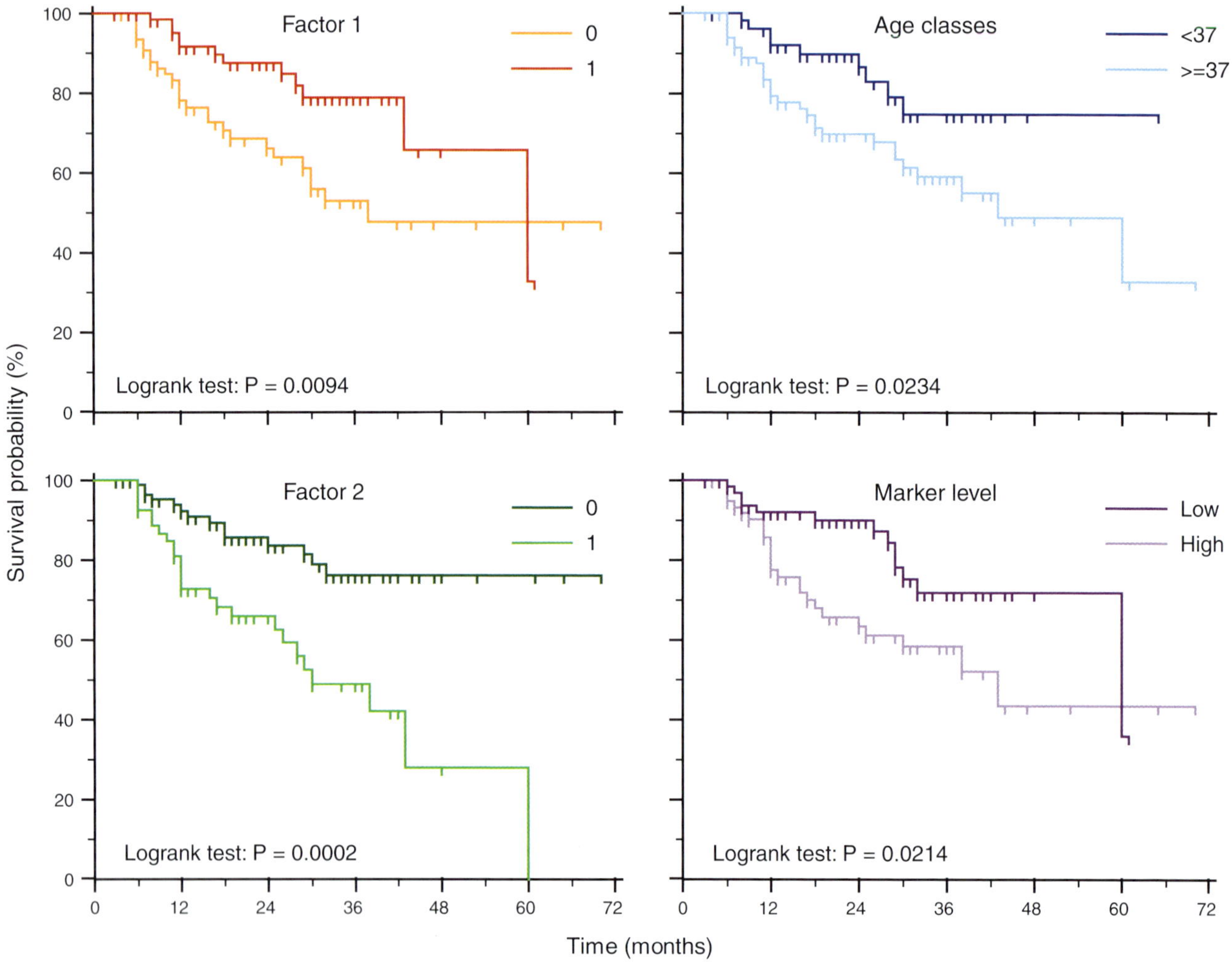

Fig. 9 Kaplan-Meier analysis of a population used as example in Sect. 4. The *factors 1* and *2* are dummy covariates, each one containing two categories (1 and 0). The numerical covariates have been used to split the whole population into two subpopulations using specific cut-off values. Each Kaplan-Meier analysis shows significant differences between the subpopulations classified according to the covariates as shown by the p-values calculated by Logrank test

could lead to unsuitable decisions if used directly for predicting further results on patients different from the ones used in the modeling dataset.

5 Assessing the Reliability of a Survival Prediction Model

In order to validate a survival model based on PHRM several techniques can be used (Iasonos et al. 2008). These methods use a comparison between a *training dataset*, that is the original one used for model definition, and one or multiple *verification dataset*. There are three methods to define the verification dataset:

(1) *Cross-validation*: this method uses the same source dataset by splitting it in subgroups that are used either for model training or validation.
(2) *Bootstrap validation*: this method (Efron and Tibshirani 1993) uses randomly chosen samples from the original dataset, that can be also re-used more than one time, in order to build verification datasets with the same number of cases as the initial one.
(3) *External validation*: cross-validation and bootstrapping are methods that can prevent over-interpretation of current data (*overfitting*), but they cannot ensure external usefulness of the model. Indeed using a model on new patients (not belonging to the primary dataset) could detect erroneous predictions just due to potential *overfitting* of the initial model. This is a very important concern that can be overcome by verifying the model on a new population and so, the use of external validation is becoming the gold-standard in oncological literature to create and validate predictive models. Whatever method is used in order to get the verification

Table 4 Results of Cox Proportional-Hazard Regression for the example given in the text

Regression method					Stepwise
Enter variable if P<					0.05
Remove variable if P>					0.1
Sample size					144
Overall model fit					
Null model-2 Log likelihood					339.097
Full model-2 Log likelihood					308.391
Chi square					30.706
DF					3
Significance level					P < 0.0001
Coefficients and standard errors					
Covariate	β	*SE*	*P*	Exp (β)	95 % CI of Exp (β)
Age	0.0487	0.01658	0.0033	1.0499	1.0165–1.0844
Factor 1 = 0	−1.1378	0.3734	0.0023	0.3205	0.1547–0.6639
Factor 2 = 0	1.4372	0.3524	<0.0001	4.2090	2.1170–8.3687
Variables not included in the model: marker level					
Baseline cumulative hazard function					
Time	Baseline cumulative hazard–$H_0(t)$			At mean of covariates	
				Cumulative hazard	Survival
6	0.002			0.022	0.978
7	0.003			0.033	0.968
8	0.005			0.050	0.952
9	0.006			0.056	0.946
10	0.007			0.062	0.940
11	0.009			0.082	0.922
12	0.012			0.117	0.889
13	0.013			0.126	0.882
16	0.015			0.144	0.866
17	0.016			0.153	0.858
18	0.018			0.173	0.841
19	0.019			0.183	0.833
24	0.021			0.195	0.823
25	0.022			0.207	0.813
26	0.023			0.220	0.802
28	0.025			0.234	0.792
29	0.027			0.261	0.770
30	0.030			0.289	0.749
32	0.032			0.308	0.735
38	0.036			0.341	0.711
43	0.043			0.411	0.663
60	0.075			0.716	0.489

The model shows a high level of significance (P < 0.0001). Looking at the covariates, age, dummy covariates Factor 1 = 0 and Factor 2 = 0 are significant, while the marker level, dummy covariates Factor 1 = 1 and Factor 2 = 1 are not. In the lower part of the table the values of baseline cumulative hazard function are shown, allowing to calculate the predicted value for a new patient having the same covariates set analyzed in the model at the given time shown in the leftmost column

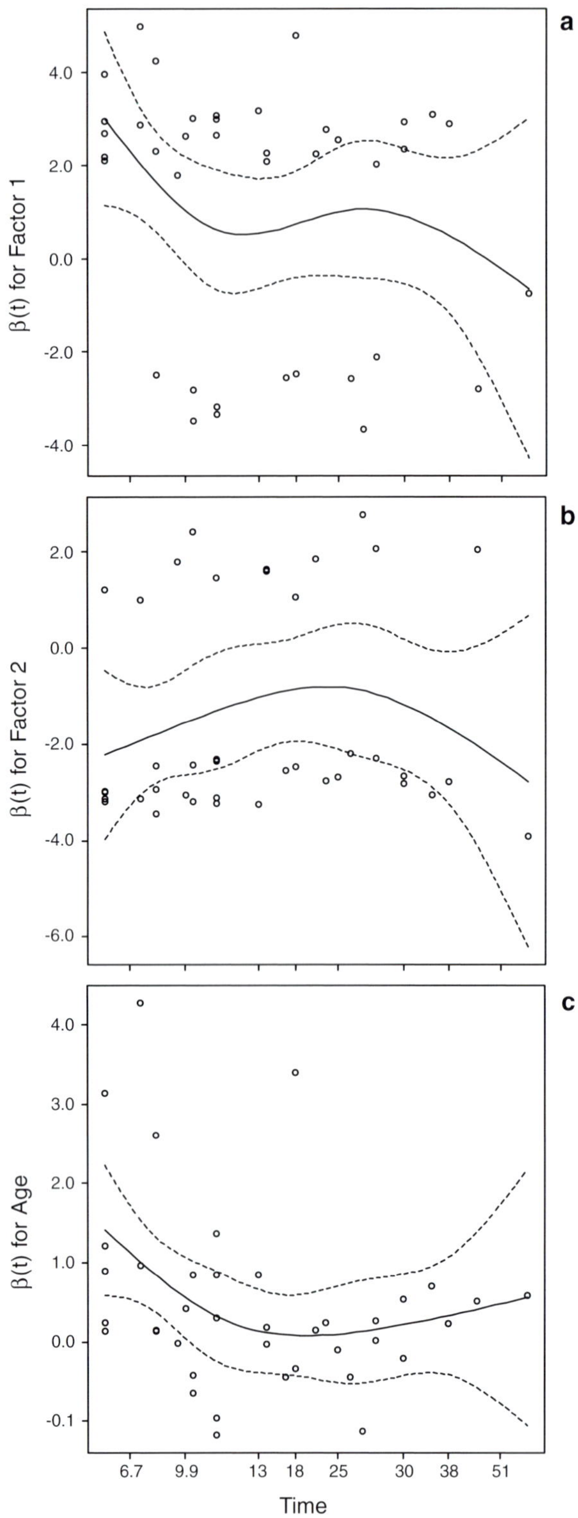

Fig. 10 Plot of scaled Schoenfeld residuals of the Cox Proportional-Hazard Regression for the example given in the text. The use of this tool is able detect if there is lack of proportionality (showing some kind of trends) among covariates. The dichotomous covariates (**a**, **b**) show the position of the scaled residuals in two groups up and down in their plots, while the scaled residuals for the age (continuous covariate) are randomly spread in the plot area (**c**)

Table 5 Results of proportional hazards test for the example in the text

	ρ	χ^2	P-value
Age	−0.2649	3.326	0.0682
Factor 1	−0.2306	2.716	0.0993
Factor 2	0.0815	0.251	0.6160
GLOBAL	NA	4.542	0.2086

Each covariate, and the global model behavior, show a P value > 0.05, meaning that there is no lack of proportional hazard over time (despite the presence of a 'trend' in lack of proportionality for covariate 'Age', showing a P value close to 0.05)

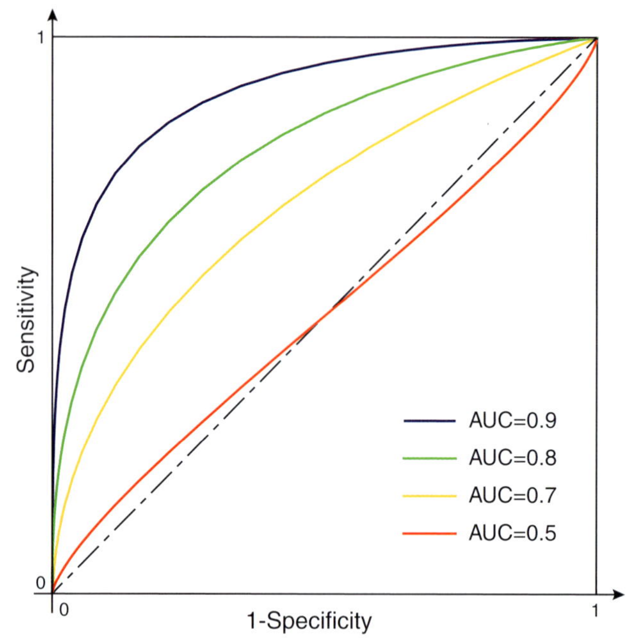

Fig. 11 Example of four ROC curves with corresponding AUC values. AUC = 0.5 corresponds to absence of predictive value for a model, the curve lies close to the *diagonal line* that represents the bisection of the square with AUC = 1; AUC = 0.7 corresponds to a model that can have some predictive value, AUC = 0.8 corresponds to a model having a good predictive value; AUC = 0.9 corresponds to a model having an excellent predictive value, but it could be affected by some kind of *overfitting*, which should be avoided. In real modeling conditions the shape of the curves can be quite different from these *smooth lines*

dataset, the first step to achieve the validation of a new model requires the analysis of the overall 'benchmark' of the model itself. For this purpose a *binary classifier* (able to discern between patients who show the *event* and patients who don't) has to be used. Usually it is the *concordance index* (*c-index*), also defined as the *receiver operating characteristic curve* (*ROC*) and its *area under the curve* (*AUC*). The ROC curve is a graph which illustrates the performance of a binary classifier system as its discrimination threshold is varied. It is created by plotting the fraction of true positives out of

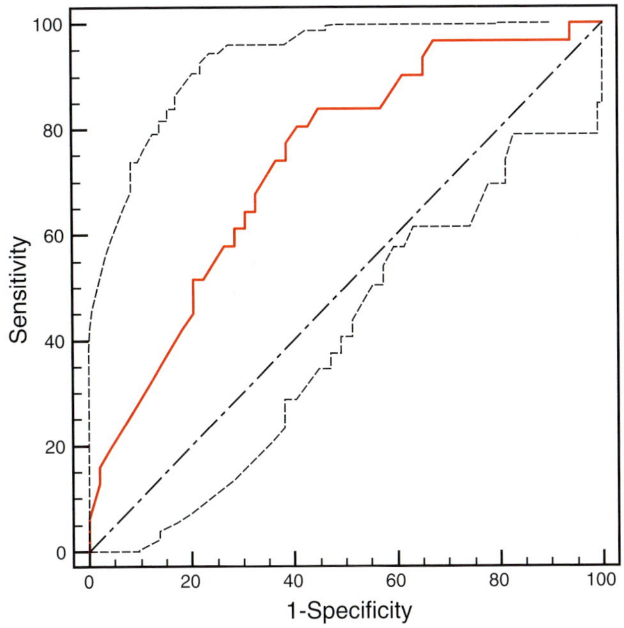

Fig. 12 ROC curve for the example model in the test. AUC = 0.7347, the ROC curve is the *red-line*, the two *thin black dashed lines* represent the 95 % confidence interval of the ROC curve, the *diagonal black dashed-dot line* represents the value of AUC = 0.5 corresponding to a model with random predictive power

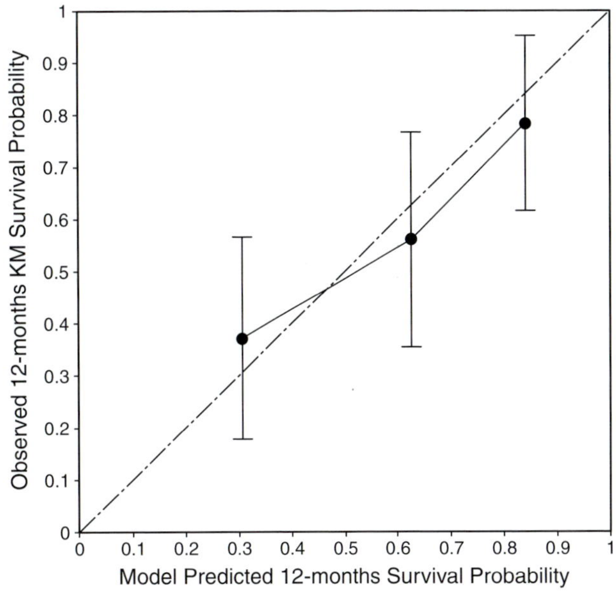

Fig. 13 Calibration plot for the example model in the text. The values of predicted probability for three groups of patients are plotted versus the observed KM survival for the follow-up time chosen in model definition (12 months). The *dots* close to the *diagonal dash-dot line* (that represents the reference of the perfect calibration) and the *bars* showing the 95 % confidence interval of KM survival overlapped to the same *diagonal dash-dot line* show a good predictive performance of the model for each examined patient subgroup

positives (TPR = true positive rate) vs. the fraction of false positives out of negatives (FPR = false positive rate), at increasing threshold settings. TPR is also known as sensitivity, and FPR is 1-specificity or true negative rate. ROC analysis provides tools to select possibly optimal models and to discard suboptimal ones, e.g. when trying to detect the accuracy of a diagnosis related to a blood parameter (interpreted as a tumor marker). The interpretation of ROC curve is easy: in Fig. 11 there are 4 different curves showing 4 different AUC levels: 0.5 (poor predictive power, same as a coin-toss: 50 % to get the correct prediction), 0.7 (lowest predictive power to consider the model prediction *reliable*), 0.8 (optimal predictive power), 0.9 (excellent predictive power but beware of the risk of *overfitting*). The areas under the curves (AUC) are proportional to the *reliability* of the prediction, thus a comparison among different models can be easily achieved by using this tool. The problem in survival statistics is that the binary outcome is not provided by a 'simple' diagnostic definition (such as in ROC used for detecting the optimal threshold of a diagnostic test) but it should take into account that the binary outcome (the survival provided by the censoring status) is spread over the observation time. One solution to this problem is to use a specific follow-up time to fix the reliability of the prediction (T_p) and defining a censor-related-to-time (CT_p) that provides a time-dependent version of

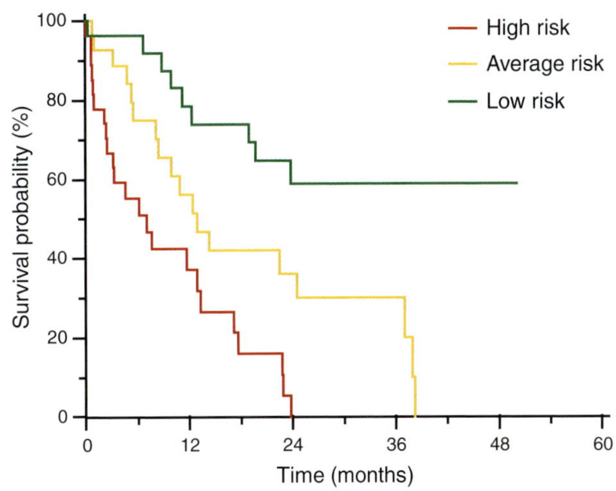

Fig. 14 Kaplan-Meier survival curves of the three subgroups of patients in the verification dataset classified according to the risk classes achieved from the calculated PHRM and used in the calibration plot of Fig. 13. Logrank test *P* value < 0.0001. The distinction among the classes is largely significant

sensitivity and specificity (Heagerty et al. 2000). In this case IF the patient shows the event (status = 1) AND the *survival* $\leq T_p$ THEN $CT_p = 1$, ELSE $CT_p = 0$. Once the list of CT_p is built, a list of survival probability at T_p ($S(T_p)$) has to be filled by using Eqs. 7 or 8. Now the AUC can be calculated by using CT_p as classification

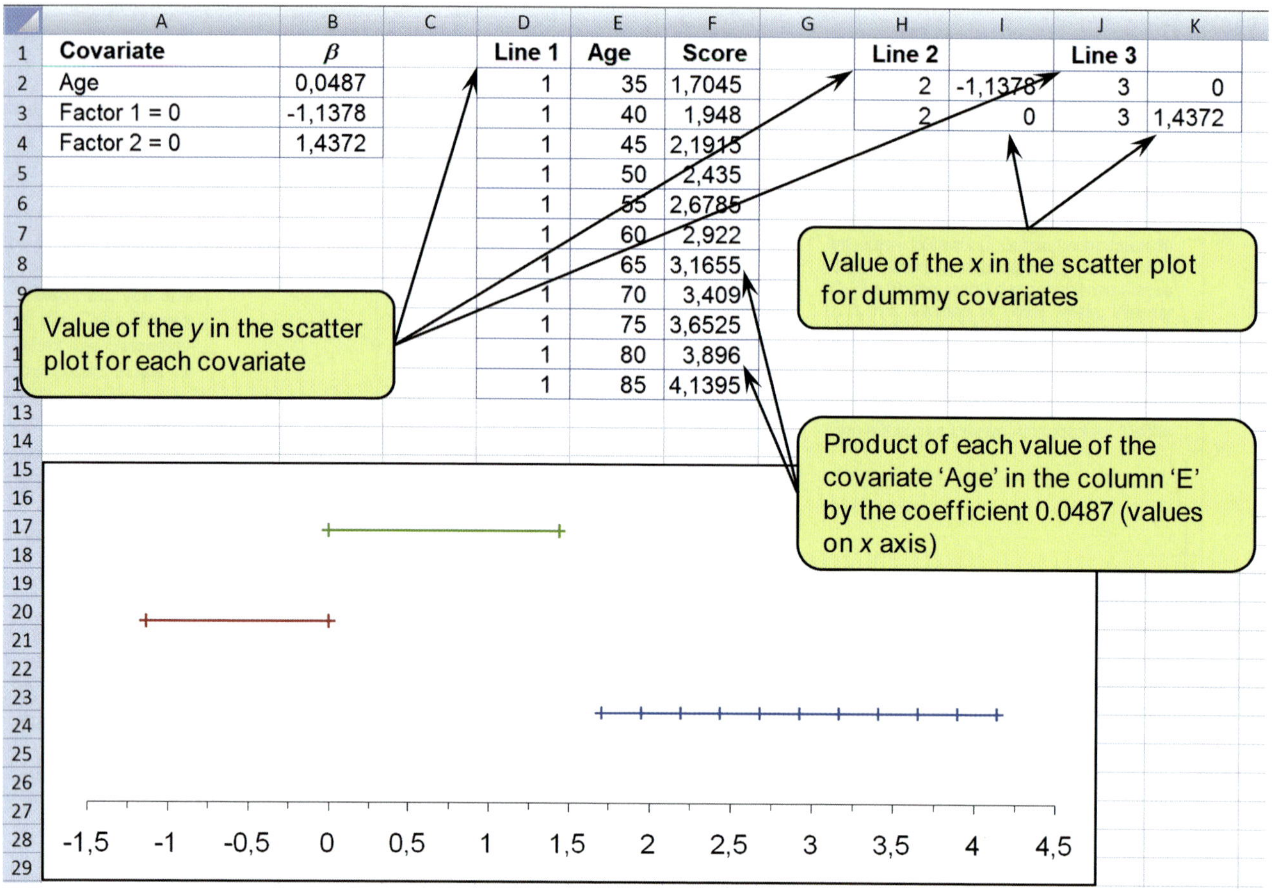

Fig. 15 First step of nomogram drawing: creation of the covariates scales using a *scatter plot with lines* that join the values of the same covariate. For the dummy covariates (Factor 1 and Factor 2) only the significant values have to be used, the not significant values have value '0'. For the continuous covariate (age) a scale containing predefined intervals has to be created by multiplying each step with the covariate coefficient. The three lines lies on three different levels (given by the *y* values of the scatter plot) and the *x* axis shows the value of the score that have to be summed to achieve the exponent of the survival equation

variable and $S(T_p)$ as *marker* in the ROC analysis. An example of the result of ROC analysis for the patient series in the example given above is shown in Fig. 12 where the AUC = 0.7347 for the survival prediction calculated at 12 months of follow up time. The calculation has been achieved over a new distribution (the *verification set*) counting 80 patients with the same covariates as the previous model. Finally the validation of a model requires another step: it is important to relate the prediction to various levels of actual outcome and verify if there are differences among them in the predicted values. In order to do this the verification set is divided into equal parts according the value of $S(T_p)$. In our example the verification set was divided in tertiles (three groups of 27, 27 and 26 patients each one) and for each one the Kaplan-Meier survival was calculated with 95 % confidence interval at 12 months. Finally a scatter plot with the KM survival on the *y* axis and the mean $S(T_p)$ for each group was drawn. It is also possible (and desirable) to plot the confidence interval of the KM survival in order to show whether the actual KM survival moves far from the predicted survival given by the model. This plot, also named *calibration plot* (Taktak et al. 2007), shows the behavior of the model for different risk-classes of patients. In our example the calibration plot is shown in Fig. 13 and the confidence intervals overlap the diagonal line representing the perfect calibration so confirming an overall good performance of the model for the different risk levels. Using the definition of risk classes it is also possible to draw KM survival curves for each class, showing the trend of survival observed in the verification (or training) dataset. Figure 14 displays the KM survival plot for the three classes in the verification dataset of our example. The Logrank test gave $p < 0.0001$ and so the separation among these three risk classes is largely statistically significant.

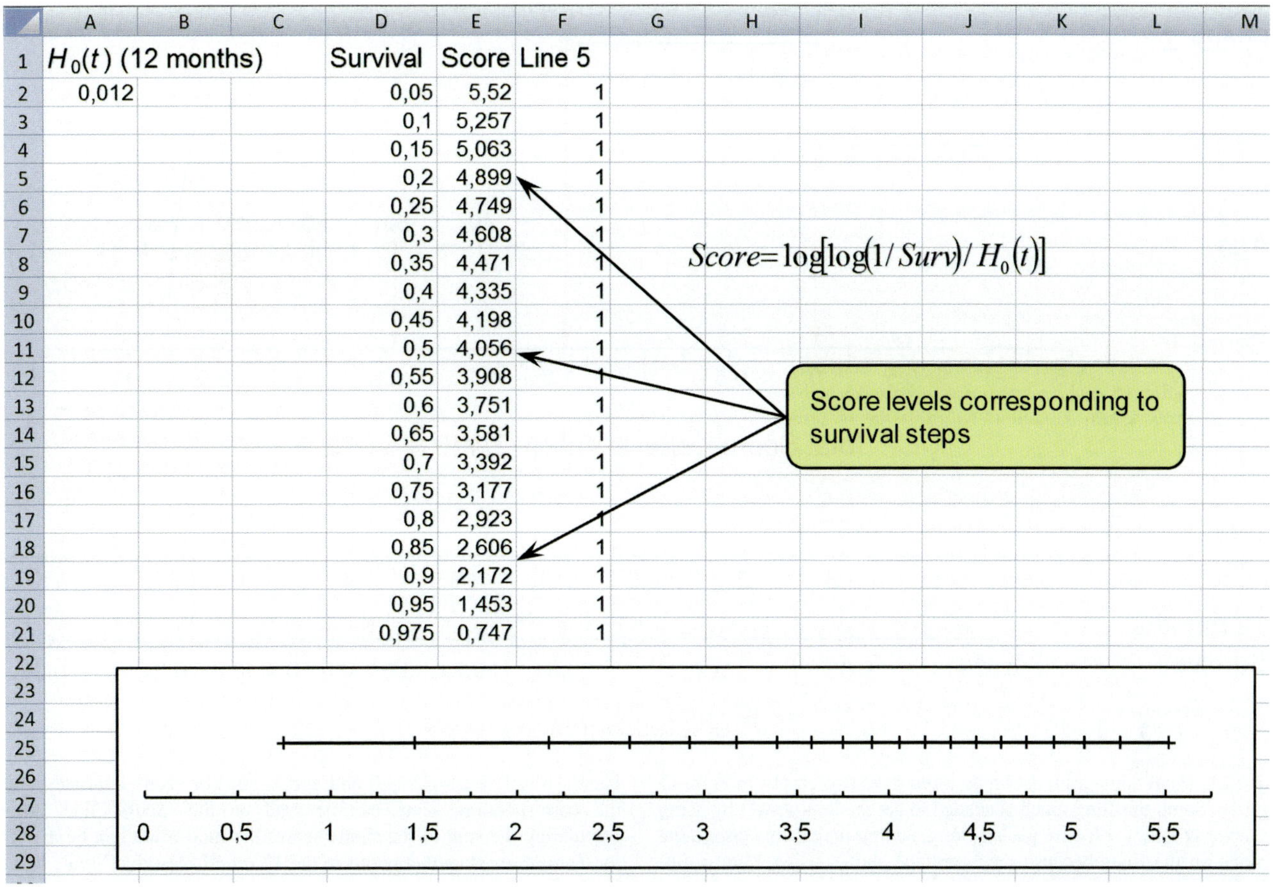

Fig. 16 Creation of the conversion scale between the total score given by the x axis and the survival steps defined by the user. The conversion is achieved by using Eq. 12 in the text

6 Model Presentation: Creating a Nomogram

The use of PHRM to predict the survival expected for a new patient starting its treatment is of course possible when information technology support for calculating the results of Eqs. 7 or 8 is available. Nevertheless in daily clinical practice the use of such kind of resources (think for example during a patient consultation) could not be so easy. This is the reason that led many authors to publish simple graphical tools that allow to calculate 'by hand', or simply using a ruler, the expected outcome. These tools are called *nomograms* and were widely used in the past to help engineers, mathematicians and physicists to calculate the solutions of complex equations very quickly (Doerfler 2009). During the last years many papers have been published presenting such kind of tools to help clinicians in the decision-making process for diagnosis (Kattan et al. 2003), for addressing patients to specific treatment protocols or predicting survival (Lee et al. 2011; Valentini et al. 2011), for predicting response to treatment (Van Stiphout et al. 2011) or for analyzing the chances of side-effects due to treatment (Bradley et al. 2007). The cited references are only a small sample of the large numbers of papers (still growing) published during the last decade and focusing on this specific topic. But which is the process that allows to translate the results of a predictive model, such as a PHRM, into a nomogram? In this section we will proceed with the creation of a nomogram summarizing the results for the example of PHRM given in the two sections above. There are several software products that allow to create nomograms starting from models created within their own environments (e.g. MATLAB®, © 1994–2013 The MathWorks, Inc.; R, project for statistical computing, http://www.r-project.org/). Of course this is a powerful solution for readers who have skills in computer programming (as these software products are mainly based on command line interface) but for readers not versed in computer programming we propose a 'hand-made' solution that uses simply Microsoft® Excel (or another spreadsheet software) and any vector graphics software (e.g. Adobe® Illustrator®, © 1987–2012 Adobe System Incorporated; InkScape, ©1989–1991 Free Software Foundation, Inc.) to 'assemble' the final plot. Starting from the results of the PHRM in our

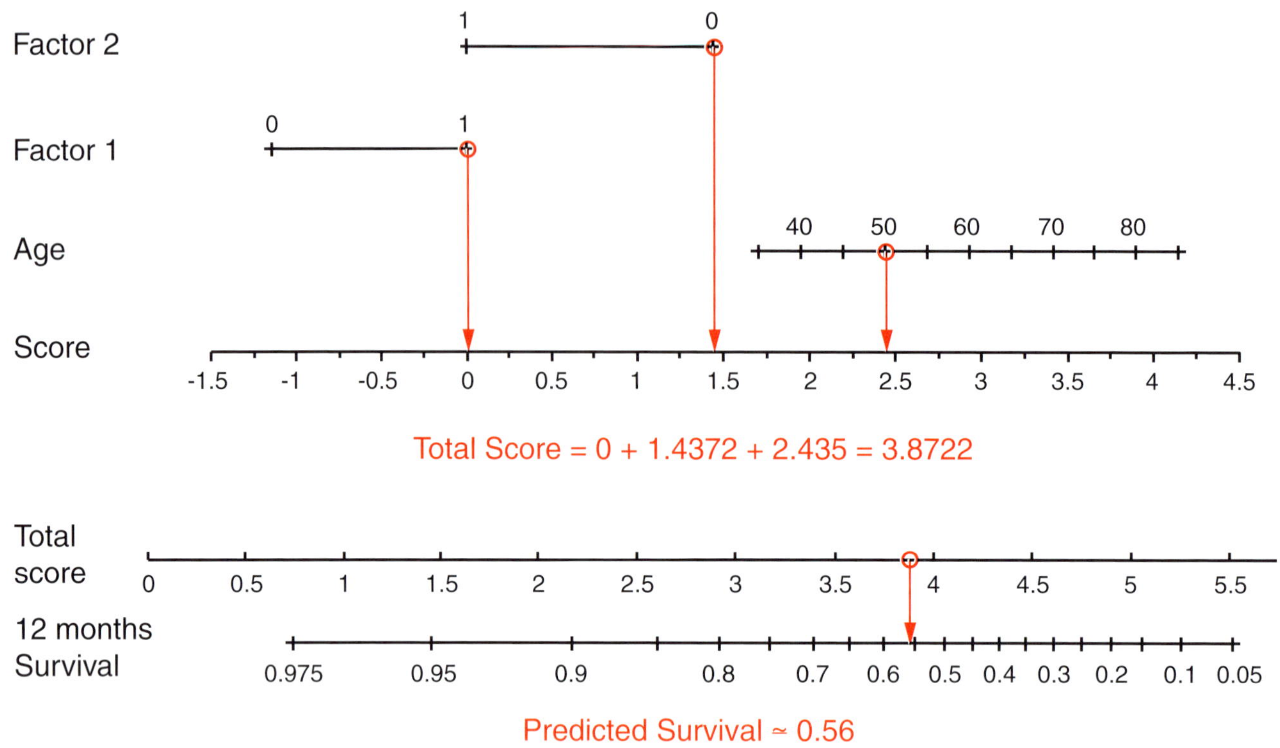

Fig. 17 Final nomogram drawn by joining the two graphs in Figs. 15 and 16. Some finishing touch is needed to get the final aspect by using a vector graphics software package (e.g. adding the labels close to the values on the lines because they can't be shown using Microsoft® Excel). An example of use is provided by using a patient having Factor 1 = 1, Factor 2 = 0 and age = 50. For each covariate value the corresponding score can be read on the '*Score*' line. After calculating the sum of the single scores the final result can be read in the *Total score*' line that points to the' 12 months Survival' scale in the bottom

example shown in Table 4 we want to calculate the predicted survival at 12 months. The result of prediction is given by the equation:

$$S_i(t) = e^{\{-H_i(t)\}} = e^{\left\{-H_0(t)\cdot e^{[x_i\beta]}\right\}} \tag{9}$$

$$\text{with } x_i\beta = 0.0487 \cdot Age - 1.1378 \cdot Factor1 + 1.4372 \cdot Factor2 \tag{10}$$

$$\text{and } H_0(t) = 0.012 \tag{11}$$

We create a scatterplot where three lines define the contribution of the three addenda in the Eq. 9 to the exponent of the function. This exponent $x_i\beta$ is usually referred as *score*. For the age, a continuous variable, a scale with different steps is created multiplying each age value with the corresponding coefficient (0.0487). It is important to use as extreme values of the scale numbers that can be found in the dataset used for verification, because the validation of the model has been achieved over a specific range of covariates levels and extrapolations could be misleading. For the not-significant values of dummy covariates the resulting addendum is null, for the significant ones it is the value of the coefficients. Figure 15 contains the screenshot of the spreadsheet with the values to be shown in the scatterplot. Of course it is useful to join the points in each plotted series (corresponding to each covariate) with a line. Finally we need to translate the score into a survival value. A second scatter plot can be created by filling a column with a series of steps related to preset survival values and the corresponding score can be calculated by solving the Eq. 7 as function of $x_i\beta$. The solution is given in the Eq. 12:

$$x_i\beta = \log\{\log[1/S_i(t)]/H_0(t)\} \tag{12}$$

The new spreadsheet with the new scatter plot is shown in Fig. 16. In order to publish the nomogram the final step is to assemble the two graphs created in the spreadsheet, by adding the labels and optimizing the final graphical result. An example of 'final product' is shown in Fig. 17. In order to calculate the survival the reader has to find in the covariates lines the values corresponding to the patient's features (in the example Factor 1 = 1, Factor 2 = 0, Age = 50 years) and then trace vertical lines from the corresponding values down to the 'Score' scale, in order to get the addenda to be summed each other for calculating the 'Total score'. Finally starting from the 'Total score' scale another vertical line has to be drawn down to the '12 months survival' scale in order to get the final result.

7 Appendix 1

#	Survival	Census	Factor_1	Factor_2	Marker level	Age	Age class	Marker class
1	3	0	1	1	27	45	Elderly	High
2	3	0	0	0	13	38	Young	Low
3	3	0	1	1	26	62	Elderly	High
4	4	0	1	1	27	39	Young	High
5	5	0	0	0	12	55	Elderly	Low
6	6	0	1	1	28	45	Elderly	High
7	6	0	1	1	27	41	Young	High
8	6	0	1	1	27	55	Elderly	High
9	6	1	1	0	26	43	Elderly	High
10	6	1	1	0	28	53	Elderly	High
11	6	1	1	0	24	44	Elderly	High
12	6	0	0	1	6	44	Elderly	Low
13	6	0	1	0	27	41	Young	High
14	6	1	1	1	21	73	Elderly	Low
15	6	1	1	0	23	50	Elderly	High
16	6	0	1	1	27	48	Elderly	High
17	7	1	1	0	27	50	Elderly	High
18	7	0	1	1	28	42	Elderly	High
19	7	1	1	1	21	83	Elderly	Low
20	8	1	1	0	17	64	Elderly	Low
21	8	1	0	0	13	49	Elderly	Low
22	8	1	1	0	25	41	Young	High
23	8	0	0	1	16	36	Young	Low
24	8	0	1	1	30	47	Elderly	High
25	8	0	1	0	26	41	Young	High
26	9	0	1	1	29	50	Elderly	High
27	9	1	1	1	24	41	Young	High
28	9	0	0	1	12	43	Elderly	Low
29	10	1	1	0	17	43	Elderly	Low
30	11	0	1	1	23	47	Elderly	High
31	11	0	0	0	16	50	Elderly	Low
32	11	1	0	1	26	43	Elderly	High
33	11	0	1	0	28	41	Young	High
34	11	1	1	0	26	47	Elderly	High
35	11	0	1	1	27	41	Young	High
36	11	0	1	1	27	38	Young	High
37	11	0	1	1	18	53	Elderly	Low
38	11	1	0	0	24	43	Elderly	High
39	12	1	1	0	26	42	Elderly	High
40	12	1	1	0	23	47	Elderly	High
41	12	0	1	1	27	41	Young	High
42	12	0	1	0	27	43	Elderly	High

(continued)

(continued)

#	Survival	Census	Factor_1	Factor_2	Marker level	Age	Age class	Marker class
43	12	1	1	1	24	54	Elderly	High
44	12	1	0	0	24	38	Young	High
45	12	0	1	1	26	57	Elderly	High
46	12	1	0	0	23	36	Young	High
47	12	0	0	1	25	41	Young	High
48	12	0	0	1	5	39	Young	Low
49	13	0	1	0	26	41	Young	High
50	13	0	0	1	18	41	Young	Low
51	13	0	0	1	20	41	Young	Low
52	13	0	0	1	9	68	Elderly	Low
53	13	0	0	1	18	44	Elderly	Low
54	13	1	1	0	23	47	Elderly	High
55	14	0	1	0	25	41	Young	High
56	14	0	0	1	8	50	Elderly	Low
57	14	0	0	1	16	45	Elderly	Low
58	16	1	1	1	26	41	Young	High
59	16	1	1	1	25	43	Elderly	High
60	16	0	0	1	13	39	Young	Low
61	17	0	0	1	24	45	Elderly	High
62	17	0	1	1	27	38	Young	High
63	17	0	1	1	24	41	Young	High
64	17	1	0	0	23	43	Elderly	High
65	17	0	1	1	26	41	Young	High
66	18	1	0	0	21	44	Elderly	Low
67	18	1	1	1	23	73	Elderly	High
68	18	0	1	1	20	46	Elderly	Low
69	19	0	0	0	5	41	Young	Low
70	19	0	1	1	20	51	Elderly	Low
71	19	1	1	1	26	42	Elderly	High
72	20	0	0	0	20	37	Young	Low
73	20	0	0	1	18	44	Elderly	Low
74	20	0	0	0	25	42	Elderly	High
75	21	0	1	1	20	36	Young	Low
76	21	0	1	1	18	59	Elderly	Low
77	21	0	1	1	27	46	Elderly	High
78	22	0	0	1	21	39	Young	Low
79	22	0	0	1	11	55	Elderly	Low
80	23	0	0	1	15	41	Young	Low
81	24	0	0	1	16	39	Young	Low
82	24	0	1	1	28	41	Young	High
83	24	0	0	1	16	37	Young	Low
84	24	1	1	0	24	41	Young	High
85	25	0	0	0	18	45	Elderly	Low
86	25	1	1	0	25	38	Young	High

(continued)

(continued)

#	Survival	Census	Factor_1	Factor_2	Marker level	Age	Age class	Marker class
87	25	0	0	0	27	46	Elderly	High
88	26	0	0	0	14	40	Young	Low
89	26	0	1	1	25	47	Elderly	High
90	26	1	0	0	15	43	Elderly	Low
91	28	0	0	1	11	38	Young	Low
92	28	1	0	1	1	39	Young	Low
93	29	0	0	1	15	38	Young	Low
94	29	1	0	0	19	50	Elderly	Low
95	29	1	1	1	21	42	Elderly	Low
96	29	0	1	1	24	41	Young	High
97	30	0	1	0	27	39	Young	High
98	30	0	0	0	22	47	Elderly	Low
99	30	1	1	0	9	45	Elderly	Low
100	30	1	1	0	25	38	Young	High
101	31	0	1	1	26	41	Young	High
102	31	0	0	1	5	38	Young	Low
103	31	0	0	0	24	59	Elderly	High
104	32	1	1	0	21	47	Elderly	Low
105	32	0	1	1	26	41	Young	High
106	32	0	0	1	27	41	Young	High
107	32	0	0	0	13	45	Elderly	Low
108	33	0	0	0	18	44	Elderly	Low
109	34	0	0	0	16	43	Elderly	Low
110	34	0	0	1	11	65	Elderly	Low
111	34	0	1	1	16	43	Elderly	Low
112	34	0	0	0	4	43	Elderly	Low
113	35	0	0	1	25	47	Elderly	High
114	36	0	0	1	13	40	Young	Low
115	36	0	1	1	25	51	Elderly	High
116	36	0	1	0	26	41	Young	High
117	36	0	1	1	23	52	Elderly	High
118	36	0	0	1	26	39	Young	High
119	37	0	1	1	26	42	Elderly	High
120	37	0	0	1	12	39	Young	Low
121	37	0	1	0	27	39	Young	High
122	37	0	1	1	27	47	Elderly	High
123	38	0	0	1	21	53	Elderly	Low
124	38	1	1	0	26	45	Elderly	High
125	38	0	0	1	24	39	Young	High
126	40	0	0	1	8	36	Young	Low
127	41	0	0	0	15	37	Young	Low
128	41	0	0	1	27	49	Elderly	High
129	42	0	0	0	16	78	Elderly	Low
130	42	0	1	0	15	41	Young	Low

(continued)

(continued)

#	Survival	Census	Factor_1	Factor_2	Marker level	Age	Age class	Marker class
131	42	0	1	1	22	46	Elderly	Low
132	42	0	1	1	17	44	Elderly	Low
133	43	1	0	1	27	52	Elderly	High
134	44	0	1	1	24	41	Young	High
135	44	0	1	0	21	43	Elderly	Low
136	45	0	0	1	19	52	Elderly	Low
137	47	0	1	1	27	38	Young	High
138	48	0	0	1	10	46	Elderly	Low
139	48	0	0	1	22	45	Elderly	Low
140	53	0	1	0	25	44	Elderly	High
141	60	1	0	0	16	50	Elderly	Low
142	61	0	0	1	21	46	Elderly	Low
143	65	0	1	1	26	38	Young	High
144	70	0	1	1	24	47	Elderly	High

References

Bradley JD, Hope A, El Naqa I, Apte A, Lindsay PE, Bosch W (2007) A nomogram to predict radiation pneumonitis, derived from a combined analysis of RTOG 9311 and institutional data. Int J Radiat Oncol Biol Phys 69(4):985–992. doi: 10.1016/j.ijrobp.2007.04.077

Cox DR (1972) Regression models and life-tables. J Roy Stat Soc B (Methodol) 34(2):187–220

Doerfler R (2009) The lost art of nomography. UMAP J 30(4):457–493. http://myreckonings.com/wordpress/wp-content/uploads/JournalArticle/The_Lost_Art_of_Nomography.pdf. Accessed 15 Mar 2013

Efron B, Tibshirani RJ (1993) An introduction to the bootstrap. Chapman & Hall, New York

Eisenhauer EA, Therasse P, Bogaerts J, Schwartz LH, Sargent D, Ford R (2009) New response evaluation criteria in solid tumours: revised RECIST guideline (version 1.1). Eur J Cancer 45(2):228–247. doi: 10.1016/j.ejca.2008.10.026

Grambsch PM, Therneau TM (1994) Proportional hazards tests and diagnostics based on weighted residuals. Biometrika 81(3): 515–526

Harrel FE (2001) Regression modeling strategies. Springer, New York

Heagerty PJ, Lumley T, Pepe MS (2000) Time-dependent ROC curves for censored survival data and a diagnostic marker. Biometrics 56(2):337–344. doi:10.1111/j.0006-341X.2000.00337.x

Iasonos A, Schrag D, Raj GV, Panageas KS (2008) How to build and interpret a nomogram for cancer prognosis. J Clin Oncol 26(8):1364–1370. doi:10.1200/JCO.2007.12.9791

Kattan MW, Eastham JA, Wheeler TM, Maru N, Scardino PT, Erbersdobler A (2003) Counseling men with prostate cancer: a nomogram for predicting the presence of small, moderately differentiated, confined tumors. J Urol 170(5):1792–1797. doi: 10.1097/01.ju.0000091806.70171.41

Lee CK, Simes RJ, Brown C, Lord S, Wagner U, Plante M et al (2011) Prognostic nomogram to predict progression-free survival in patients with platinum-sensitive recurrent ovarian cancer. Br J Cancer 105(8):1144–1150. doi:10.1038/bjc.2011.364

Machin D, Cheung YB, Parmar MKB (2006) Survival analysis: a practical approach. Wiley, Chichester

Mantel N (1966) Evaluation of survival data and two new rank order statistics arising in its consideration. Cancer Chemother Rep Part 1 50(3):163–170

Schemper M, Smith TL (1996) A note on quantifying follow-up in studies of failure time. Control Clin Trials 17(4):343–346. doi: 10.1016/0197-2456(96)00075-X

Schoenfeld D (1982) Hazards regression Partial residuals for the proportional model. Biometrika 69(1):239–241

Shuster JJ (1991) Median follow-up in clinical trials. J Clin Oncol 9(1):191–192

Van Stiphout RGPM, Lammering G, Buijsen J, Janssen MHM, Gambacorta MA, Slagmolen P (2011) Development and external validation of a predictive model for pathological complete response of rectal cancer patients including sequential PET-CT imaging. Radiother Oncol 98(1):126–133. doi: 10.1016/j.radonc.2010.12.002

Taktak AFG, Eleuteri A, Lake SP, Fisher AC (2007) Evaluation of prognostic models: discrimination and calibraation performance. Computational Intelligence in Medicine, Plymouth. http://pcwww.liv.ac.uk/~afgt/CIMED07_1.pdf. Accessed 15 Mar 2013

Valentini V, Van Stiphout RGPM, Lammering G, Gambacorta MA, Barba MC, Bebenek M (2011) Nomograms for predicting local recurrence, distant metastases, and overall survival for patients with locally advanced rectal cancer on the basis of European randomized clinical trials. J Clin Oncol 29(23):3163–3172. doi: 10.1200/JCO.2010.33.1595

Integration of Gene Signatures and Genomic Data into Radiation Oncology Practice

Maria A. Thomas, Ramachandran Rashmi, Jacqueline Payton, Imran Zoberi, and Julie K. Schwarz

Contents

M. A. Thomas · R. Rashmi · I. Zoberi · J. K. Schwarz (✉)
Department of Radiation Oncology, Washington University School of Medicine in St. Louis, 4921 Parkview Place, Box 8224, St. Louis, MO 63110, USA
e-mail: jschwarz@radonc.wustl.edu

J. Payton
Department of Pathology and Immunology, Washington University School of Medicine in St. Louis, 4921 Parkview Place, Box 8224, St. Louis, MO 63110, USA

J. K. Schwarz
Department of Cell Biology and Physiology, Washington University School of Medicine in St. Louis, 4921 Parkview Place, Box 8224, St. Louis, MO 63110, USA

Abstract

One of the goals of personalized medicine is to utilize biomarkers to sub-classify patients into risk groups that can be used to guide recommendations for therapy. In addition to classical risk factors, gene signatures and genomics are being developed as a means to biologically characterize tumors and to stratify patients according to the risk associated with the specific molecular aberrations present in their disease. Gene signatures and genomics are currently being investigated as a personalized medicine strategy for many cancers, but have been studied most extensively in breast cancer. In this disease, the results of genetic signatures have come to influence current recommendations for adjuvant chemotherapy for appropriately selected patient populations. In this chapter, we will review the use of gene signatures and genomics in the development of personalized oncology, with an emphasis on applications for breast cancer.

1 Personalized Medicine and Biomarkers

Cancer often exhibits both inter-patient and intra-tumoral genetic heterogeneity, even among patients with the same primary malignancy (Schilsky 2010; De Palma and Hanahan 2012). In order to assess an individual patient's prognosis, often clinical or pathologic features are utilized, such as age, tumor size, lymph node status, histology, grade, and margin status, among other features depending on the specific malignancy. With a steadily growing understanding of the biologic basis for the heterogeneity of cancer, there is considerable interest in biomarker development and the implementation of personalized medicine (Ely 2009; Ginsburg and Willard 2009). A biomarker is defined by the NCI as a biological molecule that is found in the blood, other body fluids, or tissue that is a sign of a condition or disease. Biomarkers have many uses in oncology, including risk

C. Nieder and L. E. Gaspar (eds.), *Decision Tools for Radiation Oncology*, Medical Radiology. Radiation Oncology,
DOI: 10.1007/174_2013_858,
Published Online: 25 June 2013

assessment (BRCA mutation analysis), screening (PSA), prognosis (Oncotype DX), and prediction of response to therapy (HER2 amplification) (Henry and Hayes 2012). In addition, several biomarkers, such as CEA, PSA, and CA 15-3, can be used to monitor response to therapy and to detect recurrent disease. An important distinction should be made regarding the difference between prognostic and predictive biomarkers. Prognostic biomarkers provide information on patient outcome, independent of treatment. Predictive biomarkers, however, can be used to predict the likelihood of a response to a given therapy. While prognostic biomarkers may be useful to determine the natural history of disease, predictive biomarkers may be better suited to provide a means to personalize therapy (La Thangue and Kerr 2011).

As many key regulators of cellular processes have been identified, including oncogenes and tumor suppressor genes, it was anticipated that normal cellular function might be restored by counteracting a specific genetic abnormality. However, the complexity of the dysregulation that develops during carcinogenesis is perhaps greater than was originally anticipated. In addition, the frequent crosstalk between pathways has sometimes hindered development of novel cancer therapies that have meaningful clinical efficacy (De Palma and Hanahan 2012; Mendelsohn et al. 2012).

The concept of personalized medicine, at first glance, might seem to imply that each individual patient would receive a unique combination of therapies specific to the genetic aberrations present in his/her malignancy. However, as a practical matter, personalized medicine in oncology often uses predictive biomarkers to identify subgroups of patients who are likely to benefit from a specific targeted therapy. With many of the recently developed targeted therapies, often only a small proportion of patients, on the order of 10–20 %, will harbor the specific molecular aberration and be expected to respond to the targeted therapy. Instead of exposing a large population of patients to additional systemic therapy, treatment efficacy could be maximized by administering this therapy only to those most likely to derive a benefit. In this way, patients who are unlikely to benefit from the therapy can avoid the additional side effects and cost. The overall goal of this strategy of personalized medicine is to define specific subgroups of patients and to tailor therapy accordingly (La Thangue and Kerr 2011). It should be emphasized that risk stratification in personalized medicine using biomarkers is currently only additive in the context of clinical/anatomic staging. Gene expression profiling is one method that has been used clinically to define patient subgroups and to administer personalized medicine. We will next review the methods and statistical issues related to gene expression profiling.

2 Introduction to Gene Expression Profiling and Associated Technologies

2.1 Methods of Gene Expression Profiling

Gene expression is the formation of a functional gene product that is created from the information contained within a gene. Gene expression profiling involves assessing the relative amounts of mRNA produced from various genes. The first step of gene expression profiling involves isolation and purification of the mRNA from the test sample. In the case of tumor samples, this is often obtained from formalin-fixed paraffin-embedded (FFPE) tissue, such as biopsy or surgical resection specimens. Although this method is feasible, formalin-fixation and processing of a tissue specimens results in chemical modification and degradation of RNA (Medeiros et al. 2007). Therefore, when possible, frozen specimens or fresh specimens stored in special RNA-preserving solution are desired, as they yield more intact RNA. Regardless of the method of preservation, delays between tissue harvesting and specimen fixation should be minimized, in order to reduce RNA degradation. Once the mRNA is isolated and purified, it is converted to complementary DNA (cDNA) by reverse transcription.

The microarray technique utilizes an array of gene-specific DNA probes or oligos, spotted onto a slide (Quackenbush 2006; Tefferi et al. 2002; Hamilton 2012). Each spot contains a specific DNA sequence corresponding to a gene. The relative level of gene expression for each gene can be determined for a sample by fluorescently-labeling the cDNA and then hybridizing the labeled cDNA with the DNA microarray. The relative fluorescence intensity, which corresponds to the level of gene expression, can then be determined for each gene (Fig. 1). The Mammaprint is an example of a microarray-based test designed to assess a woman's risk of metastasis from breast cancer, and will be discussed in more detail later in this chapter (Kim et al. 2009).

Alternatively, gene expression can be assessed with a quantitative PCR (qPCR) based approach, in which the cDNA obtained from a sample is amplified using gene-specific primers and labeled probes. This method requires creation of specific primers and probes for each gene of interest, and logistically this limits the number of genes that can be analyzed. Oncotype DX is an example of a qPCR-based test which can be used to assess recurrence risk for women with ER-positive, lymph node-negative breast cancer. The Oncotype DX assay will be discussed further later in this chapter (Kim et al. 2009).

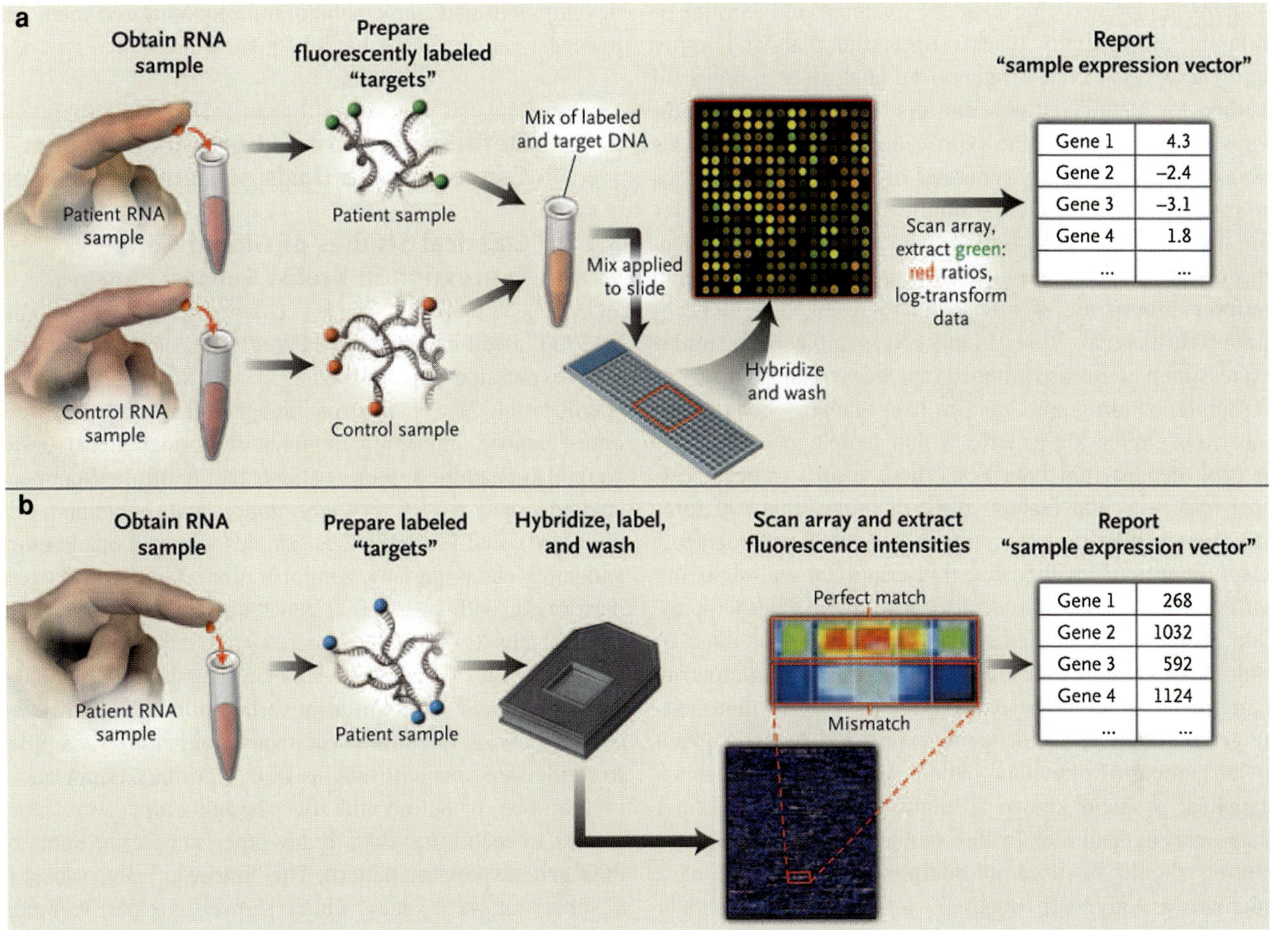

Fig. 1 Overview of microarray analysis. Reprinted with permission from Quackenbush (2006)

2.2 Validation of Gene Expression Profiling

Prior to clinical application, the use of a specific biomarker or a panel of biomarkers must be thoroughly studied and validated (Simon et al. 2009). Teutsch et al. outline three key components to evaluation of a genetic test: analytic validity, clinical validity, and (Henry and Hayes 2012; Teutsch et al. 2009). The first component, *analytic validity*, is defined as the ability of a test to accurately and reliably measure the genotype of interest. The analytic validity includes assessment of the sensitivity, specificity, precision (reproducibility), and assay robustness (resistance to small changes in assay parameters). The second component, *clinical validity*, is defined as the ability of a test to accurately and reliably predict the clinical event. This includes determination of the positive and negative predictive values of the test. Clinical validity requires analysis of an independent cohort to validate the original findings. This is often performed with an initial analysis of a "test set" and confirmation with an independent "validation set", which may be an independent cohort of patients at the same institution or, alternatively, patients at another institution. The third component in evaluating a new biomarker is *clinical utility*, which is defined as evidence of improved measurable clinical outcome, and added value to patient management decision-making compared with current management. In other words, does the use of the new biomarker provide additional information that changes patient management? Also, the extent of the effect of the biomarker is considered. For example, does the biomarker status correspond to a small percentage change in outcome or does it confer a large, several-fold difference? Is this difference enough for clinicians to change management?

Microarray data analysis enables us to monitor the expression level of genes and changes in the expression patterns with respect to pathologic conditions at a genome scale. There are two approaches to analyze the data—supervised or unsupervised analysis. In supervised analysis, distinct groups of genes or samples (i.e. patient vs. normal) are identified and differences in expression profiles between the groups are evaluated. On the other hand, in unsupervised analysis, sets of genes or samples with similar expression profiles are grouped, and their common clinical and physiological and/or biological features are identified.

If there are pre-existing clusters (patients and normal or different known tumor types), supervised analysis is more appropriate. However, unsupervised analysis is a powerful method for identifying new clusters (uncharacterized pathways of dysregulated gene expression, new tumor subtypes etc.) Clustering analysis generates distinct groups of genes or samples based on their similarity of expression profiles and may be hierarchical or non-hierarchical. In hierarchical clustering, the relationships among objects within and between groups are specified and represented as dendrograms (Hastie et al. 2009). In this way, samples with similar expression patterns are grouped together within branches of a sample dendrogram, and in like manner, genes with consistent expression patterns within sample groups cluster in gene dendrogram branches. These results indicate cellular and molecular features differentiating groups of samples, which may be important for diagnosis or prognosis, and furthermore identify key transcriptional and signaling pathways that may be targeted by new or existing therapies. One pitfall with microarray data analysis is the issue of multiple hypothesis testing. By definition, microarray experiments simultaneously test the expression of thousands of genes, often assessing gene expression using a much lower number of individual patient samples. This creates a statistical problem known as multiple hypothesis testing. Data analysis solutions to this problem exist, but extreme caution should be used in interpreting the results of a microarray study with relatively low numbers of patient samples (<25), thousands of gene probes and a single patient/tumor data set. The false discovery rate (FDR), which is a modified p value used to adjust for multiple comparisons, is often reported when groups of patient samples are compared for gene expression using microarrays. In general, FDR values <0.05 are acceptable for statistical significance in microarray studies, and most current studies employ additional methods to reduce the false positive rate (Benjamini and Hochberg 1995; Storey and Tibshirani 2003). In addition, a number of more advanced statistical methods are currently available for data analysis, many of which evaluate biologically meaningful gene sets or pathways (Hastie et al. 2009; Tseng et al. 2012).

In summary, prior to implementation of a new biomarker or gene signature into clinical practice, it must be evaluated for analytic validity, clinical validity, and clinical utility. Large validation studies are required. The highest level of evidence for a new genetic signature would be a prospective clinical study that is designed with assessment of the biomarker as the primary objective of the trial (Henry and Hayes 2012). This would minimize bias in subject selection and standardize sample handling and assay conditions. Gene expression profiling has been perhaps most extensively studied in breast cancer. We will next review the development and implementation of personalized medicine in breast cancer on the basis of gene expression.

3 Defining Patient Subgroups in Breast Cancer on the Basis of Gene Expression

3.1 Classical Studies of Global Gene Expression in Breast Cancer

In 2000, a seminal paper by Perou et al. characterized the gene expression patterns for 42 women with breast cancer (Perou et al. 2000). Most of the specimens analyzed were breast cancer, but a few samples of normal breast tissue were also examined. Some patients had multiple specimens studied, such as the primary tumor and a lymph node metastasis, and in some cases samples were obtained before and after chemotherapy administration. Microarrays were performed, with over 8,000 genes analyzed. Using a hierarchical clustering method, genes were grouped based on the similarity of their patterns of expression. The authors found that there was significant variation in gene expression patterns among the tumor specimens. Interestingly, samples from the same patient, such as from a primary tumor and a lymph node, or before and after chemotherapy, were more similar to each other than to any other sample, in terms of their gene expression pattern. The "intrinsic" gene subset is a subset of 496 genes which showed greater variation between unrelated samples than was seen between samples from the same patient. This subset of genes includes specific clusters of genes, such as the luminal cluster, HER2 (Erb-B2) cluster, proliferation cluster, and basal cluster. The "molecular portraits" of gene expression examined in this study led to identification of the intrinsic subtypes of breast cancer. In the first publication, the subtypes identified were ER+/luminal-like, basal-like, Erb-B2+, and normal breast (Perou et al. 2000). Further investigation led to the finding that the luminal subtype could potentially be divided into two or three subgroups, termed luminal A, luminal B, and luminal C, each with a unique gene expression pattern (Sorlie et al. 2001). Alternatively, two luminal subgroups, luminal A and luminal B, could be described. Importantly, the clinical outcome of patients was evaluated for each of the subtypes, including luminal A, luminal B, luminal C, normal breast-like, Erb-B2+, and basal-like. Significant differences were seen in both relapse-free survival and overall survival, with basal-like and Erb-B2+ subtypes having the worst outcome and luminal A subtype showing the best outcome (Fig. 2). In a subsequent analysis of 115 breast cancers, the subtypes were further refined (Sorlie et al. 2003), to include the luminal A, luminal B, basal, Erb-B2+, and normal breast-like subtypes. The cluster dendrogram for tumors, when divided into these five subtypes

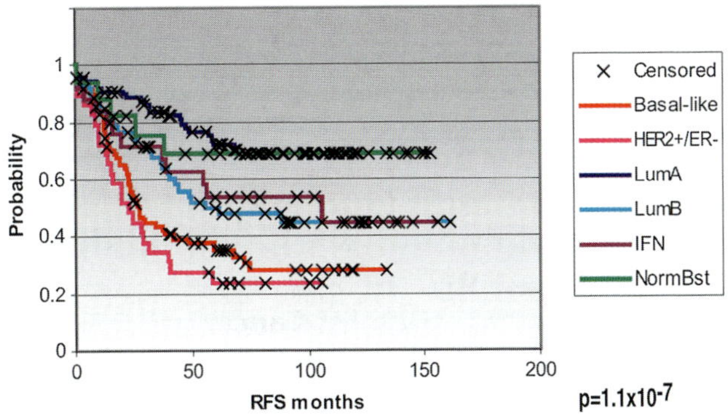

Fig. 2 Clinical outcome for patients based on tumor subtype. Kaplan-Meier survival curves demonstrate the relapse-free survival (RFS) for breast cancer patients, as classified by tumor subtype. Reprinted with permission from Hu et al. (2006)

(luminal A, luminal B, normal breast-like, Erb-B2+, and basal-like), can be seen in Fig. 3. Also, the full cluster diagram and gene expression patterns can be seen in Fig. 4. Subtype characterization was confirmed by cluster analyses performed on independent data sets of cohorts of patients from other institutions. The clinical outcomes of different subtypes were assessed and revealed differences in overall survival and time to distant metastases. One other interesting finding from this work was that *BRCA1* mutation was strongly associated with predisposition to the basal tumor phenotype.

More recently, a new breast cancer intrinsic gene list containing 1300 genes was evaluated and validated in independent data sets (Hu et al. 2006). This analysis stratified patients into five subtypes, luminal A, luminal B, basal-like, HER2+, and normal breast-like, using a 105 tumor training set and validation set of 311 tumor samples (compiled from three independent studies). Clinical outcomes for the subtypes were significantly different in terms of relapse-free and overall survival. Multivariate analysis demonstrated that tumor subtype was prognostic of relapse-free, disease-specific, and overall survival, independent of standard clinical factors such as tumor size, lymph node status, and tumor grade.

3.2 Implications of Breast Cancer Subtype for Systemic Therapy Selection

Determination of breast tumor subtype is clinically valuable, as the subtype (often clinically defined by immunohistochemical profile) frequently guides decisions for systemic therapy. For example, women with luminal A or luminal B (ER positive) breast cancer, are known to derive benefit from adjuvant hormone therapy (Davies et al. 2011), and therefore most will receive anti-estrogen therapy in the form of tamoxifen or an aromatase inhibitor. Patients with the Erb-B2+(HER2+) subtype will often receive Herceptin (trastuzumab), which is a monoclonal antibody against the HER2/neu receptor. Women with HER2-positive breast cancer who are either lymph node-positive or high-risk node negative have been found to benefit from Herceptin therapy (Smith et al. 2007; Perez et al. 2011) and many current studies are exploring combinations of anti-HER2 targeted therapies for these patients (Gianni et al. 2012). The basal subtype or the overlapping subtype known as "triple negative breast cancer" continues to receive significant research attention due to its relative poor prognosis and lack of targeted therapeutic strategies. Information provided by the intrinsic subtypes (using an immunohistochemical approach) has been adopted by 2011 St. Gallen Consensus Conference (Goldhirsch et al. 2011) (Table 1).

4 Gene Signatures and Clinical Decision Making in Breast Cancer

Fortunately, the majority of women diagnosed with breast cancer do not have metastatic disease at the time of diagnosis, and are in a clinically curable situation. However, after surgery, all women have some degree of risk of relapse, at local, regional, and distant sites. The magnitude of the risk of relapse can be quite different depending on the individual woman, and can be assessed using clinical, pathologic, and treatment-related variables. Over the past decade, gene signatures for women with breast cancer have provided significant additional prognostic information. The greatest clinical impact of these assays has been risk stratification in relatively low risk patient populations (ER positive and node negative). Specifically, Mammaprint is a commercially available gene expression assay that has been used to predict recurrence in patients with node negative cancers. Oncotype DX is a commercially available, clinically validated gene expression assay that is used to guide recommendations for the use of systemic chemotherapy in addition to anti-estrogen therapy for patients with ER positive, node negative disease. It is important to note that clinical use of any gene signature should be considered only for independently validated assays performed on large datasets, and care should be taken to apply use of the signature only to patients for whom the assay has been validated. Currently, clinical use of Oncotype DX in node positive and/or ER negative disease is considered experimental.

4.1 Mammaprint

One of the earliest gene signatures for breast cancer was the Mammaprint, or the Amsterdam 70-gene prognostic

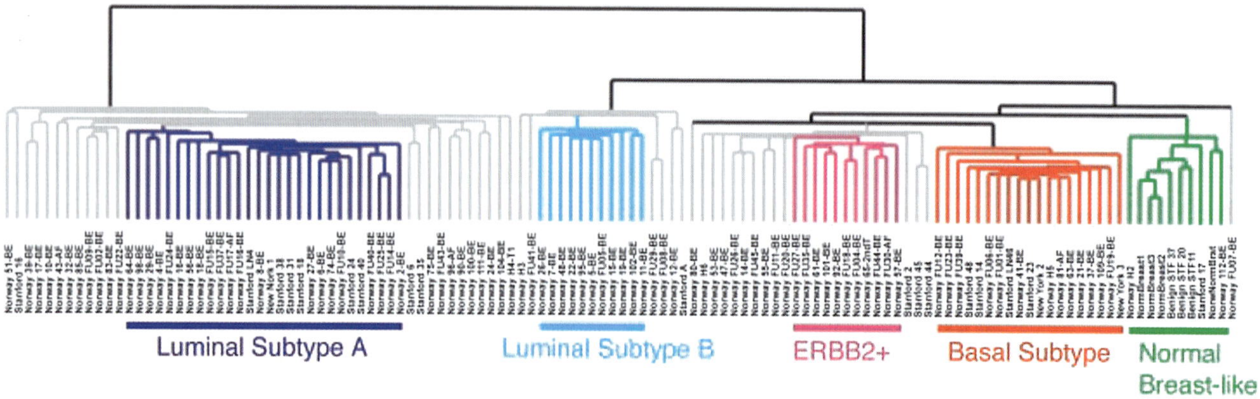

Fig. 3 Cluster dendrogram demonstrating tumor subtypes. This dendogram shows the clustering of the tumors into five tumor subgroups. Branches for tumors with low correlation to any tumor subtype are shown in gray. Reprinted with permission from Sorlie et al. (2003)

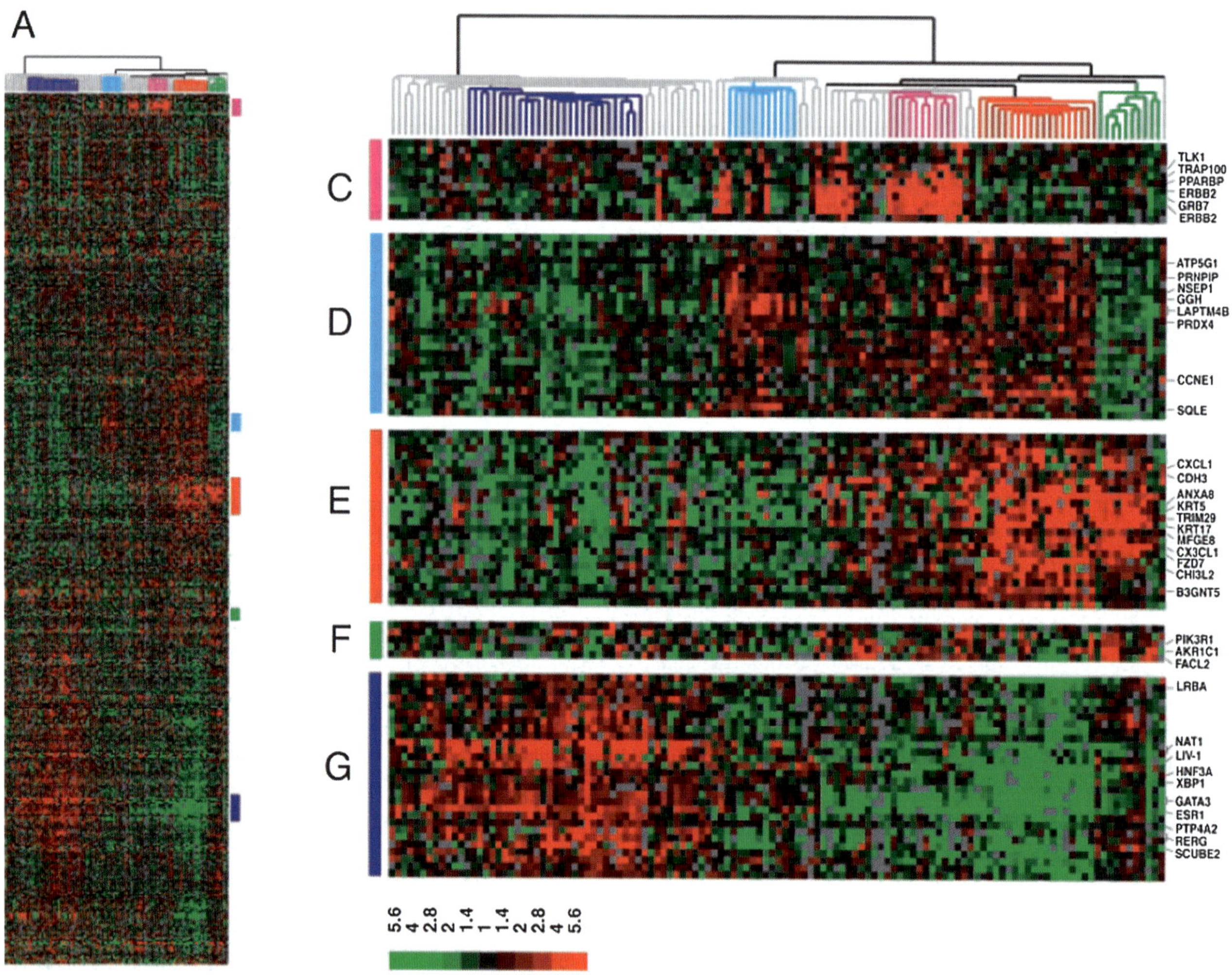

Fig. 4 Hierarchical clustering of breast tumors using the intrinsic gene set, with full cluster (*left*) and specific gene clusters shown in more detail (*right*), including the Erb B2+ (*C*), luminal B (*D*), basal (*E*), normal breast-like (*F*), and luminal A (*G*) clusters. Reprinted with permission from Sorlie et al. (2003)

Table 1 2011 St Gallen consensus recommendations of systemic treatment

IHC Subtype	Definition	Type of adjuvant therapy
Luminal A	HR+/HER2-/Ki67 low	Endocrine therapy alone[a]
Luminal B	HR+/HER2−/Ki67 high	Endocrine therapy ± cytotoxic therapy
HER2-positive	HR-/HER2+	Cytotoxics + anti-HER2 therapy
Triple-negative	HR−/HER2−	Cytotoxics

[a] A few patients require cytotoxics (such as high nodal status or other indicator of risk)
HR hormone receptor
Source This table reprinted with permission from Prat et al. (2011) summarizes current treatment recommendations for systemic therapy based upon breast cancer subtype

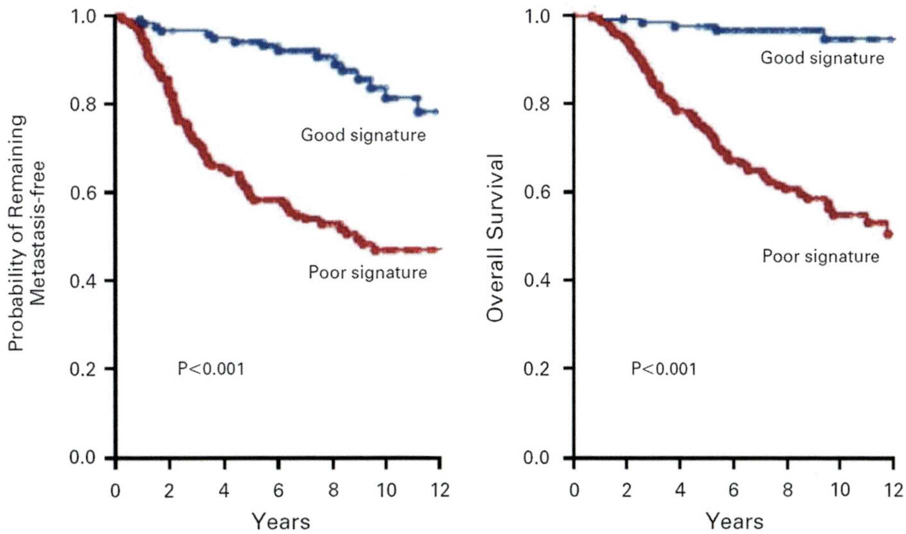

Fig. 5 Patient outcome based on Mammaprint signature. The metastasis-free survival (*left panel*) and overall survival (*right panel*) of breast cancer patients with good prognosis signature and poor prognosis signature are shown. Reprinted with permission from van de Vijver et al. (2002)

signature. This signature was initially characterized in a cohort of 98 primary breast cancer patients, which included 34 women that developed distant metastatic disease within 5 years and 44 women who did not (van't Veer et al. 2002). There were also 20 patients with BRCA1 or BRCA2 germline mutations included in the analysis. For the sporadic cases, all women were <55 years old, had a tumor size <5 cm, and were lymph node negative. RNA was isolated from frozen tumor samples and supervised analysis of the microarray data identified a set of 70 genes that allowed discrimination between patients with good and poor prognosis, with an accuracy of 83 %. The Mammaprint allows a binary classification, either a good prognosis or poor prognosis signature (Fig. 5). Women in the poor prognostic group based on this signature have a significantly increased risk of developing distant metastatic disease within 5 years (odds ratio, OR = 28). On multivariate analysis including classical prognostic factors, the Mammaprint signature was an independent predictor of outcome.

Further validation of the Mammaprint gene signature was performed in a cohort of 295 patients (van de Vijver et al. 2002). All patients were less than 53 years old, had a primary tumor size of less than 5 cm, and in this cohort 151 were lymph node negative, while 144 were lymph node positive. Overall survival at 10 years was 95 % for those with good prognosis signature and was 55 % for those with poor prognosis signature. Probability of remaining free of distant metastases was 85 % for those with good prognosis signature and 51 % for those with poor prognosis signature. However, it should be noted that 61 patients in this study were also members of the original cohort used to develop the signature. Independent validation studies were subsequently conducted, including an analysis of 302 patients from five European centers (Buyse et al. 2006). Patients included in this analysis were <61 years old, lymph node negative, tumor size <5 cm, and did not receive adjuvant systemic therapy. Median follow-up was 13.6 years. The 70-gene prognostic signature remained an independent prognostic factor for development of distant metastases and overall survival, with unadjusted hazard ratios of 2.32 and 2.79, respectively.

There is also interest in assessing risk of distant metastatic disease in older women, who may not tolerate chemotherapy well. Identification of older women that have a low risk of distant metastatic disease might allow avoidance of the considerable toxicity associated with chemotherapy in this group of women. The Mammaprint gene signature has also been evaluated for women between the ages of 55 and 70 (Mook et al. 2010). In this analysis, frozen tumor specimens from 148 women, aged 55–70 years old with tumor size <5 cm and negative lymph nodes, were analyzed and assigned either good or poor prognosis based on their 70-gene signature. The 70-gene prognosis signature was prognostic of breast cancer-specific survival ($P = 0.036$). Distant metastasis-free survival at 5 years was 93 % for patients with a good prognosis signature and 72 % for those with poor prognosis signature, but this difference was not statistically different in this cohort ($P = 0.07$).

Currently, there are several ongoing clinical trials designed to further characterize the utility of Mammaprint. MINDACT (Microarray In Node-negative and 1–3 positive lymph node Disease may Avoid ChemoTherapy; EORTC 10041), is a Phase III prospective randomized study comparing Mammaprint with clinical-pathological assessment (Adjuvant! Online) in selecting patients with 0–3 positive lymph nodes for adjuvant chemotherapy. In the trial, women with discordant prognostic assessment on Mammaprint and Adjuvant! Online will be randomized for the decision of adjuvant chemotherapy based on either Mammaprint or Adjuvant! Online risk status. All women with high risk scores on both Mammaprint and Adjuvant! Online will receive chemotherapy and all women with low risk scores on both will not receive chemotherapy. Accrual of 6,600 patients has been achieved, with results currently pending.

Other ongoing trials include PROMIS, which is a prospective registry study to assess the impact of Mammaprint on systemic therapy decision making for patients with an intermediate Oncotype DX score. NBRST, is a prospective registry study designed to measure outcomes based on molecular subgroups, determined by Mammaprint and other profiles, for patients undergoing neoadjuvant chemotherapy or endocrine therapy. Similarly, MINT I, is a study designed to test the ability of Mammaprint (in combination with other factors) to predict response to neoadjuvant chemotherapy. Of note, initial studies using Mammaprint were conducted on frozen tissue, but currently the assay can be performed on fresh, frozen, or formalin-fixed paraffin-embedded specimens.

4.2 Oncotype DX

The Oncotype DX is a real-time quantitative reverse-transcriptase-polymerase-chain-reaction (RT-PCR) assay of 21 prospectively selected genes designed for use in fixed, paraffin-embedded tumor specimens. Paik and colleagues first developed a real-time RT-PCR assay to quantify gene expression of 250 candidate genes and subsequently

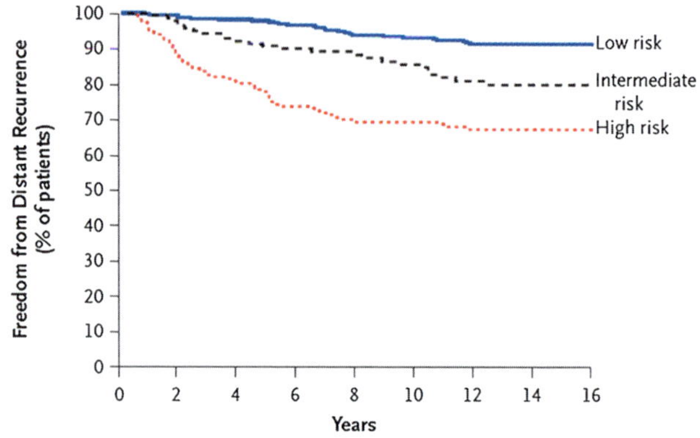

No. at Risk									
Low risk	338	328	313	298	276	258	231	170	38
Intermediate risk	149	139	128	116	104	96	80	66	16
High risk	181	154	137	119	105	91	83	63	13

Fig. 6 Stratification of patient outcome based on Oncotype DX risk group. The freedom from distant recurrence is shown for patients in the low, intermediate, and high risk groups. Reprinted with permission from Paik et al. (2004)

analyzed the relation between breast cancer recurrence and gene expression in a preliminary inquiry of 447 patients (Paik et al. 2004). From this analysis, they selected a panel of 16 cancer-related genes and five reference genes. The cancer-related genes included those involved in proliferation and invasion, among others. An algorithm was designed to calculate a Recurrence Score (RS) based on the levels of expression of these genes. The RS ranged from 0 to 100, with higher scores reflecting greater likelihood of distant recurrence. Patients were divided into three risk categories based on their RS: low-risk (RS < 18), intermediate-risk (RS 18–30), and high-risk (RS > 30). Paik et al. demonstrated the ability of the Oncotype DX assay to predict the likelihood of distant recurrence for women with ER-positive, lymph node-negative breast cancer (Paik et al. 2004). In this analysis, tumor samples from 668 women treated with tamoxifen on NSABP B-14 were evaluated. NSABP B-14 was a clinical trial of ER-positive, node-negative breast cancer, in which women were randomized to tamoxifen versus placebo. The rate of distant recurrence at 10 years was 7 % for those with low-risk RS, 14 % for intermediate-risk RS, and 31 % for high-risk RS (Fig. 6). Recurrence score was found to be an independent prognostic factor on multivariate analysis. RS was also predictive of overall survival. The risk of distant recurrence can be predicted using the RS as a continuous function (Fig. 7).

Determination of the RS from the Oncotype DX assay was also found to predict the magnitude of benefit from chemotherapy. An analysis was performed of tumor samples from the NSABP B-20 trial, in which women with ER-positive, node negative breast cancer were randomized to tamoxifen with or without chemotherapy. RT-PCR was

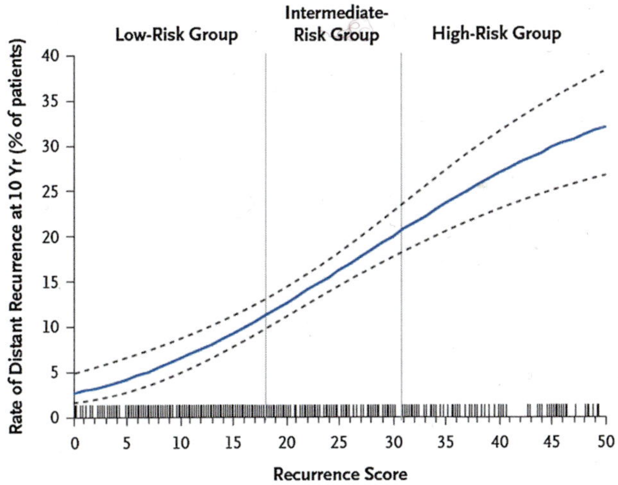

Fig. 7 Rate of distant metastases as a function of Recurrence Score, determined by Oncotype DX analysis. The risk of distant metastasis at 10 years can be estimated for any given recurrence score, using the continuous function shown here. Reprinted with permission from Paik et al. (2004)

successful in the majority (97 %) of blocks that had sufficient remaining specimen and were therefore included in this analysis (n = 651). In NSABP B-20, there was a benefit with the addition of chemotherapy, in terms of local, regional, and distant recurrence. In the current study, the magnitude of benefit from chemotherapy was greatest among patients with high risk RS, and patients in intermediate or low risk groups demonstrated no significant benefit from chemotherapy (Paik et al. 2006). In another study, the Oncotype DX-derived RS was found to be predictive of pathologic complete response (pCR) in patients receiving neoadjuvant chemotherapy (Gianni et al. 2005). Patients with higher RS had a greater probability of having a pCR after completion of neoadjuvant chemotherapy. Based on the findings above, the randomized Phase III TAILORx trial for women with ER-positive, node-negative breast cancer was designed. Women enrolled on this trial with an Oncotype DX RS <11 receive hormone therapy only, and those with a RS >25 receive chemotherapy followed by hormone therapy. Women with RS of 11–25 are randomized to either hormone therapy alone or in combination with chemotherapy. Enrollment has been completed and results are currently pending.

Two preliminary studies have reported on the utility of the Oncotype DX assay in lymph-node positive patients (Dowsett et al. 2010; Albain et al. 2010). Dowsett et al. evaluated the Oncotype DX assay on specimens from the ATAC (Arimidex, Tamoxifen, Alone or in Combination) trial (Dowsett et al. 2010). The ATAC trial compared the efficacy of arimidex, tamoxifen, or both for post-menopausal women. In this analysis, Oncotype DX assay was performed for samples of patients on the single agent arms (arimidex only or tamoxifen only; n = 1,372). Prognostic value of Oncotype-based RS was seen both in patients treated with tamoxifen and confirmed for patients treated with arimidex. In addition, RS was predictive of distant recurrence for lymph node negative (n = 872) and also for lymph node positive patients (n = 306). Similarly, Albain et al. investigated the utility of the Oncotype DX assay for post-menopausal women with node-positive, ER-positive breast cancer (Albain et al. 2010). In this retrospective analysis, 367 samples from the Phase III SWOG-8814 trial, in which women were randomized to tamoxifen with or without the addition of chemotherapy, were analyzed. Patients with high-risk RS showed a significant benefit in disease-free survival with the addition of chemotherapy, whereas those with intermediate- or low-risk RS did not. An ongoing Phase III trial, SWOG RxPONDER (S1007), has been initiated to prospectively evaluate the benefit of chemotherapy for women with 1–3 positive lymph nodes, ER-positive, HER2-negative breast cancer with RS of 25 or less. Women meeting eligibility criteria will be randomized to receive endocrine therapy with or without the addition of chemotherapy. The primary endpoint is disease-free survival and enrollment is ongoing.

Oncotype DX assessment is incorporated in the ASCO recommendations for use of tumor markers in breast cancer and in NCCN guidelines to predict the risk of recurrence for women with ER-positive, HER2-negative, node-negative breast cancer treated with tamoxifen. The NCCN panel considers Oncotype DX an option, to be taken into consideration only in the context of other elements of patient risk stratification. Other applications at this time are investigational and require further validation prior to inclusion in clinical decision-making.

Recently there has been interest in molecular characterization of ductal carcinoma in situ, DCIS. DCIS is a non-invasive form of breast cancer that has the potential to develop into invasive disease over time. Adjuvant radiation therapy has been shown to decrease the risk of both non-invasive and invasive recurrence after partial mastectomy for DCIS. There is ongoing interest in identifying women with DCIS with a low risk of recurrence after surgery who would likely derive a small absolute benefit from adjuvant therapy. However, the use of clinical and pathologic factors to identify women with low risk DCIS is not entirely straightforward. Even patients with low or intermediate grade DCIS and negative margins have a measurable risk of recurrence. Solin et al. reported DCIS risk stratification utilizing 12 of the 21 genes in the Oncotype DX assay (Solin et al. 2012). In data presented at the San Antonio Breast Cancer Symposium in 2011, the Oncotype DX assay has been proposed as a means to stratify risk of recurrence in patients with DCIS who have undergone partial mastectomy alone. For this analysis, the Oncotype DX was performed for 327 women (approximately 50 % of patients) enrolled on the ECOG E-5194 study. Women in this study had relatively low risk DCIS, with either low or intermediate grade DCIS $\leq$ 2.5 cm or high grade DCIS $\leq$ 1 cm. The "DCIS Score" was determined and women were grouped into three categories: high, intermediate, and low. They found that the DCIS Score obtained from the Oncotype DX assay was a significant independent predictor of ipsilateral breast events (either invasive or DCIS) on multivariate analysis. It was proposed that the DCIS Score could be used to estimate a woman's risk of recurrence after partial mastectomy for DCIS and potentially guide individual recommendations for adjuvant therapy. However, even the low risk group had a 12 % risk of any breast event (either invasive or non-invasive recurrence). Also, further validation is necessary before this is applied to routine clinical practice.

4.3 Other Novel Gene Signature Assays

Other gene signatures are being developed, including the Breast Cancer Index (BCI), MapQuant DX Genomic Grade Index (GGI), among others (Prat et al. 2011). The Breast Cancer Index (BCI) is an assay for women with ER-positive, node-negative breast cancer, which may assist in prediction of the risk of distant recurrence. Two prognostic quantitative real-time PCR assays, the HOXB13:IL17BR two-gene ratio and the molecular grade index (MGI), are incorporated in the BCI. *HOXB13* is an antiapoptotic gene associated with increased risk of recurrence and the IL-17 receptor B is associated with decreased risk of recurrence. The combination of the HOXB13:IL17BR and MGI were found to be prognostic of outcome (Ma et al. 2008). MapQuant DX, also known as Genomic Grade Index or GGI, is a microarray based assay that defines two molecular subgroups that have distinct clinical outcomes (Loi et al. 2007). Early comparisons of the various gene signatures show high rates of concordance in predicting outcome (Fan et al. 2006).

4.4 Gene Expression and Radiation Therapy

The primary purpose and utility of the previously discussed gene signatures was to stratify patients based on risk of distant recurrence. There are several questions regarding gene expression in breast cancer that are more relevant to radiation therapy, and we will review the existing data for each of these questions here. Haffty and Buchholz (2010) have recently written an excellent editorial on recent publications concerning gene expression and local recurrence in breast cancer, and interested readers are encouraged to review their findings (Haffty and Buchholz 2010). In brief, the authors define the following questions regarding gene expression and radiation therapy: (1) Is there a group of women at sufficiently low risk of local recurrence after lumpectomy alone that can be spared radiation therapy? (2) Alternatively, can gene expression signatures be used to identify a group of women at sufficiently high risk of local or regional recurrence after breast conservation (BCT)? Would these patients be better served with dose escalation or the use of radiosensitizers? (3) As breast conservation treatments evolve to include accelerated regimens, hypofractionation and partial breast volumes, can the results of gene expression assist in selection of patients for altered radiotherapy regimens? (4) With respect to postmastectomy irradiation, are our current guidelines oversimplified with respect to tumor biology? Can gene expression profiling be used to identify patients at risk for local regional recurrence after mastectomy?

Over the past few years, several groups have assessed the Oncotype DX and other gene expression signatures for their association with risk of locoregional recurrence. In one study the Oncotype DX RS was shown to predict risk of locoregional recurrence in a cohort of women with node-negative ER-positive breast cancer (Mamounas et al. 2010). In contrast, a similar study evaluated the RS for patients treated with breast conserving surgery, chemotherapy, and radiation therapy on ECOG E2197 (Solin et al. 2012). In this analysis, RS was determined for patients with 1–3 positive lymph nodes or negative lymph nodes with tumor size greater than 1.0 cm. Neither the intrinsic biologic subtype nor the RS was predictive of local or regional recurrence in this cohort, suggesting inability to define a subset of patients that may not require adjuvant radiation as part of breast conservation. Voduc et al. (2010) used an immunohistochemical panel (ER, PR, HER2, EGFR, CK5/6 and Ki-67) and a tissue microarray to classify 2,985 tumors into intrinsic subtypes (luminal A, luminal B, luminal-HER2, Her2 enriched, basal-like or triple negative phenotype non basal) (Voduc et al. 2010) (Fig. 8). A multivariate analysis was then performed to determine the risk of local or regional relapse associated with the intrinsic subtypes after adjusting for standardized risk factors. Luminal A tumors were found to have the lowest risk of locoregional recurrence, and 10-year local relapse-free survival after breast conserving surgery was 92 % (95 % confidence interval (CI) 90–95 %) for this patient population. For patients with HER2-enriched and basal subtypes, the 10-year local relapse-free survival after breast conserving surgery was reduced to 79 % (95 % CI 69–89 %) and 86 % (95 % CI 80–93 %), respectively. Haffty and Buchholz noted that these data were generated prior to the trastuzumab era, and caution that the HER2-enriched data may not be as clinically relevant today as recent data have

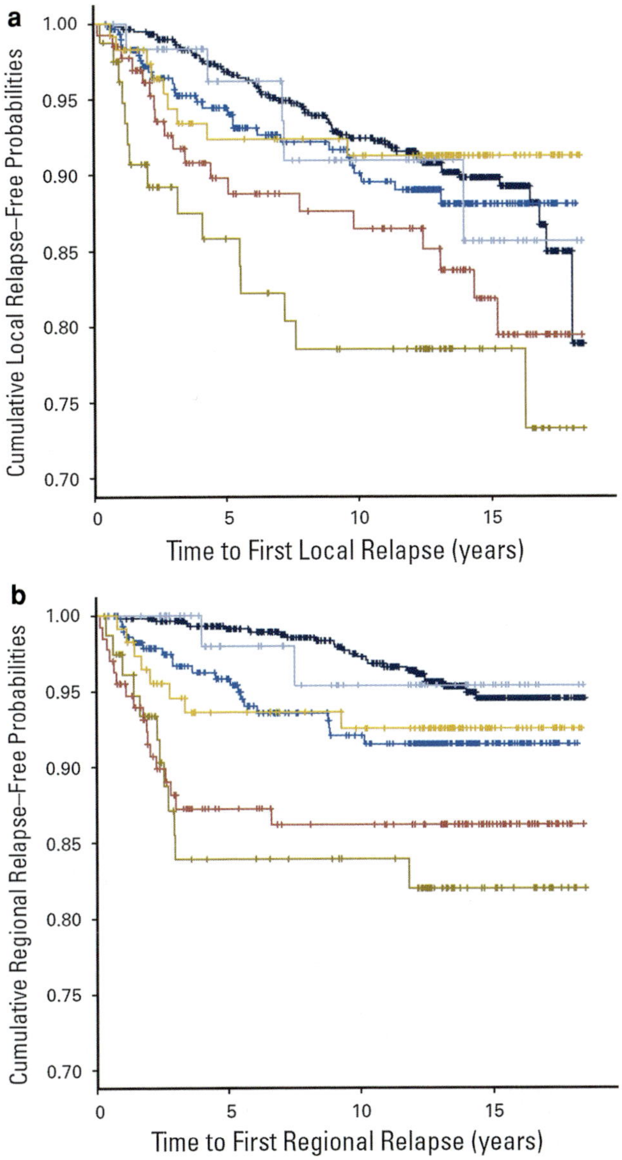

Fig. 8 Local (**a**) and regional (**b**) relapse rates, by intrinsic subtype. *Violet line*, luminal A; *light blue*, luminal human epidermal growth factor receptor 2 (HER2); *dark blue*, luminal B; *yellow*, five-marker negative phenotype; *red, basal; beige*, HER2 enriched. Reprinted with permission from Voduc et al. (2010)

shown that the addition of trastuzumab is associated with a significant improvement in local control (Haffty and Buchholz 2010). Perhaps the most useful piece of data from this analysis is the fact that luminal A tumors have an excellent prognosis and very low rates of local recurrence after breast conservation treatment.

More recently, Abdulkarim et al. (2011) reported that patients with T1-T2 triple negative breast cancers treated with breast conserving surgery followed by irradiation had a 5-year actuarial locoregional recurrence rate of 4 % compared to 10 % after mastectomy alone ($P = 0.027$) (Abdulkarim et al. 2011). These results suggest that in field effects of local irradiation are important for control of triple negative breast cancer and provide clinical evidence that tumor biology may influence response to local radiation (Pignol et al. 2011). Most importantly, these results call into question our previous assumption that breast conservation and mastectomy are equivalent treatments for biologically aggressive breast cancer. In this patient population, it appears that minimal surgery followed by local radiotherapy is more effective than a more radical surgery. Finally, we must also revisit our recommendations regarding postmastectomy radiation. These results suggest that our guidelines should be modified to include intrinsic subtype. Additional study will be needed to determine whether postmastectomy radiation can improve local control for triple negative breast cancers (Pignol et al. 2011).

Do we need to develop new gene expression signatures to directly address response to radiation in breast cancer? Initial studies showed relatively little difference in global gene expression profiles from primary breast tumors that recurred locally after breast conservation therapy versus tumors that did not (Kreike et al. 2006). Based on the hypothesis that gene expression patterns related to wound healing would be important for cancer invasion and metastasis, Chang et al. developed the "core serum response" (CSR) gene signature in vitro and then tested the ability of this gene signature to predict outcome in 295 patients treated for early breast cancer (Chang et al. 2004, 2005). In this patient population, the increased expression of the CSR genes (also known as the "wound response signature") was associated with decreased overall and distant metastasis-free survival. Nuyten et al. then trained ($n = 81$) and validated ($n = 80$) a classifier for local recurrence after breast conservation therapy (BCT) using the wound response signature (Nuyten 2006). Most recently, Kreike et al. have compared gene expression profiles from 56 primary breast cancers that recurred after BCT versus 109 primary breast cancers that did not recur after BCT (Kreike et al. 2009). Both supervised and unsupervised methods of classification were used to separate patients based on local recurrence after treatment. In addition, the authors tested many other published gene signatures for the ability to predict local recurrence, including their previously developed wound response signature. In this analysis, the five molecular subtypes [as most recently defined by Hu et al. (2006)] were associated with local recurrence after BCT. Luminal B type and HER2-like tumors had significantly increased local recurrence after BCT versus the other subtypes including the basal/triple negative subtype. Repeat testing of the wound response signature in this data set did not accurately predict local recurrence, emphasizing the importance of multiple validation studies prior to clinical implementation. In a supervised analysis, the authors developed a new 111 gene signature for the prediction of local recurrence after BCT and subsequently validated this signature using separate dataset of 161 patients. The results of these studies are compelling and could potentially allow for treatment intensification for patients at a high risk of local recurrence after BCT. Although these results are promising, rigorous clinical validation studies will be needed before we can consider incorporating these results into clinical practice.

It has been hypothesized that gene expression profiling could be used to develop a signature predictive of response to radiotherapy, although the genetic diversity observed in solid tumors may obscure these effects. Numerous studies have analyzed gene expression patterns before and after radiotherapy, and most of these studies have used in vitro or in vivo model systems (Ogawa et al. 2007). Not surprisingly, many categories of genes are upregulated in response to radiation treatment, and many of these genes regulate cellular responses to stress, cell cycle progression and DNA repair. Torres-Roca et al. (2005) developed a gene signature for radiosensitivity using a panel of 35 cancer cell lines and the results of clonogenic survival assays after 2 Gy (SF2) (Torres-Roca et al. 2005). Gene selection was based upon an fit to a linear regression model of gene expression versus cellular radiosensitivity. Genes selected were then used to build a multivariate model to predict SF2. The initial study identified novel genes implicated in the radiation response (*RBAP48* and *RGS19*). The same group then integrated gene expression and cellular radiosensitivity data from 48 cell lines and used a systems-biology based approach to develop a 10 gene network (*AR, cJun, STAT1, PKC, RelA, cABL, SUMO1, CDK1, HDAC1*, and *IRF1*) associated with cellular radiosensitivity (Eschrich et al. 2009a, b). The radiosensitivity index (RSI) is a linear function of expression of the ten genes. The RSI is inversely proportional to the radiosensitivity of the tumor (i.e. a low RSI indicates a more radiosensitive tumor). The RSI has been clinically tested in three datasets (rectal, esophageal, head and neck) for total of 118 patients (Eschrich et al. 2009a, b). Eschrich et al. (2012) recently published the results of RSI testing in two breast cancer datasets that included patients treated with breast conservation and mastectomy (Eschrich et al. 2012). In the first dataset, patients treated with radiotherapy and predicted to be radiosensitive (RS) on the basis of RSI were found to have improved 5-year relapse-free survival versus patients predicted to be radioresistant (RR) (95 vs. 75 %, n = 77). In the second data set, patients treated with radiotherapy and RS on the basis of RSI were found to have improved 5-year distant metastasis free survival versus RR patients (77 vs. 64 %), and RSI was found to be an independent predictor of outcome in ER positive patients treated with radiotherapy. Piening et al. developed a gene signature for radiation induced (RI) and radiation repressed (RR) genes using 12 human lymphoblast cell lines exposed to 5 Gy (Piening et al. 2009). The RI and RR gene sets were then compared to published gene signatures and used to predict outcome after treatment in two published breast cancer patient data sets. The authors note that while many RR genes overlap with the previously well characterized proliferation signature, the RI genes add prognostic information, and the combination of RR and RI genes was able to predict outcome in the published data sets tested. Additional study, including clinical validation and clinical utility studies, will be needed to determine whether RR and RI genes can be used independently to predict outcome to radiotherapy in breast cancer.

Very few studies have explored gene expression differences before and after irradiation in breast cancer using clinical samples. Helland et al. analyzed gene expression from tumor samples from 19 stage III/IV breast cancer patients before and after radiotherapy with 20 Gy (Helland et al. 2006). In that study, several genes were upregulated in irradiated tumors including *GPX1*, *DDB2*, *GDF15* and *CDKN1A*. The authors noted that the tumor suppressor gene *TP53* was mutated in 39 % of their samples, and gene expression profiles were, not surprisingly, influenced by *TP53* mutational status. It should also be noted that this relatively small patient dataset was quite hetereogeneous for biomarker expression (ER/PR/HER2) and instrinsic subtype analysis was not performed.

In summary, recent studies have shown that intrinsic breast cancer subtypes do influence local control after radiation treatment in breast cancer. In general, the luminal A subtype has the lowest risk of local recurrence after radiotherapy. Patients with early stage triple negative breast cancers have improved local control when radiation is used as part of breast conserving therapy compared to similar patients treated with mastectomy. In the research setting, several groups have developed gene signatures associated with radiation response in breast cancer. Additional validation and utility studies will be needed before we can use these signatures in the clinic.

5 Genetic Variation in Cancer and Targeted Therapy

5.1 Nature of Genetic Variation in Cancer

Cancer is classically considered to be a genetic disorder which develops as an evolutionary process, consisting of serial acquisition of somatic mutations and subsequent natural selection. Clones of abnormal cells arise from this process and continue to evolve during oncogenesis. With successive cell divisions, subclones with varying capabilities of proliferation, survival, invasion, and metastasis develop. Some subclones will emerge as dominant, while others will acquire deleterious mutations and are outcompeted by more dominant clones. Depending on the severity of the deleterious mutations, these clones may die or continue to exist as small remnants of the evolutionary history of the malignant process. The somatic mutations may include insertions, deletions, base substitutions, rearrangements, copy number alterations, or epigenetic changes.

Somatic mutations are acquired over one's lifetime and are randomly distributed in the genome. In addition, germline mutations can also affect one's susceptibility to cancer. There is some variation in genome sequence among humans, representing approximately 0.1 % of the genome. This genetic variation may range from single nucleotide changes to gross karyotype alterations. Single nucleotide polymorphisms (SNPs) are the most common type of variation representing approximately 90 % of human genome variation, but there are also structural variants (insertions, deletions, inversions, copy number variations), rare variants, and epigenetic differences. One's risk of cancer may be influenced both by the inherent genetic variation and germline mutations as well as the somatic mutations that occur over one's lifetime, which may be modulated by lifestyle and environmental factors (Stratton 2011; Stratton et al. 2009).

Although mutations occur throughout the genome, those that by chance occur in certain regions of the genome may be more likely to promote oncogenesis. "Driver mutations" are those that tend to occur in a subset of genes known as the "cancer genes". Driver mutations confer a growth advantage to the cell and directly contribute to cancer development. Passenger mutations, on the other hand, are those that happen along the way but do not give the cell a growth advantage. Passenger mutations may be detected in a cancer genome, but have not contributed to oncogenesis (Stricker et al. 2011). Some estimates suggest that several, perhaps approximately five, key mutations are required to generate cancer (Stratton 2011; Stratton et al. 2009).

Cancer genes may be functionally classified as dominant or recessive, in terms of their behavior at the cellular level. Dominant cancer genes, or oncogenes, require only one allele to be mutated and often result in constitutive activation. Oncogenes promote cell survival and proliferation. The majority (>80 %) of known of cancer genes are dominantly acting. Recessive cancer genes, or tumor suppressor genes, require both alleles to be altered in order for an effect to be seen. Tumor suppressor genes often play a role in cell cycle regulation, DNA repair, and apoptosis. If only one copy of the tumor suppressor gene is mutated or lost, the other copy can function normally. Examples of tumor suppressor genes include retinoblastoma protein *RB1*, *TP53*, *BRCA1*, and *BRCA2*. Mutations that affect the DNA repair process may result in an increase in the rate of somatic mutations in the cancer cell lineage (Stratton 2011; Stratton et al. 2009).

5.2 Methods Used to Study Genetic Variation

Initial studies of the genetics of cancer involved cytogenetic studies of chromosomes, with characterization of chromosomal translocations and abnormalities of chromosome copy number. The development of recombinant DNA technology later provided the ability to isolate and sequence portions of the genome associated with frequent rearrangements. In 2000, a draft sequence of the human genome was completed (Lander et al. 2001; Venter et al. 2001). This was a monumental step, which has facilitated further sequencing of cancer genomes, including whole gene families and most protein-coding exons. Nearly one decade after the human genome sequence was announced, the first completely sequenced cancer genomes were published in January 2010 (Pleasance et al. 2010a, b). Many more cancer genomes are being sequenced, and it is estimated that tens of thousands of cancer genomes will be sequenced over the next several years (Fig. 9). Efforts are being led by the International Cancer Genome Consortium and the Cancer Genome Atlas project in the United States.

The primary techniques used to study cancer genomics include: whole genome sequencing, targeted genome sequencing, cancer genotyping, and genome-wide association studies . Whole genome sequencing, as the name implies, determines the entire DNA sequence of a genome. First generation DNA sequencing techniques included Maxam–Gilbert chemical sequencing (Maxam and Gilbert 1977) and Sanger (chain-termination) sequencing (Sanger et al. 1977). Sanger sequencing is very accurate, but is limited by its high cost and low throughput. Newer sequencing methods, termed next-generation sequencing (NGS), have since been developed that have higher throughput and are more economical. Examples of next-generation sequencing techniques include massively parallel signature sequencing (MPSS), pyrosequencing, Illumina sequencing (sequencing by synthesis), SOLiD sequencing, ion semiconductor sequencing, and single molecule real-time (SMRT) sequencing (Tran et al. 2012). With these and other novel sequencing techniques, whole genome sequencing is becoming more affordable and feasible to perform. We have come a long way from the sequencing of the first human genome which cost nearly $3 billion and took a decade to complete, with current cost of approximately $10,000 per genome (Fig. 10).

Targeted genomic sequencing uses a similar approach, but limits sequencing efforts to specific regions or genes of interest. By sequencing only specific portions of the genome, targeted genomic sequencing is both efficient and

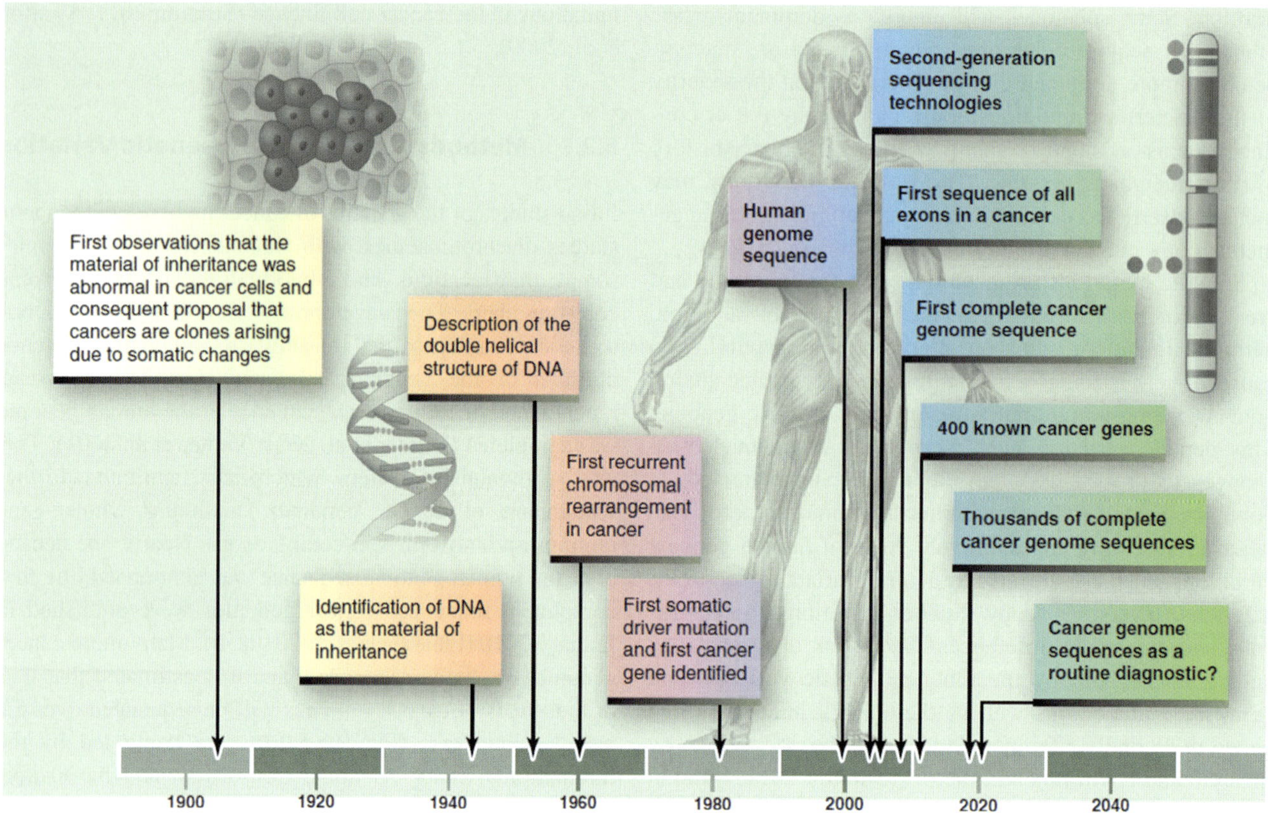

Fig. 9 Timeline of key events in cancer genomics. Reprinted with permission from Stratton (2011)

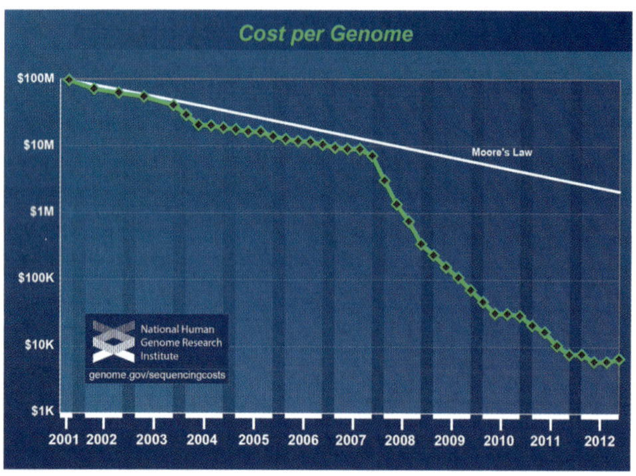

Fig. 10 Cost of genome sequencing over time. Reprinted with permission from Wetterstrand, http://www.genome.gov/sequencingcosts

cost-effective. The regions of interest may be a limited number of genes, the whole exome (portion of the genome formed by exons), or the cancer genome (portion of the genome containing the cancer genes). Data analysis is also simplified, as only segments of the genome are sequenced and subsequently analyzed (Tran et al. 2012). Our institution is among the institutions that now offer targeted genomic sequencing of multiple cancer genes available for clinical use.

Cancer genotyping refers to a method of determining whether a specific known cancer gene mutation is present in a tumor. As common mutations of cancer genes are continually being identified, it can be relatively straightforward to assess whether these specific mutations are present in a patient's tumor. Genotyping of clinical specimens is performed with high-throughput genotyping platforms, such as Taqman OpenArray Genotyping, Affymetrix genotyping arrays, and MassARRAY (Tran et al. 2012).

Another method of studying genetic variation is through genome-wide association study (GWAS). In this type of analysis, typically two cohorts are studied, those with the disease of interest (cases) and those without the disease (controls). GWAS looks for associations between single-nucleotide polymorphisms (SNPs) and a disease (Manolio 2010). A SNP is considered to be associated with a disease if it is more common in those with the disease than in the control population. GWAS data is often displayed in a Manhattan plot, which shows the relative association for various SNPs across the genome (Fig. 11). GWAS analysis has some limitations, including the issue of multiple hypothesis testing and the fact that most SNPs identified by GWAS thus far have been typically associated with only a

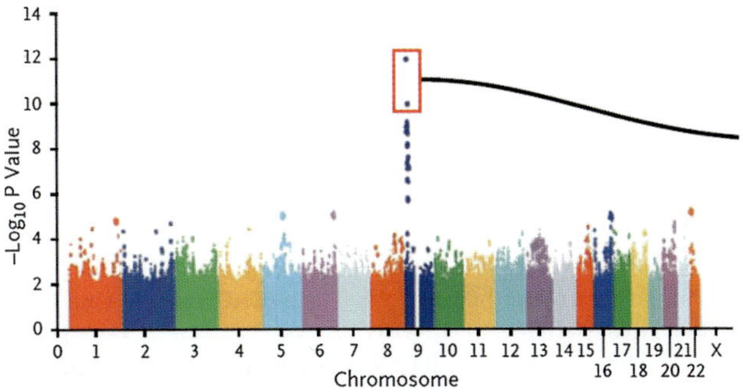

Fig. 11 Genome-wide association studies (GWAS). A sample Manhattan plot is shown, which displays the P values for all genotyped single-nucleotide polymorphisms (SNPs). Reprinted with permission from Manolio (2010)

small increase in the risk of disease, with a median odds ratio of 1.33 (Manolio 2010).

5.3 Clinical Cancer Genomics

A human breast cancer genome was sequenced and published in April 2010, only a few months after the first cancer genomes were published (Ding et al. 2010). In this publication the investigators sequenced four samples from a patient with metastatic basal-like breast cancer, including the primary tumor, peripheral blood, a brain metastasis and a xenograft derived from the primary tumor. Several interesting findings were reported, including a number of mutations contained in the primary tumor that were found to be enriched in the metastatic tumor.

Several publications in *Nature* in 2012 highlighted breast cancer genomics studies, demonstrating considerable progress in our understanding (Comprehensive Molecular Portraits of Human Breast Tumours 2012; Ellis et al. 2012; Curtis et al. 2012; Stephens et al. 2012; Shah et al. 2012; Banerji et al. 2012). Stephens and colleagues examined somatic mutations in 100 breast cancer genomes. They found driver mutations in several known cancer genes and also identified several new cancer genes based on nonrandom clustering of mutations (Stephens et al. 2012). Shah and colleagues studied mutations in 104 triple negative breast cancers (Shah et al. 2012). They found that the most frequently mutated gene was *TP53*, which had mutations in 62 % of patients with basal triple negative breast cancer, and 43 % of non-basal triple negative disease. Other genes with frequent mutations included *PIK3CA*, *USH2A*, *PTEN*, and *RB1*. Interestingly, they discovered that for most tumors, mutations in tumor suppressor genes such as *TP53* tended to occur in the highest clonal frequency, suggestive of an early event in the clonal evolution of the tumor. By comparing RNA sequencing with the genome data, they also found that only 36 % of single nucleotide variants were expressed. Curtis et al. (2012) examined the genomes and transcriptomes of nearly 2,000 breast cancers and based on joint clustering of copy number and gene expression data, identified 10 patient subgroups with a range of breast cancer outcomes. Banerji and colleagues determined the sequence of whole exomes for 103 breast cancer patients in Mexico and Vietnam, as well as whole genome sequences for 22 breast cancer/normal pairs. They found frequent mutations in many known breast cancer genes, as well as identified mutations in the *CBFB* transcription factor gene and a *MAGI3-AKT3* fusion which results in constitutive *AKT* activation (Banerji et al. 2012).

Koboldt et al. from The Cancer Genome Atlas Network studied several hundred patients, 463 of whom were evaluated on five different platforms, including mRNA expression microarrays, DNA methylation chips, SNP arrays, miRNA sequencing, and whole-exome sequencing (Comprehensive Molecular Portraits of Human Breast Tumours 2012). Somatic mutations in only three genes (*TP53*, *PIK3CA* and *GATA3*) occurred at >10 % incidence across breast cancers. Characteristic mutations were found within breast cancer subtypes, including common mutations in *GATA3*, *PIK3CA* and *MAP3K1* in the luminal A subtype. *TP53* was mutated in 84 % of basal-like breast cancers, and copy number analysis demonstrated many similarities between basal-like breast cancers and serous ovarian cancers, including widespread genomic instability, common gains of 1q, 3q, 8q and 12p, and common losses of 4q, 5q and 8p. Integrated analysis of protein phosphorylation and mRNA data identified two subgroups within the HER2+ group. Only 50 % of HER2+ cancers were categorized as *HER2* overexpressing by mRNA analysis; the remaining 50 % of HER2+ cancers were within the luminal subtypes. When both HER2 protein and mRNA were overexpressed, increased expression of EGFR, pEGFR, HER2 and pHER2 was observed. Ellis and colleagues conducted either whole exome or whole genome sequencing for 77 patients with ER positive breast cancer from two trials of neoadjuvant aromatase inhibition (Ellis et al. 2012). In patients with aromatase inhibitor resistance, some pathways including *TP53*, DNA replication, and mismatch repair, were found to be enriched relative to patients sensitive to aromatase inhibition.

In summary, genomics has provided additional insight into the molecular mechanisms that drive breast cancer development. Only a very few genes are mutated at a high frequency across all breast cancers. Characteristic mutations are common within breast cancer subtypes and may help to guide targeted therapy in the future. Many of these mutations are within pathways that regulate the radiation response. Additional study will be needed to determine if individual gene mutations can serve as biomarkers for breast cancer response to radiation.

6 Conclusion

Through remarkable scientific innovation, we have witnessed elaborate gene expression profiling studies as well as the sequencing of entire cancer genomes over the past decade, which provides intricate knowledge about oncogenesis and the drivers of this process. As we gain further understanding of the molecular processes involved, novel therapeutics may be developed and subsequently utilized for the patients most likely to derive a benefit. Considerable progress has been made in this regard in the fields of breast cancer, non-small cell lung cancer, and melanoma, among others, and will likely play an increasing role in the treatment of these and other malignancies in the future.

References

Abdulkarim BS, Cuartero J, Hanson J, Deschenes J, Lesniak D, Sabri S (2011) Increased risk of locoregional recurrence for women with T1–2N0 triple-negative breast cancer treated with modified radical mastectomy without adjuvant radiation therapy compared with breast-conserving therapy. J Clin Oncol 29(21):2852–2858

Albain KS, Barlow WE, Shak S et al (2010) Prognostic and predictive value of the 21-gene recurrence score assay in postmenopausal women with node-positive, oestrogen-receptor-positive breast cancer on chemotherapy: a retrospective analysis of a randomised trial. Lancet Oncol 11(1):55–65

Banerji S, Cibulskis K, Rangel-Escareno C et al (2012) Sequence analysis of mutations and translocations across breast cancer subtypes. Nature 486(7403):405–409

Benjamini Y, Hochberg Y (1995) Controlling the false discovery rate: a practical and powerful approach to multiple testing. J R Stat Soc B 57(1):289–300

Buyse M, Loi S, van't Veer LJ et al (2006) Validation and clinical utility of a 70-gene prognostic signature for women with node-negative breast cancer. J Natl Cancer Inst 98(17):1183–1192

Chang HY, Sneddon JB, Alizadeh AA et al (2004) Gene expression signature of fibroblast serum response predicts human cancer progression: similarities between tumors and wounds. PLoS Biol 2(2):E7

Chang HY, Nuyten DS, Sneddon JB et al (2005) Robustness, scalability, and integration of a wound-response gene expression signature in predicting breast cancer survival. Proc Natl Acad Sci USA 102(10):3738–3743

Comprehensive Molecular Portraits of Human Breast Tumours (2012) Nature 490(7418): 61–70

Curtis C, Shah SP, Chin SF et al (2012) The genomic and transcriptomic architecture of 2,000 breast tumours reveals novel subgroups. Nature 486(7403):346–352

Davies C, Godwin J, Gray R et al (2011) Relevance of breast cancer hormone receptors and other factors to the efficacy of adjuvant tamoxifen: patient-level meta-analysis of randomised trials. Lancet 378(9793):771–784

De Palma M, Hanahan D (2012) The biology of personalized cancer medicine: facing individual complexities underlying hallmark capabilities. Mol Oncol 6(2):111–127

Ding L, Ellis MJ, Li S et al (2010) Genome remodelling in a basal-like breast cancer metastasis and xenograft. Nature 464(7291): 999–1005

Dowsett M, Cuzick J, Wale C et al (2010) Prediction of risk of distant recurrence using the 21-gene recurrence score in node-negative and node-positive postmenopausal patients with breast cancer treated with anastrozole or tamoxifen: a TransATAC study. J Clin Oncol 28(11):1829–1834

Ellis MJ, Ding L, Shen D et al (2012) Whole-genome analysis informs breast cancer response to aromatase inhibition. Nature 486(7403): 353–360

Ely S (2009) Personalized medicine: individualized care of cancer patients. Transl Res 154(6):303–308

Eschrich S, Zhang H, Zhao H et al (2009a) Systems biology modeling of the radiation sensitivity network: a biomarker discovery platform. Int J Radiat Oncol Biol Phys 75(2):497–505

Eschrich SA, Pramana J, Zhang H et al (2009b) A gene expression model of intrinsic tumor radiosensitivity: prediction of response and prognosis after chemoradiation. Int J Radiat Oncol Biol Phys 75(2):489–496

Eschrich SA, Fulp WJ, Pawitan Y et al (2012) Validation of a radiosensitivity molecular signature in breast cancer. Clin Cancer Res 18(18):5134–5143

Fan C, Oh DS, Wessels L et al (2006) Concordance among gene-expression-based predictors for breast cancer. N Engl J Med 355(6):560–569

Gianni L, Zambetti M, Clark K et al (2005) Gene expression profiles in paraffin-embedded core biopsy tissue predict response to chemotherapy in women with locally advanced breast cancer. J Clin Oncol 23(29):7265–7277

Gianni L, Pienkowski T, Im YH et al (2012) Efficacy and safety of neoadjuvant pertuzumab and trastuzumab in women with locally advanced, inflammatory, or early HER2-positive breast cancer (NeoSphere): a randomised multicentre, open-label, phase 2 trial. Lancet Oncol 13(1):25–32

Ginsburg GS, Willard HF (2009) Genomic and personalized medicine: foundations and applications. Transl Res 154(6):277–287

Goldhirsch A, Wood WC, Coates AS, Gelber RD, Thurlimann B, Senn HJ (2011) Strategies for subtypes–dealing with the diversity of breast cancer: highlights of the St. Gallen international expert consensus on the primary therapy of early breast cancer 2011. Ann Oncol 22(8):1736–1747

Haffty BG, Buchholz TA (2010) Molecular predictors of locoregional recurrence in breast cancer: ready for prime time? J Clin Oncol 28(10):1627–1629

Hamilton SR (2012) Molecular pathology. Mol Oncol 6(2):177–181

Hastie T, Tibshirani R, Friedman J (2009) The elements of statistical learning, 2nd ed. Springer Series

Helland A, Johnsen H, Froyland C et al (2006) Radiation-induced effects on gene expression: an in vivo study on breast cancer. Radiother Oncol 80(2):230–235

Henry NL, Hayes DF (2012) Cancer biomarkers. Mol Oncol 6(2):140–146

Hu Z, Fan C, Oh DS et al (2006) The molecular portraits of breast tumors are conserved across microarray platforms. BMC Genomics 7:96

Kim C, Taniyama Y, Paik S (2009) Gene expression-based prognostic and predictive markers for breast cancer: a primer for practicing pathologists. Arch Pathol Lab Med 133(6):855–859

Kreike B, Halfwerk H, Kristel P et al (2006) Gene expression profiles of primary breast carcinomas from patients at high risk for local

recurrence after breast-conserving therapy. Clin Cancer Res 12(19):5705–5712
Kreike B, Halfwerk H, Armstrong N et al (2009) Local recurrence after breast-conserving therapy in relation to gene expression patterns in a large series of patients. Clin Cancer Res 15(12): 4181–4190
La Thangue NB, Kerr DJ (2011) Predictive biomarkers: a paradigm shift towards personalized cancer medicine. Nat Rev Clin Oncol 8(10):587–596
Lander ES, Linton LM, Birren B et al (2001) Initial sequencing and analysis of the human genome. Nature 409(6822):860–921
Loi S, Haibe-Kains B, Desmedt C et al (2007) Definition of clinically distinct molecular subtypes in estrogen receptor-positive breast carcinomas through genomic grade. J Clin Oncol 25(10): 1239–1246
Ma XJ, Salunga R, Dahiya S et al (2008) A five-gene molecular grade index and HOXB13:IL17BR are complementary prognostic factors in early stage breast cancer. Clin Cancer Res 14(9):2601–2608
Mamounas EP, Tang G, Fisher B et al (2010) Association between the 21-gene recurrence score assay and risk of locoregional recurrence in node-negative, estrogen receptor-positive breast cancer: results from NSABP B-14 and NSABP B-20. J Clin Oncol 28(10): 1677–1683
Manolio TA (2010) Genomewide association studies and assessment of the risk of disease. N Engl J Med 363(2):166–176
Maxam AM, Gilbert W (1977) A new method for sequencing DNA. Proc Natl Acad Sci USA 74(2):560–564
Medeiros F, Rigl CT, Anderson GG, Becker SH, Halling KC (2007) Tissue handling for genome-wide expression analysis: a review of the issues, evidence, and opportunities. Arch Pathol Lab Med 131(12):1805–1816
Mendelsohn J, Ringborg U, Schilsky RL (2012) Personalized cancer—a strategy to counteract an increasing cancer challenge. Mol Oncol 6(2):109–110
Mook S, Schmidt MK, Weigelt B et al (2010) The 70-gene prognosis signature predicts early metastasis in breast cancer patients between 55 and 70 years of age. Ann Oncol 21(4):717–722
Nuyten D, Kreike B, Hart A et al (2006) Predicting a local recurrence after breast-conserving therapy by gene expression profiling. Breast Cancer Res 8(5):R62
Ogawa K, Murayama S, Mori M (2007) Predicting the tumor response to radiotherapy using microarray analysis (Review). Oncol Rep 18(5):1243–1248
Paik S, Shak S, Tang G et al (2004) A multigene assay to predict recurrence of tamoxifen-treated, node-negative breast cancer. N Engl J Med 351(27):2817–2826
Paik S, Tang G, Shak S et al (2006) Gene expression and benefit of chemotherapy in women with node-negative, estrogen receptor-positive breast cancer. J Clin Oncol 24:3726–3734
Perez EA, Romond EH, Suman VJ et al (2011) Four-year follow-up of trastuzumab plus adjuvant chemotherapy for operable human epidermal growth factor receptor 2-positive breast cancer: joint analysis of data from NCCTG N9831 and NSABP B-31. J Clin Oncol 29(25):3366–3373
Perou CM, Sorlie T, Eisen MB et al (2000) Molecular portraits of human breast tumours. Nature 406(6797):747–752
Piening BD, Wang P, Subramanian A, Paulovich AG (2009) A radiation-derived gene expression signature predicts clinical outcome for breast cancer patients. Radiat Res 171(2):141–154
Pignol JP, Rakovitch E, Olivotto IA (2011) Is breast conservation therapy superior to mastectomy for women with triple-negative breast cancers? J Clin Oncol 29(21):2841–2843
Pleasance ED, Stephens PJ, O'Meara S et al (2010a) A small-cell lung cancer genome with complex signatures of tobacco exposure. Nature 463(7278):184–190
Pleasance ED, Cheetham RK, Stephens PJ et al (2010b) A comprehensive catalogue of somatic mutations from a human cancer genome. Nature 463(7278):191–196
Prat A, Ellis MJ, Perou CM (2011) Practical implications of gene-expression-based assays for breast oncologists. Nat Rev Clin Oncol 9(1):48–57
Quackenbush J (2006) Microarray analysis and tumor classification. N Engl J Med 354(23):2463–2472
Sanger F, Nicklen S, Coulson AR (1977) DNA sequencing with chain-terminating inhibitors. Proc Natl Acad Sci USA 74(12): 5463–5467
Schilsky RL (2010) Personalized medicine in oncology: the future is now. Nat Rev Drug Discov 9(5):363–366
Shah SP, Roth A, Goya R et al (2012) The clonal and mutational evolution spectrum of primary triple-negative breast cancers. Nature 486(7403):395–399
Simon RM, Paik S, Hayes DF (2009) Use of archived specimens in evaluation of prognostic and predictive biomarkers. J Natl Cancer Inst 101(21):1446–1452
Smith I, Procter M, Gelber RD et al (2007) 2-year follow-up of trastuzumab after adjuvant chemotherapy in HER2-positive breast cancer: a randomised controlled trial. Lancet 369(9555): 29–36
Solin LJ, Gray R, Goldstein LJ et al (2012) Prognostic value of biologic subtype and the 21-gene recurrence score relative to local recurrence after breast conservation treatment with radiation for early stage breast carcinoma: results from the eastern cooperative oncology group E2197 study. Breast Cancer Res Treat 134(2): 683–692
Sorlie T, Perou CM, Tibshirani R et al (2001) Gene expression patterns of breast carcinomas distinguish tumor subclasses with clinical implications. Proc Natl Acad Sci U S A 98(19): 10869–10874
Sorlie T, Tibshirani R, Parker J et al (2003) Repeated observation of breast tumor subtypes in independent gene expression data sets. Proc Natl Acad Sci USA 100(14):8418–8423
Stephens PJ, Tarpey PS, Davies H et al (2012) The landscape of cancer genes and mutational processes in breast cancer. Nature 486(7403):400–404
Storey JD, Tibshirani R (2003) Statistical significance for genomewide studies. Proc Natl Acad Sci U S A 100(16):9440–9445
Stratton MR (2011) Exploring the genomes of cancer cells: progress and promise. Science 331(6024):1553–1558
Stratton MR, Campbell PJ, Futreal PA (2009) The cancer genome. Nature 458(7239):719–724
Stricker T, Catenacci DV, Seiwert TY (2011) Molecular profiling of cancer—the future of personalized cancer medicine: a primer on cancer biology and the tools necessary to bring molecular testing to the clinic. Semin Oncol 38(2):173–185
Tefferi A, Bolander ME, Ansell SM, Wieben ED, Spelsberg TC (2002) Primer on medical genomics. Part III: microarray experiments and data analysis. Mayo Clin Proc 77(9):927–940
Teutsch SM, Bradley LA, Palomaki GE et al (2009) The evaluation of genomic applications in practice and prevention (EGAPP) initiative: methods of the EGAPP working group. Genet Med 11(1):3–14
Torres-Roca JF, Eschrich S, Zhao H et al (2005) Prediction of radiation sensitivity using a gene expression classifier. Cancer Res 65(16):7169–7176
Tran B, Dancey JE, Kamel-Reid S et al (2012) Cancer genomics: technology, discovery, and translation. J Clin Oncol 30(6): 647–660
Tseng GC, Ghosh D, Feingold E (2012) Comprehensive literature review and statistical considerations for microarray meta-analysis. Nucleic Acids Res 40(9):3785–3799

van de Vijver MJ, He YD, van't Veer LJ et al (2002) A gene-expression signature as a predictor of survival in breast cancer. N Engl J Med 347(25):1999–2009

van't Veer LJ, Dai H, van de Vijver MJ et al (2002) Gene expression profiling predicts clinical outcome of breast cancer. Nature 415(6871): 530–536

Venter JC, Adams MD, Myers EW et al (2001) The sequence of the human genome. Science 291(5507):1304–1351

Voduc KD, Cheang MC, Tyldesley S, Gelmon K, Nielsen TO, Kennecke H (2010) Breast cancer subtypes and the risk of local and regional relapse. J Clin Oncol 28(10):1684–1691

Wetterstrand KA, DNA Sequencing Costs: Data from the NHGRI Genome Sequencing Program (GSP). http://www.genome.gov/sequencingcosts. Accessed March 29 2013

Brain Tumors

Stephanie E. Weiss and Lynn Chang

Contents

Abstract

Glial tumors represent a class of primary brain tumor that includes neoplasms of astrocytic, oligodendritic and ependymal origin. The majority of adult gliomas are grade II–IV astrocytomas and oligodendrogliomas or are mixed with components of both (oligoastrocytoma) (CBTRUS 2010; Robertson et al. 2011; Brat et al. 2008) (Table 1). Histo-pathology and grading have been the historical cornerstones of diagnosis and therapeutic recommendation in the treatment of glioma (Weller et al. 2012). Nevertheless, prognosis and response to treatment is widely variable even among patients diagnosed with the same histo-pathologic disease entity and grade (Robertson et al. 2011). Modern techniques in gene and enzyme analysis have led to the recent proliferation of predictive and prognostic markers available for study. Some of these play a role in explaining the variable outcomes for glioma patients while others provide tantalizing prospects for potential future therapies. This chapter will provide a current review of the treatment of adult primary glioma including high and low grade astrocytoma, oligodendroglioma and oligoastrocytoma. There is an emphasis on predictive and prognostic models that have been published in recent years as applies to radiation oncologists. An evaluation of confidence levels in the literature will be provided.

1 Biomarkers

Diagnosis and treatment of glioma is rapidly shifting away from a purely histopathologic paradigm towards one that incorporates and may ultimately be replaced by biomarkers for diagnosis, prognosis, and selection of therapy. Indeed while the current buzzwords "personalized medicine" belie a long medical tradition to seek better, more out understanding of targeted treatments, biotechnology has advanced sufficiently that molecular medicine has become considerably

S. E. Weiss (✉)
Department of Radiation Oncology Fox Chase Cancer Center, Chief of Adult Brain Tumors Radiotherapy and Radiosurgery, 333 Cottman Ave, Philadelphia, PA 19111, USA
e-mail: sweissmd@yahoo.com

L. Chang
Department of Radiation Oncology, Fox Chase Cancer Center, 333 Cottman Ave, Philadelphia, PA 19111, USA

C. Nieder and L. E. Gaspar (eds.), *Decision Tools for Radiation Oncology*, Medical Radiology. Radiation Oncology,
DOI: 10.1007/174_2013_929, © Springer-Verlag Berlin Heidelberg 2013
Published Online: 24 October 2013

Table 1 World health organization primary brain tumor and glioma classification

Classification	WHO grade
Astrocytic[a]	
Pilocytic	I
Diffuse	II
Anaplastic	III
Glioblastoma	IV
Oligodendroglial and oligoastrocytic[a]	
Oligodendroglioma	II
Oligoastrocytoma	II
Anaplastic oligodendroglioma	III
Anaplastic oligoastrocytoma	III
Glioblastoma with oligodendroglioma component	IV
Ependymal[a]	I–III
Choroid plexus	I, III
Neuronal and mixed neuronal-glial	I–II
Pineal parenchymal	II, IV
Embryonal	IV
Meningeal	I–III

[a] Glial tumors
(Robertson et al. 2011; Brat et al. 2008)

more granular. We can correlate new biomarkers with previously known imaging features, histopathologic findings, and patient outcomes. We may to determine if a marker is diagnostic, prognostic and/or predictive to available therapies. Often because we know long standing therapies based on older histopathologic classification empirically work, ethical consideration make it difficult to establish how newly discovered biomarkers might alter therapeutic approach. We identify an interesting genetic marker but remain in the dark with regard to what protein it codes for and wonder if it is a potential molecular target of therapy. For these reasons the current study of glioma is fascinating and frustrating (Tables 2, 3).

1.1 1p/19 q

Co-deletion of chromosomal arms 1p and 19q is a genetic signature found in approximately 65 % of high-grade and 85 % of low-grade oligodendrogliomas (LGG). It is less commonly observed in mixed glioma or astrocytomas. The higher incidence of co-deletion in low grade glioma may suggest an early event in tumor formation (Smith et al. 2000; Barbashina et al. 2005). While histopathological interpretation is still necessary for subtyping of glial tumor, 1p/19q co-deletion can be used to support a *diagnosis* of oligodendroglioma where histology is ambiguous or in the event of inter-observer disagreement (Aldape et al. 2007). While the role of the gene product is undetermined, co-deletion in anaplastic oligodendroglioma is both *predictive* and *prognostic*; that is, co-deleted tumors are more responsive to chemo- and radiotherapy and have a more favorable prognosis regardless of treatment than lesions without co-deletion (Robertson et al. 2011; Hofer and Lassman 2010; Cairncross et al. 1998; Bauman et al. 2000; Wick et al. 2009b, Intergroup Radiation Therapy Oncology Group Trial 9402 et al. 2006; van den Bent et al. 2013).

Data regarding the value of 1p/19q in low-grade glioma is beginning to emerge but is not definitive. Some suggest that in the absence of adjuvant cytoxic therapy, 1p/19q status loses its prognostic impact for LGG while neuroradiologic monitoring studies suggest a slower natural growth rate for untreated co-deleted lesions. (Robertson et al. 2011; Weller et al. 2009; Ricard et al. 2007). The Clinical Cooperation Unit Neuropathology in Germany evaluated markers including 1p/19q deletion and their relationship to progression free survival (PFS) in LGG cohorts who either did or did not receive adjuvant radio- or chemotherapy. In this study no biomarker was prognostic for PFS in the absence of adjuvant therapy while 1p/19q co-deletion was associated with both PFS and overall survival (OS) for patients receiving either adjuvant chemotherapy or radiotherapy (Smith et al. 2000; Hartmann et al. 2011; Barbashina et al. 2005). This report is interesting but limited as a retrospective study of relatively small numbers.

The impact of a single arm deletion is not definitively understood. Preliminary data from EORTC 22033–26033 trial was presented at ASCO in 2013. High-risk low-grade glioma patients were randomized to radiotherapy versus temozolomide (TMZ) and were stratified by 1p status. 1p deletion was confirmed to be a positive prognostic factor regardless of treatment. Patients with intact 1p treated with TMZ were observed to have a non-significant trend towards inferior progression-free survival. Overall survival may be superior with 1p deletion (Aldape et al. 2007; Baumert et al. 2013). However maturation of the data and analysis of 1p/19q co-deletion is required before any definitive assessment of response to therapy by these biomarkers. Results are pending from E3F05 in which patients were receiving radiotherapy ± TMZ for LGG. The study will include an analysis of 1p/19q status as it correlates to outcome (NCT 00978458).

1.2 MGMT

O6-methylguanylmethyltransferace (MGMT) is a DNA repair protein that removes alkyl groups from the O6 position of guanine. The mechanism of the anti-tumor activity of temozolomide (TMZ) is believed to be through tumor DNA-alkylation most frequently at the N7 and O6 position of the

Table 2 Prognostic biomarkers in glioma

	Dx	A	Oligo	OA	AA	AO	AOA	GBM
1p/19q	+	NA	+[a]	+[a]	NA	+	+	NA
MGMT	–	?	?	?	+	+	+	+
IDH	+	+	+	+	+	+	+	+[a]

Prognostic biomarkers: *Dx* is diagnosis; + Biomarker is prognostic; −Biomarker is not prognostic; + [a] Some evidence for prognostic role but inconclusive; ? Unknown; *NA* Not applicable. *A* astrocytoma; *Oligo* oligodendroglioma; *AA* anaplastic astrocytoma; *AO* anaplastic oligodendroglioma; *AOA* anaplastic oligoastrocytoma; *GBM* glioblastoma

Table 3 Predictive biomarkers in glioma

	A	O	Mixed	AA	AO	AOA	GBM
1p/19q	NA	+[a]	+[a]	NA	+	+	NA
MGMT	?	?	?	?	?	?	+[a]
IDH	?	?	?	?	?	?	?

Predictive biomarkers: + Biomarker is predictive of response to therapy; – Biomarker is not predictive of response to therapy; + [a] Some evidence for predictive role but inconclusive; ? Unknown; *NA* Not applicable. *A* astrocytoma; *Oligo* oligodendroglioma; *Mixed* mixed Oligoastrocytoma; *AA* anaplastic astrocytoma; *AO* anaplastic oligodendroglioma; *AOA* anaplastic oligoastrocytoma; *GBM* glioblastoma

guanine moiety. Epigenetic silencing of MGMT by promoter methylation (MGMT-met) is associated with a loss of enzymatic expression and subsequent diminished DNA repair activity. Therefore tumor in which MGMT is silenced (i.e. methylated) is expected to be more sensitive to TMZ than unmethylated lesions (MGMT-unmet).

The powerful predictive and prognostic role of MGMT promoter methylation in glioblastoma was illustrated in a classic EORTC-NCIC study of GBM patients treated with radiation with and without concomitant and adjuvant temozolomide (Stupp et al. 2005; Hegi et al. 2005). In that study, patients whose tumors were MGMT methylated had a more favorable overall survival than those whose tumors were MGMT unmethylated. This finding could signify a more favorable natural outcome for MGMT-met GBM, or reflect a more favorable response to both RT and TMZ than MGMT-unmet. An analysis was not performed comparing outcomes by methylation status for patients receiving radiotherapy only. Examination of the survival curves for patients receiving RT alone demonstrates an appreciable separation by MGMT methylation status. When both treatment assignment and MGMT methylation status were considered, the most favorable outcome was found in MGMT-met patients receiving combined therapy. It is interesting to note that OS trended towards significance for combined therapy even when tumors were MGMT-unmet, arguing that alkylation of the O6 moiety on the MGMT promoter is not the sole mediator of TMZ efficacy (Hegi et al. 2005).

Because temozolomide was frequently used for salvage after progression in the radiotherapy only arm, the authors looked at the interaction of treatment assignment and MGMT status on progression-free survival to better assess the predictive nature of MGMT methylation to therapy. For patients with MGMT-met tumors, PFS was superior for patients receiving combined therapy than compared to those receiving radiotherapy alone. PFS with combined therapy was also superior for patients with MGMT-unmet tumors again suggesting alternate pathways for the efficacy of temozolomide. This study could not address whether MGMT status predicts response to RT alone (Hegi et al. 2005).

The NOA-04 trial prospectively randomized patients with grade III glioma- anaplastic oligodendroglioma (AO), anaplastic oligoastrocytoma (AOA) and anaplastic astrocytoma (AA)- to RT versus either a combination of procarbazine, lomustine and vincristine (PCV) or TMZ chemotherapy. MGMT promoter methylation was associated with PFS for both chemotherapy and radiotherapy confirming its prognostic relevance. However the trial did not support the hypothesis that MGMT methylation simply predicted response to alkylating chemotherapy (Wick et al. 2009b). Unlike the EORTC-NCIC trial of GBM, an analysis of MGMT status in the radiotherapy alone arm was performed. MGMT methylation conferred a clear and significant PFS benefit for patients receiving RT alone. The authors concluded that in anaplastic glioma, MGMT promoter hypermethylation was (1) a prognostic marker for patients treated with RT or (2) a predictive for response to RT itself (Wick et al. 2009b). The EORTC 26951 study of anaplastic oligodendroglial tumors makes for an interesting companion study. EORTC 26951 randomly assigned patients to either RT or RT followed by adjuvant PCV. MGMT promoter methylation was prognostic for both PFS and OS in both arms and did not have predictive significance for response to PCV. Interestingly in lesions identified as GBM on central review in this study no prognostic role for MGMT methylation was observed (van den Bent et al. 2013).

The Methusalem trial demonstrated that for the elderly with malignant astrocytoma (AA or GBM), MGMT-met is associated with improved OS. In the event of promoter methylation, event-free survival is improved for patients assigned to TMZ compared to those who receive RT. In the absence of methylation however, event free survival was superior for patients assigned to the radiotherapy group. There was no arm of patients receiving combined therapy (Wick et al. 2012).

The data is conflicted with regard to the value of MGMT in the prediction of response to therapy and prognostication in low-grade glioma. An association of MGMT promoter methylation with overall survival has been demonstrated. Correlation of MGMT-met with the putative prognostic marker 1p/19q co-deletion has been postulated as an explanation for this finding (Kesari et al. 2009; Leu et al. 2013). Other studies however contradict these observations (Tosoni et al. 2008). There is a paucity of data to suggest a predictive relationship between methylation status of MGMT and response to TMZ (Hartmann et al. 2011; Kesari et al. 2009; Groenendijk et al. 2011).

1.3 IDH1/IDH2

Parsons et al. used high-density oligonucleotide DNA array to detect the presence of amplifications and deletions among 20,661 coding genes in GBM samples. Recurrent mutations at codon 132 in the active site of isocitrate dehydrogenase 1 (IDH1) were noted with an incidence of 12 % (Parsons et al. 2008). The mutation was associated with younger patients, secondary GBM and improved survival. This may explain long observed association between younger age at diagnosis and improved outcome in glioma (Scott et al. 1998). Subsequent work has identified an association between IDH mutations and grade II and III astrocytoma, oligodendroglioma and oligoastrocytoma, and has identified IDH2 (codon 172) which is primarily associated with oligodendroglioma (Yan et al. 2009; Hartmann et al. 2009). IDH mutations are quite rare in de novo GBM and absent in pilocytic astrocytoma.

IDH mutations are tightly correlated with other biomarkers and histologic subtype. For instance IDH mutation is associated with 1p/19q co-deletion in oligodendroglial tumor and TP53 in astrocytoma, but seems to be mutually exclusive with EGFR and PTEN abnormalities. Combined IDH1 and IDH2 mutation is rare (Yan et al. 2009; Gupta and Salunke 2012; Sanson et al. 2009). It has been observed that IDH remains an independent favorable prognostic marker after adjustment for grade and MGMT status (Sanson et al. 2009).

In the cell IDH catalyzes oxidative decarboxylation of isocitrate to α-ketoglutarate (α-KG) in the citric acid cycle. The enzyme products of IDH1/2 utilize NADP +, which is transformed into NADPH with the generation of α-KG. These products normally protect against oxidative damage (Gupta and Salunke 2012). Both "loss of function" (production of α-KG and NADPH) and "gain of function" (accumulation of D-2-hydroxyglutarate (D2HG)) hypotheses have been put forwards to explain the mechanisms by which IDH mutation mediates oncogenesis. IDH1 mutations are tightly associated with CpG island methylator phenotype across tumor grade, raising the hypothesis that mutation may predispose cells to large-scale epigenetic disruption (Gupta and Salunke 2012; Noushmehr et al. 2010).

IDH has meaningful diagnostic potential and can be used in the clinic to increase confidence in differentiating between grade II glioma and IDH-wild type lesions such as pilocytic astrocytoma, pleomorphic xanthroastrocytoma or medulloblastoma. An IDH mutant oligodendroglial tumor may be distinguished from neurocytoma or dysembryoplastic neuroepithelial tumors and secondary GBM from de novo GBM (Gupta et al. 2011; Yan et al. 2009; Capper et al. 2011).

IDH mutation has been associated with better overall prognosis for glioma across multiple studies among several subtypes. IDH appears to have prognostic value in multivariate analysis even when controlling for other favorable variables such as low grade, young age, 1p/19q co-deletion and MGMT promoter methylation (Metellus et al. 2010; Alexander and Mehta 2011; Parsons et al. 2008; Sanson et al. 2009; Wick et al. 2009b; van den Bent et al. 2010; Weller et al. 2009; Houillier et al. 2010). IDH mutation status may have more powerful prognostic value in high-grade glioma than standard histopathologic classification. An analysis of NOA-04 demonstrated that IDH mutation status may override grade in malignant glioma in terms of prognostication (Hartmann et al. 2010; Alexander and Mehta 2011).

While several studies have demonstrated an association between mutated IDH and improved survival in glioma patients, there is as of yet no robust evidence that an IDH mutation predicts response to any therapy (Yan et al. 2009; Parsons et al. 2008; van den Bent et al. 2010; Hartmann et al. 2010). In a clinical study IDH mutation has been associated with improved response to TMZ, however this observation may be due to its association with 1p/19q (Houillier et al. 2010).

1.4 Imaging biomarkers

Imaging biomarkers (an evolution of what was previously called "Roentgen signs" in prior generations) can be useful in the diagnosis and grading of glioma however as yet cannot be considered pathognomonic for a particular pathologic sub-type of glioma or grade. Nevertheless a constellation of imaging features may direct diagnostic assessment and subsequent management. The standardization of biomarkers is evolving and their utility is appreciated. As such a rigorous criteria for imaging biomarkers as surrogate endpoints has been developed for use in clinical trials (Schatzkin and Gail 2002).

1. The presence of the biomarker is closely coupled or linked to the condition.
2. The detection and/or quantitative measurement of the biomarker is accurate, reproducible and feasible over time.
3. The measured changes over time in the imaging biomarker are closely coupled or linked to the success or failure of the therapeutic effect and the true end-point sought for the medical therapy being evaluated.

Low-grade glioma tends to appear bright on magnetic resonance imaging (MRI) T2/Flair imaging and hypodense on T1-weighted images and typically do not enhance with the addition of IV contrast. An exception is grade 1 pilocytic astrocytoma which usually presents in the posterior fossa and enhances with contrast (Lee et al. 1989). The presence of even trace or wispy amounts of enhancement on T1 weighted images should raise suspicion for an at least partially high-grade lesion. If definitive resection cannot be achieved the surgeon should attempt biopsy of the enhancing region if possible in order to establish the highest-grade component of the lesion. Failure to indentify high-grade tumor in a region of enhancement by a small sample may be the result of sampling error and may not definitively rule out the possibility of the presence of malignant glioma (Pignatti 2002; Bauman et al. 1999).

Oligodendroglial tumors have a greater propensity for the frontal and temporal lobes, and more frequently present with calcifications and hemorrhage than do astrocytomas (Lee and Van Tassel 1989). Positron-emission tomography (PET) may help to clarify clinical diagnosis. Glucose hypometabolism on PET supports a diagnosis of LGG whereas hypermetabolic activity is consistent with the presence of a high-grade lesion. Magnetic resonance spectroscopy, PET and L-(methyl-11C) methionine (MET-PET), can all contribute to direct guided biopsy of areas suspicious for malignancy (Pirotte et al. 2004; McKnight et al. 2002).

2 Low Grade Glioma

The designation low-grade glioma represents a heterogeneous population of primary tumors. For our purposes we will confine discussion to the relatively common astrocytic and oligodendroglial sub-types.

LGG often come to attention due to new on-set seizure activity (Lote et al. 1998). The acute and dramatic nature of seizure typically results in a short interval between initial symptom and diagnosis. However symptoms of LGG can often be insidious. Patients may report a vague, chronic history of headache for which they have previously received medical attention. The pain pattern is widely variable and may even remit from time to time or be at least initially responsive to conservative medical therapy. Focal neurologic deficits may develop depending upon the location of the lesion and will frequently precipitate neurologic imaging.

The gold standard for diagnosis of LGG is histo-pathologic examination of tumor. However tissue sampling may be limited by neurosurgical accessibility of the lesion and the resulting specimen non-diagnostic. Perhaps more frequently, biopsy sampling is sufficient to make a diagnosis of glioma but not to adequately grade it, the consequence of which being the potential under-treatment of a high-grade lesion. Thus in the absence of adequate tissue for full diagnosis, we rely upon other potential biomarkers as noted in the above section.

2.1 Initial Treatment. Postoperative Radiotherapy: Adjuvant or Delayed?

As there is evidence for improved survival, we recommend maximal safe resection at time of diagnosis (Smith et al. 2008; Keles et al. 2001). The role and selection of adjuvant therapy in the immediate post-operative setting is dependent upon risk factors, predictive biomarkers and neurologic status (Van den Bent et al. 2005; Pignatti 2002; Shaw 2002).

The EORTC 22845 trial assigned patients to receive RT either immediately following resection or at the time of progression. While immediate postoperative RT significantly prolonged PFS (5.4 versus 3.7 years), overall survival was not affected (7.4 versus 7.2 years) (Van den Bent et al. 2005). Importantly, this study demonstrated that malignant transformation was not more likely in patients having received post-operative radiotherapy. This study also demonstrates the efficacy of radiotherapy for treatment of low-grade glioma. Though the incidence of seizure at baseline between the two arms was comparable, at one year seizure incidence was significantly lower in patients undergoing immediate postoperative RT (25 versus 41 %) and is a justification for the use of RT for LGG patients with refractory seizure (Van den Bent et al. 2005).

Low-grade glioma patients at high risk for early and rapid progression after surgery alone have been identified. Multivariate analysis has shown that age >/= 40, pure astrocytoma subtype, diameter >/= 6 cm, tumor crossing midline and neurologic deficit prior to surgery are unfavorable prognostic features for OS. The presence of three or more high-risk features identifies patients who may warrant immediate adjuvant radiotherapy (Pignatti 2002; Shaw 2002).

2.2 Radiation Dose-Escalation

Both the EORTC and the RTOG have conducted multicenter prospective randomized trials comparing 45–50.4 Gy in conventional fraction to higher total doses of 59.4–64.8 Gy in an attempt to improve outcomes of LGG through dose-escalation. Both trials failed to demonstrate benefit and severe radionecrosis was doubled in the highest dose arm. Thus doses of 45–54 Gy remain the standard of care for low-grade glioma (Karim et al. 1996; Shaw 2002).

2.3 Adjuvant Chemotherapy?

The role of postoperative chemotherapy for LGG is still being investigated. RTOG 9802 examined patients deemed high-risk by virtue of age >/= 40 or subtotal resection. Patients were randomized to postoperative RT with or without six cycles of adjuvant PCV. Recent early reports demonstrate no difference in overall survival, however a trend at 5 years was noticed favoring the combined therapy arm. For patients surviving at least 2 years, the probability of surviving an additional 5 years was 74 % versus 59 % significantly favoring the combined therapy arm (Shaw et al. 2012). There are several caveats in applying the results from RTOG 9802 to the clinic. First, this data has yet to mature as median survival has not yet been reached. Further, in this initial analysis outcomes by histopathology and molecular status of 1p/19q have not been reported. Clinical decision-making would benefit from this more granular approach to the data. A bigger challenge in applying this data however is the definition of "high-risk" defined by RTOG 9802 that differs from the robust EORTC model which was published subsequent to 9802's opening. The EORTC used their dataset from Trial 22844 to construct their model and Trial 22845 served to validate it (Pignatti 2002). Clinically, the EORTC criteria, rather than the RTOG definition of subtotal resection or age >/= 40 alone, is used in the US as a rationale for immediate postoperative adjuvant therapy. Therefore how the results of RTOG 9802 ought to be applied in terms of the timing of chemo radiation -i.e. immediate adjuvant versus salvage at progression-remains uncertain. Finally RTOG 9802 used PCV for cytoxic chemotherapy. Since the design of this trial the more easily tolerated oral agent temozolomide has been routinely substituted in the clinic where glioma chemotherapy is warranted. In *anaplastic* astrocytoma, efficacy for TMZ is equivalent to PCV chemotherapy, is better tolerated, and is significantly less frequently discontinued prematurely due to toxicity (0 versus 37 %) (Brandes et al. 2008; Wick et al. 2009a. On the other hand an international retrospective study of 1000 patients with *anaplastic* oligodendroglioma found that time to progression was longer after treatment with PCV than with TMZ, an observation that remained significant on multivariate analysis (Lassman et al. 2011). However, these trials examined high-grade tumors and the latter was a retrospective review. The choice of optimal drug where combined therapy is indicated in terms of both efficacy and side effect profile for LGG thus has yet to be determined.

We await the maturation of RTOG 0424 that used the EORTC definition of *high-risk low-grade glioma* to evaluate patients treated on a single arm in the fashion of the standard GBM regimen of RT + TMZ followed by adjuvant TMZ. The EORTC high-risk low grade glioma data was used as historical control for comparison. At ASCO in 2013, median OS has not yet been reached, however 3 year OS was 73 %, significantly improved from historical controls and the study hypothesis of 65 %. The number of risk factors (3, 4 or 5) was not significant. 3-year PFS was 59.2 % and grade 3 and 4 adverse events were 43 and 10 %, predominantly related to temozolomide (Fisher et al. 2013).

In the clinic in the setting of a pure oligodendroglial lesion, the approach to adjuvant therapy may be modified by knowledge of the natural history of the disease and by biomarkers. 1p/19q deleted tumors appear to have a slower natural growth rate compared to lesions without codeletion (Ricard et al. 2007). After resection, the generally more favorable natural history of co-deleted low grade oligodendroglioma, evidence that delayed adjuvant therapy does not impinge on overall survival and a desire to avoid treatment related side effects supports active surveillance as a very reasonable therapeutic approach in the absence of other high-risk features (Van den Bent et al. 2005; Pignatti 2002; Ricard et al. 2007).

For patients with high-risk oligodendroglioma as defined by the EORTC, or with persistent symptoms including refractory seizure, adjuvant therapy is typically indicated. In the setting of 1p/19q co-deletion, either chemotherapy or RT alone may be considered (Hartmann et al. 2011; Peyre et al. 2010; Stege et al. 2005; Mason et al. 1996). Chemotherapy appears to be associated with a prolonged response in appropriately selected patients. Often this may be seen in a delayed fashion even after active therapy is discontinued. The role of combined chemoradiotherapy is still being elucidated. RTOG 9802 suggests a there is a benefit to combined therapy over RT alone, but as detailed above the specifics of patient selection and the optimal chemotherapeutic agents have yet to be elucidated (Shaw et al. 2012).

For patients without 1p/19q codeletion, radiotherapy is typically the treatment of choice for high-risk patients or for patients at progression with oligodendroglioma.

We do not recommend the routine administration of immediate adjuvant chemotherapy for diffuse astrocytoma. RTOG 9802 did not report outcomes based on histology (Shaw et al. 2012).

3 High-Grade Glioma

3.1 Glioblastoma

The gold standard for treatment of GBM was established with the publication of the joint EORTC/NCIC trial in 2005 (Stupp et al. 2005). The addition of temozolomide chemotherapy concomitant with, and adjuvant to, radiotherapy in the postoperative setting demonstrated a superior median survival compared to radiotherapy alone (14.6 versus 12.1 months). Importantly, overall survival for combined therapy compared favorably with radiotherapy alone at 2 years (27.2 versus 10.9 %) and 5 years (Stupp et al. 2009) (9.8 versus 1.9 %) (Stupp et al. 2005, 2009). For MGMT promoter methylated patients 5-year OS was 13.8 and 5.2 %, and for MGMT-unmet 8.3 and 0 %. As noted in the section on biomarkers, MGMT patients appear to have a more favorable prognosis in either arm, and temozolomide seems to demonstrate some benefit even for MGMT-unmet patients. Given the generally favorable side-effect profile, we routinely offer temozolomide for all patients regardless of MGMT status unless otherwise contraindicated.

Two randomized trials attempting to address the role of anti-angiogenic drugs in the upfront treatment of GBM were recently presented at ASCO 2013. The results have muddied the waters. Both RTOG 0825 and the Roche-funded AVAglio trial added bevacizumab (BVZ) to gold standard radiotherapy with temozolomide compared with the standard of care alone. Neither study could demonstrate an overall survival benefit with the addition of BVZ. Progression free survival was improved in both studies. However while PFS was numerically improved in RTOG 0825, the pre-defined threshold of a 30 % reduction in the hazard of failure was not met. Quality of life data was also contradictory. Quality of life seemed to improve with bevacizumab in the AVAglio trial while it was inferior in the RTOG trial. Further, BVZ is associated with an increase in grade III and IV adverse events (Gilbert et al. 2013; Wick et al. 2013; Wefel et al. 2013; Armstrong et al. 2013; Henriksson et al. 2013). The Federal Drug Administration (FDA) is currently reviewing the data but for the time being there does not appear to be a role for the routine administration of BVZ to patients with newly diagnosed GBM (Goldberg 2013). Given the ability for BVZ to close down the blood-brain-barrier and reduce edema, we reserve its use for patients who continue to have symptoms of mass effect and require prolonged high steroid use, and in the setting of recurrence (Ellingson et al. 2011; Reardon et al. 2011; Wen et al. 2010).

Outcomes for GBM do not seem to be improved over the EORTC-NCIC regimen by administering alternative regimens of TMZ such as in a dose-dense schedule (Gilbert et al. 2011) or by exchanging TMZ for PVC (Stupp et al. 2005, 2009; Brada et al. 2010).

Attempts were made to develop nomograms predicting survival of patients with GBM (Gorlia et al. 2008). However, recent data question the validity of this model and caution against its use without further validation (Parks et al. 2013).

3.2 Anaplastic Astrocytoma

Post-operative radiotherapy for anaplastic astrocytoma (AA) has long been the standard of care in the treatment of these lesions. The role for adjuvant chemotherapy for AA is less well defined. Most clinical practices extrapolate from the EORTC data on GBM and deliver concomitant temozolomide at 75 mg/m^2 with radiation to approximately 60 Gy followed by 6–12 months of adjuvant TMZ at 200 mg/m^2 for 5 days on a 28 day cycle (Stupp et al. 2005). A retrospective analysis of two consecutive trials demonstrated that in anaplastic astrocytoma, adjuvant temozolomide was as effective as and less toxic than PCV, and was discontinued prematurely less often (0 versus 37 %) (Brandes et al. 2008).

The question of optimal sequencing of chemotherapy and radiotherapy in all subtypes of anaplastic glioma has been examined in a prospective fashion. The NOA-04 trial randomly assigned patients to RT versus either procarbazine, lomustine and vincristine (PCV) or TMZ chemotherapy (See Fig. 1). At progression, patients in the RT arm were randomized to either PCV or TMZ chemotherapy while patients in the chemotherapy arms who achieved an initial response or stable disease and completed the full course were re-treated by the same agent. Chemotherapy patients who progressed during their initial drug regimen were transitioned to RT. At time of 2nd progression, the RT group switched to the novel drug (PCV or TMZ) while in the CT group the remaining novel available modality was initiated (either RT for patients having progressed after two challenges of the same chemotherapy, or the novel chemo for patients who had progressed early through their first chemo and had then received RT). *There was no arm with concomitant chemoradiation.* There was no overall difference in time to treatment failure (i.e. have progressed through both radiation and chemotherapy in whatever

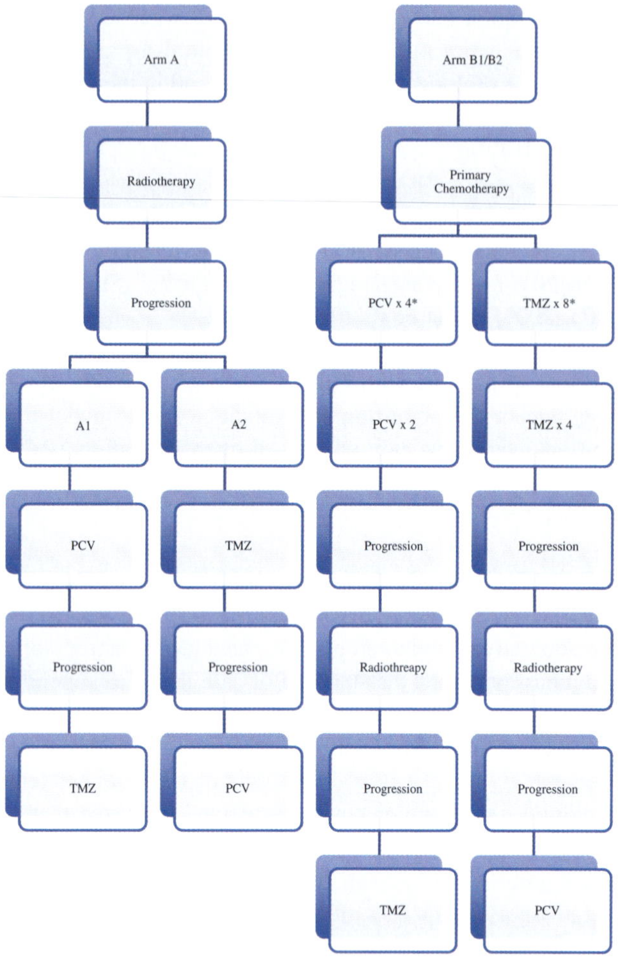

Fig. 1 NOA-04 trial design. Adapted from (Wick et al. 2009) * In Arm B, patients with progression after response or stable disease at completion of initial chemotherapy are rechallenged with same agent. If progression during initial therapy, transition to RT

sequence) between treatment arms. *There was no difference in time to treatment failure between PCV and temozolomide*. Time to treatment failure for anaplastic astrocytoma was substantially worse than for AO or AOA but was not dependent upon treatment sequence. (Wick et al. 2009a). NOA-04 failed to demonstrate superiority of either treatment sequence or of drug for patients with anaplastic glioma.

3.3 Anaplastic Oligodendroglial Lesions

Grade III oligodendroglial tumors fare better than their anaplastic counterparts. Historically it was felt that mixed anaplastic oligoastrocytoma would have an intermediate outcome but this was not noted in NOA-04 (Wick et al. 2009b. Contemporary researchers recognize that not all grade III glioma behave similarly, and the importance of biomarkers for diagnosis, treatment stratification and prognostication (IRTOGT et al. 2006; van den Bent 2006) (see section on biomarkers above). The ideal sequencing and selection of adjuvant therapy for anaplastic oligodendroglioma is not well defined however there are several robust studies that can help guide treatment.

Two cooperative group trials provide evidence that sequential adjuvant radiation and chemotherapy is associated with improved outcomes over single agent therapy alone. The order of sequencing (i.e. radiotherapy or chemotherapy first) does not seem to have an impact. The EORTC 26951 trial randomized patients to receive RT with or without sequential adjuvant PCV (van den Bent et al. 2013). Exploratory analysis of the correlation between 1p/19q status and survival was included. Overall survival for sequential treatment was superior to RT alone (42.3 versus 30.6 months). In the patients with 1p/19q co-deletion OS was increased with a non-significant trend towards a benefit from adjuvant PCV (median OS not reached versus. 112 months). In this study TMZ was not studied and there was no arm to evaluate combined therapy (van den Bent et al. 2013). In the RTOG 9402 trial patients were randomized to either PCV chemotherapy preceding radiotherapy or to radiotherapy alone. In the initial report progression free survival was increased with sequential therapy compared to RT alone (2.1 versus 1.7 years) although the difference in OS was not significant. At 11 year median follow-up, *the molecular characteristics drove outcome*. With 1p/19q co-deletion, overall survival was significantly prolonged in the sequential therapy group (14.7 versus 7.3 years). In the absence of co-deletion prognosis was worse and treatment arm did not impact overall survival (2.6 versus 2.7 years) (Cairncross et al. 2013, Intergroup Radiation Therapy Oncology Group Trial 9402 et al. 2006). As detailed in the section on anaplastic astrocytoma, the German-Swiss NOA-04 group randomized patients to radiation followed by chemotherapy with either PCV or TMZ at progression versus chemotherapy followed by RT at progression. There was no difference in time to treatment failure between arms or by choice of chemotherapy.

Taken as a whole this data suggests that sequential therapy for AO and AOA may be superior to radiotherapy alone particularly in patients with 1p/19q co-deleted tumors. Whether concomitant chemoradiation to 60 Gy followed by adjuvant chemotherapy as is delivered for GBM is superior to sequential treatment for AO/AOA has not been definitively addressed. Temozolomide is probably equivalent to PCV for first line therapy though no randomized study comparing PCV to TMZ alone is available. An international review of 1000 patients with anaplastic oligodendroglioma found that time to progression was longer after treatment with PCV than with TMZ, an observation that remained significant on multivariate analysis. However this study is limited as a retrospective review (Lassman et al. 2011). The authors speculate that TMZ may be less durable with fewer complete responses than PCV, however these inferences were gleaned by comparing outcomes across selected studies (Cairncross et al. 1994; Vogelbaum et al. 2009; Weller 2010). The authors also concede that their findings may be the result of a diagnostic shift that occurred over the time-period of their investigation. This may have resulted in a clustering of PCV use more frequently in cases of chemo-sensitive classical oligodendroglial histology during the earlier part of the study period where TMZ was not available (Lassman et al. 2011). In the end there is no robust evidence that either drug has superior efficacy. Temozolomide is associated with a more favorable side-effect profile than PCV. Further, in patients without co-deletion outcomes are typically worse and the relative benefit of adjuvant chemotherapy is less certain thus the risk/benefit ratio of any given chemotherapy may shift accordingly and be considered in this context.

We await outcomes for two trials investigating anaplastic glioma by 1p/19q status; the on-going CATNON Intergroup trial is randomizing patients with non-1p/19q deleted anaplastic glioma to radiotherapy alone, RT + concurrent TMZ, RT + adjuvant TMZ and RT + concurrent and adjuvant TMZ. The RTOG 1071 intergroup study which randomized patients to radiotherapy alone versus TMZ alone versus concomitant and adjuvant chemo RT with TMZ for 1p/19q co-deleted anaplastic glioma recently closed without meeting accrual. The lack of accrual was likely due to the reluctance to put 1p/19q co-deleted patients on the radiation therapy only arm.

3.4 High Grade Glioma in Elderly Patients

Because of the relatively poor survival of elderly patients with high-grade glioma, physicians and patients have questioned the advantage of aggressive, time consuming and potentially toxic therapy in this population. The role for routine radiotherapy with best supportive care over best supportive care alone in elderly patients with GBM was examined in a multi-institutional randomized trial. Median survival was superior for patients receiving RT (29 versus 16.9 weeks). Equally important were the findings regarding quality of life measures. Overall there was no difference between patients receiving radiotherapy and those receiving supportive care. However compared with supportive care alone, patients in the radiation arm did not demonstrate a detriment in cognitive function (Keime-Guibert et al. 2007).

An argument can be made that 6 weeks of daily therapy requiring clinic visits is itself a quality of life issue, potentially representing a substantial portion of median life expectancy in this population. Roa et al. demonstrated in a randomized study that 3 weeks of hypofractionated radiotherapy at a dose of 267 cGy to a total dose of 4005 cGy provides comparable control to conventional 6-week therapy. No chemotherapy was used in this trial (Roa 2004). The Nordic group compared TMZ alone with hypofractionated radiotherapy (34 Gy in 3.4 Gy fractions over 2 weeks) and standard radiotherapy to 60 Gy in patients over 60 years of age. There was no combined therapy group. In a three-way comparison of OS, temozolomide was superior to conventional RT but not hypofractionated RT. For patients over 70 years, survival with TMZ and hypofractionation was superior to standard RT. MGMT-met was associated with longer survival for patients treated with TMZ but not for those treated with radiotherapy (Malmstrom et al. 2012). The European NOA-08 group randomized patients over 65 years and a good performance status (KPS) to week-on week-off temozolomide at 100 mg/m^2 or conventional radiotherapy. This study demonstrated the equivalence of TMZ to RT in terms of OS (8.6 versus 9.6 mos). In findings reflecting those of the Nordic group, patients with MGMT-met lesions had improved event free survival if they received TMZ compared to RT. However if MGMT was unmethylated, event free survival was worse for patients receiving TMZ (Wick et al. 2012). This study did not compare combined modality therapy or hypofractionation. Other data suggests that MGMT promoter methylation maybe be particularly prognostic in the elderly population (Combs et al. 2011).

There is data that hypofractionation with concomitant TMZ is safe and efficacious. An early trial by Weiss et al. reported on a series of patients receiving hypofractionation with concomitant and adjuvant TMZ and found good outcomes compared with historical data (Weiss et al. 2010). A larger trial by Minetti and colleagues confirms these findings (Minetti et al. 2012).

The appropriate selection of therapy for elderly patients with GBM depends upon a balance of efficacy, side effects and quality of life issues as they impact on patients with generally poor prognosis. However physicians should be cautious of an overly fatalistic approach to this population. Many patients can do surprisingly well and aggressive therapy is warranted for well-selected patients and should not be ruled out based on age alone.

3.5 Assessing Response to Treatment of High-Grade Glioma

Assessing response to definitive therapy in the treatment of high-grade glioma can be challenging. The classic criteria for imaging assessment relies on an at least 25 % increase in contrast-enhancing lesion as a surrogate for tumor progression. It should be kept in mind that enhancement is in fact a measure of the permeability of the blood-brain barrier and as

Table 4 The response assessment in neuro-oncology (RANO) working group

	CR	PR	SD	PD
T1 enhancing	None	≥50 % ↓	<50 % ↓ but <25 % ↑	≥25 % ↑[a]
T2/FLAIR	Stable or ↓	Stable or ↓	Stable or ↓	↑[a]
New lesion	None	None	None	Present[a]
Corticosteroids	None	Stable or ↓	Stable or ↓	NA+
Clinical status	Stable or ↑	Stable or ↑	Stable or ↓	↓[a]
Requirement for response	All	All	All	Any[a]

Adapted from (Wen et al. 2010) *CR* complete response; *PR* partial response; *SD* stable disease; *PD* progressive disease; *FLAIR* fluid-attenuated inversion recovery; *NA* not applicable. [a] Progression occurs when this criterion present; +Increase in corticosteroids alone will not be taken into account in determining progression in the absence of persistent clinical deterioration

such changes in the extent of contrast may also reflect changes in steroid dose, the use of anti-angiogenic drugs and the natural inflammatory response of the body to efficacious therapy (Watling et al. 1994; Wen et al. 2010). For instance enhancement will be increased in approximately 30 % of the first post-radiotherapy MRIs of patients receiving gold standard treatment for GBM, and will subsequently subside without intervention. This phenomenon of "pseudoprogression" often results from temporarily increased permeability of vasculature after chemoradiation with (and without) temozolomide. Pseudoprogression appears to be more common in patients with MGMT promoter methylated tumors (Brandes et al. 2008). Conversely, a "pseudoresponse" phenomenon occurs with the administration of biologic agents that target vascular endothelial growth factor pathway, such as bevacizumab. In this instance modification of the permeable blood brain barrier occurs with apparent "improvement" of enhancement on neuroradiologic imaging. Over time however worsening disease is typically noted by changes on T2 and FLAIR images suggesting progressive infiltrative disease even in the absence of post-contrast enhancement on T1 weighted images. (Norden et al. 2008; Narayana et al. 2008). To account for these confounding mechanisms in the interpretation of post-therapy monitoring of high-grade glioma the international Response Assessment in Neuro-Oncology (RANO) working group established new standardized response criteria (Wen et al. 2010). The new criteria employs a more granular assessment of MRI interpretation, taking into account both T1 + contrast and T2/FLAIR findings as well as relevant clinical factors such as recent radiotherapy, chemotherapy and antiangiogenic administration, changes in steroid administration and clinical status (See Table 4).

4 Future Directions

Medical therapy of glioma will increasingly rely on molecular and other biomarkers. Presently they are used in the clinic to support diagnosis, select therapy and to prognosticate. It is likely that future classification systems for glioma will rely on novel biomarkers. The ultimate goal is the rational design of biologic therapies directed by information gleaned by biomarkers. We look forward to the success of researchers in developing a clearer understanding of the mechanism of tumor formation and progression. For instance it has been postulated that HIF-1α up-regulation of target genes related to α-ketoglutarate depletion is a driving force in glioma formation. Therefore agents that can mimic αKG might be designed to reverse the effect. Several other potential therapeutic strategies to target IDH mutated tumors have been forwarded (Alexander and Mehta 2011; Zhao et al. 2009). If breast cancer can be looked to as an early model of the successful use of biomarkers for individualized medicine, translational research in glioma can be viewed as a field ripe for study.

References

Aldape K, Burger PC, Perry A (2007) Clinicopathologic aspects of 1p/19q loss and the diagnosis of oligodendroglioma. Arch Pathol Lab Med 131(2):242–251

Alexander BM, Mehta MP (2011) Role of isocitrate dehydrogenase in glioma. Expert Rev Neurother 11(10):1399–1409

Armstrong TS et al (2013) Comparative impact of treatment on patient reported outcomes (PROs) in patients with glioblastoma (GBM) enrolled in RTOG 0825. ASCO Meet Abst 31(15):2003

Barbashina V et al (2005) Allelic losses at 1p36 and 19q13 in gliomas: correlation with histologic classification, definition of a 150-kb minimal deleted region on 1p36, and evaluation of CAMTA1 as a candidate tumor suppressor gene. Clin Cancer Res: Off J Am Assoc Cancer Res 11(3):1119–1128

Bauman G et al (1999) Pretreatment factors predict overall survival for patients with low-grade glioma: a recursive partitioning analysis. Radiat Oncol Biol 45(4):923–929

Bauman GS et al (2000) Allelic loss of chromosome 1p and radiotherapy plus chemotherapy in patients with oligodendrogliomas. Radiat Oncol Biol 48(3):825–830

Baumert BG et al (2013) Temozolomide chemotherapy versus radiotherapy in molecularly characterized (1p loss) low-grade glioma: a randomized phase III intergroup study by the EORTC/NCIC-CTG/TROG/MRC-CTU (EORTC 22033–26033). ASCO Meet Abs 31(15):2007

Brada M et al (2010) Temozolomide versus procarbazine, lomustine, and vincristine in recurrent high-grade glioma. J Clin Oncol: Offi J Am Soc Clin Oncol 28(30):4601–4608

Brandes AA et al (2008) MGMT promoter methylation status can predict the incidence and outcome of pseudoprogression after concomitant radiochemotherapy in newly diagnosed glioblastoma patients. J Clin Oncol : Off J Am Soc Clin Oncol 26(13):2192–2197

Brat DJ et al (2008) Diagnosis of malignantglioma: role of neuropathology. J Neurooncol 89(3):287–311

Cairncross G et al (1994) Chemotherapy for anaplastic oligodendroglioma. National Cancer Institute of Canada Clinical Trials Group. J Clin Oncol: Off J Am Soc Clin Oncol 12(10):2013–2021

Cairncross G et al (2013) Phase III trial of chemoradiotherapy for anaplastic oligodendroglioma: long-term results of RTOG 9402. J Clin Oncol: Off J Am Soc Clin Oncol 31(3):337–343

Cairncross JG et al (1998) Specific genetic predictors of chemotherapeutic response and survival in patients with anaplastic oligodendrogliomas. J Natl Cancer Inst 90(19):1473–1479

CBTRUS (2010) http://www.cbtrus.org/2010-NPCR-SEER/CBTRUS-WEBREPORT-Final-3-2-10.pdf

Combs SE et al (2011) Prognostic significance of IDH-1 and MGMT inpatients with glioblastoma: one step forward, and one step back? Radiat Oncol 6(1):115

Capper D, Reuss D, Schittenhelm J, Hartmann C, Bremer J, Sahm F, Harter PN, Jeibmann A, von Deimling A (2011) Mutation-specific IDH1 antibody differentiates oligodendrogliomas and oligoastrocytomas from other brain tumors with oligodendroglioma-like morphology. Acta Neuropathol 121(2):241–252

Ellingson BM et al (2011) Quantitative volumetric analysis of conventional MRI response in recurrent glioblastoma treated with bevacizumab. Neuro-Oncol 13(4):401–409

Fisher BJ et al (2013) A phase II study of a temozolomide-based chemoradiotherapy regimen for high-risk low-grade gliomas: preliminary results of RTOG 0424. ASCO Meet Abs 31(15):2008

Goldberg P http://www.cancerletter.com/articles/20130614_1. Accessed 14 June 2013

Gilbert MR et al (2011) RTOG 0525: a randomized phase III trial comparing standard adjuvant temozolomide (TMZ) with a dose-dense (dd) schedule in newly diagnosed glioblastoma (GBM). ASCO Meet Abs 29(15):2006

Gilbert MR et al (2013) RTOG 0825: phase III double-blind placebo-controlled trial evaluating bevacizumab (Bev) in patients (Pts) with newly diagnosed glioblastoma (GBM). ASCO Meet Abs 31(15):1

Gorlia T, van den Bent MJ, Hegi ME, Mirimanoff RO, Weller M, Cairncross JG, Eisenhauer E, Belanger K, Brandes AA, Allgeier A, Lacombe D, Stupp R (2008) Nomograms for predicting survival of patients with newly diagnosed glioblastoma: prognostic factor analysis of EORTC and NCIC trial 26981–22981/CE.3. Lancet Oncol 9(1):29–38

Groenendijk FH, Taal W, Dubbink HJ, Haarloo CR, Kouwenhoven MC, van den Bent MJ, Kros JM, Dinjens WN (2011) MGMT promoter hypermethylation is a frequent, early, and consistent event in astrocytoma progression, and not correlated with TP53 mutation. J Neurooncol 101(3):405–417

Gupta K, Salunke P (2012) Molecular markers of glioma: an update on recent progress and perspectives. J Cancer Res Clin Oncol 138(12):1971–1981

Gupta R et al (2011) Isocitrate dehydrogenase mutations in diffuse gliomas: clinical and aetiological implications. J Clin Pathol 64(10):835–844

Hartmann C et al (2009) Type and frequency of IDH1 and IDH2 mutations are related to astrocytic and oligodendroglial differentiation and age: a study of 1,010 diffuse gliomas. Acta Neuropathol 4:469–474

Hartmann C et al (2010) Patients with IDH1 wild type anaplastic astrocytomas exhibit worse prognosis than IDH1-mutated glioblastomas, and IDH1 mutation status accounts for the unfavorable prognostic effect of higher age: implications for classification of gliomas. Acta Neuropathol 120(6):707–718

Hartmann C et al (2011) Molecular markers in low-grade gliomas: predictive or prognostic? Clin Cancer Res 17(13):4588–4599

Hegi ME et al (2005) MGMT gene silencing and benefit from temozolomide in glioblastoma. N Engl J Med 352(10):997–1003

Henriksson R et al (2013) Progression-free survival (PFS) and health-related quality of life (HRQoL) in AVAglio, a phase III study of bevacizumab (Bv), temozolomide (T), and radiotherapy (RT) in newly diagnosed glioblastoma (GBM). ASCO Meet Abs 31(15): 2005

Hofer S, Lassman AB (2010) Molecular markers in gliomas: impact for the clinician. Targeted Oncol 5(3):201–210

Houillier C et al (2010) IDH1 or IDH2 mutations predict longer survival and response to temozolomide in low-grade gliomas. Neurology 75(17):1560–1566

Intergroup Radiation Therapy Oncology Group Trial 9402 et al (2006) Phase III trial of chemotherapy plus radiotherapy compared with radiotherapy alone for pure and mixed anaplastic oligodendroglioma: Intergroup Radiation Therapy Oncology Group Trial 9402. J Clin Oncol: Off J Am Soc Clin Oncol 24(18):2707–2714

Karim AB et al (1996) A randomized trial on dose-response in radiation therapy oflow-gradecerebralglioma: European Organization for Research and Treatment of Cancer (EORTC) Study 22844. Int J Radiat Oncol Biol Phys 36(3):549–556

Keime-Guibert F et al (2007) Radiotherapy for glioblastoma in the elderly. N Engl J Med 356(15):1527–1535

Keles GE, Lamborn KR, Berger MS (2001) Low-grade hemispheric gliomas in adults: a critical review of extent of resection as a factor influencing outcome. J Neurosurg 95(5):735–745

Kesari S et al (2009) Phase II study of protracted daily temozolomide for low-grade gliomas in adults. Clin Cancer Res 15(1):330–337

Lassman AB et al (2011) International retrospective study of over 1000 adults with anaplastic oligodendroglial tumors. Neuro-Oncol 13(6):649–659

Lee YY et al (1989) Juvenile pilocytic astrocytomas: CT and MR characteristics. AJR Am J Roentgenol 152(6):1263–1270

Lee YY, Van Tassel P (1989) Intracranial oligodendrogliomas: imaging findings in 35 untreated cases. AJR Am J Roentgenol 152(2):361–369

Leu S, von Felten S, Frank S, Vassella E, Vajtai I, Taylor E, Schulz M, Hutter G, Hench J, Schucht P, Boulay JL, Mariani L (2013) IDH/MGMT-driven molecular classification of low-grade glioma is a strong predictor for long-term survival. Neuro Oncol 15(4): 469–479

Lote K et al (1998) Prevalence and prognostic significance of epilepsy in patients with gliomas. Eur J Cancer 34(1):98–102

Malmstrom A et al (2012) Temozolomide versus standard 6-week radiotherapy versus hypofractionated radiotherapy in patients older than 60 years with glioblastoma: the Nordic randomised, phase 3 trial. Lancet Oncol 13(9):916–926

Mason WP, Krol GS, DeAngelis LM (1996) Low-grade oligodendroglioma responds to chemotherapy. Neurology 46(1):203–207

McKnight TR et al (2002) Histopathological validation of a three-dimensional magnetic resonance spectroscopy index as a predictor of tumor presence. J Neurosurg 97(4):794–802

Metellus P, Coulibaly B, Colin C, de Paula AM, Vasiljevic A, Taieb D, Barlier A, Boisselier B, Mokhtari K, Wang XW, Loundou A, Chapon F, Pineau S, Ouafik L, Chinot O, Figarella-Branger D (2010) Absence of IDH mutation identifies a novel radiologic and molecular subtype of WHO grade II gliomas with dismal prognosis. Acta Neuropathol 120(6):719–729

Minetti D et al (2012) Phase II study of short-course radiotherapy plus concomitant and adjuvant temozolomide in elderly patients with glioblastoma. Radiat Oncol Biol 83(1):93–99

Narayana A et al (2008) Bevacizumab therapy in recurrent high grade glioma: impact on local control and survival. ASCO Meet Abs 26(15):13000

NCT 00978458 http://clinicaltrials.gov/show/NCT00978458

Norden AD, Drappatz J, Wen PY (2008) Rapid review. Lancet Neurol 7(12):1152–1160

Noushmehr H et al (2010) Identification of a CpG island methylator phenotype that defines a distinct subgroup of glioma. Cancer Cell 17(5):510–522

Parks C, Heald J, Hall G, Kamaly-Asl I (2013) Can the prognosis of individual patients with glioblastoma be predicted using an online calculator? Neuro Oncol 15(8):1074–1078

Parsons DW et al (2008) An integrated genomic analysis of human glioblastoma multiforme. Science 321(5897):1807–1812

Peyre M et al (2010) Prolonged response without prolonged chemotherapy: a lesson from PCV chemotherapy in low-grade gliomas. Neuro Oncol 12(10):1078–1082

Pignatti F (2002) Prognostic factors for survival in adult patients with cerebral low-grade glioma. J Clin Oncol 20(8):2076–2084

Pirotte B et al (2004) Combined use of 18F-fluorodeoxyglucose and 11C-methionine in 45 positron emission tomography-guided stereotactic brain biopsies. J Neurosurg 3:476–483

Reardon DA et al (2011) A review of VEGF/VEGFR-targeted therapeutics for recurrent glioblastoma. J Natl Compr Canc Netw 9(4):414–427

Ricard D et al (2007) Dynamic history of low-grade gliomas before and after temozolomide treatment. Ann Neurol 61(5):484–490

Roa W (2004) Abbreviated course of radiation therapy in older patients with glioblastoma multiforme: a prospective randomized clinical trial. J Clin Oncol: Off J Am Soc Clin Oncol 22(9):1583–1588

Robertson T, Koszyca B, Gonzales M (2011) Overview and recent advances in neuropathology. Part 1: central nervous system tumours. Pathology 43(2):88–92

Sanson M et al (2009) Isocitrate dehydrogenase 1 codon 132 mutation is an important prognostic biomarker in gliomas. J Clin Oncol: Off J Am Soc Clin Oncol 27(25):4150–4154

Schatzkin A, Gail M (2002) The promise and peril of surrogate endpoints in cancer research. Nat Rev Cancer 2:19–27

Scott CB et al (1998) Validation and predictive power of Radiation Therapy Oncology Group (RTOG) recursive partitioning analysis classes for malignant glioma patients: a report using RTOG 90–06. Radiat Oncol Biol 40(1):51–55

Shaw E (2002) Prospective randomized trial of low- versus high-dose radiation therapy in adults with supratentorial low-grade glioma: initial report of a north central cancer treatment group/radiation therapy oncology group/eastern cooperative oncology group study. J Clin Oncol 20(9):2267–2276

Shaw EG et al (2012) Randomized trial of radiation therapy plus procarbazine, lomustine, and vincristine chemotherapy for supratentorial adult low-grade glioma: initial results of RTOG 9802. J Clin Oncol: Off J Am Soc Clin Oncol 30(25):3065–3070

Smith JS et al (2000) Alterations of chromosome arms 1p and 19q as predictors of survival in oligodendrogliomas, astrocytomas, and mixed oligoastrocytomas. J Clin Oncol 18(3):636–645

Smith JS et al (2008) Role of extent of resection in the long-term outcome of low-grade hemispheric gliomas. J Clin Oncol: Off J Am Soc Clin Oncol 26(8):1338–1345

Stege EM et al (2005) Successful treatment of low-grade oligodendroglial tumors with a chemotherapy regimen of procarbazine, lomustine, and vincristine. Cancer 103(4):802–809

Stupp R et al (2009) Effects of radiotherapy with concomitant and adjuvant temozolomide versus radiotherapy alone on survival in glioblastoma in a randomised phase III study: 5-year analysis of the EORTC-NCIC trial. Lancet Oncol 10(5):459–466

Stupp R et al (2005) Radiotherapy plus concomitant and adjuvant temozolomide for glioblastoma. N Engl J Med 352(10):987–996

Tosoni A, Franceschi E, Ermani M, Bertorelle R, Bonaldi L, Blatt V, Brandes AA (2008) Temozolomide three weeks on and one week off as first line therapy for patients with recurrent or progressive low grade gliomas. J Neurooncol 89(2):179–85

Van den Bent M et al (2005) Long-term efficacy of early versus delayed radiotherapy for low-grade astrocytoma and oligodendroglioma in adults: the EORTC 22845 randomised trial. The Lancet 366(9490):985–990

van den Bent MJ (2006) Adjuvant procarbazine, lomustine, and vincristine improves progression-free survival but not overall survival in newly diagnosed anaplastic oligodendrogliomas and oligoastrocytomas: a randomized European organisation for research and treatment of cancer phase III trial. J Clin Oncol: Off J Am Soc Clin Oncol 24(18):2715–2722

van den Bent MJ et al (2013) Adjuvant procarbazine, lomustine, and vincristine chemotherapy in newly diagnosed anaplastic oligodendroglioma: long-term follow-up of EORTC brain tumor group study 26951. J Clin Oncol: Off J Am Soc Clin Oncol 31(3):344–350

van den Bent MJ et al (2010) IDH1 and IDH2 mutations are prognostic but not predictive for outcome in anaplastic oligodendroglial tumors: a report of the European organization for research and treatment of cancer brain tumor group. Clin Cancer Res: Off J Am Assoc Cancer Res 16(5):1597–1604

Vogelbaum MA et al (2009) Phase II trial of preirradiation and concurrent temozolomide in patients with newly diagnosed anaplastic oligodendrogliomas and mixed anaplastic oligoastrocytomas: RTOG BR0131. Neuro-Oncol 11(2):167–175

Watling CJ et al (1994) Corticosteroid-induced magnetic resonance imaging changes in patients with recurrent malignant glioma. J Clin Oncol: Off J Am Soc Clin Oncol 12(9):1886–1889

Wefel JS et al (2013) Neurocognitive function (NCF) outcomes in patients with glioblastoma (GBM) enrolled in RTOG 0825. ASCO Meet Abs 31(15):2004

Weiss SE, Cheung A, Drappatz J (2010) Hypofractionated radiotherapy with temozolomide for elderly patients with glioblastoma. Int J Radiat Oncol, Biol, Phys 78(3):S271 EP

Weller M (2010) Chemotherapy for low-grade gliomas: when? How? how long? Neuro-Oncol 12(10):1013

Weller M et al (2009) Molecular predictors of progression-free and overall survival in patients with newly diagnosed glioblastoma: a prospective translational study of the German glioma network. J Clin Oncol: Off J Am Soc Clin Oncol 27(34):5743–5750

Weller M, Stupp R, Hegi ME, van den Bent M, Tonn JC, Sanson M, Wick W, Reifenberger G (2012) Personalized care in neuro-oncology coming of age: why we need MGMT and 1p/19q testing for malignant glioma patients in clinical practice. Neuro Oncol 14:4

Wen PY et al (2010) Updated response assessment criteria for high-grade gliomas: response assessment in neuro-oncology working group. J Clin Oncol: Off J Am Soc Clin Oncol 28(11):1963–1972

Wick W et al (2012) Temozolomide chemotherapy alone versus radiotherapy alone for malignant astrocytoma in the elderly: the NOA-08 randomised, phase 3 trial. Lancet Oncol 13(7):707–715

Wick W et al (2013) Tumor response based on adapted Macdonald criteria and assessment of pseudoprogression (PsPD) in the phase III AVAglio trial of bevacizumab (Bv) plus temozolomide (T) plus radiotherapy (RT) in newly diagnosed glioblastoma (GBM). ASCO Meet Abs 31(15):2002

Wick W, Hartmann C, Engel C, Stoffels M, Felsberg J, Stockhammer F, Sabel MC, Koeppen S, Ketter R, Meyermann R, Rapp M, Meisner C, Kortmann RD, Pietsch T, Wiestler OD, Ernemann U, Bamberg M, Reifenberger G, Deimling von A, Weller M (2009a)

NOA-04 randomized phase III trial of sequential radiochemotherapy of anaplastic glioma with procarbazine, lomustine, and vincristine or temozolomide. J Clin Oncol: Off J Am Soc Clin Oncol 27(35):5874–5880

Wick W, Hartmann C, Engel C, Stoffels M, Felsberg J, Stockhammer F, Sabel MC, Koeppen S, Ketter R, Meyermann R, Rapp M, Meisner C, Kortmann RD, Pietsch T, Wiestler OD, Ernemann U, Bamberg M, Reifenberger G, Deimling von A, Weller M (2009b) NOA-04 randomized phase III trial of sequential radiochemotherapy of anaplastic glioma with procarbazine, lomustine, and vincristine or temozolomide. J Clin Oncol: OffJ Am Soc Clin Oncol 27(35):5874–5880

Yan H et al (2009) IDH1 and IDH2 mutations in gliomas. N Engl J Med 360(8):765–773

Zhao S et al (2009) Glioma-derived mutations in IDH1 dominantly inhibit IDH1 catalytic activity and induce HIF-1alpha. Science 324(5924):261–265

Head and Neck Squamous Cell Cancer

Carsten Nieder

Contents

C. Nieder (✉)
Department of Oncology and Palliative Medicine, Nordland Hospital, Bodø, Norway
e-mail: Carsten.Nieder@nordlandssykehuset.no

C. Nieder
Faculty of Health Sciences, Institute of Clinical Medicine, University of Tromsø, Tromsø, Norway

Abstract

Patients with head and neck squamous cell cancer are a very heterogeneous group with regard to aetiology, age and other host factors, disease stage and biology, and treatment approaches and outcome. Given the major implications of both tumour and treatment on quality of life and functional status, comprehensive pre-treatment assessments and multidisciplinary approaches are recommended. Models and tools facilitating decision making such as staging systems and nomograms are discussed in this chapter, which is dedicated to Kie Kian Ang, an outstanding leader in the field of head and neck cancer, who passed away much too early. During a post doctoral fellowship at the University of Texas M.D. Anderson Cancer Center Dr. Ang taught me the art and science of writing reviews and book chapters.

1 Introduction

Radiotherapy plays a pivotal role in the curative treatment of head and neck squamous cell carcinoma (HNSCC). Currently, the majority of patients with HNSCC have locally advanced disease and are treated with radiotherapy with or without other modalities, such as surgery, chemotherapy and/or biological targeting agents. Despite the advances made in the primary treatment of HNSCC, still 30–50 % of all curatively treated patients will develop a loco-regional recurrence (Brockstein et al. 2004; Pignon et al. 2009). In addition, for those who survive, there is a constant threat of the development of a new head and neck tumour (field cancerisation, for example related to smoking). In a meta-analysis, the incidence of second primary tumours (SPTs) was 14 % (Haughey et al. 1992). In most cases high-dose radiation is needed, with doses close to the generally accepted tolerance limits of the normal tissues. Not all patients are candidates for such aggressive treatment. Decision making has become complex,

C. Nieder and L. E. Gaspar (eds.), *Decision Tools for Radiation Oncology*, Medical Radiology. Radiation Oncology,
DOI: 10.1007/174_2013_934, © Springer-Verlag Berlin Heidelberg 2013
Published Online: 2 November 2013

has to integrate quality of life (QoL) and functional outcome considerations, and requires close collaboration of many medical disciplines. Some of the questions relevant during pre-treatment discussion, e.g. in tumour boards, are summarised in Table 1.

2 Recent Developments

In the last decades, major progress has been made in the treatment of patients with HNSCC. In particular, the addition of concomitant chemotherapy (Langendijk et al. 2004; Pignon et al. 2000, 2009) to radiation and the introduction of altered fractionation schedules (Bourhis et al. 2006) have resulted in a significant improvement of loco-regional tumour control and overall survival. These new treatment regimens have gained conceptual acceptance and are now considered standard among patients with HNSCC in the organ preservation as well as in the unresectable setting. Moreover, the results of recent studies also indicate that new induction chemotherapy regimens (Hitt et al. 2005; Posner et al. 2007; Vermorken et al. 2007) and the addition of cetuximab to radiation (Bonner et al. 2006) may further improve outcome after non-surgical treatment, at least for selected patients. Since the publication of the results of two prospective randomised studies, an increasing number of patients are now treated with postoperative concomitant chemoradiation instead of postoperative radiotherapy alone (Bernier et al. 2004; Cooper et al. 2004). In this setting extracapsular extension and positive surgical margins are important predictors of loco-regional control and survival.

Human papilloma virus (HPV) status has been shown to predict outcomes (loco-regional control, metastases-free survival, survival) in several series (Fakhry et al. 2008; Lassen et al. 2009; Rischin et al. 2010; Oguejiofor et al. 2013; Rades et al. 2013a). Positivity might be assessed by in situ hybridisation and/or positive p16 immunostaining. In Radiation Therapy Oncology Group (RTOG) studies median pack-years of tobacco smoking were lower among p16-positive than p16-negative patients with oropharyngeal cancer in both trials (RTOG 9003: 29 v 46 pack-years; $p = 0.02$; RTOG 0129: 10 v 40 pack-years; $p < 0.001$) (Gillison et al. 2012). After adjustment for p16 and other factors, risk of progression or death increased by 1 % per pack-year (for both, hazard ratio [HR], 1.01; 95 % CI, 1.00 to 1.01; $p = 0.002$) or 2 % per year of smoking (for both, HR, 1.02; 95 % CI, 1.01 to 1.03; $p < 0.001$) in both trials. In RTOG 9003, risk of death doubled (HR, 2.19; 95 % CI, 1.46 to 3.28) among those who smoked during radiotherapy after accounting for pack-years and other factors, and risk of second primary tumours increased by 1.5 % per pack-year (HR, 1.015; 95 % CI, 1.005–1.026). Despite the association with more advanced nodal stage, patients with HPV positive oropharyngeal cancers have better outcomes. A study by Hong et al. suggested that the prognostic significance of the conventional staging system in tonsillar cancer is modified by HPV (Hong et al. 2013). Ongoing studies will determine whether or not future treatment strategies should be different for the two patient groups with or without HPV positivity.

Table 1 Decision making regarding treatment indication, disease extent, outcomes and side effects: what do we wish to predict?

Questions to address
Should a given patient receive radiotherapy, as opposed to for example surgery?
Should we combine radiotherapy with systemic agents?
What is the optimal regimen for a given patient?
What is the true disease extent in the presence of given imaging findings?
What is the biology/aetiology of the tumour?
What do we need to delineate on treatment planning scans?
How does the optimal dose distribution look like?
Is there a role for dose intensification to subvolumes?
Do we need adaptive replanning during radiotherapy?
Can we predict response early during treatment?
Is there a need for salvage surgery?
What is the risk of severe acute toxicity?
Are preventive measures indicated, such as feeding tubes?
What is the risk of significant late toxicity?
What is the anticipated functional outcome and need for rehabilitation?
What is the risk of a second primary tumour?

3 Prognostic Factors for Survival and Predictors for Recurrence

In general, prognosis depends on the biological aggressiveness of the tumour, e.g. its ability to metastasise and to withstand non-surgical treatment attempts. Host characteristics play an important role because they determine whether aggressive treatment is possible. A large analysis of 1,093 participants in two RTOG trials (9003, 9111) showed that age, performance status, marital status and cigarette smoking significantly predicted survival (Coyne et al. 2007). Prognosis and primary treatment approach vary with anatomical site and disease extent staged according to the AJCC TNM system.

3.1 Nasopharyngeal Cancer

For nasopharyngeal cancer the AJCC TNM staging system is shown in Tables 2 and 3. Besides T category (local invasion), tumour volume is of prognostic significance,

Table 2 AJCC TNM classification of carcinoma of the nasopharynx

Stage	Description
Primary tumor (T)	
TX	Primary tumor cannot be assessed
T0	No evidence of primary tumor
Tis	Carcinoma in situ
T1	Tumor confined to the nasopharynx, or tumor extends to oropharynx and/or nasal cavity without parapharyngeal extension (i.e., posterolateral infiltration of tumor)
T2	Tumor with parapharyngeal extension (i.e., posterolateral infiltration of tumor)
T3	Tumor involves bony structures of skull base and/or paranasal sinuses
T4	Tumor with intracranial extension and/or involvement of cranial nerves, hypopharynx, or with extension to the infratemporal fossa/masticator space
Regional lymph nodes (N)	
NX	Regional lymph nodes cannot be assessed
N0	No regional lymph node metastasis
N1	Unilateral (including ipsilateral) metastasis in cervical lymph node(s), ≤6 cm in greatest dimension, above the supraclavicular fossa, and/or unilateral or bilateral, retropharyngeal lymph nodes, ≤6 cm in greatest dimension
N2	Bilateral metastasis in cervical lymph node(s), ≤6 cm in greatest dimension, above the supraclavicular fossa
N3a	Metastasis in a lymph node(s) >6 cm in dimension
N3b	Metastasis in a lymph node(s) to the supraclavicular fossa
Distant metastasis (M)	
M0	No distant metastasis
M1	Distant metastasis (including seeding of the peritoneum and positive peritoneal cytology)

Source Edge et al. (2009)

Table 3 Stage grouping of carcinoma of the nasopharynx

Stage grouping				
	T1	T2	T3	T4
N0	I	II	III	IVA
N1	II	II	III	IVA
N2	III	III	III	IVA
N3	IVB	IVB	IVB	IVB
M1	IVC	IVC	IVC	IVC

Source Edge et al. (2009)

especially when attempting to kill cancer cells by radio- and chemotherapy as opposed to complete surgical resection (cell number, increasing likelihood of hypoxia in larger tumours) (Sze et al. 2004; Chen et al. 2009; Guo et al. 2012). Other staging systems have been developed by different groups. In general, T classification predominantly affects local control, while N classification predicts neck and distant control. Epstein-Barr virus DNA (less than versus equal to or greater than 1,500 copies/ml) is a prognostic biomarker that predicts overall and relapse-free survival. Other markers such as serum lactate dehydrogenase (LDH) (Zhou et al. 2012; Wan et al. 2013), vascular endothelial growth factor (VEGF) and osteopontin have been suggested and should be studied further (Lv et al. 2011).

3.2 Cancer of the Oral Cavity and Oropharynx

For cancer of the oral cavity and oropharynx the AJCC TNM staging system is shown in Tables 4 and 5. In these diseases, male gender, cigarette smoking and poor performance status are adverse prognostic factors. Patients who are p16 positive have improved survival. After surgical resection for oral cavity carcinoma, adjuvant radiotherapy may be recommended for patients at higher risk for loco-regional recurrence, but it can be difficult to predict whether a particular patient will benefit. Wang et al. constructed several types of survival models using a set of 979 patients with oral cavity squamous cell carcinoma treated in the United States and Brazil (Wang et al. 2013). Covariates were age, sex, tobacco use, stage, grade, margins, and subsite. The best performing model was externally validated on a set of 431 patients from Princess Margaret Hospital, Toronto, Canada. The primary outcome measure of interest was loco-regional recurrence-free survival. An online nomogram was built from this model that estimates loco-regional failure-free survival with and without postoperative radiotherapy. However, none of the patients had received postoperative radiochemotherapy. Information on extracapsular extension, lymphovascular space invasion, and perineural invasion were not available in this data set, also limiting its general use. The prediction model indicated that patients with positive margins and/or N2–N3 disease will derive the most benefit from adjuvant radiotherapy, although the relative magnitude of this benefit will vary depending on the other patient and tumour characteristics entered into the model. Histologic grade was also an independent predictor of prognosis in stage I or II oral cavity carcinoma in the Surveillance, Epidemiology, and End Results (SEER) database of the National Cancer Institute (Thomas et al. 2013). Among patients age 20–65 with AJCC stage I or II cancer, the adjusted risk of death was 2.7 times greater (95 % CI 1.7 to 4.1) if the tumour was poorly differentiated or undifferentiated than it was if the tumour was well differentiated. Among patients age 66–94, the risk of death was 3.0 (95 % CI 2.0–4.5) times greater. For those over age 65, moderately differentiated tumours also conferred an estimated 42 % increased risk of death, which was borderline significant ($p = 0.05$).

It is hypothesised that molecular biomarkers might improve current decision models. Protein 53 (p53), insulin-like growth factor II mRNA-binding protein 3 (IMP3),

Table 4 AJCC TNM classification of carcinoma of the oral cavity and oropharynx

Stage	Description
Primary tumor (T)	
TX	Primary tumor cannot be assessed
T0	No evidence of primary tumor
Tis	Carcinoma in situ
T1	Tumor ≤2 cm in greatest dimension
T2	Tumor >2 cm but ≤4 cm in greatest dimension
T3	Tumor >4 cm in greatest dimension
T4 (lip)	Tumor invades through cortical bone, inferior alveolar nerve, floor of mouth, or skin of face, chin, or nose
T4a (oral cavity)	Tumor invades through cortical bone, into deep (extrinsic) muscle of tongue, maxillary sinus, or skin of face
T4b (oral cavity)	Tumor involves masticator space, pterygoid plates, or skull base, and/or encases internal carotid artery
T4a (oropharynx)	Tumor invades the larynx, deep, extrinsic muscle of tongue/medial pterygoid/hard palate, or mandible
T4b (oropharynx)	Tumor involves lateral pterygoid muscle, pterygoid plates, lateral nasopharynx, skull base, and/or encases internal carotid artery
Regional lymph nodes (N)	
NX	Regional lymph nodes cannot be assessed
N0	No regional lymph node metastasis
N1	Metastasis in a single ipsilateral lymph node, ≤3 cm in greatest dimension
N2a	Metastasis in a single ipsilateral lymph node, >3 cm but ≤6 cm in greatest dimension
N2b	Metastasis in multiple ipsilateral lymph nodes, none >6 cm in greatest dimension
N2c	Metastasis in bilateral or contralateral lymph nodes, none >6 cm in greatest dimension
N3	Metastasis in a lymph node, >6 cm in greatest dimension
Distant metastasis (M)	
M0	No distant metastasis
M1	Distant metastasis (including seeding of the peritoneum and positive peritoneal cytology)

Source Edge et al. (2009)

cyclooxygenase 2 (COX2), and HuR were analysed by immunohistochemistry in 96 patients with primary oral squamous cell cancer who underwent surgical resection at the Yonsei Dental Hospital in Seoul, Korea (Kim et al. 2012). On univariate and multivariate analysis, the expression of IMP3 was significantly associated with the risk of death. P53 was also significantly associated with survival in the case of negative IMP3 and the prediction accuracy was improved by including these 2 factors in the prediction

Table 5 Stage grouping of carcinoma of the oral cavity and oropharynx

Stage grouping					
	T1	T2	T3	T4a	T4b
N0	I	II	III	IVA	IVB
N1	III	III	III	IVA	IVB
N2	IVA	IVA	IVA	IVA	IVB
N3	IVB	IVB	IVB	IVB	IVB
M1	IVC	IVC	IVC	IVC	IVC

Source Edge et al. (2009)

model. The latter nomogram included age, sex, presence of lymph node metastases, T stage, tumour site, p53 and IMP3. In general, such tools need external validation in sufficiently large databases before widespread implementation.

3.3 Cancer of the Larynx and Hypopharynx

For cancer of the larynx and hypopharynx the AJCC TNM staging system is shown in Table 6. Egelmeer et al. performed a population-based cohort study on 994 laryngeal carcinoma patients, treated with radiotherapy from 1977 until 2008 (Egelmeer et al. 2011). Two nomograms were developed and validated. Performance of the models was expressed as the area under the curve (AUC). Unfavourable prognostic factors for overall survival were low haemoglobin level, male sex, high T status, nodal involvement, older age, lower EQD(2T) (total radiation dose corrected for fraction dose and overall treatment time), and non-glottic tumour. All factors except tumour location were predictive for local control. The AUCs were 0.73 for overall survival and 0.67 for local control. External validation of the survival model yielded AUCs of 0.68, 0.74, 0.76 and 0.71 for cohorts from Leuven (n = 109), VU Amsterdam (n = 178), Manchester (n = 403) and Amsterdam (n = 205), respectively, while the validation procedure for the local control model resulted in AUCs of 0.70, 0.71, 0.72 and 0.62. The resulting nomograms were made available on the website www.predictcancer.org. Further evidence from multivariate analyses suggests that tumour volume also influences local control and survival in T2 tumours (Rutkowski et al. 2013) and T3-4 tumours (Hoebers et al. 2013).

Wang et al. (2013) analyzed the impact of the lymph node ratio (LNR, ratio of metastatic to examined nodes) on the prognosis of hypopharyngeal cancer patients. SEER registered hypopharyngeal cancer patients with lymph node metastasis were evaluated using multivariate Cox regression analysis to identify the prognostic role of the LNR. The categorical LNR was compared with the continuous LNR and pN classifications to predict cause-specific and overall survival (n = 916). T classification, N classification,

Table 6 AJCC TNM classification of carcinoma of the larynx and hypopharynx

Stage	Description
Primary tumor (T)	
TX	Primary tumor cannot be assessed
T0	No evidence of primary tumor
Tis	Carcinoma in situ
Supraglottis	
T1	Tumor limited to 1 subsite of supraglottis, with normal vocal cord mobility
T2	Tumor invades mucosa of more than 1 adjacent subsite of supraglottis or glottis or region outside the supraglottis, without fixation of the larynx
T3	Tumor limited to larynx with vocal cord fixation and/or invades any of the following: postcricoid area, preepiglottic space, paraglottic space, and/or inner cortex of thyroid cartilage
T4a	Moderately advanced local disease: Tumor invades through the thyroid cartilage and/or invades tissues beyond the larynx
T4b	Very advanced local disease: Tumor invades prevertebral space, encases carotid artery, or invades mediastinal structures
Glottis	
T1a	Tumor limited to 1 vocal cord (may involve anterior or posterior commissure) with normal mobility
T1b	Tumor involves both vocal cords (may involve anterior or posterior commissure) with normal mobility
T2	Tumor extends to supraglottis and/or subglottis, and/or with impaired vocal cord mobility
T3	Tumor limited to the larynx with vocal cord fixation and/or invasion of paraglottic space, an/or inner cortex of the thyroid cartilage
T4a	Moderately advanced local disease: Tumor penetrates the outer cortex of the thyroid cartilage and/or invades tissues beyond the larynx
T4b	Very advanced local disease: Tumor invades prevertebral space, encases carotid artery, or involves mediastinal structures
Subglottis	
T1	Tumor limited to the subglottis
T2	Tumor extends to vocal cord(s) with normal or impaired mobility
T3	Tumor limited to larynx with vocal cord fixation
T4a	Moderately advanced local disease: Tumor invades cricoid or thyroid cartilage and/or invades tissues beyond the larynx
T4b	Very advanced local disease: Tumor invades prevertebral space, encases carotid artery, or involves mediastinal structures
Hypopharynx	
T1	Tumor limited to 1 subsite of hypopharynx and/or $\leq$2 cm in greatest dimension
T2	Tumor invades more than 1 subsite of hypopharynx or an adjacent site, or measures >2 cm but $\leq$4 cm in greatest dimension
T3	Tumor >4 cm in greatest dimension or with fixation of hemilarynx or extension to esophagus
T4a	Moderately advanced local disease: Tumor invades thyroid/cricoid cartilage, hyoid bone, thyroid gland, or central compartment soft tissue includes prelaryngeal strap muscles and subcutaneous fat
T4b	Very advanced local disease: Tumor invades prevertebral fascia, encasescarotid artery, or involves mediastinal structures
Regional lymph nodes (N)	
NX	Regional lymph nodes cannot be assessed
N0	No regional lymph node metastasis
N1	Metastasis in a single ipsilateral lymph node, $\leq$3 cm in greatest dimension
N2a	Metastasis in a single ipsilateral lymph node, >3 cm but $\leq$6 cm in greatest dimension
N2b	Metastasis in multiple ipsilateral lymph nodes, none >6 cm in greatest dimension
N2c	Metastasis in bilateral or contralateral lymph nodes, none >6 cm in greatest dimension
N3	Metastasis in a lymph node, >6 cm in greatest dimension
Distant metastasis (M)	
M0	No distant metastasis
M1	Distant metastasis

M classification, the number of regional lymph nodes examined, the continuous LNR (Hazard ratio 2.4, 95 % CI 1.7–3.4, $p < 0.001$) were among prognostic variables that were associated with cause-specific survival. The categorical LNR showed a higher C-index and lower Akaike information criterion (AIC) value than the continuous LNR. When patients were classified into four risk groups according to LNR, R0 (LNR = 0), R1 (LNR $\leq$ 0.05), R2 (LNR 0.05–0.3) and R3 (LNR > 0.3), the Cox regression model for both endpoints using the R classification had a higher C-index value and lower AIC value than the model using the pN classification. In conclusion, using the cutoff points 0.05/0.3, the R classification was more accurate than the pN classification in predicting survival.

4 Haemoglobin and Oxygenation

Tumour perfusion and oxygenation have long been of interest in head and neck cancer research. Identification of potential surrogate markers and dynamics during treatment are subject of numerous recent studies. Low haemoglobin is associated with inferior loco-regional control and survival in multivariate analyses of mixed populations (Rades et al. 2013b: stage III/IV, postoperative radiotherapy; McCloskey et al. 2009: definitive chemoradiation; Agarwala et al. 2007: definitive chemoradiation). Correction of pre-treatment low haemoglobin by blood transfusion and/or erythropoietin (EPO) stimulating agents does, however, not improve the outcome (Hoff 2012). Smoking leads to a decrease in effective haemoglobin and poorer treatment outcome. Smoking should be avoided in order to improve the therapeutic efficacy of radiotherapy and development of other smoking-related diseases and/or secondary cancers. A study on postoperative radiotherapy with multivariate analysis suggested that improved loco-regional control was significantly associated with no EPO expression of tumour cells (risk ratio [RR] 3.7; 95 % CI 1.35–15.4; $p = 0.008$) (Seibold et al. 2013). Improved metastases-free survival was also significantly associated with no EPO expression (RR 5.45; 95 % CI 1.1–97.8; $p = 0.031$). The same holds true for improved survival.

The concentration of osteopontin (SPP1) in plasma is associated with tumour hypoxia. The Danish Head and Neck Cancer group DAHANCA 5 trial found that the hypoxia radiosensitiser nimorazole significantly improved the outcome of radiotherapy for patients with head and neck cancer compared with placebo. However, whether all patients benefit from such modification of hypoxia is unclear. DAHANCA researchers aimed to assess whether the concentration of plasma osteopontin could predict response to the hypoxia radiosensitiser in 320 patients randomised in the DAHANCA 5 trial (Overgaard et al. 2005). Samples were grouped into tertiles according to high, intermediate or low concentrations of plasma osteopontin, and analysed for loco-regional tumour control and disease-specific survival at 5 years. Overall, loco-regional tumour failure and disease-specific mortality were more frequent in patients assigned placebo than in those assigned nimorazole. Loco-regional tumour failure was more frequent in patients with high concentrations of osteopontin assigned placebo than in those with high concentrations assigned nimorazole, as was disease-specific mortality. However, neither loco-regional tumour failure nor disease-specific mortality differed between groups for patients with low concentrations of plasma osteopontin or for those with intermediate concentrations. This study suggested that high plasma concentrations of osteopontin are associated with a poor outlook after radiotherapy for patients with head and neck cancer, but can be improved by use of nimorazole.

TROG researchers sought to confirm the prognostic and predictive significance of osteopontin in patients treated on a large international trial (stage III/IV, randomised to receive definitive radiotherapy concurrently with cisplatin or cisplatin plus the hypoxic cell cytotoxin tirapazamine (n = 578) (Lim et al. 2012). Osteopontin concentrations were analyzed for overall survival and loco-regional failure, adjusting for known prognostic factors. Additional analysis was carried out in patients with available tumour p16 staining status. High osteopontin levels were not associated with worse outcome. There was no interaction between osteopontin and treatment arm for either endpoint. Thus, there is no conclusive evidence that high plasma osteopontin levels are associated with an adverse prognosis, or are predictive of benefit with hypoxia targeting therapy. The same TROG dataset suggested that elevated plasma interleukin (IL)-8 level is an independent prognostic factor for survival irrespective of treatment (Le et al. 2012).

A different study from the Netherlands (based on a randomised trial in patients with laryngeal cancer) reported that only in tumours with a low EGFR fraction (immunohistochemical staining), adding hypoxia modification to accelerated radiotherapy has an additive beneficial effect on outcome (Nijkamp et al. 2013). EGFR expression appears to be a predictive biomarker for the selection of patients that will or will not respond to carbogen and nicotinamide (ARCON), a hypoxia targeting strategy that is thought to counteract enhanced tumour cell proliferation- and hypoxia-related radioresistance. Hypoxia gene expression signatures are another developing strategy to assess and categorise hypoxia (Toustrup et al. 2012). This method has evolved along with the development of complementary DNA microarray analysis and classifies tumours in accordance to the expression of specific hypoxia-responsive genes in the tumour biopsy. Thus, tumours are classified and categorised in terms of the biological behaviour to hypoxic conditions in the microenvironment. Ongoing research will determine the clinical applicability of gene expression signatures, also with regard to other endpoints such as normal tissue toxicity.

A recent DAHANCA study evaluated (18)F-fluoroazomycin arabinoside (FAZA) positron emission tomography (PET)/CT hypoxia imaging as a prognostic factor in HNSCC patients receiving radiotherapy (Mortensen et al. 2012). Forty patients were included. Static FAZA PET/CT imaging was conducted prior to irradiation. The hypoxic volume (HV) was delineated. In 13 patients, a repetitive FAZA PET/CT scan was conducted during the radiotherapy treatment. A hypoxic volume could be identified in 25 (63 %) of the 40 tumours. FAZA PET HV varied considerably with a range from 0 to 31 (median: 0.3) cm^3. The distribution of hypoxia among the HPV positive and negative tumours was not significantly different. In the FAZA PET/CT scans performed during radiotherapy, hypoxia could be detected in six of the 13 patients. For these six patients the location of HV remained stable in location during radiotherapy treatment, though the size of the HV decreased. In 30 patients a positive correlation was detected between maximum FAZA uptake in the primary tumour and the lymph node. During a median follow up of 19 months a significant difference in disease-free survival rate with 93 % for patients with non-hypoxic tumours and 60 % for patients with hypoxic tumours could be detected. The definitive role of FAZA PET/CT imaging as a suitable assay with prognostic potential for detection of hypoxia should be determined in confirmatory trials. Other tracers and imaging methods (dynamic contrast-enhanced magnetic resonance imaging (DCE-MRI), DCE computed tomography, and diffusion-weighted MRI, measuring for example distribution of tumour blood volume and blood flow) are also under prospective evaluation (Quon and Brizel 2012).

5 Other Aspects of PET/CT

PET/CT might improve staging of HNSCC and is recommended in the M and bilateral nodal staging of all patients where conventional imaging is equivocal, or where treatment may be significantly modified (Yoo et al. 2013). PET is recommended in all patients after conventional imaging and in addition to, or prior to, diagnostic panendoscopy where the primary site is unknown (Nieder et al. 2001). Besides staging and target volume delineation, other advantages of PET have been discussed in the literature [prognostic and predictive information, monitoring of response, adaptive radiotherapy (Garg et al. 2012)]. All these potential indications require additional evidence from prospective trials. However, examples from the literature are presented here. Metabolic tumour volume (MTV) of (18)F-FDG PET/CT is a volumetric measurement of tumour cells with increased 18F-FDG uptake. Park et al. evaluated the prognostic value of MTV in 81 patients with locoregionally advanced laryngeal and hypopharyngeal cancer (Park et al. 2013). On multivariate analysis, MTV was an independent prognostic factor for both loco-regional control and survival. Comparable findings were made by Tang et al. in 83 patients (Tang et al. 2012). A different study included 69 patients with SCC of the tonsil who underwent pretreatment FDG PET/CT with measurement of maximum standardized uptake value (SUV(max)), MTV, total lesion glycolysis (TLG), and asymmetry indices (of SUV(max), MTV, and TLG) (Moon et al. 2013). The prognostic significance of these parameters and clinical variables was assessed by multivariate Cox proportional hazards regression analysis with adjustments for age, sex, and AJCC stage. This study showed that only TLG (HR 1.02, 95 % CI 1.003–1.037, $p = 0.023$) was an independent prognostic factor associated with decreased overall survival.

An ongoing multi-centre trial aims to improve outcome in two ways. Firstly, by redistribution of the radiation dose to the metabolically most FDG avid part of the tumour (Heukelom et al. 2013). Hereby, a biologically more effective dose distribution might be achieved while simultaneously sparing normal tissues. Secondly, by improving patient selection. Both cisplatin and EGFR antibodies like cetuximab in combination with radiotherapy are effective in enhancing tumour response. However, it is unknown which patients will benefit from either agent in combination with irradiation. The plan is to analyse the predictive value of biological markers and (89)Zr-cetuximab uptake for treatment outcome of chemoradiation with cetuximab or cisplatin to improve patient selection. The so-called ART-FORCE study is a randomized phase II trial for 268 patients with a factorial 2 by 2 design: cisplatin versus cetuximab and standard versus redistributed radiotherapy. Adaptation of treatment for anatomical changes in the third week of treatment is planned. Patients with locally advanced squamous cell carcinoma of the oropharynx, oral cavity or hypopharynx are eligible. Primary endpoints are: loco-regional recurrence-free survival at 2 years, correlation of the median (89)Zr-cetuximab uptake and biological markers with treatment specific outcome, and toxicity (clinicaltrials.gov, identifier: NCT01504815).

6 Further Recent Biomarker Studies

Table 7 shows a brief summary of study results. Attempts to identify biomarkers that could improve current predictive and prognostic models are necessary, given that outcome is not satisfactory in some stages of head and neck cancer while other subgroups might benefit from less aggressive

Table 7 Recently studied biomarkers (selected examples, multivariate analysis performed)

Authors	Biomarker	Patient population (n)	Correlated with
Balermpas et al. (2013)	NF-κB/p65 nuclear immunoreactivity	101, locally advanced, primary CRT	OS, PFS, and DMFS
Semrau et al. (2013)	EGFR, survivin	52, primary CRT	No correlation
Snietura et al. (2012)	PTEN	147, postoperative RT, subgroup from a randomised trial	LRC, tumours with a high intensity of PTEN staining had significant gain in LRC from 7-days-a-week RT
Le et al. (2009)	Lysyl oxidase	306, subgroup from RTOG trials	OS, DMFS, TTP
Dos Santos et al. (2012)	HIF-1 alpha	66, oral cavity	Local control, OS after RT
Schrijvers et al. (2012)	FADD	92, T1-T2 glottic carcinoma, RT	Local control
Nichols et al. (2012)	Ki-67, EGFR, Bcl-2	75, T1-T2 glottic carcinoma, RT	DFS (Ki-67 only)
Ang et al. (2002)	EGFR	155, primary RT	OS, LRC
Eriksen et al. (2005)	EGFR	803, randomised DAHANCA trials	Tumours with high EGFR and well/moderate differentiation did benefit from moderate acceleration of treatment regarding LRC and DSS, no such effect in tumours with low EGFR and/or poor differentiation

CRT chemoradiotherapy, *OS* overall survival, *PFS* progression-free survival, *DMFS* distant metastases-free survival, *DFS* disease-free survival, *DSS* disease-specific survival, *LRC* loco-regional control, *TTP* time to progression, *RTOG* Radiation Therapy Oncology Group, *DAHANCA* Danish Head and Neck Cancer Group, *EGFR* epidermal growth factor receptor, *FADD* Fas-associated death domain

treatment in terms of reduced toxicity and better functional status. The challenges of biomarker research, at least when it comes to generalisation of findings from single studies, have been addressed in the first chapters of this textbook. In brief, methods such as tissue preparation, immunohistochemistry, molecular analyses or imaging protocols require standardisation in order to obtain reproducible results across institutions. Readers of published studies must be able to understand the methodology, including how multivariate analyses were performed. If already established prognosticators are not included, new biomarkers might not necessarily provide added value. For example such biomarkers might just be a surrogate or replacement for known parameters associated with tumour aggressiveness like histologic grade, vascular or perineural invasion, haemoglobin and others (Table 8). Rigorous large scale validation studies are essential before incorporating new biomarkers into current algorithms.

Cisplatin concomitant to radiotherapy is a preferred standard for locally advanced HNSCC. However, the cisplatin-attributable survival benefit is limited and toxicity substantial. A biomarker of cisplatin resistance could guide treatment selection and spare morbidity. The ERCC1-XPF nuclease is critical to DNA repair pathways resolving cisplatin-induced lesions. In a phase II trial, patients with stage III-IVb HNSCC were randomised to combined cisplatin and radiotherapy with/without erlotinib. Archived primary tumours were available from 90 of 204 patients for a planned substudy (Bauman et al. 2013). Semi-quantitative ERCC1 protein expression was determined using antibodies. The primary analysis evaluated the relationship between continuous ERCC1 protein expression and progression-free survival. Secondary analyses included two pre-specified ERCC1 cut-points and performance in HPV-associated disease. Higher ERCC1 expression was associated with inferior progression-free survival. Patients with increased versus decreased/normal ERCC1 expression experienced inferior progression-free survival. This threshold remained prognostic in HPV-associated disease. Sun et al. used immunohistochemistry to examine the expression of ERCC1 in nasopharyngeal tumour tissue of patients treated with concurrent cisplatin-based chemoradiation (Sun et al. 2011). Patients ($n = 77$) were categorized into either a resistant or sensitive group depending on their treatment response outcome. The resistant and sensitive groups included 25 and 52 patients, respectively. ERCC1 expression was positive in the tumour tissue for 39 of the 77 patients (51 %). Significantly more ERCC1-negative tumours were in the sensitive group than in the resistant group ($p = 0.035$). In terms of survival outcome, univariate analysis determined that patients with ERCC1-negative tumours had longer disease-free survival and overall survival ($p = 0.013$) than patients with ERCC1-positive tumours. Multivariate analysis confirmed that negative ERCC expression in tumours was an independent predictor for prolonged overall survival (hazard ratio, 0.14; 95 % CI, 0.03–0.71).

Table 8 Hypothetical multivariate analysis of prognostic factors for survival after radiotherapy in patients with locally advanced larynx/hypopharynx cancer: the aim is to determine whether potential biomarkers add value to existing models

Established factors based on 994 patients published by Egelmeer et al. (2011)	Other factors that could be considered for inclusion based on different datasets discussed in this chapter	Biomarkers of interest (arbitrary selection)[a]
Low haemoglobin level	Tumour volume	EGFR
Male sex	Hypoxic subvolume	Ki-67
Older age	Histologic grade	FADD
Advanced T category	Lymph node ratio	HIF-1alpha
Nodal involvement	Comorbidity index	
Non-glottic tumour	Smoking	
Biologically effective radiation dose	Performance status	
	Marital status	
	Body mass index	

[a] Consider the complexity of adding such variables either as continuous or categorical variables (what is the optimal cut-off?), remember to include sufficiently large patient numbers (at least 10 events per variable in the multivariate model)
EGFR epidermal growth factor receptor, *FADD* Fas-associated death domain

7 Comorbidity and Nutritional Status

A retrospective nationwide population-based study of all Danish HNSCC patients diagnosed from 1992 to 2008 was recently published (Bøje et al. 2013). A total of 12,623 patients were identified through the DAHANCA database. By linking to the Danish registers, information on somatic comorbidity present prior to the HNSCC diagnosis was obtained and adapted to the Charlson Comorbidity Index (CCI). The influence of comorbidity on overall survival and cancer-specific death was evaluated and the type and prevalence of comorbidity described. In total, 36 % of patients had comorbidity according to CCI. Increasing age was significantly associated with increasing CCI. In multivariate analyses, the CCI score remained a strong independent prognostic factor for overall survival, the HR being 1.16 (95 % CI 1.08–1.25), 1.34 (1.22–1.46), and 1.63 (1.51–1.80) for patients with CCI score 1, 2, and 3+ , respectively. The CCI score did not influence cancer specific death, suggesting that patients die from their comorbidities rather than their cancer.

In patients who received definitive chemoradiation, multivariate analysis indicated that pre-treatment percentage of ideal body weight (%IBW) ($p = 0.04$) was statistically significantly associated with loco-regional failure (Platek et al. 2011). A larger study with more than 1,500 patients found that higher pre-treatment body mass index (BMI) positively influenced survival outcomes (Pai et al. 2012). Comparable results were seen in 400 patients with locoregionally advanced nasopharyngeal carcinoma treated with combination of chemotherapy and radiotherapy (Huang et al. 2013). The patients were divided into four groups of underweight, normal weight, overweight or obese according to the World Health Organization classifications for Asian populations. The 5-year failure-free survival rates for the underweight, normal weight, overweight and obese groups were 44, 61, 68 and 73 %, respectively ($p = 0.014$), and the 5-year overall survival rates were 51, 68, 80 and 72 % ($p = 0.001$), respectively. BMI was a significant prognostic factor of overall survival and failure-free survival in a Cox regression model.

8 Toxicity Prediction

Radiation-induced side effects mainly depend on total dose and volume irradiated, illustrated by numerous reports on Normal Tissue Complication Probability (NTCP) models for different late side effects such as xerostomia and swallowing dysfunction. To achieve a reduction of the irradiated volume of normal tissues, two main strategies have been applied, including attempts to redefine the clinical target volume (CTV) and the use of advanced and emerging radiation delivery techniques. Elective nodal treatment, either by surgery or radiotherapy, is commonly applied in the primary treatment of HNSCC in case the probability of occult nodal metastases is 20 % or higher (Weiss et al. 1994, Gregoire et al. 2000). This threshold of 20 % is more or less arbitrarily determined taking into account the expected treatment-related morbidity in reference to the expected improvement of regional control which can be achieved with elective treatment of the regional lymph node areas. Given the known dose-effect relationships for tumour control, both dose-escalation in the target volume and maximal reduction of the dose distribution in OARs is important. In this respect, the use of advanced radiation delivery techniques becomes increasingly relevant. Intensity modulated radiotherapy (IMRT) is a radiation technique in which the intensity of multiple beams can be optimized in order to conform the radiation dose to the target volumes, while reducing the dose to adjacent critical structures. The initial experiences with IMRT have provided encouraging results regarding loco-regional tumour control, overall survival and in particular reduction of side effects (Lee et al. 2006, McMillan et al. 2006, Pow et al. 2006, Vergeer et al. 2009). As IMRT permits increased possibilities to conform the dose to the target volume, it promises to both reduce toxicity and improve loco-regional tumour control. One of the advantages of using stereotactic radiation techniques could be the use of image-guided high precision repositioning in order to be able to safely reduce the margins from CTV to PTV.

Tribius et al. (2012) examined 95 patients with locally advanced tumours treated with curative intent (IMRT to 60–70 Gy). (Chemo)radiotherapy was either definitive or adjuvant. Patients completed the EORTC QLQ-C30 and HNC-specific HN35 module before and at the end of (chemo)radiotherapy and 6–8 weeks after therapy completion. At baseline, patients reported significantly lower global health status, functioning, and symptom scale scores than a reference German population (all $p < 0.001$). At the end of (chemo)radiotherapy, patients had significantly lower QoL scores versus baseline on all functioning scales ($p < 0.05$). Most symptom and HN35 scores worsened during (chemo)radiotherapy but many recovered 6–8 weeks post-treatment. QoL deteriorated more in patients with high versus low baseline QoL; no clinical or sociodemographic characteristics of patients most likely to experience a significant deterioration in QoL during treatment were identified.

Nourrisat et al. (2010) focused on weight loss in a study that was part of a phase 3 chemoprevention trial. A total of 540 patients (stage I or II) were randomised. The patients were weighed before and after radiotherapy. The mean weight loss was 2.2 kg (standard deviation, 3.4). Five factors were associated with a greater weight loss: all HN cancer sites other than the glottic larynx ($p < 0.001$), higher pre-treatment body weight ($p < 0.001$), stage II disease ($p = 0.002$), dysphagia and/or odynophagia before radiotherapy ($p = 0.001$), and a lower Karnofsky performance score ($p = 0.028$). There was no association with baseline lifestyle habits, diet, or QoL. The bootstrapping method confirmed the reliability of this predictive model. The area under the curve was 71 % (95 % CI, 66–77), which represents an acceptable ability of the model to predict critical weight loss.

Dysphagia and xerostomia are dose-dependent side effects that might cause measurable and relevant QoL deterioration. Significant factors in predicting swallowing problems are age, follow-up duration, tumour site, chemotherapy, surgery of the primary tumour and neck, and dose (Teguh et al. 2013). For dry mouth, the significant factors were age, gender, tumour site, N stage, chemotherapy, and bilateral irradiation in this study of 434 patients from the Netherlands (randomised trial on hyperbaric oxygen). The authors developed a predictive risk model that could be used to select patients for hyperbaric oxygen treatment to prevent or reduce severe late side effects. Table 9 shows further data on factors that might predict toxicity risk. Langendijk et al. (2009) performed a prospective study with 529 patients with HNSCC treated with curative (chemo)radiation. In all patients, acute and late radiation-induced morbidity (RTOG Acute and Late Morbidity Scoring System) was scored prospectively. Multivariate logistic regression analyses were carried out with grade 2 or higher RTOG swallowing dysfunction at 6 months as the primary (SWALL(6 months)) endpoint. The model was validated by comparing the predicted and observed complication rates and by testing if the model also predicted acute dysphagia and late dysphagia at later time points (12, 18 and 24 months). The following factors turned out to be independent predictive factors for SWALL (6 months): T3–T4, bilateral neck irradiation, weight loss prior to radiation, oropharyngeal and nasopharyngeal tumours, accelerated radiotherapy and concomitant chemoradiation. By summation of the regression coefficients derived from the multivariate model, the Total Dysphagia Risk Score (TDRS) could be calculated. In the logistic regression model, the TDRS was significantly associated with SWALL(6 months) ($p < 0.001$). Subsequently, the authors defined three risk groups based on the TDRS. The rate of SWALL(6 months) was 5, 24 and 46 % in case of low-, intermediate- and high-risk patients, respectively. These observed percentages were within the 95 % confidence intervals of the predicted values. The TDRS risk group classification was also significantly associated with acute dysphagia ($p < 0.001$ at all time points) and with late swallowing dysfunction at 12, 18 and 24 months ($p < 0.001$ at all time points). A smaller Japanese study (47 patients treated with definitive chemoradiation) validated the TDRS model (Koiwai et al. 2010).

Another large multicentre prospective cohort study was reported by Christianen et al. (2012). These researchers wanted to identify which dose volume histogram parameters and pre-treatment factors were most important to predict physician-rated and patient-rated swallowing dysfunction in order to develop predictive models (curative (chemo)radiotherapy). The study population consisted of 354 patients. The primary endpoint was grade 2 or more swallowing dysfunction according to the RTOG/EORTC late radiation morbidity scoring criteria at 6 months after (CH)RT. The secondary endpoints were patient-rated swallowing complaints as assessed with the EORTC QLQ-H&N35 questionnaire. To select the most predictive variables a multivariate logistic regression analysis with bootstrapping was used. At 6 months after (CH)RT the bootstrapping

Table 9 Recent toxicity prediction analyses (selected examples, multivariate analysis performed)

Authors	Side effect	Patient population (n)	Correlated with
Self et al. (2013)	Oropharyngeal haemorrhage	139, CRT without surgery	Advanced T stage
Monnier et al. (2011)	Mandibular osteoradionecrosis	73, oral cavity/oropharynx, including postoperative RT	Mandibular surgery
Lee et al. (2009)	Mandibular osteoradionecrosis	198, oral cavity/oropharynx	Mandibular surgery, higher biologically effective radiation dose
Dorth et al. (2013)	Carotid artery stenosis	224, majority with stage III/IV and cisplatin-based CRT	Framingham risk factors, radiation dose
Teguh et al. (2008)	Trismus	81, oropharyngeal cancer	Mean dose in masseter and pterygoid muscles
Su et al. (2013)	Temporal lobe necrosis	870, nasopharynx cancer, IMRT	Percent of temporal lobes receiving 40 Gy and absolute volume receiving 40 Gy
Machtay et al. (2012)	Chronic grade 3-4 pharyngeal/laryngeal toxicity and/or requirement for a feeding tube $\geq$2 years after registration and/or potential treatment-related death within 3 years	154, 3 RTOG chemoradiation trials	Older age, radiation dose received by the inferior hypopharynx >60 Gy
Ghadjar et al. (2012)	Late RTOG $\geq$ grade 3 toxicity and/or potential treatment-related death within 3 years	213, hyperfractionated RT $\pm$ concomitant cisplatin (randomised trial)	Advanced N-classification, technically unresectable disease, weight loss ratio, severe acute dysphagia
Beetz et al. (2012)	Xerostomia at 6 months	167, 3-D (C)RT	Mean parotid dose, age and baseline xerostomia
Mortensen et al. (2013)	Late dysphagia	259, primary IMRT	Objective measurements and observer-assessed dysphagia correlated with dose to pharyngeal constrictor muscles, whereas QoL endpoints correlated with DVH parameters in the glottis/supraglottic larynx

CRT chemoradiotherapy, *IMRT* intensity-modulated radiotherapy, *QoL* quality of life, *DVH* dose-volume histogram, *RTOG* Radiation Therapy Oncology Group

procedure revealed that a model based on the mean dose to the superior pharyngeal constrictor muscle (PCM) and mean dose to the supraglottic larynx was most predictive. For the secondary endpoints different predictive models were found: for problems with swallowing liquids the most predictive factors were the mean dose to the supraglottic larynx and radiation technique (3D-CRT versus IMRT). For problems with swallowing soft food the mean dose to the middle PCM, age (18–65 vs. >65 years), tumour site (naso/oropharynx versus other sites) and radiation technique (3D-CRT versus IMRT) were the most predictive factors. For problems with swallowing solid food the most predictive factors were the mean dose to the superior PCM, the mean dose to the supraglottic larynx and age (18–65 vs. >65 years). And for choking when swallowing the V60 of the oesophageal inlet muscle and the mean dose to the supraglottic larynx were the most predictive factors. These data suggest that separate predictive models are needed for different endpoints and factors other than dose volume histogram parameters are important as well.

Sensori-neural hearing loss (SNHL) is a complication to radiation therapy in the upper head and neck region. Honoré et al. (2002) estimated the dose response relationship for SNHL with adjustment for pre-therapeutic risk factors. The pre- and post-therapeutic hearing levels were recorded in 20 patients receiving radiotherapy for nasopharyngeal carcinoma. The dose to the inner ear of these patients was estimated with a CT based treatment planning system. SNHL increased significantly with increasing dose to the cochlea. Increasing patient's age and decreasing pre-therapeutic hearing level were statistically significantly associated with an increased risk of SNHL. A nomogram was presented for estimating individualised dose constraints of potential use in treatment planning.

9 Patient Selection for Re-irradiation

As re-irradiation, with or without other modalities, is associated with a considerable risk of severe acute and late treatment-related side effects, proper selection of patients is essential to optimise the therapeutic ratio (Spencer et al. 1999, 2001, 2008; Nieder et al. 2000; Schaefer et al. 2000; De Crevoisier et al. 1998, 2001, Kasperts et al. 2005; Langer et al. 2007; Janot et al. 2008; Sulman et al. 2009). There are a number of methodological problems with regard to the identification and validation of prognostic factors in the re-irradiation setting, including (1) differences in eligibility criteria and subsequent heterogeneity of the study populations among the different studies; (2) the retrospective design of most studies; (3) the relatively limited number of patients included with a too low power to detect clinically relevant prognostic factors, and (4) the large variety of treatment regimens used. Nevertheless, despite these methodological shortcomings, there are a limited number of prognostic factors that seem to be important. Recently, Tanvetyanon et al. (2009) reported on a retrospective analysis of prognostic factors for survival among patients treated with curatively intended salvage re-irradiation for head and neck cancer. The study population was composed of patients with recurrent tumours as well as second primaries, and 46 out of 103 patients underwent salvage surgery and postoperative re-irradiation. These authors developed a nomogram for the prediction of death within 24 months after re-irradiation, including a combination of prognostic factors such as co-morbid disease based on the Charlson index, organ dysfunction prior to re-irradiation, isolated neck recurrence, tumour bulk (i.e., sum of the maximal diameter of tumour at the neck plus measurable mucosal tumour at salvage surgery) and time interval between completion of previous therapy and initiation of re-irradiation. The performance of this nomogram showed good agreement between predicted and observed outcomes, with a C-index of 0.75. The factors included in this nomogram generally reflect the most frequently reported prognostic factors in the re-irradiation setting. However, other potential prognostic factors such as recurrent versus second primary tumour, total dose of radiation, previous chemoradiation and radiation technique were not identified as significant prognostic factors. Nevertheless, the nomogram could be a useful tool to select patients with favourable outcome for the more intensified (chemo) re-irradiation strategies. An important finding of this study was that comorbidity and pre-existing organ dysfunction were the most important prognostic factors. More specifically, the median overall survival among patients with neither significant comorbidity nor pre-treatment organ dysfunction was 59.6 months which was markedly better compared to those with both comorbidity and organ dysfunction, in whom the median survival was only 5.5 months with no survivors beyond 2 years of follow-up ($p < 0.001$). These two factors are probably important because they may increase the risk of cancer-related death due to poor treatment tolerance and compliance and/or increase the risk of non-cancer-related death. Moreover, organ dysfunction, which is mainly due to radiation-induced toxicity from the previous treatment, may also be a surrogate marker of a more aggressive biological behaviour of the tumour. Hence, given the large impact on overall survival, both factors may interact negatively with (chemo) re-irradiation, but may also be a competing risk of death. A limited validation study with 28 Japanese patients was published (Shikama et al. 2013). Twenty-two patients were treated with stereotactic body radiotherapy using a median total dose of 30 Gy in 1–7 fractions and six patients were treated with conventional external beam radiotherapy. The 2-year overall survival was 22 %. The 2-year overall survival in 20 patients with unfavourable prognosis (median 2-year survival probability, 5.5 %) and in 8 patients with favourable prognosis (median 2-year survival probability, 45 %) were 11 and 46 %, respectively. Larger and more sophisticated statistical analyses are necessary to confirm the validity of the nomogram.

References

Agarwala SS, Cano E, Heron DE, Johnson J, Myers E, Sandulache V et al (2007) Long-term outcomes with concurrent carboplatin, paclitaxel and radiation therapy for locally advanced, inoperable head and neck cancer. Ann Oncol 18:1224–1229

Ang KK, Berkey BA, Tu X, Zhang HZ, Katz R, Hammond EH et al (2002) Impact of epidermal growth factor receptor expression on survival and pattern of relapse in patients with advanced head and neck carcinoma. Cancer Res 62:7350–7356

Balermpas P, Michel Y, Wagenblast J, Seitz O, Sipek F, Rödel F et al (2013) Nuclear NF-κB expression correlates with outcome among patients with head and neck squamous cell carcinoma treated with primary chemoradiation therapy. Int J Radiat Oncol Biol Phys 86:785–790

Bauman JE, Austin MC, Schmidt R, Kurland BF, Vaezi A, Hayes DN et al (2013) ERCC1 is a prognostic biomarker in locally advanced head and neck cancer: results from a randomised, phase II trial. Br J Cancer. doi:10.1038/bjc.2013.576

Beetz I, Schilstra C, Burlage FR, Koken PW, Doornaert P, Bijl HP et al (2012) Development of NTCP models for head and neck cancer patients treated with three-dimensional conformal radiotherapy for xerostomia and sticky saliva: the role of dosimetric and clinical factors. Radiother Oncol 105:86–93

Bernier J, Domenge C, Ozsahin M, Matuszewska K, Lefebvre JL, Greiner RH et al (2004) Postoperative irradiation with or without concomitant chemotherapy for locally advanced head and neck cancer. N Engl J Med 350:1945–1952

Bøje CR, Dalton SO, Grønborg TK, Primdahl H, Kristensen CA, Andersen E et al (2013) The impact of comorbidity on outcome in 12 623 Danish head and neck cancer patients: a population based study from the DAHANCA database. Acta Oncol 52:285–293

Bonner JA, Harari PM, Giralt J, Azarnia N, Shin DM, Cohen RB et al (2006) Radiotherapy plus cetuximab for squamous-cell carcinoma of the head and neck. N Engl J Med 354:567–578

Bourhis J, Overgaard J, Audry H, Ang KK, Saunders M, Bernier J et al (2006) Hyperfractionated or accelerated radiotherapy in head and neck cancer: a meta-analysis. Lancet 368:843–854

Brockstein B, Haraf DJ, Rademaker AW, Kies MS, Stenson KM, Rosen F et al (2004) Patterns of failure, prognostic factors and survival in locoregionally advanced head and neck cancer treated with concomitant chemoradiotherapy: a 9-year, 337-patient, multi-institutional experience. Ann Oncol 15:1179–1186

Chen KW, Lin JF, Jan JS, Chao JY, Lin JC (2009) The effect of primary tumor volume measured by MR imaging on T stage, local control, and survival in patients with advanced nasopharyngeal carcinoma. Therapeut Radiol Oncol 16:1–13

Christianen ME, Schilstra C, Beetz I, Muijs CT, Chouvalova O, Burlage FR et al (2012) Predictive modelling for swallowing dysfunction after primary (chemo)radiation: results of a prospective observational study. Radiother Oncol 105:107–114

Cooper JS, Pajak TF, Forastiere AA, Jacobs J, Campbell BH, Saxman SB et al (2004) Postoperative concurrent radiotherapy and chemotherapy for high-risk squamous-cell carcinoma of the head and neck. N Engl J Med 350:1937–1944

Coyne JC, Pajak TF, Harris J, Konski A, Movsas B, Ang KK et al (2007) Emotional well-being does not predict survival in head and neck cancer patients: a Radiation Therapy Oncology Group study. Cancer 110:2568–2575

De Crevoisier R, Bourhis J, Domenge C, Wibault P, Koscielny S, Lusinchi A et al (1998) Full-dose reirradiation for unresectable head and neck carcinoma: experience at the Gustave-Roussy Institute in a series of 169 patients. J Clin Oncol 16:3556–3562

De Crevoisier R, Domenge C, Wibault P, Koscielny S, Lusinchi A, Janot F et al (2001) Full dose reirradiation combined with chemotherapy after salvage surgery in head and neck carcinoma. Cancer 91:2071–2076

Dorth JA, Patel PR, Broadwater G, Brizel DM (2013) Incidence and risk factors of significant carotid artery stenosis in asymptomatic survivors of head and neck cancer after radiotherapy. Head Neck. doi:10.1002/hed.23280

Dos Santos M, Mercante AM, Louro ID, Gonçalves AJ, de Carvalho MB, da Silva EH et al (2012) HIF1-alpha expression predicts survival of patients with squamous cell carcinoma of the oral cavity. PLoS One 7:e45228

EdgeSB, Byrd DR, Compton CC et al (2009) American Joint Committee on Cancer, American Cancer Society. AJCC cancer staging manual, 7th edn. Springer, Berlin

Egelmeer AG, Velazquez ER, de Jong JM, Oberije C, Geussens Y, Nuyts S et al (2011) Development and validation of a nomogram for prediction of survival and local control in laryngeal carcinoma patients treated with radiotherapy alone: a cohort study based on 994 patients. Radiother Oncol 100:108–115

Eriksen JG, Steiniche T, Overgaard J (2005) Danish Head and Neck Cancer study group (DAHANCA). The influence of epidermal growth factor receptor and tumor differentiation on the response to accelerated radiotherapy of squamous cell carcinomas of the head and neck in the randomized DAHANCA 6 and 7 study. Radiother Oncol 74:93–100

Fakhry C, Westra WH, Li S, Cmelak A, Ridge JA, Pinto H et al (2008) Improved survival of patients with human papillomavirus-positive head and neck squamous cell carcinoma in a prospective clinical trial. J Natl Cancer Inst 100:261–269

Garg MK, Glanzman J, Kalnicki S (2012) The evolving role of positron emission tomography-computed tomography in organ-preserving treatment of head and neck cancer. Semin Nucl Med 42:320–327

Ghadjar P, Simcock M, Zimmermann F, Betz M, Bodis S, Bernier J et al (2012) Predictors of severe late radiotherapy-related toxicity after hyperfractionated radiotherapy with or without concomitant cisplatin in locally advanced head and neck cancer. Secondary retrospective analysis of a randomized phase III trial (SAKK 10/94). Radiother Oncol 104:213–218

Gillison ML, Zhang Q, Jordan R, Xiao W, Westra WH, Trotti A et al (2012) Tobacco smoking and increased risk of death and progression for patients with p16-positive and p16-negative oropharyngeal cancer. J Clin Oncol 30:2102–2111

Gregoire V, Coche E, Cosnard G, Hamoir M, Reychler H (2000) Selection and delineation of lymphnode target volumes in head and neck conformal radiotherapy. Proposal for standardizing terminology and procedure based on the surgical experience. Radiother Oncol 56:135–150

Guo R, Sun Y, Yu XL, Yin WJ, Li WF, Chen YY et al (2012) Is primary tumor volume still a prognostic factor in intensity modulated radiation therapy for nasopharyngeal carcinoma? Radiother Oncol 104:294–299

Haughey BH, Gates GA, Arfken CL, Harvey J (1992) Meta-analysis of second malignant tumors in head and neck cancer: the case for an endoscopic screening protocol. Ann Otol Rhinol Laryngol 101:105–112

Heukelom J, Hamming O, Bartelink H, Hoebers F, Giralt J, Herlestam T et al (2013) Adaptive and innovative Radiation Treatment FOR improving Cancer treatment outcomE (ARTFORCE); a randomized controlled phase II trial for individualized treatment of head and neck cancer. BMC Cancer 13:84

Hitt R, Lopez-Pousa A, Martinez-Trufero J, Escrig V, Carles J, Rizo A et al (2005) Phase III study comparing cisplatin plus fluorouracil to paclitaxel, cisplatin, and fluorouracil induction chemotherapy followed by chemoradiotherapy in locally advanced head and neck cancer. J Clin Oncol 23:8636–8645

Hoebers F, Rios E, Troost E, van den Ende P, Kross K, Lacko M et al (2013) Definitive radiation therapy for treatment of laryngeal carcinoma : impact of local relapse on outcome and implications for treatment strategies. Strahlenther Onkol 189:834–841

Hoff CM (2012) Importance of hemoglobin concentration and its modification for the outcome of head and neck cancer patients treated with radiotherapy. Acta Oncol 51:419–432

Hong AM, Martin A, Armstrong BK, Lee CS, Jones D, Chatfield MD et al (2013) Human papillomavirus modifies the prognostic significance of T stage and possibly N stage in tonsillar cancer. Ann Oncol 24:215–219

Honoré HB, Bentzen SM, Møller K, Grau C (2002) Sensori-neural hearing loss after radiotherapy for nasopharyngeal carcinoma: individualized risk estimation. Radiother Oncol 65:9–16

Huang PY, Wang CT, Cao KJ, Guo X, Guo L, Mo HY et al (2013) Pretreatment body mass index as an independent prognostic factor in patients with locoregionally advanced nasopharyngeal carcinoma treated with chemoradiotherapy: findings from a randomised trial. Eur J Cancer 49:1923–1931

Janot F, De Raucourt D, Benhamou E, Ferron C, Dolivet G, Bensadoun RJ et al (2008) Randomized trial of postoperative reirradiation combined with chemotherapy after salvage surgery compared with salvage surgery alone in head and neck carcinoma. J Clin Oncol 26:5518–5523

Kasperts N, Slotman B, Leemans CR, Langendijk JA (2005) A review on re-irradiation for recurrent and second primary head and neck cancer. Oral Oncol 41:225–243

Kim KY, Li S, Cha JD, Zhang X, Cha IH (2012) Significance of molecular markers in survival prediction of oral squamous cell carcinoma. Head Neck 34:929–936

Koiwai K, Shikama N, Sasaki S, Shinoda A, Kadoya M (2010) Validation of the Total Dysphagia Risk Score (TDRS) as a predictive measure for acute swallowing dysfunction induced by chemoradiotherapy for head and neck cancers. Radiother Oncol 97:132–135

Langendijk JA, Leemans CR, Buter J, Berkhof J, Slotman BJ (2004) The additional value of chemotherapy to radiotherapy in locally advanced nasopharyngeal carcinoma: a meta-analysis of the published literature. J Clin Oncol 22:4604–4612

Langendijk JA, Doornaert P, Rietveld DH, Verdonck-de Leeuw IM, Leemans CR, Slotman BJ (2009) A predictive model for swallowing dysfunction after curative radiotherapy in head and neck cancer. Radiother Oncol 90:189–195

Langer CJ, Harris J, Horwitz EM, Nicolaou N, Kies M, Curran W et al (2007) Phase II study of low-dose paclitaxel and cisplatin in combination with split-course concomitant twice-daily reirradiation in recurrent squamous cell carcinoma of the head and neck:

results of Radiation Therapy Oncology Group Protocol 9911. J Clin Oncol 25:4800–4805
Lassen P, Eriksen JG, Hamilton-Dutoit S, Tramm T, Alsner J, Overgaard J (2009) Effect of HPV-associated p16INK4A expression on response to radiotherapy and survival in squamous cell carcinoma of the head and neck. J Clin Oncol 27:1992–1998
Le QT, Harris J, Magliocco AM, Kong CS, Diaz R, Shin B et al (2009) Validation of lysyl oxidase as a prognostic marker for metastasis and survival in head and neck squamous cell carcinoma: Radiation Therapy Oncology Group trial 90–03. J Clin Oncol 27:4281–4286
Le QT, Fisher R, Oliner KS, Young RJ, Cao H, Kong C et al (2012) Prognostic and predictive significance of plasma HGF and IL-8 in a phase III trial of chemoradiation with or without tirapazamine in locoregionally advanced head and neck cancer. Clin Cancer Res 18:1798–1807
Lee NY, de Arruda FF, Puri DR, Wolden SL, Narayana A, Mechalakos J et al (2006) A comparison of intensity-modulated radiation therapy and concomitant boost radiotherapy in the setting of concurrent chemotherapy for locally advanced oropharyngeal carcinoma. Int J Radiat Oncol Biol Phys 66:966–974
Lee IJ, Koom WS, Lee CG, Kim YB, Yoo SW, Keum KC et al (2009) Risk factors and dose-effect relationship for mandibular osteoradionecrosis in oral and oropharyngeal cancer patients. Int J Radiat Oncol Biol Phys 75:1084–1091
Lim AM, Rischin D, Fisher R, Cao H, Kwok K, Truong D et al (2012) Prognostic significance of plasma osteopontin in patients with locoregionally advanced head and neck squamous cell carcinoma treated on TROG 02.02 phase III trial. Clin Cancer Res 18:301–307
Lv X, Xiang YQ, Cao SM, Qian CN, Li NW, Guo L et al (2011) Prospective validation of the prognostic value of elevated serum vascular endothelial growth factor in patients with nasopharyngeal carcinoma: more distant metastases and shorter overall survival after treatment. Head Neck 33:780–785
Machtay M, Moughan J, Farach A, Martin-O'Meara E, Galvin J, Garden AS et al (2012) Hypopharyngeal dose is associated with severe late toxicity in locally advanced head-and-neck cancer: an RTOG analysis. Int J Radiat Oncol Biol Phys 84:983–989
McCloskey SA, Jaggernauth W, Rigual NR, Hicks WL Jr, Popat SR, Sullivan M et al (2009) Radiation treatment interruptions greater than one week and low hemoglobin levels (12 g/dL) are predictors of local regional failure after definitive concurrent chemotherapy and intensity-modulated radiation therapy for squamous cell carcinoma of the head and neck. Am J Clin Oncol 32:587–591
McMillan AS, Pow EH, Kwong DL, Wong MC, Sham JS, Leung LH, Leung WK (2006) Preservation of quality of life after intensity-modulated radiotherapy for early-stage nasopharyngeal carcinoma: results of a prospective longitudinal study. Head Neck 28:712–722
Monnier Y, Broome M, Betz M, Bouferrache K, Ozsahin M, Jaques B (2011) Mandibular osteoradionecrosis in squamous cell carcinoma of the oral cavity and oropharynx: incidence and risk factors. Otolaryngol Head Neck Surg 144:726–732
Moon SH, Choi JY, Lee HJ, Son YI, Baek CH, Ahn YC et al (2013) Prognostic value of 18F-FDG PET/CT in patients with squamous cell carcinoma of the tonsil: comparisons of volume-based metabolic parameters. Head Neck 35:15–22
Mortensen LS, Johansen J, Kallehauge J, Primdahl H, Busk M, Lassen P et al (2012) FAZA PET/CT hypoxia imaging in patients with squamous cell carcinoma of the head and neck treated with radiotherapy: results from the DAHANCA 24 trial. Radiother Oncol 105:14–20
Mortensen HR, Jensen K, Aksglæde K, Behrens M, Grau C (2013) Late dysphagia after IMRT for head and neck cancer and correlation with dose-volume parameters. Radiother Oncol 107:288–294
Nichols AC, Whelan F, Basmaji J, Dhaliwal S, Dowthwaite S, Chapeskie C et al (2012) Ki-67 expression predicts radiotherapy failure in early glottic cancer. J Otolaryngol Head Neck Surg 41:124–130
Nieder C, Milas L, Ang KK (2000) Tissue tolerance to reirradiation. Semin Radiat Oncol 10:200–209
Nieder C, Gregoire V, Ang KK (2001) Cervical lymph node metastases from occult squamous cell carcinoma: cut down a tree to get an apple? Int J Radiat Oncol Biol Phys 50:727–733
Nijkamp MM, Span PN, Terhaard CH, Doornaert PA, Langendijk JA, van den Ende PL et al (2013) Epidermal growth factor receptor expression in laryngeal cancer predicts the effect of hypoxia modification as an additive to accelerated radiotherapy in a randomised controlled trial. Eur J Cancer 49:3202–3209
Nourissat A, Bairati I, Samson E, Fortin A, Gélinas M, Nabid A et al (2010) Predictors of weight loss during radiotherapy in patients with stage I or II head and neck cancer. Cancer 116:2275–2283
Oguejiofor KK, Hall JS, Mani N, Douglas C, Slevin NJ, Homer J et al (2013) The prognostic significance of the biomarker p16 in oropharyngeal squamous cell carcinoma. Clin Oncol (R Coll Radiol) 25:630–638
Overgaard J, Eriksen JG, Nordsmark M, Alsner J, Horsman MR (2005) Danish Head and Neck Cancer Study Group. Plasma osteopontin, hypoxia, and response to the hypoxia sensitiser nimorazole in radiotherapy of head and neck cancer: results from the DAHANCA 5 randomised double-blind placebo-controlled trial. Lancet Oncol 6:757–764
Pai PC, Chuang CC, Tseng CK, Tsang NM, Chang KP, Yen TC et al (2012) Impact of pretreatment body mass index on patients with head-and-neck cancer treated with radiation. Int J Radiat Oncol Biol Phys 83:e93–e100
Park GC, Kim JS, Roh JL, Choi SH, Nam SY, Kim SY (2013) Prognostic value of metabolic tumor volume measured by 18F-FDG PET/CT in advanced-stage squamous cell carcinoma of the larynx and hypopharynx. Ann Oncol 24:208–214
Pignon JP, Bourhis J, Domenge C, Designe L (2000) Chemotherapy added to locoregional treatment for head and neck squamous-cell carcinoma: three meta-analyses of updated individual data. MACH-NC Collaborative Group. Meta-analysis of chemotherapy on head and neck cancer. Lancet 355:949–955
Pignon JP, le Maitre A, Maillard E, Bourhis J (2009) Meta-analysis of chemotherapy in head and neck cancer (MACH-NC): an update on 93 randomised trials and 17,346 patients. Radiother Oncol 92:4–14
Platek ME, Reid ME, Wilding GE, Jaggernauth W, Rigual NR, Hicks WL Jr et al (2011) Pretreatment nutritional status and locoregional failure of patients with head and neck cancer undergoing definitive concurrent chemoradiation therapy. Head Neck 33:1561–1568
Posner MR, Hershock DM, Blajman CR, Mickiewicz E, Winquist E, Gorbounova V et al (2007) Cisplatin and fluorouracil alone or with docetaxel in head and neck cancer. N Engl J Med 357:1705–1715
Pow EH, Kwong DL, McMillan AS, Wong MC, Sham JS, Leung LH, Leung WK (2006) Xerostomia and quality of life after intensity-modulated radiotherapy vs. conventional radiotherapy for early-stage nasopharyngeal carcinoma: initial report on a randomized controlled clinical trial. Int J Radiat Oncol Biol Phys 66:981–991
Quon H, Brizel DM (2012) Predictive and prognostic role of functional imaging of head and neck squamous cell carcinomas. Semin Radiat Oncol 22:220–232
Rades D, Seibold ND, Schild SE, Gebhard MP, Noack F (2013a) Androgen receptor expression: prognostic value in locally advanced squamous cell carcinoma of the head and neck. Strahlenther Onkol 189:849–855
Rades D, Seibold ND, Gebhard MP, Noack F, Thorns C, Schild SE (2013b) Impact of the HPV-positivity definition on the prognostic value of HPV status in patients with locally advanced squamous cell carcinoma of the head and neck. Strahlenther Onkol 189:856–860

Rischin D, Young RJ, Fisher R, Fox SB, Le QT, Peters LJ et al (2010) Prognostic significance of p16INK4A and human papillomavirus in patients with oropharyngeal cancer treated on TROG 02.02 phase III trial. J Clin Oncol 28:4142–4148

Rutkowski T, Wygoda A, Składowski K, Hejduk B, Rutkowski R, Kołosza Z, Maciejewski B (2013) Prognostic role of tumor volume for radiotherapy outcome in patient with T2 laryngeal cancer. Strahlenther Onkol 189:861–866

Schaefer U, Micke O, Schueller P, Willich N (2000) Recurrent head and neck cancer: retreatment of previously irradiated areas with combined chemotherapy and radiation therapy-results of a prospective study. Radiology 216:371–376

Schrijvers ML, Pattje WJ, Slagter-Menkema L, Mastik MF, Gibcus JH, Langendijk JA et al (2012) FADD expression as a prognosticator in early-stage glottic squamous cell carcinoma of the larynx treated primarily with radiotherapy. Int J Radiat Oncol Biol Phys 83:1220–1226

Seibold ND, Schild SE, Gebhard MP, Noack F, Rades D (2013) Prognosis of patients with locally advanced squamous cell carcinoma of the head and neck. Impact of tumor cell expression of EPO and EPO-R. Strahlenther Onkol 189:559–565

Self EM, Bumpous J, Ziegler C, Wilson L, Potts K (2013) Risk factors for hemorrhage after chemoradiation for oropharyngeal squamous cell carcinoma. JAMA Otolaryngol Head Neck Surg 139:356–361

Semrau R, Duerbaum H, Temming S, Huebbers C, Stenner M, Drebber U et al (2013) Prognostic impact of human papillomavirus status, survivin, and epidermal growth factor receptor expression on survival in patients treated with radiochemotherapy for very advanced nonresectable oropharyngeal cancer. Head Neck 35:1339–1344

Shikama N, Kumazaki Y, Tsukamoto N, Ebara T, Makino S, Abe T et al (2013) Validation of nomogram-based prediction of survival probability after salvage re-irradiation of head and neck cancer. Jpn J Clin Oncol 43:154–160

Snietura M, Jaworska M, Mlynarczyk-Liszka J, Goraj-Zajac A, Piglowski W, Lange D et al (2012) PTEN as a prognostic and predictive marker in postoperative radiotherapy for squamous cell cancer of the head and neck. PLoS One 7:e33396

Spencer SA, Wheeler RH, Peters GE, Beenken SW, Meredith RF, Smith J, Conner W, Salter MM (1999) Concomitant chemotherapy and reirradiation as management for recurrent cancer of the head and neck. Am J Clin Oncol 22:1–5

Spencer SA, Harris J, Wheeler RH, Machtay M, Schultz C, Spanos W et al (2001) RTOG 96–10: reirradiation with concurrent hydroxyurea and 5-fluorouracil in patients with squamous cell cancer of the head and neck. Int J Radiat Oncol Biol Phys 51:1299–1304

Spencer SA, Harris J, Wheeler RH, Machtay M, Schultz C, Spanos W et al (2008) Final report of RTOG 9610, a multi-institutional trial of reirradiation and chemotherapy for unresectable recurrent squamous cell carcinoma of the head and neck. Head Neck 30:281–288

Su SF, Huang SM, Han F, Huang Y, Chen CY, Xiao WW et al (2013) Analysis of dosimetric factors associated with temporal lobe necrosis (TLN) in patients with nasopharyngeal carcinoma (NPC) after intensity modulated radiotherapy. Radiat Oncol 8:17

Sulman EP, Schwartz DL, Le TT, Ang KK, Morrison WH, Rosenthal DI et al (2009) IMRT reirradiation of head and neck cancer-disease control and morbidity outcomes. Int J Radiat Oncol Biol Phys 73:399–409

Sun JM, Ahn MJ, Park MJ, Lee HY, Ahn JS, Lee S et al (2011) Expression of excision repair cross-complementation group 1 as predictive marker for nasopharyngeal cancer treated with concurrent chemoradiotherapy. Int J Radiat Oncol Biol Phys 80:655–660

Sze WM, Lee AW, Yau TK, Yeung RM, Lau KY, Leung SK et al (2004) Primary tumor volume of nasopharyngeal carcinoma: prognostic significance of local control. Int J Radiat Oncol Biol Phys 59:21–27

Tang C, Murphy JD, Khong B, La TH, Kong C, Fischbein NJ et al (2012) Validation that metabolic tumor volume predicts outcome in head-and-neck cancer. Int J Radiat Oncol Biol Phys 83:1514–1520

Tanvetyanon T, Padhya T, McCaffrey J, Zhu W, Boulware D, Deconti R, Trotti A (2009) Prognostic factors for survival after salvage reirradiation of head and neck cancer. J Clin Oncol27:1983–1991

Teguh DN, Levendag PC, Voet P, van der Est H, Noever I, de Kruijf W et al (2008) Trismus in patients with oropharyngeal cancer: relationship with dose in structures of mastication apparatus. Head Neck 30:622–630

Teguh DN, Levendag PC, Ghidey W, van Montfort K, Kwa SL (2013) Risk model and nomogram for dysphagia and xerostomia prediction in head and neck cancer patients treated by radiotherapy and/or chemotherapy. Dysphagia 28:388–394

Thomas B, Stedman M, Davies L (2013) Grade as a prognostic factor in oral squamous cell carcinoma: A population based analysis of the data. Laryngoscope. doi:10.1002/lary.24357

Toustrup K, Sørensen BS, Alsner J, Overgaard J (2012) Hypoxia gene expression signatures as prognostic and predictive markers in head and neck radiotherapy. Semin Radiat Oncol 22:119–127

Tribius S, Reemts E, Prosch C, Raguse M, Petersen C, Kruell A et al (2012) Global quality of life during the acute toxicity phase of multimodality treatment for patients with head and neck cancer: can we identify patients most at risk of profound quality of life decline? Oral Oncol 48:898–904

Vergeer MR, Doornaert PA, Rietveld DH, Leemans CR, Slotman BJ, Langendijk JA (2009) Intensity-modulated radiotherapy reduces radiation-induced morbidity and improves health-related quality of life: results of a nonrandomized prospective study using a standardized follow-up program. Int J Radiat Oncol Biol Phys 74:1–8

Vermorken JB, Remenar E, van Herpen C, Gorlia T, Mesia R, Degardin M et al (2007) Cisplatin, fluorouracil, and docetaxel in unresectable head and neck cancer. N Engl J Med 357:1695–1704

Wan XB, Wei L, Li H, Dong M, Lin Q, Ma XK et al (2013) High pretreatment serum lactate dehydrogenase level correlates with disease relapse and predicts an inferior outcome in locally advanced nasopharyngeal carcinoma. Eur J Cancer 49:2356–2364

Wang YL, Feng SH, Zhu J, Zhu GP, Li DS, Wang Y et al (2013a) Impact of lymph node ratio on the survival of patients with hypopharyngeal squamous cell carcinoma: a population-based analysis. PLoS One 8:e56613

Wang SJ, Patel SG, Shah JP, Goldstein DP, Irish JC, Carvalho AL et al (2013b) An oral cavity carcinoma nomogram to predict benefit of adjuvant radiotherapy. JAMA Otolaryngol Head Neck Surg 139:554–559

Weiss MH, Harrison LB, Isaacs RS (1994) Use of decision analysis in planning a management strategy for the stage N0 neck. Arch Otolaryngol Head Neck Surg 120:699–702

Yoo J, Henderson S, Walker-Dilks C (2013) Evidence-based guideline recommendations on the use of positron emission tomography imaging in head and neck cancer. Clin Oncol (R Coll Radiol) 25:e33–e66

Zhou GQ, Tang LL, Mao YP, Chen L, Li WF, Sun Y et al (2012) Baseline serum lactate dehydrogenase levels for patients treated with intensity-modulated radiotherapy for nasopharyngeal carcinoma: a predictor of poor prognosis and subsequent liver metastasis. Int J Radiat Oncol Biol Phys 82:e359–e365

Breast Cancer

Christine M. Fisher and Rachel A. Rabinovitch

Contents

Abstract

Numerous prognostic and predictive tools have been developed to help guide breast cancer counseling on outcomes, treatment decisions, and toxicity. Key prognostic and predictive factors remain estrogen and progesterone status as well as HER2 overexpression. Prognostic tools include Adjuvant! Online, which incorporates validated clinical prognostic factors to provide survival data, as well as Oncotype DX, which uses a 21 gene assay to derive a prognostic recurrence score and is also predictive for chemotherapy response, and Mammaprint, a 70 gene assay. Predictive tools including nomograms have been developed to help with many breast cancer clinical scenarios, including ductal carcinoma in situ, risk of sentinel node positivity, risk of non-sentinel node positivity in the setting of positive sentinel node, risk of brain metastases, and others. Tools to help predict toxicity have been developed, but are currently more sophisticated at predicting toxicity from systemic therapy than radiation therapy. These individualized decision making tools continue to advance breast cancer care and should be incorporated into patient discussions and decision making on validation.

1 Breast Cancer Epidemiology

Breast cancer is the most common non-hematologic cancer in women in the United States, and remains the second most common cause of cancer death in US women. There were 229,060 estimated new cases of breast cancer in 2012, comprising predominantly female patients (226,070) with a minority of male patients (2190). 39,920 deaths were estimated for 2012, with 39,510 women and 410 men estimated to die of the disease. Lifetime risk remained relatively stable at 1 of 8 women from birth to death (Siegel et al. 2012).

C. M. Fisher (✉) · R. A. Rabinovitch
University of Colorado Cancer Center,
Campus Mail Stop F-706, 1665 Aurora Court,
Aurora, CO 80045, USA
e-mail: Christine.fisher@ucdenver.edu

C. Nieder and L. E. Gaspar (eds.), *Decision Tools for Radiation Oncology*, Medical Radiology. Radiation Oncology,
DOI: 10.1007/174_2013_876, © Springer-Verlag Berlin Heidelberg 2013
Published Online: 17 November 2013

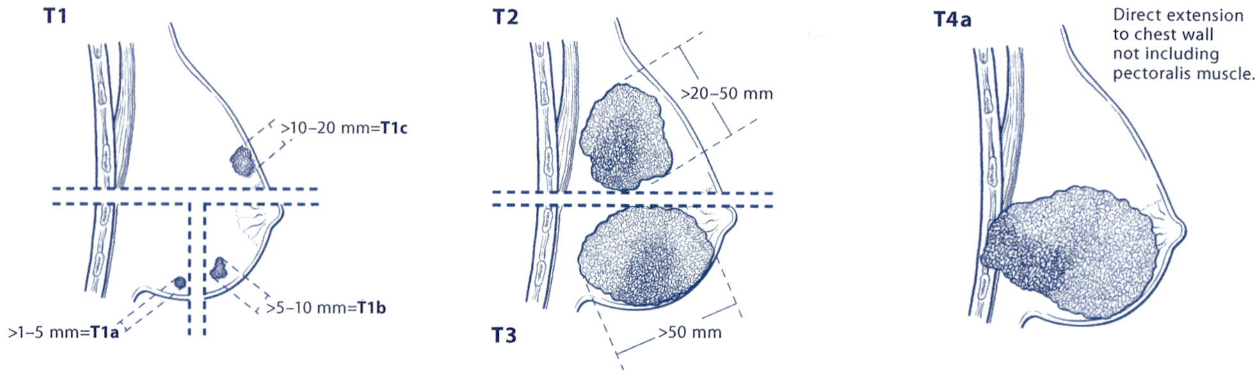

Primary Tumor (T)

- TX Primary tumor cannot be assessed
- T0 No evidence of primary tumor
- Tis Carcinoma in situ
- Tis (DCIS) Ductal carcinoma in situ
- Tis (LCIS) Lobular carcinoma in situ
- Tis (Paget's) Paget's disease of the nipple NOT associated with invasive carcinoma and/or carcinoma in situ (DCIS and/or LCIS) in the underlying breast parenchyma. Carcinomas in the breast parenchyma associated with Paget's disease are categorized based on the size and characteristics of the parenchymal disease, although the presence of Paget's disease should still be noted
- T1 Tumor ≤ 20 mm in greatest dimension
- T1mi Tumor ≤ 1 mm in greatest dimension
- T1a Tumor > 1 mm but ≤ 5 mm in greatest dimension
- T1b Tumor > 5 mm but ≤ 10 mm in greatest dimension
- T1c Tumor > 10 mm but ≤ 20 mm in greatest dimension
- T2 Tumor > 20 mm but ≤ 50 mm in greatest dimension
- T3 Tumor > 50 mm in greatest dimension
- T4 Tumor of any size with direct extension to the chest wall and/or to the skin (ulceration or skin nodules)
  Note: Invasion of the dermis alone does not qualify as T4
- T4a Extension to the chest wall, not including only pectoralis muscle adherence/invasion
- T4b Ulceration and/or ipsilateral satellite nodules and/or edema (including peau d'orange) of the skin, which do not meet the criteria for inflammatory carcinoma
- T4c Both T4a and T4b
- T4d Inflammatory carcinoma (see "Rules for Classification")

Distant Metastases (M)

- M0 No clinical or radiographic evidence of distant metastases
- cM0(i+) No clinical or radiographic evidence of distant metastases, but deposits of molecularly or microscopically detected tumor cells in circulating blood, bone marrow, or other nonregional nodal tissue that are no larger than 0.2 mm in a patient without symptoms or signs of metastases
- M1 Distant detectable metastases as determined by classic clinical and radiographic means and/or histologically proven larger than 0.2 mm

ANATOMIC STAGE/PROGNOSTIC GROUPS

Stage 0	Tis	N0	M0
Stage IA	T1*	N0	M0
Stage IB	T0	N1mi	M0
	T1*	N1mi	M0
Stage IIA	T0	N1**	M0
	T1*	N1**	M0
	T2	N0	M0
Stage IIB	T2	N1	M0
	T3	N0	M0
Stage IIIA	T0	N2	M0
	T1*	N2	M0
	T2	N2	M0
	T3	N1	M0
	T3	N2	M0
Stage IIIB	T4	N0	M0
	T4	N1	M0
	T4	N2	M0
Stage IIIC	Any T	N3	M0
Stage IV	Any T	Any N	M1

Notes

- * T1 includes T1mi.
- ** T0 and T1 tumors with nodal micrometastases only are excluded from Stage IIA and are classified Stage IB.
- M0 includes M0(i+).
- The designation pM0 is not valid; any M0 should be clinical.
- If a patient presents with M1 prior to neoadjuvant systemic therapy, the stage is considered Stage IV and remains Stage IV regardless of response to neoadjuvant therapy.
- Stage designation may be changed if postsurgical imaging studies reveal the presence of distant metastases, provided that the studies are carried out within 4 months of diagnosis in the absence of disease progression and provided that the patient has not received neoadjuvant therapy.
- Postneoadjuvant therapy is designated with "yc" or "yp" prefix. Of note, no stage group is assigned if there is a complete pathologic response (CR) to neoadjuvant therapy, for example, ypT0ypN0cM0.

Fig. 1 7th edition AJCC breast cancer staging. AJCC staging reprinted with kind permission, Springer Publications

2 Breast Cancer Staging

Staging in this article is based on the seventh edition of the AJCC Staging manual (Edge et al. 2009). Breast cancer staging divides patients into ductal carcinoma in situ, early breast cancer, locally advanced breast cancer, and metastatic breast cancer. Figure 1 illustrates the current (7th edition) staging manual of the AJCC for breast cancer, which will be used in further discussion in this chapter.

3 Prognostic Factors in Breast Cancer

3.1 Clinical Factors

Until recently, clinical factors have largely guided treatment decision-making and discussions about prognosis with individual patients. Factors that can increase the risk for breast cancer include female gender, family history of breast cancer, genetic mutations, particularly BRCA1 and BRCA 2 mutations, and increasing age. Increasing exposure to estrogens, including early menarche, late menopause, nulliparity or older age at first childbirth, and exogenous hormone replacement therapy are all associated with an increasing risk of breast cancer (Carlson et al. 2013). Lobular carcinoma in situ is a risk factor for development of invasive breast cancer in either breast of greater than 20 % at 15 years (Haagensen et al. 1981). Pleomorphic lobular carcinoma in situ has been reported as a more aggressive variant with higher propensity to develop into invasive breast cancer, and these are typically managed with surgical excision when found on biopsy (Anderson et al. 2006). Age is one of the most important clinical factors, as numerous reports have shown that younger patients have a higher risk of breast cancer recurrence (Zhou et al. 2004). On recursive partitioning analysis of prognostic factors for breast cancer outcomes, age is the first split in the tree (Freedman et al. 2002). Location of the tumor within the breast does not affect outcomes, though it can have an effect on cosmesis (Freedman et al. 2002).

Axillary nodal status on clinical staging portends a worse clinical outcome (Carter et al. 1989). The staging described earlier divides pathological disease in the axilla into numerous categories, with published papers showing a worse outcome for node positive patients (Dent 1996) as well as greater nodal burden (Cabanes et al. 1992) versus nodal negative patients (Jatoi et al. 1999). Axillary surgical staging is recognized as a diagnostic and therapeutic procedure (Moore and Kinne 1997). While this was debated for some time as to whether it showed a lead time bias in catching node positive cancers later in their natural history, it is now clear that these tumors are biologically different than node negative cancers (Mittra 1993).

Clinical stage is correlated with outcome, with higher tumor and nodal stage having worse clinical outcomes. Inflammatory breast cancer, described in the staging as T4d, shows a poor outcome regardless of other prognostic factors at the time of diagnosis (Chang et al. 1998). With the poorer outcomes for inflammatory breast cancer based on clinical factors, management involves tri-modality therapy consisting of radiation therapy with dose escalation to decrease recurrence (Liao et al. 2000), cytotoxic chemotherapy, and mastectomy with axillary nodal dissection in all cases where feasible (Cristofanilli et al. 2003).

3.2 Pathologic Factors

The pathology report after breast-conserving surgery or mastectomy remains a crucial driver of adjuvant treatment and outcomes. The effect of margin status remains hotly debated after decades of papers and discussions in the breast cancer literature. Some define a negative margin as no tumor at ink, and this has been the standard in all National Surgical Adjuvant Breast and Bowel Program (NSABP) trials that have driven clinical practice (Wapnir et al. 2011). Tumor at ink has been shown to correlate with recurrence rates (Macmillan et al. 1997). Others chose 2 mm as the definition of a negative margin, and papers published show this associated with a very low risk of ipsilateral breast tumor recurrence after breast conservation, while those with a smaller margin are at a similar risk to those with tumor at ink (Freedman et al. 1999). More recent papers, taking into account better biologic understanding and systemic therapy of tumors, conclude that no tumor at ink is a sufficient negative margin in most clinical scenarios, similar to the NSABP practice (Morrow et al. 2012).

Margin status has also been investigated closely in ductal carcinoma in situ, with wider margins associated with fewer recurrences in some studies (MacDonald et al. 2005). Grade has proven to be an important factor in the recurrence of ductal carcinoma in situ. For high grade patients who have lumpectomy without radiation, the observed recurrence rate is 15.3 % at 5 years, or over 3 % per year. In patients with low to intermediate grade ductal carcinoma in situ, the rate is closer to 1 % per year (Hughes et al. 2009).

Tumor markers are important in breast cancer prognosis. Estrogen receptor status, including the amount of estrogen receptor positivity and the percentage of cells staining positive, should be reported on the pathology report after breast conservation surgery and mastectomy. Estrogen receptor quantity is prognostic for survival from breast cancer (Shek et al. 1989). Estrogen receptor status by immunohistochemistry is superior to ligand binding (Harvey et al. 1999). Estrogen receptor status is linked to long term survival prognosis (Crowe et al. 1991) and is an established prognostic factor in breast cancer (Speirs and Kerin 2008). Progesterone receptor status will be similarly reported, and this usually but not always mimics estrogen receptor expression. Progesterone is also a clinical prognostic factor (Liu et al. 2010).

HER2/*neu* oncogene amplification is a recognized prognostic factor in both recurrence and survival (Slamon et al. 1987). This oncogene is a member of the Epidermal Growth Factor Receptor (EGFR) family (Yamamoto et al. 1986) and retains significant prognostic power after multivariate analysis. This family is known to play an important role in cancer progression (Holbro et al. 2003). Node positive patients have inferior survival with HER2/*neu* oncogene amplification (Borg et al. 1990). In multivariate analysis, gene amplification was the second most important prognostic factor after axillary nodal status (Paik et al. 1990).

Nodal staging has undergone significant changes in the AJCC staging system (American Joint Committee on Cancer 2002). One of the major areas of debate is how to handle cells that are found on immunohistochemistry or molecular testing and whether this merits full axillary dissection (Teng et al. 2000). They have now been found to behave more similarly to node negative patients (Cote et al. 1999) and the updated breast staging reflects this by the designation as N0(i +) or N0(mol +) (American Joint Committee on Cancer 2009). Pathologic tumor size and nodal status remain significant predictors of locoregional recurrence after mastectomy (Buchholz et al. 2002).

Triple negative breast cancers are a less common subtype that are negative for estrogen receptors, progesterone receptors, and HER2/*neu* oncogene amplification. These tumors have a worse prognosis than tumors with tumor marker positivity. Prognostic factors in these triple negative tumors include lymph node status and tumor size, while other parameters that did not reach significance on multivariate analysis include age, histological grade, tumor size, and vascular invasion (Rakha et al. 2007). Triple negative breast cancers have been shown to have elevated intratumoral levels of Vascular Endothelial Growth Factor (VEGF) expression which is correlated with poorer survival (Linderholm et al. 2009).

Recurrent breast cancer represents an unfavorable subset (Lee et al. 2006), yet prognostic factors can be identified within this group to help differentiate outcomes (Pater et al. 1981). Estrogen and progesterone status play an important role in survival from recurrent breast cancer (Howat et al. 1985). Nodal status also plays an important role in survival from recurrent breast cancer (Shek et al. 1987).

3.3 Adjuvant! Online

Numerous prognostic factors have been identified and published in the breast cancer literature. The most robust non-genomic prognostic tool to incorporate this vast literature is Adjuvant! Online, an online tool that allows oncologists to determine quantitative data for their patients in order to make medical decision-making, based initially off of the SEER database (Ravdin et al. 2001). This has been separately validated in the British Columbia Tumor Registry (Olivotto et al. 2005) and is in frequent clinical use and cited in the NCCN guidelines for management of breast cancer (Carlson et al. 2013).

Strengths of Adjuvant! Online is its ease of use and accessibility to clinicians anywhere with internet access. It can be easily opened at consultations and help reassure the patient about outcomes and guide the conversation. One major limitation is the lack of incorporation of HER2 status, which is a major prognostic factor, into its model. For radiation oncologists, it cannot be used as a predictive tool to look at survival with and without radiation, as can some of the nomograms presented later in this chapter.

An example is illustrated for a 65 year old woman with minor medical comorbidities with a pT1cN0 ER + Grade 1 breast cancer. Looking at the 10 year risk for mortality, one calculates a 84.7 % chance of the patient being alive in 10 years, with a 2.8 % risk of dying of disease and 12.5 % risk of dying of other causes. The data was based off of mortality data, and this remains the most robust use of this tool, though it can also be used to look at recurrence.

3.4 Oncotype DX

The Oncotype DX is a 21 gene assay that produces a recurrence score for women based on 16 cancer genes and five reference genes (Paik et al. 2004). The ability to use paraffin embedded tissue to extract these 21 genes was separately validated (Esteva et al. 2005). The assay was developed for use in estrogen receptor positive, node negative invasive, non-metastatic breast cancer and validated in numerous populations including SWOG 8814 (Albain et al. 2010).

The use of the Oncotype DX has subsequently expanded into different populations. It has now been validated in the node positive population, allowing novel approaches to this group who have traditionally all been offered chemotherapy (Dowsett et al. 2010).

Advantages of the Oncotype DX are that one can use paraffin-embedded tissue, which is easier to attain or send post-operatively than fresh tissues. It provides a more individualized picture of each patient's recurrence score than the Adjuvant! Online, and does incorporate HER2 overexpression as one of the genes investigated, unlike Adjuvant! Online. Prior to the advent of the Oncotype DX assay, chemotherapy for node negative, estrogen receptor positive women was commonly given to those with a tumor size of 1 cm or greater, whereas now many of these women are spared chemotherapy that will have little to no benefit in low Oncotype DX recurrence score patients.

Disadvantages include that many patients fall into an intermediate score category, where the predictive value for chemotherapy benefit is less certain than a low score where anti-estrogen therapy alone is likely sufficient or a high score where the margin of benefit of chemotherapy is much greater. The Trial Assessing IndividuaLized Options for Treatment (TAILORx) investigated this population with intermediate Oncotype DX scores, randomizing individuals to either anti-endocrine therapy alone or with the addition of

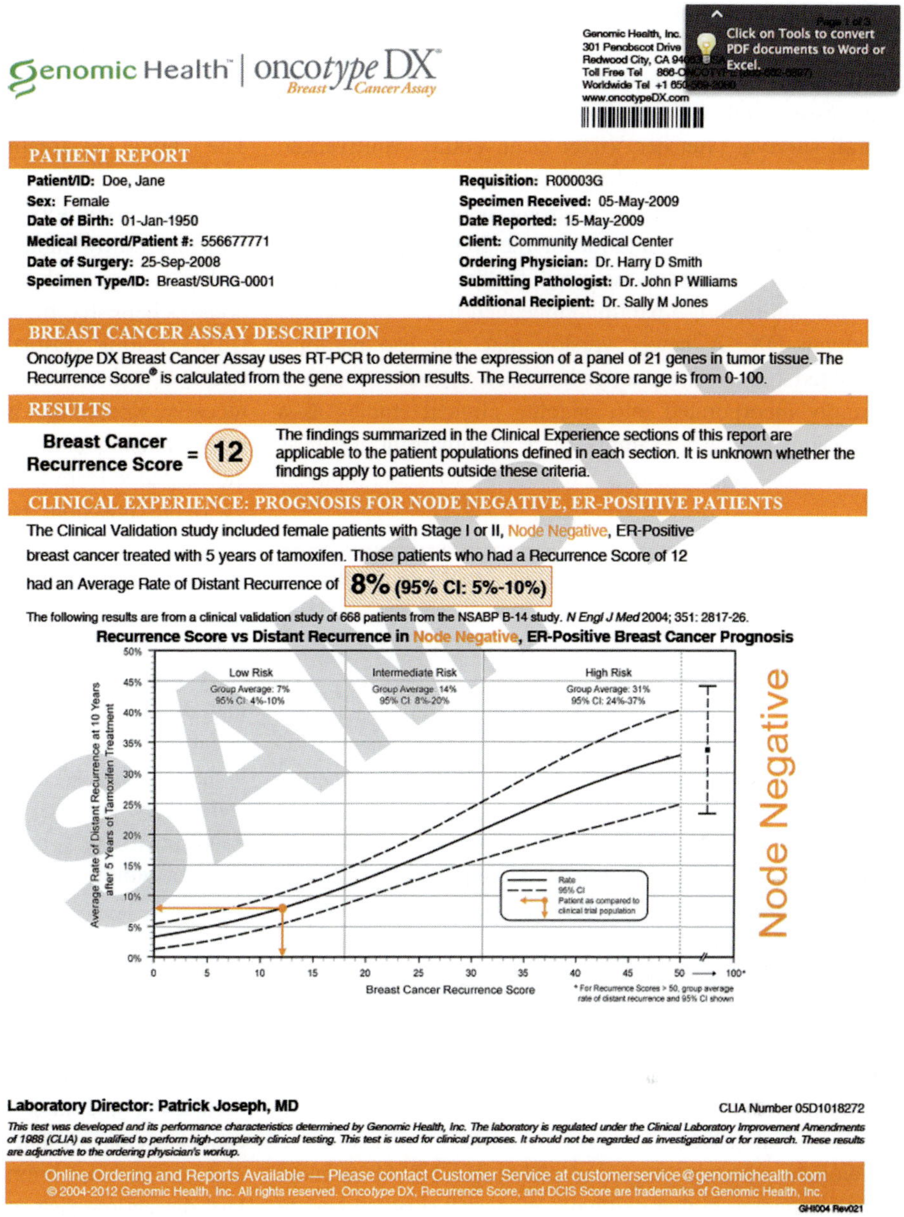

Genomic Health™ | oncotype DX® Breast Cancer Assay

Genomic Health, Inc.
301 Penobscot Drive
Redwood City, CA 94063 USA
Toll Free Tel 866-ONCOTYPE
Worldwide Tel +1 650-569-2080
www.oncotypeDX.com

Click on Tools to convert PDF documents to Word or Excel.

PATIENT REPORT

Patient/ID: Doe, Jane
Sex: Female
Date of Birth: 01-Jan-1950
Medical Record/Patient #: 556677771
Date of Surgery: 25-Sep-2008
Specimen Type/ID: Breast/SURG-0001

Requisition: R00003G
Specimen Received: 05-May-2009
Date Reported: 15-May-2009
Client: Community Medical Center
Ordering Physician: Dr. Harry D Smith
Submitting Pathologist: Dr. John P Williams
Additional Recipient: Dr. Sally M Jones

BREAST CANCER ASSAY DESCRIPTION

Onco*type* DX Breast Cancer Assay uses RT-PCR to determine the expression of a panel of 21 genes in tumor tissue. The Recurrence Score® is calculated from the gene expression results. The Recurrence Score range is from 0-100.

RESULTS

Breast Cancer Recurrence Score = 12

The findings summarized in the Clinical Experience sections of this report are applicable to the patient populations defined in each section. It is unknown whether the findings apply to patients outside these criteria.

CLINICAL EXPERIENCE: PROGNOSIS FOR NODE NEGATIVE, ER-POSITIVE PATIENTS

The Clinical Validation study included female patients with Stage I or II, Node Negative, ER-Positive breast cancer treated with 5 years of tamoxifen. Those patients who had a Recurrence Score of 12 had an Average Rate of Distant Recurrence of **8% (95% CI: 5%-10%)**

The following results are from a clinical validation study of 668 patients from the NSABP B-14 study. *N Engl J Med* 2004; 351: 2817-26.

Laboratory Director: Patrick Joseph, MD CLIA Number 05D1018272

This test was developed and its performance characteristics determined by Genomic Health, Inc. The laboratory is regulated under the Clinical Laboratory Improvement Amendments of 1988 (CLIA) as qualified to perform high-complexity clinical testing. This test is used for clinical purposes. It should not be regarded as investigational or for research. These results are adjunctive to the ordering physician's workup.

Online Ordering and Reports Available — Please contact Customer Service at customerservice@genomichealth.com
© 2004-2012 Genomic Health, Inc. All rights reserved. Onco*type* DX, Recurrence Score, and DCIS Score are trademarks of Genomic Health, Inc.
GHI004 Rev021

Fig. 2 Oncotype report for node negative breast cancer. Oncotype report reprinted with kind permission, genomic health 2013

chemotherapy but results are not yet available (Zujewski and Kamin 2008).

Oncotype DX has also been shown to predict for loco-regional recurrence when used on patients from the NSABP trials B-14 and B-20. In particular, the mastectomy patients treated without radiation had excellent predictive value, suggesting that adjuvant radiation therapy could potentially be tailored to individual patient risk in this group (Mamounas et al. 2010).

Oncotype DX for ductal carcinoma in situ is also available to help guide recurrence risk in this population. Similarly to the Oncotype DX for invasive breast cancer, a tissue specimen is used to look at 21 genes and predict a local recurrence score from 0 to 100 for ductal carcinoma in situ or an invasive recurrence based on the results. The Oncotype DX for ductal carcinoma in situ was validated in a population of women from the ECOG E5194 trial (Hughes et al. 2009), presented in 2011 (Solin et al. 2011), and is now clinically available to help guide decision making. The low score (0–38) predicts a 12 % risk of local recurrence in the next 10 years, an intermediate score (39–54) predicts a 24.5 % recurrence rate, and a high score (55 or higher) predicts a 27.3 % risk of a local recurrence in 10 years. From the validation group in ECOG E5194, 75 % of women ended up in the low risk group (Solin et al. 2011). This test is useful to help quantify the risk of recurrence and potentially guide treatment decisions (Fig. 2).

3.5 Mammaprint as a Prognostic Tool

Mammaprint has subsequently been introduced as a 70 gene assay and validated to have prognostic value in overall survival (van der Vijver et al. 2002). Multivariate analyses show that even when controlling for other clinical factors, the assay remains a strong predictor of overall survival. One major limitation of the Mammaprint in the United States has been the need for fresh tissue, rather than the ability to use paraffin-embedded tissue as with the Oncotype DX. A newer version that can use paraffin-embedded tissue, Symphony, has been introduced and is currently incorporated into ongoing clinical studies as a prognostic tool. An example of a mammaprint result is shown below (Fig. 3).

4 Predictive Factors and Tools in Breast Cancer

4.1 Clinical Factors

Imaging has proven useful to determine stage as well as potential treatment options. Magnetic resonance imaging (MRI) has been extensively studied, and has been shown to alter the surgical options in up to one-third of women who undergo MRI of the breast (Houssami et al. 2008). However, there is no prospective trial data showing a difference in clinical outcomes when MRI is used and retrospective studies do no suggest a difference (Solin et al. 2008).

Radiation has been demonstrated to change the failure pattern when used in the post-mastectomy setting, decreasing locoregional failures including chest wall (Nielsen et al. 2006).

Women who are staged as pathologic N2 (4 or more lymph nodes) or higher will have an overall survival benefit from post-mastectomy radiation. There is some suggestion that the survival benefit is greatest in those with the appropriate biological equivalent dose of 40–60 Gy in 2 Gy fractions and appropriate controls and targeting for radiation delivery (Gebski et al. 2006).

4.2 Pathologic Factors

All breast cancer pathology reports should include estrogen and progesterone receptor status and quantification as well as HER2 overexpression. These three markers remain the most important in guiding choice of adjuvant systemic therapy, as well as being important prognostic tools. They are all incorporated into genomic tools including Oncotype DX and Mammaprint. Patients with estrogen responsive tumors should benefit from anti-endocrine therapy as their final adjuvant treatment for at least 5 years, though some data suggests that longer treatment may have further benefit. The choice of treatment for premenopausal women is tamoxifen, and for women without functional ovaries, aromatase inhibitors are first line therapy. Both of these typically follow radiation therapy.

For women with HER2 overexpression of 3+ by immunohistochemistry or on fluorescence in situ hybridization (FISH) testing, trastuzumab is typically used in addition to cytotoxic chemotherapy (Romond et al. 2005). Until recently, women that had some degree of overexpression by immunohistochemistry (1+ −2+) did not realize any predictive value from this as trastuzumab is used only in HER2 3+ overexpression. However, these tumors that are node positive and 1+ −2+ are now eligible for Neuvax, a peptide vaccine targeting the HER2 protein that has demonstrated efficacy in women with overexpression (Peoples et al. 2005).

Axillary nodal status remains the top pathologic factor that drives adjuvant treatment choices. In clinically node negative patients, the standard procedure to accompany breast surgery is sentinel lymph node biopsy, as long as technically successful. Much of the data for predicting nodal positivity is based on axillary dissections prior to the sentinel lymph node trial results.

4.3 Introduction to Nomograms in Breast Cancer Management

Nomograms have been developed to predict risks of recurrence and help guide treatment in numerous breast cancer scenarios. They include estimation risk of sentinel and non-sentinel lymph node positivity to help guide axillary dissection, risk of recurrence from DCIS, early breast cancer, advanced breast cancer, and even metastatic disease. There are also powerful predictive tools to help guide systemic therapy based on individual tumor genetic markers that have rapidly changed the breast cancer landscape. We will look at management decisions for in situ carcinomas, early invasive carcinomas, advanced carcinomas, and metastatic disease separately. Many predictive tools to help guide treatment decisions and outcome discussions have been developed in breast cancer.

Different predictive tools have been developed and broadly classified into nomograms. Kattan defined a nomogram more narrowly as a graphical calculation instrument that can be based on any type of function, such as logistic regression or Cox hazard ratio regression models (Kattan 2001).

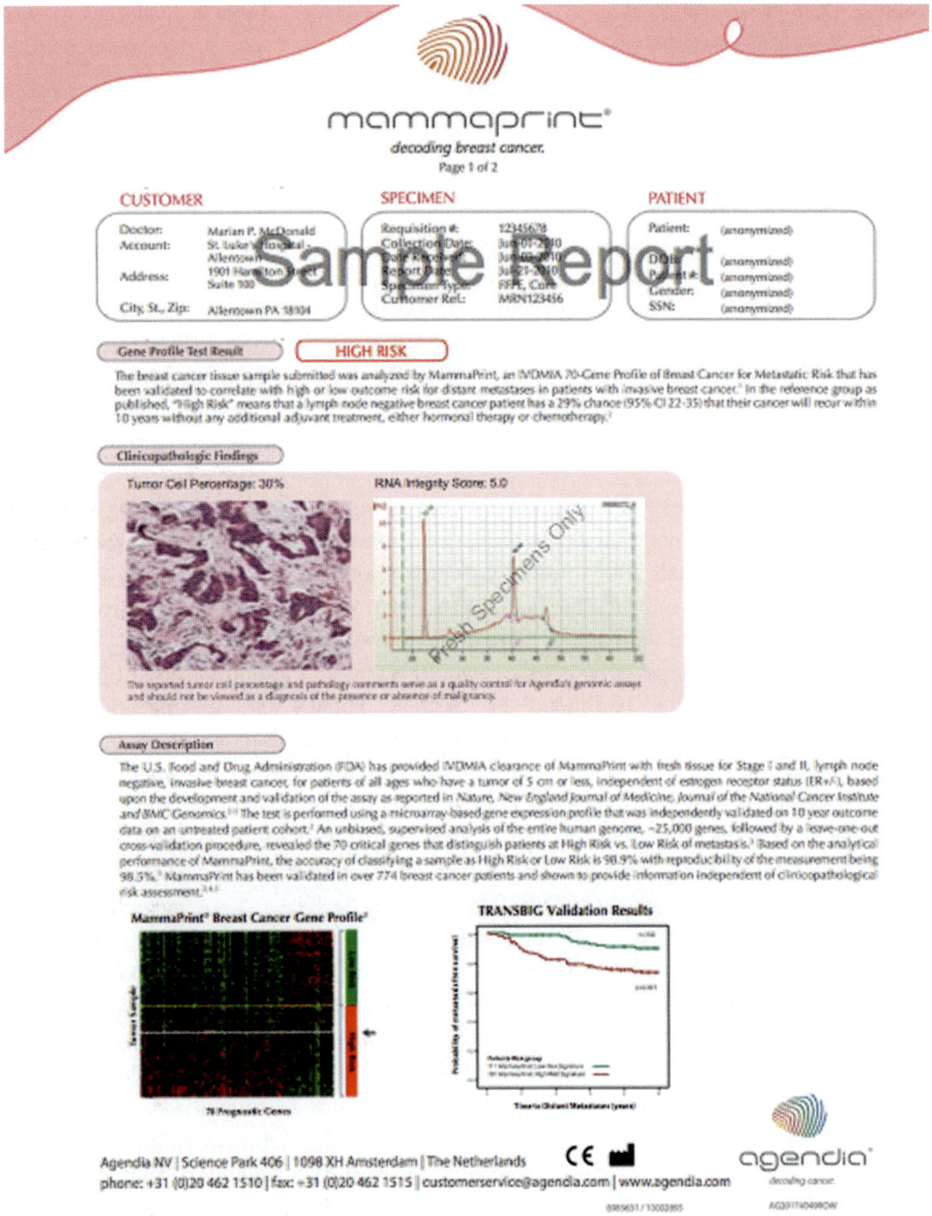

Fig. 3 Mammaprint report for a high risk patient. Mammaprint report provided with kind permission, Agendia 2013

4.4 Nomograms for Predicting Outcomes and Guiding Treatment in Ductal Carcinoma In situ

Breast cancer cells that are lining the ductal system, commonly causing signature calcifications, but have not invaded the basement membrane are known as ductal carcinomas in situ (DCIS) (Rudloff 2010).

Memorial Sloan Kettering physicians developed a DCIS recurrence nomogram that quantifies, based on known risks factors, the risk of a DCIS recurrence. Factors that are included in this nomogram are listed in (Table 1).

Since this nomogram includes potential adjuvant treatments, one can quantify five and 10 year recurrence rates for patients with different possible treatment scenarios. For instance, a 50 year old woman with one surgery showing negative margins, no family history, and intermediate grade DCIS with a radiologic presentation in 2012 can have her risk of recurrence quantified with and without radiation therapy and with and without endocrine therapy. This flexibility is very helpful for clinicians trying to individualize care for each patient.

Table 1 DCIS nomogram factors

Age at diagnosis (25–90)	Family history of breast cancer
Presentation (physical exam or imaging)	Year of surgery
Use of adjuvant radiation therapy	Use of adjuvant endocrine therapy
Nuclear grade	Association of necrosis with DCIS
Surgical margins	Number of surgical excisions

4.5 Nomograms for Predicting Sentinel Lymph Node Involvement

Large randomized studies have been done investigating the equivalence of sentinel node biopsy to axillary lymph node dissection (Veronesi et al. 2003). Initial concerns over the sentinel node procedure included the fact that the recurrence rate might be higher than with axillary nodal dissection, but this is not the case in large series (Naik et al. 2004).

Predictive factors for likelihood of axillary nodal involvement have been published and are incorporated into nomograms predicting likelihood of sentinel node involvement (Gann et al. 1999). This has also been reported in early breast cancer patients, limited to T1a and T1b tumors to help determine who might have the highest likelihood of axillary nodal metastases (Rivadeneira et al. 2000). Large series have also been published looking at what factors women with axillary nodal metastases and early breast tumors have in common (Maibenco et al. 1999). Histopathology has been shown to play a role in the likelihood of early breast tumors with positive lymph nodes (Mustafa et al. 1997).

The likelihood of an involved sentinel lymph node has become an important predictor for prognosis with implications for systemic therapy and its sequencing, particularly with consideration of neoadjuvant systemic therapy. Neoadjuvant cytotoxic therapy has been used in randomized clinical trials to allow some additional patients to undergo breast conservation therapy rather than mastectomy, and ongoing trials are evaluating the role of neoadjuvant hormonal therapy. Many clinicians are not obtaining a pre-treatment sentinel node in a patient with a clinically negative axilla, so predictive tools play a crucial role in this population (Jackson et al. 2000).

Bevilacqua and colleagues have developed a tool that can predict the probability of tumor spread to sentinel lymph nodes. The factors utilized in this tool are listed in (Table 2) (Bevilacqua et al. 2007).

Strengths of this nomogram include the fact that all data can be used pre-operatively. The model was developed based on a cohort of 3,786 women and validated on a separate cohort of 1,545 women with sentinel node biopsies.

Table 2 Nomogram for sentinel node involvement

Patient age	Tumor size
Tubular, colloid/mucinous, or medullary	Location in upper inner quadrant only
LVSI	Multifocality
Tumor type (lobular vs. ductal)	If ductal, histologic grade (I–III)
Estrogen receptor status	Progesterone receptor status

This yielded an area under the receiver operating curve of 0.754. This information is very useful to radiation oncologists and surgeons in deciding how to assess the nodal risk of tumor involvement and make decisions regarding local therapy.

4.6 Determining Risks of Non-sentinel Lymph Node Positivity in Women with a Positive Sentinel Node

Sentinel node biopsy has become an accepted standard of care for the clinically node-negative axilla to detect and remove the node or nodes at highest risk for tumor spread from the breast. Trials such as ACOSOG Z11 have raised questions about the best way to manage patients with positive sentinel nodes, and whether they all need completion axillary dissection.

Van Zee and colleagues developed a nomogram to predict the likelihood of further lymph node metastases in the event that a positive node is found, incorporating published predictive factors (Rahusen et al. 2001) (Turner et al. 2000). This nomogram is not applicable in patients who have had neoadjuvant systemic or radiation therapy. As is true for the sentinel node procedure in general, the patient must have a clinically node negative axilla. The nomogram incorporates numerous clinical factors listed in Table 3 (Van Zee et al. 2003) (Fig. 4).

The nomogram above from Van Zee et al (Fig. 4) is pictured here. Each factor listed has an assigned number of points, which are determined by a vertical line to the points line at the top of the nomogram. The total points are then added up and this total is located on the Total Points line. Finally, a vertical line is drawn from the Total Points line down to the Predicted Probability of positive (+) Non-SLN line to determine the likelihood of non-sentinel lymph nodes that are involved with disease.

A strength of this nomogram is that it does not overestimate the risk of further positive nodes. Other predictive tools have been published, and are useful at picking out patients at high risk for further nodes, but are unable to identify the patients who will have no further lymph nodes positive (Wong et al. 2001). In the era of ACOSOG Z11 where some patients are not getting further dissection in the

Table 3 Predicting additional positive nodes

Frozen section performed	Tumor size
Tumor type (ductal vs. lobular)	Nuclear grade of ductal carcinomas
Number of positive sentinel nodes	Method of detection in sentinel nodes
Number of negative sentinel nodes	Lymphovascular space invasion
Tumor multifocality	Estrogen receptor status

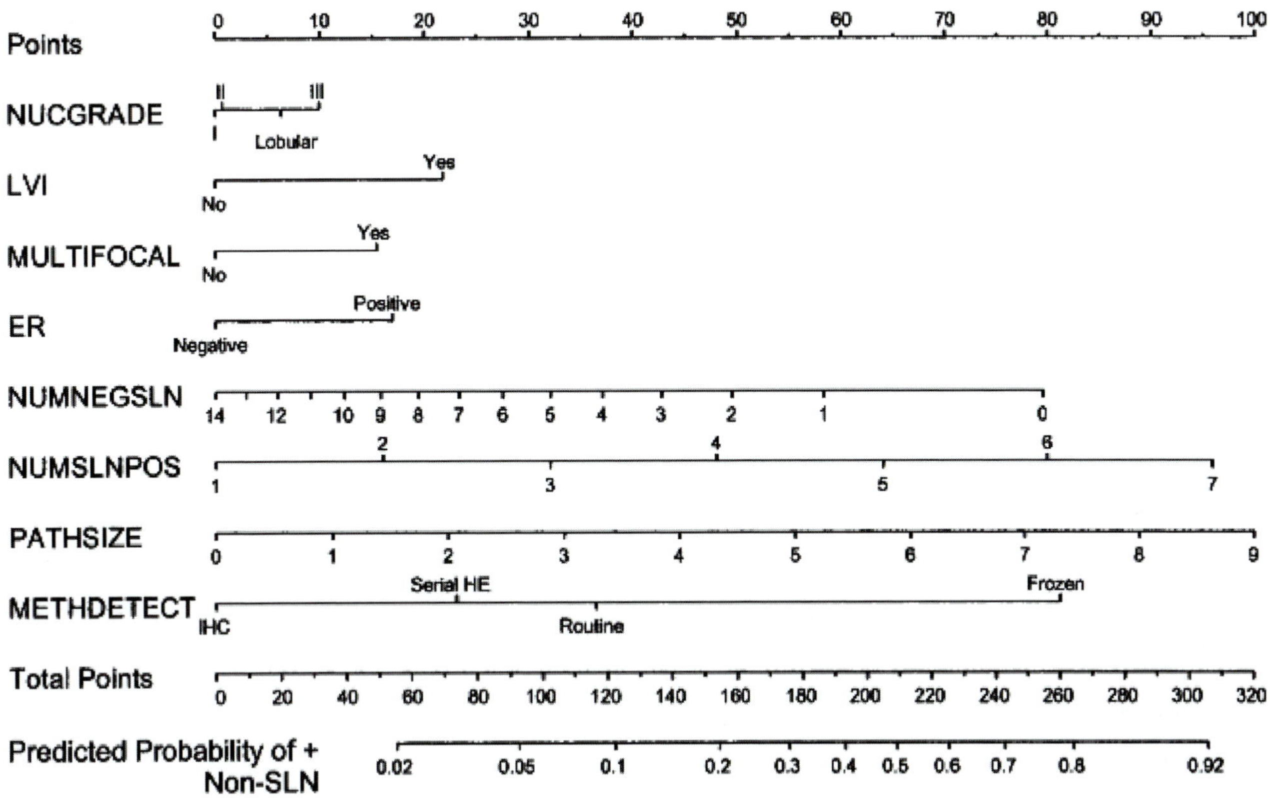

Fig. 4 The nomogram above from Van Zee et al. Reprinted with kind permission from springer science and business media

setting of positive sentinel node or nodes, this nomogram is very useful to estimate further disease burden.

Clinicians were compared to the nomogram by Specht et al. (2005). The clinicians were presented clinical cases and asked to predict the likelihood of additional sentinel nodes, before seeing the results of the nomogram (Fig. 5).

The receiver operator curve above shows the performance of clinicians in the dotted line and the nomogram in the solid line. The area under the curve assesses the ability of a test to determine an outcome, with an area under the curve of 1.0 a perfect test and an area under the curve of 0.5 a test with no predictive ability. The area under the curve for the clinicians was 0.54 and the nomogram was 0.72, suggesting that nomograms can be beneficial to improve clinical decision-making, such as whether to complete an axillary dissection or target undissected nodes with radiation.

4.7 Predicting Brain Metastases

Metastatic disease in the brain is typically a fatal event, and this occurs in numerous breast cancer patients. In order to select patients at high risk for development of brain disease, and help guide therapeutic targets that will include blood brain barrier penetration, a nomogram was developed by Graesslin and colleagues (2010). They looked at a set of metastatic breast cancer patients at a single institution, and of the 2136 women, 236 developed brain metastases. Using multivariate logistic regression analysis, they identified factors of significance including number of metastatic sites, disease free survival, age, grade, estrogen receptor negative disease. Together, the nomogram was found to be predictive for patients developing metastatic disease to the brain, and it outperformed

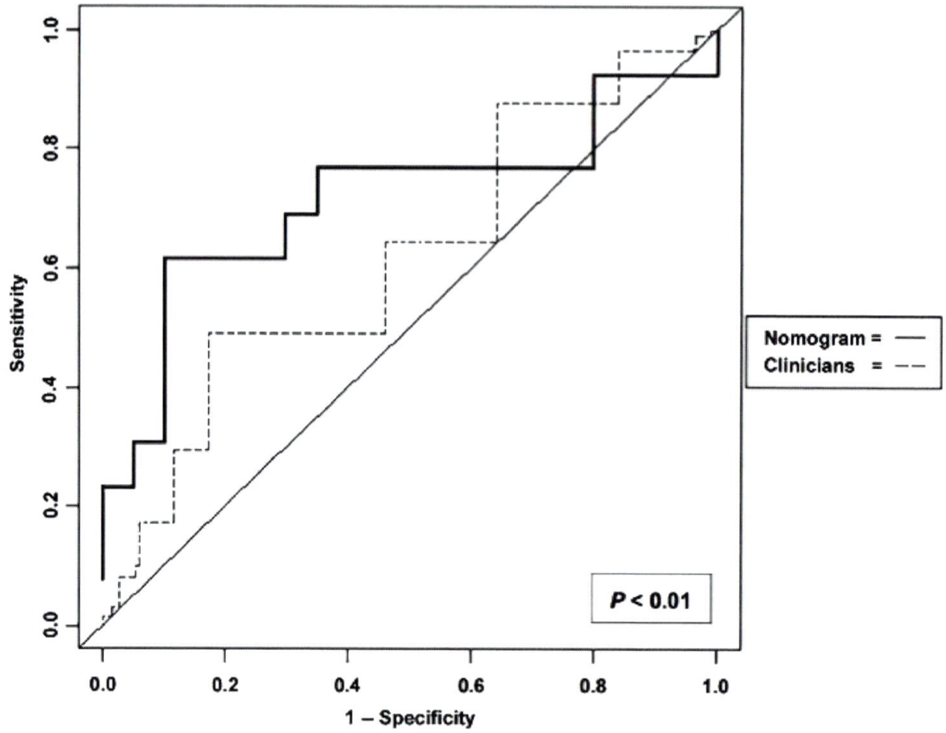

Fig. 5 The receiver operating curve. Reprinted with kind permission from Springer science and business media

Table 4 RTOG pneumonitis grading

1	Mild symptoms of dry cough or dyspnea on exertion
2	Persistent cough requiring narcotic antitussive agent or dyspnea with minimal effort but not at rest
3	Severe cough unresponsive to narcotic antitussive agent or dyspnea at rest. Intermittent oxygen or steroids may be required
4	Severe respiratory insufficiency. Continuous oxygen or assisted ventilation
5	Fatal

Table 5 Factors for increased risk of toxicity from systemic therapy

Increased risk of toxicity with chemotherapy
Increased diastolic blood pressure
Elevated LDH
Published toxicity of the chemotherapy regimen
Bone marrow invasion by tumor

existing tools such as recursive partitioning analysis with an area under the curve of 0.74 in the validation set (Graesslin et al. 2010).

5 Predicting Toxicity in Breast Cancer Patients

5.1 Predicting Toxicity Related to Radiation Therapy

Radiation therapy for breast cancer is generally well-tolerated, but both acute, subacute, and late toxicities develop in patients undergoing treatment. Of these, late and subacute cause the most concern, and it is largely in regards to these toxicities that dose volume histogram (DVH) parameters have been developed to try to limit toxicity.

Cardiac toxicity is the most potentially life threatening late effect following breast or chest wall irradiation. Attempts to derive the appropriate "safe" dose to the heart show that even with a small volume of heart irradiated, a potential risk of radiation-induced cardiac disease is present. A V25 of <10 % at 2 Gy per fraction is offered in the QUANTEC paper on cardiac effects of radiation as having a risk of cardiac mortality <1 % (Gagliardi et al. 2010). However, the incidence of non-fatal cardiac disease will be higher. No excellent predictive model exists for radiation-induced cardiac disease at this time, but this will certainly be an area of further study.

Pulmonary effects of thoracic radiation include early and late toxicity (Marks 1994). Clinical radiation pneumonitis is generally considered a subacute toxicity, and presents initially with mild symptoms of dry cough with Radiation Therapy Oncology Group (RTOG) pneumonitis grading presented (Table 4).

While mean lung dose (MLD) is used in lung cancer toxicity prediction, V20 seems a more reasonable choice in breast cancer. Much of the data is still derived from lung studies, and Graham et al. demonstrated that V20 can be used to estimate risk (Graham et al. 1999).

Specific patient populations are at higher risk for toxicity from radiation therapy. Any pregnant patient is ineligible for radiation therapy, due to risk of harm to the fetus. Patients with connective tissue disease, particularly active lupus and scleroderma, have had severe reactions to radiation therapy described in the literature and radiation should be avoided whenever possible in this population (Carlson et al. 2013). In a systematic review of radiation therapy in connective tissue diseases, the pooled relative risk in patients with connective tissue diseases was 2.0, indicating a twofold increase in complications compared to patients without connective tissue diseases (Holscher et al. 2006).

5.2 Predicting Toxicity Related to Systemic Therapy

Much work has been done to predict what patients may experience the greatest toxicity from systemic therapy, thus allowing a more accurate assessment of the risk to benefit ratio for any treatment, as well as different treatment regimens. Factors identified on initial prospective investigation associated with higher chemotherapy toxicity are listed in (Table 5) (Extermann et al. 2002; 2010). Factors account for decreased physiologic reserve in organs including bone marrow and liver, as well as potential underlying serious disease.

This was honed into the MAX2 index, which considers both hematologic and non-hematologic toxicity and shows an excellent correlation with the incidence of severe toxicity in all patients as well as the elderly (age >70) population (Extermann et al. 2004).

References

Albain KS, Barlow WE, Shak S et al (2010) Prognostic and predictive value of the 21-gene recurrence score assay in postmenopausal women with node-positive, oestrogen-receptor-positive breast cancer on chemotherapy: a retrospective analysis of a randomised trial. Lancet Oncol 11:55–65

American Joint Committee on Cancer (2002) Breast. AJCC cancer staging manual, 6th edn. Springer, New York, pp 221–240

American Joint Committee on Cancer (2009) Breast. AJCC cancer staging manual, 7th edn. Springer, New York, pp 345–376

Anderson BO, Calhoun KE, Rosen EL (2006) Evolving concepts in the management of lobular neoplasia. J Natl Compr Canc Netw 4:511–522

Bevilacqua JL, Kattan MW, Fey JV et al (2007) Doctor, what are my chances of having a positive sentinel node? a validated nomogram for risk estimation. J Clin Oncol 25:3670–3679

Borg A, Tandon AK, Sigurdsson H et al (1990) HER-2/neu amplification predicts poor survival in node-positive breast cancer. Cancer Res 50:4332–4337

Buchholz TA, Katz A, Strom EA et al (2002) Pathologic tumor size and lymph node status predict for different rates of locoregional recurrence after mastectomy for breast cancer patients treated with neoadjuvant versus adjuvant chemotherapy. Int J Radiat Oncol Biol Phys 53:880–888

Cabanes PA, Salmon RJ, Vilcoq JR et al (1992) Value of axillary dissection in addition to lumpectomy and radiotherapy in early breast cancer. Lancet 339:1245–1248

Carlson RW, McCormick B et al (2013) NCCN clinical practice guidelines in oncology: breast cancer. National comprehensive cancer network. NCCN.org, Version 1.2013

Carter CL, Allen C, Henson DE (1989) Relation of tumor size, lymph node status, and survival in 24,740 breast cancer cases. Cancer 63:181–187

Chang S, Parker SL, Pham T et al (1998) Inflammatory breast cancer incidence and survival. The surveillance epidemiology and end results (SEER) program of the national cancer institute, 1975–1992. Cancer 82:2366–2372

Cote RJ, Peterson HF, Chaiwun B et al (1999) Role of immunohistochemical detection of lymph node metastases in management of breast cancer. Int Breast Cancer Study Group Lancet 354:896–900

Cristofanilli M, Buzdar AU, Hortobagyi GN (2003) Update on the management of inflammatory breast cancer. Oncologist 8:141–148

Crowe JP Jr, Gordon NH, Hubay CA et al (1991) Estrogen receptor determination and long term survival of patients with carcinoma of the breast. Surg Gynecol Obstet. 173:273–278

Dent DM (1996) Axillary lymphadenectomy for breast cancer. Arch Surg 131:1125–1127

Dowsett M, Cuzick J, Wale C et al (2010) Prediction of risk of distant recurrence using the 21-gene recurrence score in node-negative and node-positive postmenopausal breast cancer patients treated with anastrozole or tamoxifen: a transatac study. J Clin Oncol 28:1829–1834

Edge SE, Byrd DR, Compton CC et al (2009) AJCC cancer staging manual, 7th edn. Springer, New York

Esteva FJ, Sahin AA, Cristofanilli M et al (2005) Prognostic role of a multigene reverse transcriptase-PCR assay in patients with node-negative breast cancer not receiving adjuvant systemic therapy. Clin Cancer Res 11:3315–3319

Extermann M, Chen H, Cantor AB et al (2002) Predictors of tolerance to chemotherapy in older cancer patients: a prospective pilot study. Eur J Cancer 38:1466–1473

Extermann M, Bonetti M, Sledge GW et al (2004) MAX2—a convenient index to estimate the average per patient risk for chemotherapy toxicity; validation in ECOG trials. Eur J Cancer 40:1193–1198

Extermann M, Boler I, Reich R et al (2010) The CRASH score (chemotherapy risk assessment scale for high-age patients): design and validation. 2010 ASCO annual meeting. Chicago, IL (Abstract 9000)

Freedman GM, Fowble BL, Hanlon A et al (1999) Patients with early stage invasive cancer with close or positive margins treated with conservative surgery and radiation have an increased risk of breast recurrence that is delayed by adjuvant systemic therapy. Int J Radiat Oncol Biol Phys 44:1005–1015

Freedman GM, Hanlon AL, Fowble BL et al (2002) Recursive partitioning identifies patients at high and low risk for ipsilateral tumor recurrence after breast conserving surgery and radiation. J Clin Oncol 20:4015–4021

Gagliardi G, Constine L, Moiseenko V et al (2010) Radiation dose-volume effects in the heart. Int J Radiat Oncol Biol Phys 76:S77–S85

Gann PH, Colilla SA, Gapstur SM et al (1999) Factors associated with axillary lymph node metastasis from breast carcinoma: descriptive and predictive analyses. Cancer 86:1511–1519

Gebski V, Lagleva M, Keech A et al (2006) Survival effects of postmastectomy adjuvant radiation therapy using biologically equivalent doses: A clinical perspective. J Natl Cancer Inst 98:26–38

Graesslin O, Abdulkarim BS, Coutant C et al (2010) Nomogram to predict subsequent brain metastasis in patients with metastatic breast cancer. J Clin Oncol 28:2032–2037
Graham MV, Purdy JA, Emami B et al (1999) Clinical dose-volume histogram analysis for pneumonitis after 3D treatment for non-small cell lung cancer (NSCLC). Int J Radiat Oncol Biol Phys 45:323–329
Haagensen CD, Bodian C, Haagensen DE Jr (1981) Breast carcinoma. Risk and detection. Diseases of the breast, 2nd edn. WB Saunders, Philadelphia
Harvey JM, Clark GM, Osborne CK et al (1999) Estrogen receptor status by immunohistochemistry is superior to the ligand-binding assay for predicting response to adjuvant endocrine therapy in breast cancer. J Clin Oncol 17:1474–1481
Holbro T, Civenni G, Hanes NE (2003) The ErbB receptors and their role in cancer progression. Exp Cell Res 284:99–110
Holscher T, Bentzen S, Baumann M (2006) Influence of connective tissue diseases on the expression of radiation side effects: a systematic review. Radiother Oncol 78:123–130
Houssami N, Ciatto S, Macaskill P et al (2008) Accuracy and surgical impact of magnetic resonance imaging in breast cancer staging: systematic review and meta-analysis in detection of multifocal and multicentric cancer. J Clin Oncol 26:3248–3258
Howat JMT, Harris M, Swindell R et al (1985) The effect of oestrogen and progesterone receptors on recurrence and survival in patients with carcinoma of the breast. Br J Cancer 51:262–270
Hughes LL, Wang M, Page DL et al (2009) Local excision alone without irradiation for ductal carcinoma in situ of the breast: a trial of the eastern cooperative oncology group. J Clin Oncol 27:5319–5324
Jackson JS, Olivotto IA, Wai MD et al (2000) A decision analysis of the effect of avoiding axillary lymph node dissection in low risk women with invasive breast carcinoma. Cancer 88:1852–1862
Jatoi I, Hilsenbeck SG, Clark GM et al (1999) Significance of axillary lymph node metastasis in primary breast cancer. J Clin Oncol 17:2334–2340
Kattan M (2001) Expert systems in medicine. In: Smelser NJ, Baltes PB (eds) International encyclopedia of the social and behavioral sciences. Pergamon, Oxford, pp 5135–5139
Lee LA, Silverstein MJ, Chung CT et al (2006) Breast cancer-specific mortality after invasive local recurrence in patients with ductal carcinoma-in situ of the breast. Am J Surg 192:416–419
Liao Z, Strom EA, Buzdar AU et al (2000) Locoregional irradiation for inflammatory breast cancer: effectiveness of dose escalation in decreasing recurrence. Int J Radiat Oncol Biol Phys 47:1191–1200
Linderholm BK, Hellborg H, Johansson U et al (2009) Significantly higher levels of vascular endothelial growth factor (VEGF) and shorter survival times for patients with primary operable triple-negative breast cancer. Ann Oncol 10:1639–1646
Liu S, Chia SK, Mehl E et al (2010) Progesterone receptor is a significant factor associated with clinical outcomes and effect of adjuvant tamoxifen therapy in breast cancer patients. Breast Cancer Res Treat 119:53–61
MacDonald HR, Silverstein MJ, Mabry H et al (2005) Local control in ductal carcinoma in situ treated by excision alone: incremental benefit of larger margins. Am J Surg 190:521–525
Macmillan RD, Purushotham AD, Mallon E et al (1997) Tumor bed positivity predicts outcome after breast conserving surgery. Br J Surg 84:1559–1562
Maibenco DC, Weiss LK, Pawlish KS et al (1999) Axillary lymph node metastases associated with small invasive breast carcinomas. Cancer 85:1530–1536
Mamounas EP, Tang G, Fisher B et al (2010) Association between the 21-gene recurrence score assay and risk of locoregional recurrence in node-negative, estrogen receptor-positive breast cancer: results from NSABP B-14 and NSABP B-20. J Clin Oncol 28:1677–1683
Marks LB (1994) The pulmonary effects of thoracic radiation. Oncology 8:89–106
Mittra I (1993) Axillary lymph node metastasis in breast cancer: prognostic indicator or lead-time bias? Eur J Cancer 29:300–302
Moore MP, Kinne DW (1997) Axillary lymphadenectomy: a diagnostic and therapeutic procedure. J Surg Oncol 66:2–6
Morrow M, Harris JR, Schnitt SJ (2012) Surgical margins in lumpectomy for breast cancer—bigger is not better. N Engl J Med 367:79–82
Mustafa IA, Cole B, Wanebo HJ et al (1997) The impact of histopathology on nodal metastases in minimal breast cancer. Arch Surg 132:384–390
Naik AM, Fey J, Gemignani M et al (2004) The risk of axillary relapse after sentinel lymph node biopsy for breast cancer is comparable with that of axillary lymph node dissection: a follow-up study of 4008 procedures. Ann Surg 240:462–468
Nielsen HM, Overgaard M, Grau C et al (2006) Study of failure pattern among high-risk breast cancer patients with or without postmastectomy radiotherapy in addition to adjuvant systemic therapy: long-term results from the danish breast cancer cooperative group DBCG 82 b and c randomized studies. J Clin Oncol 24:2268–2275
Olivotto IA, Bajdik CD, Ravdin PM et al (2005) Population-based validation of the prognostic model ADJUVANT! for early breast cancer. J Clin Oncol 23:2716–2722
Paik S, Hazan R, Fisher ER et al (1990) Pathologic findings from the national surgical adjuvant breast and bowel project: prognostic significance of erbB-2 protein overexpression in primary breast cancer. J Clin Oncol 8:103–112
Paik S, Shak S, Tang G et al (2004) A multigene assay to predict recurrence of tamoxifen-treated, node-negative breast cancer. N Engl J Med 351:2817–2826
Pater JL, Mores D, Loeb M (1981) Survival after recurrence of breast cancer. Can Med Assoc J 124:1591–1595
Peoples GE, Gurney JM, Hueman MT et al (2005) Clinical trial results of a HER2/*neu* (E75) vaccine to prevent recurrence in high-risk breast cancer patients. J Clin Oncol 23:7536–7545
Rahusen FD, Torrenga H, van Diest PJ et al (2001) Predictive factors for metastatic involvement of nonsentinel nodes in patients with breast cancer. Arch Surg 136:1059–1063
Rakha EA, El-Sayed AE, Green AR et al (2007) Prognostic markers in triple negative breast cancer. Cancer 109:25–32
Ravdin PM, Siminoff LA, Davis GJ et al (2001) Computer program to assist in making decisions about adjuvant therapy for women with early breast cancer. J Clin Oncol 19:980–991
Rivadeneira DE, Simmons RM, Christos PJ et al (2000) Predictive factors associated with axillary lymph node metastases in T1a and T1b breast carcinomas: analysis in more than 900 patients. J Am Coll Surg 191:1–6
Romond EH, Perez EA, Bryant J et al (2005) Trastuzumab plus adjuvant chemotherapy for operable HER2-positive breast cancer. N Engl J Med 353:1673–1684
Rudloff U, Jacks LM, Goldberg JI et al (2010) Nomogram for predicting the risk of local recurrence after breast-conserving surgery for ductal carcinoma in situ. J Clin Oncol 28:3762–3769
Shek LL, Godolphin W, Spinelli JJ et al (1987) Oestrogen receptors, nodes and stage as predictors of post-recurrence survival in 457 breast cancer patients. Br J Cancer 56:825–829
Shek LL, Godolphin W (1989) Survival with breast cancer: the importance of estrogen receptor quantity. Eur J Cancer Clin Oncol 25:243–250
Siegel R, Naishadham D, Jemal A (2012) Cancer statistics, 2012. CA Cancer J Clin 62:10–29

Slamon DJ, Clark GM, Wong SG et al (1987) Human breast cancer: correlation of recurrence and survival with amplification of the HER2/neu oncogene. Science 287:177–182

Solin LJ, Orel SG, Hwang WT et al (2008) Relationship of breast magnetic resonance imaging to outcome after breast-conservation treatment with radiation for women with early-stage invasive breast carcinoma or ductal carcinoma in situ. J Clin Oncol 26:386–391

Solin L, Gray R, Baehner F et al (2011) A quantitative multigene RT-PCR assay for predicting recurrence risk after surgical excision alone without irradiation for ductal carcinoma in situ (DCIS): a prospective validation study of the DCIS Score from ECOG E5194. In: Presented at: 34th annual san antonio breast cancer symposium, San Antonio, TX, 6–10 Dec 2011 (Abstract S4-6)

Specht MC, Kattan MW, Gonen M et al (2005) Predicting nonsentinel node status after positive sentinel node biopsy for breast cancer: clinicians versus nomogram. Ann Surg Oncol 8:654–659

Speirs V, Kerin MJ (2008) Prognostic significance of oestrogen receptor beta in breast cancer. Br J Surg 87:405–409

Teng S, Dupont E, McCann C et al (2000) Do cytokeratin-positive-only sentinel lymph nodes warrant complete axillary lymph node dissection in patients with invasive breast cancer? Am Surg 66:574–578

Turner RR, Chu KU, Qi K et al (2000) Pathologic features associated with nonsentinel lymph node metastases in patients with metastatic breast carcinoma in a sentinel lymph node. Cancer 89:574–581

Van der Vijver MJ, He YD, V'ant Veer LJ et al (2002) A gene-expression signature as a predictor of survival in breast cancer. N Engl J Med 347:1999–2009

Van Zee KJ, Manasseh DM, Bevilacqua JL et al (2003) A nomogram for predicting the likelihood of additional nodal metastases in breast cancer patients with a positive sentinel node biopsy. Ann Surg Oncol 10:1140–1151

Veronesi U, Paganelli G, Viale G et al (2003) A randomized comparison of sentinel-node biopsy with routine axillary dissection in breast cancer. N Engl J Med 349:546–553

Wapnir IL, Dignam JJ, Fisher B et al (2011) Long-term outcomes of invasive ipsilateral breast tumor recurrences after lumpectomy in NSABP B-17 and B-24 randomized clinical trials for DCIS. J Natl Cancer Inst 103:478–488

Wong SL, Edwards MJ, Chao C et al (2001) Predicting the status of the non-sentinel axillary nodes. Arch Surg 136:563–568

Yamamoto T, Ikawa S, Akiyama T et al (1986) Similarity of protein encoded by the human c-erb-B-2 gene to epidermal growth factor receptor. Nature 319:230–234

Zhou P, Recht A (2004) Young age and outcome for women with early stage invasive breast cancer. Cancer 101:1264–1274

Zujewski JA, Kamin L (2008) Trial assessing individualized options for treatment for breast cancer: the TAILORx trial. Future Oncol 4:603–610

Lung Cancer

Hale Basak Caglar, Francesc Casas, Luhua Wang, Nenad Filipovic, and Branislav Jeremic

Contents

Abstract

In addition to investigation of various treatment approaches to optimize outcome, identification of both prognostic and predictive factors should be attempted due to its key role in the treatment decision-making process, as the current therapeutic approach utilizes a risk stratification paradigm. Of a series of patient-, tumour- and treatment-related factors, the most consistent ones independently influencing outcomes in both non-small cell (NSCLC) and small cell lung cancer (SCLC) were performance status, weight loss, stage and concurrent radiotherapy and chemotherapy as well as prophylactic cranial irradiation in small cell lung cancer. While age and gender are probably not important prognosticators, further investigations are needed to clarify the role of tumour location and histology. Due to widespread practice of using induction (neoadjuvant) therapy before surgery in locally advanced NSCLC, predictors of survival were investigated. Mediastinal nodal clearance seems to be the strongest predictor of improved survival, while right pneumonectomy seems to be the major predictor of postoperative morbidity and mortality. Finally, a number of patient-, comorbidity- and dosimetry-related factors or biomarkers as predictors of treatment-related toxicity were investigated. Although no firm evidence exists that any of these clearly predicts toxicity in NSCLC, evidence exists in SCLC. Two commonly used dosimetric factors are mean lung dose and V20. More studies investigating the important aspects of optimization of the use of radiotherapy or radiochemotherapy in lung cancer patients are urgently needed.

1 Introduction

Lung cancer is the leading cause of cancer related death in the world. An estimated 226,000 new cases of lung and bronchial cancer will be diagnosed per year and 160,000

H. B. Caglar
Department of Radiation Oncology, Acibadem University, Istanbul, Turkey

F. Casas
Department of Radiation Oncology, University Clinic, Barcelona, Spain

L. Wang
Department of Radiation Oncology, Chinese Medical Academy of Sciences, Beijing, China

N. Filipovic
BioIRC Centre for Bioengineering, Kragujevac, Serbia

B. Jeremic (✉)
Division of Radiation and Clinical Oncology, Stellenbosch University and Tygerberg Hospital, Cape Town, South Africa
e-mail: bjeremic@sun.ac.za

C. Nieder and L. E. Gaspar (eds.), *Decision Tools for Radiation Oncology*, Medical Radiology. Radiation Oncology,
DOI: 10.1007/174_2013_838, © Springer-Verlag Berlin Heidelberg 2013
Published Online: 24 April 2013

patients will die of their disease (Siegel et al. 2012). After 5 years from diagnosis only 16 % of the patients are alive according to the SEER Cancer Statistics. Many improvements have been made in management of this disease in the last 10–15 years. Among these improvements screening, minimally invasive diagnostic and surgical techniques, targeted therapies and evolution of radiotherapy (RT) should be highlighted. Due to these different advancements, survival has gradually improved. Compared to other malignancies, outcomes are still disappointing for many stages. Clearly lung cancer remains a complex and heterogeneous disease.

The primary risk factor of lung cancer is smoking and it accounts for the majority (85–90 %) of the lung cancer related deaths. The risk for lung cancer increases with the number of packs and the number of years individuals continue to smoke (Alberg et al. 2007). Radon gas, asbestos, other carcinogens, recurring lung inflammation, lung scarring secondary to tuberculosis and family history are other factors increasing the risk of lung cancer (Straif et al. 2009).

In addition to investigation of various treatment approaches to optimize outcome, identification of prognostic factors should be attempted due to its key role in the treatment decision-making process as the current therapeutic approach utilizes a risk stratification paradigm. Prognostic factors facilitate risk assessment, guide decisions on whether to initiate therapy, and influence the choice of therapy. The use of one or more of these factors, however, has in part become confusing, with conflicting results from different studies. Some prognostic factors may also be significant by random chance alone, and their importance cannot be firmly evaluated without verification in multiple studies. Furthermore, several patient characteristics can influence the clinical course (Glatstein and Makuch 1984; Simon 1984). Finally, the magnitude of differences in outcome for categories of the strongest prognostic factors can be larger than those for the type of therapy used in various studies (Curran et al. 1993). Hence, prognostic factors are used to divide the population into subgroups in order to realize the benefits of prognostic stratification (Feinstein 1972), improved medical decision making (Brundage et al. 2001), improved personal decision making beyond the treatment decision, more appropriate research design and analysis, and more appropriate health policy development (Mackillop 2001).

There is an increasing amount of literature on prognostic factors in lung cancer, however, this has brought inherent problems with their integration and clinical application due to heterogeneity for a number of factors (Buccheri and Ferrigno 1994; Brundage et al. 2002), variable quality of published reports (Watine 1998), and extensive and growing breadth of factors studied. The scope of some factors evaluated in individual studies is often inappropriate, and with the exception of a few predictive factors, the literature demonstrates conflicting evidence of the prognostic power of each factor. In addition, few studies attempt to integrate newly described factors with significant factors identified in earlier studies, and correct for evolution in staging modalities and systems. For example, the use of PET-CT often leads to up-staging of patients initially judged to have localized disease. Finally, there is still bias among researchers favouring survival over other endpoints which may be important for patients and their physicians. It also appears that relatively little research has focused on patients at time points beyond their initial presentation.

Various factors have been evaluated upon their influence on overall survival (OS), local progression-free survival (LPFS) and distant metastasis-free survival (DMFS) and occasional studies also included other endpoints such as cause-specific survival (CSS), disease-free survival (DFS) or relapse-free survival (RFS). They can broadly be divided into patient-, tumour- and treatment-related factors, with additional subgrouping within each of these.

2 Prognostic Factors in Early (I–II) Stage NSCLC

Table 1 shows the AJCC TNM classification of lung cancers and Table 2 shows stage grouping (7th edition), i.e. currently used tools to define early stage disease. Accumulating evidence shows that gender is not a prognosticator in patients with early stage NSCLC (Sandler et al. 1990; Hayakawa et al. 1992; Rosenthal et al. 1992; Slotman and Karim 1994; Gauden et al. 1995; Hayakawa et al. 1996; Jeremic et al. 1997a, b, 1999a, b; Morita et al. 1997; Yamada et al. 2003; Jeremic et al. 2005; Zhao et al. 2007), although few studies indicated an advantage for females (Chen et al. 2006; Fang et al. 2006). In addition, evidence from different studies showed no influence of age on treatment outcome (Morrison et al. 1963; Noordijk et al. 1988; Sandler et al. 1990; Hayakawa et al. 1992; Rosenthal et al. 1992; Kaskowitz et al. 1993; Slotman and Karim 1994; Slotman et al. 1996; Gauden et al. 1995; Hayakawa et al. 1996; Jeremic et al. 1999a, b; Cheung et al. 2000; Firat et al. 2002a, b; Yamada et al. 2003; Chen et al. 2006; Fang et al. 2006; Jeremic et al. 2006; Zhao et al. 2007). Contrasting these, occasional reports (Morita et al. 1997; Fang et al. 2006; Sibley et al. 1998; Lagerwaard et al. 2002) showed a detrimental effect of advanced age on OS, and occasionally on CSS (Sibley et al. 1998). Since no study provided any explanation or hypothesis for such findings we are left without clear documentation of the nature of its potential influence. Even when adverse influence of advanced age was observed on OS and/or CSS (Firat et al. 2002a, b), it was not found on LRFS and DMFS, implying

Table 1 AJCC tumor, node, and metastasis (TNM) classification of lung cancers

Stage	Description
Primary Tumor (T)	
Tx	Primary tumor cannot be assessed
T1	≤3 cm tumor, surrounded by lung parenchyma
T1a	≤2 cm tumor
T1b	2.1–3 cm tumor
T2	>3–7 cm tumor, involvement of visceral pleura, invading mainstem bronchus >2 cm from carina, or causing atelectasis to a single lobe of the lung
T2a	3.1–5 cm tumor
T2b	5.1–7 cm tumor
T3	>7 cm tumor, tumor invading mainstem bronchus <2 cm from carina, invasion of diaphragm, chest wall, pericardium, mediastinal pleura, or associated atelectasis or obstructive pneumonitis of entire lung, or satellite nodule in the same lobe
T4	Invasion of great vessels or adjacent organs, or nodules in separate lobe in the ipsilateral lung
Regional Lymph Nodes (N)	
Nx	Regional lymph nodes cannot be assessed
N0	No regional lymph nodes metastasis
N1	Ipsilateral hilar or peribronchial nodes
N2	Ipsilateral mediastinal or subcarinal nodes
N3	Any supraclavicular/scalene node or contralateral mediastinal/hilar nodes
Distant Metastasis (M)	
M1a	Malignant pleural effusion, pericardial nodules/effusions, or lung nodules in contralateral lung
M1b	Metastasis to distant organs

Source Edge et al. (2009)

Table 2 Stage grouping International Association for the Study of Lung Cancer 2007

Stage grouping	T	N	M
Occult carcinoma	Tx	N0	M0
Stage 0	Tis	N0	M0
Stage IA	T1a, b	N0	M0
Stage IB	T2a	N0	M0
Stage IIA	T1a, b	N1	M0
	T2a	N1	M0
	T2b	N0	M0
Stage IIB	T2b	N1	M0
	T3	N0	M0
Stage IIIA	T1, T2	N2	M0
	T3	N1, N2	M0
	T4	N0, N1	M0
Stage IIIB	T4	N2	M0
	Any T	N3	M0
Stage IV	Any T	Any N	M1a, b

that perhaps toxicity may have played a role in poorer outcome for elderly patients. When analyses were focused on elderly (Furuta et al. 1996; Hayakawa et al. 1999; Gauden and Tripcony 2001) no difference was found among different age groups. When toxicity, including RT-related deaths was added to various analyses, it was similar among all age groups (Gauden et al. 1995; Hayakawa et al. 1999; Gauden and Tripcony 2001).

Some authors (Slotman and Karim 1994; Gauden et al. 1995; Hayakawa et al. 1996; Cheung et al. 2000; Yamada et al. 2003; Chen et al. 2006; Fang et al. 2006; Zhao et al. 2007) found no influence of Karnofsky Performance Status (KPS) and/or weight loss on either OS or DFS/CSS or even LRFS (Chen et al. 2006; Fang et al. 2006), while others (Hayakawa et al. 1992; Rosenthal et al. 1992; Jeremic et al. 1999a, b; Jeremic et al. 2006; Zhao et al. 2007; Firat et al. 2002a, b; Lagerwaard et al. 2002; Kupelian et al. 1996; Jeremic et al. 2005) noted its effect on either OS or DFS/RFS as well as on DMFS (Jeremic et al. 2005, 2006). Clear explanation for the lack of stronger evidence of influence of both PS and weight loss is missing, possibly because there is frequent interdependence of the two. The magnitude of the effect of these two factors is usually a consequence of the existing disease, i.e. tumour burden. In early stage NSCLC, with the least tumour burden, it is likely that the effect of these two factors should be less pronounced than in locally advanced NSCLC. In current studies, however, they appear to be the strongest predictors of outcome, an important finding for future research.

We have previously (Jeremic et al. 2005, 2006) investigated influence of tumor location and observed improved OS for patients having peripheral tumours. Similarly, Chen et al. (2006) found improved OS for peripheral tumours, but no impact on CSS or LRFS. In patients treated with hyperfractionated (Hfx) RT alone (Jeremic et al. 2006), peripheral tumour location also independently predicted improved LRFS, but not DMFS. It remains unknown what may be the cause of this discrepancy, although perhaps central tumour location may lead to more regional and/or distant seeding. As an indirect evidence, Emami et al. (2003) suggested that irradiation of hilar regions may contribute to some improvement in survival in these patients. However, other studies found no such difference (Ono et al. 1991; Hayakawa et al. 1992; Slotman and Karim 1994; Slotman et al. 1996; Cheung et al. 2000; Yamada et al. 2003). Based on recent data, we are unable to confirm an independent influence of tumour location on treatment outcome. A possible explanation may lie in a presumed low incidence of regional or distant spread in peripheral tumours. In addition, tumour location did not influence

DMFS presumably, again, because of the small metastatic potential of early stage NSCLC.

While some investigators observed independent influence of T stage (Kaskowitz et al. 1993; Gauden et al. 1995; Graham et al. 1995; Jeremic et al. 1997a, b; Zhao et al. 2007), others did not (Morita et al. 1997; Cheung et al. 2000; Jeremic et al. 2005, 2006), and in some studies the results remained unchanged when tumour volume was additionally investigated. Kupelian et al. (1996) could not document that T stage influenced OS, DSS or LRFS, but found that tumours >5 cm had better DSS and those >4 cm had better LRFS. Yamada et al. (2003) found independent influence of tumour size (<3 cm vs. >3 cm) on LRFS but not on CSS. In addition to that, Hayakawa et al. (1996) found that maximal tumour diameter <5 cm independently predicted improved OS. In the study of Fang et al. (2006), tumour size (>3 and >4 cm, respectively) did not independently influence OS. However, T2 tumours predicted poor OS and LRFS, while tumours >4 cm predicted poor DMFS. If there is an influence of T stage/size on the outcome, this should happen first at local (T) level. Then, through improved LRFS, possible improvements of OS could be achieved, providing a causal relationship between LC and OS, especially in tumours with low metastatic potential.

As described previously (Jeremic et al. 2006), stage grouping (stage I vs. stage II, i.e. N0 vs. N1) did not influence any endpoint in our study. The same was observed when other investigators looked at different endpoints (Hayakawa et al. 1992, 1996; Yamada et al. 2003). Although N component (N0 vs. N1) should play a role in determining outcome, this may occur first at the level of isolated regional recurrence free survival (RRFS) or perhaps combined local–regional recurrence free survival, then on OS and/or DMFS. However, RRFS may not be an important endpoint since there is very low incidence of isolated nodal recurrences, 0–7 % in a comprehensive review of the literature (Jeremic et al. 2002). Unfortunately, also the vast majority of series concentrated on stage I NSCLC exclusively, while those including both stages did not undertake additional subgroup (N status) analysis.

Regarding histology, Sibley et al. (1998) found an improvement in CSS for squamous cell carcinoma (SCC). Gauden et al. (1995) observed improved OS and RFS for the mixed (adenocarcinoma (ADC)/SCC) histology, while Lagerwaard et al. (2002) observed an independent and favourable influence of unknown histology (vs. SCC and non-SCC) on OS. Our previous analysis (Jeremic et al. 2006) showed that SCC favourably predicted both OS and LRFS, but not DMFS. In the study of Fang et al. (2006) non-SCC histology did not independently predict OS, but predicted improved LRFS. Ishikawa et al. (2006) showed no effect of histology on OS, but ADC had better LRFS and worse DMFS than SCC. Unfortunately, no multivariate analysis was done to confirm the adverse influence of ADC. All other studies observed no such effect (Sandler et al. 1990; Hayakawa et al. 1992; Rosenthal et al. 1992; Dosoretz et al. 1992; Dosoretz et al. 1993; Slotman and Karim 1994; Slotman et al. 1996; Hayakawa et al. 1996; Jeremic et al. 1997a, b; Firat et al. 2002a, b; Jeremic et al. 2005; Chen et al. 2006). SCC had long been suspected of being more localized and having somewhat lower metastatic potential, when compared with other NSCLC. This was already brought to attention in locally advanced tumours (Cox et al. 1999); SCC was more likely to progress at the primary site than large cell carcinoma (LC), whereas ADC and LC progressed more frequently in the brain. Treatment intensification led to better OS, CSS and LRFS, but not DMFS. This may have been due to predominantly local failures in these patients, but also due to fewer events in the DMFS analysis. Higher RT doses were frequently shown to independently predict improved outcome of patients with early stage NSCLC (Cooper et al. 1985; Hayakawa et al. 1992; Dosoretz et al. 1992; Graham et al. 1995; Hafty et al. 1988; Zhang et al. 1989), although not unequivocally (Sandler et al. 1990; Kaskowitz et al. 1993; Slotman and Karim 1994; Slotman et al. 1996; Kupelian et al. 1996; Morita et al. 1997; Sibley et al. 1998). This was presumably due to somewhat narrow dose ranges used in some studies, as well as due to a mixture of different RT doses and tumour sizes/volumes in some reports. Some studies found an improvement in OS for higher RT doses, but the influence was marginally insignificant either on CSS or LRFS (Lagerwaard et al. 2002; Yamada et al. 2003; Chen et al. 2006). Similarly to own study findings, the addition of chemotherapy (CHT) to RT did not yield a benefit in the CSS analysis in the study of Yamada et al. (2003). Table 3 shows recent data from stereotactic radiotherapy trials. Such treatment results in high local control rates, even in patients with considerable comorbidity who are not candidates for surgery, and is currently being investigated in randomized clinical studies.

3 Prognostic Factors in Locally Advanced (Stage III) NSCLC

Of patient-related factors, age as prognostic factor was evaluated using multivariate analysis with conflicting results. While two Radiation Therapy Oncology Group (RTOG) data base evaluations (Komaki et al. 1998; Werner-Wasik et al. 2000a, b) showed that age > 70 years is an adverse prognostic factor for survival, some studies (Socinski et al. 2004; Basaki et al. 2006) did not find any influence, including one of our own studies which used 60 years as cut-off point. Contrary to this our first analysis

Table 3 Prognostic factors from the literature of stereotactic body radiotherapy (SBRT) for stage I non-small cell lung cancer

Author	Number of patients	SBRT regimen	Analysis	Prognostic factors
Matsuo et al. (2011)	101, histologically confirmed	4 fractions	Multivariate	Tumour diameter (LP, DP, OS) Age (DP) Gender (OS)
Fakiris et al. (2009)	70, histologically confirmed	3 fractions	Univariate	No impact of tumour volume, T stage or localisation (OS)
Andratschke et al. (2011)	92, histologically confirmed	3–5 fractions	Multivariate	No impact of tumour volume, T stage or localisation (OS) T stage (LP)

LP local progression, *DP* disease progression, *OS* overall survival

(Jeremic et al. 1995) showed that age < 60 years (vs. > 60 years.) carried better prognosis, which was confirmed in our later study (Jeremic et al. 1996). Interestingly, subsequent analysis of RTOG 9410 (Langer et al. 2001) showed better survival for elderly, and subgroup analysis of a large meta-analysis (Auperin et al. 2006) confirmed this finding. In the absence of proven influence on increased treatment-related toxicity and given the current lack of any information suggesting that tumours may have different biological characteristics and clinical course in elderly versus non-elderly, age cannot be considered as important prognosticator in this disease. Investigation of gender as prognostic factor also brought conflicting results. While CALGB (Socinski et al. 2004) and RTOG analyses (Komaki et al. 1998; Werner-Wasik et al. 2000a, b) did not find any influence, another RTOG analysis which focused on patients with supraclavicular node metastasis treated with combined modality therapy showed that female gender carried improved prognosis (Machtay et al. 1999). This was also a consistent finding in our own studies (Jeremic et al. 1995, 1996). Again, this prognostic factor can be considered a weak one, especially in the absence of any explanation why this disease could be easier to cure in females. Performance status seems to be the most frequently investigated prognostic factor. While initial observations of its importance were made more than 30 years ago (Edmonson et al. 1976; Stanley 1980), subsequent studies regardless of the stage of the disease or treatment used, generally confirmed these observations. In particular, in two major RTOG studies using recursive partitioning analysis (RPA), performance status was always the strongest prognosticator which then was used to develop classes (Komaki et al. 1998; Werner-Wasik et al. 2000a, b). In the largest analysis so far, performance status confirmed its leading role in predicting survival of patients treated with RT and/or CHT in 1999 patients enrolled in several studies (Werner-Wasik et al. 2000a, b). Data from CALGB (Socinski et al. 2004) also showed its strong independent influence on survival, as did studies by Firat et al. (2002a, b) and Jeremic et al. (1995, 1996). Compared to other parameters, PS is likely the most important determinant of outcome (Pfister et al. 2004), frequently reflected in the fact that clinical trials designed in the last decades usually use it to stratify patients treated with different approaches, including RT-CHT. Another factor, which has frequently been evaluated, is weight loss. Different cut-off values were used such as 5 or 8 %. While Stanley (1980) identified weight loss as an important prognostic factor in 5000 patients with lung cancer, some contemporary studies failed to observe this correlation (Socinski et al. 2004; Ball et al. 2002). The majority, however, did so (Komaki et al. 1998; Werner-Wasik et al. 2000a, b; Pfister et al. 2004), including our previous studies (Jeremic et al. 1995, 1996).

Among tumour-related factors, stage was frequently investigated. Similarly to our previous findings (Jeremic et al. 1995, 1996) more recent studies showed improved survival for stage IIIA patients. This can be seen as indirect confirmation of earlier observations by Stanley (1980), although a CALGB study (Socinsky et al. 2004) surprisingly showed better outcome for stage IIIB patients. As the authors correctly pointed out, even current staging systems and stage groupings are not perfect, for example regarding the dependence on size and not volume of the tumour and/or nodes in the designation process. In addition, tumour volume may actually be a more important means of investigating the potential influence of T and N components and, therefore stage. It was clearly shown that both total tumour volume or primary tumour volume (Basaki et al. 2006) can be considered as independent prognostic factors for survival. However, in that study other endpoints (local/regional PFS) were not used to prove such relationship in a causal way, as improvement in local/regional control should lead to an improved OS. The most recent staging classification of the International Association for the Study of Lung Cancer (Goldstraw et al. 2007) (Table 2) provides a new framework for further evaluation of the T, N, and M stages as well as stage grouping. While still being imperfect, it represents an ongoing effort of the community of thoracic oncologists to revise stage groupings based on a large body of data. One of the tumour-related factors that have occasionally been investigated upon its independent influence on survival is histology. While one RTOG study (Machtay et al. 1999) showed no influence of histology, similarly to the observation by Basaki et al. (2006), another RTOG study (Werner-Wasik et al. 2000a, b) clearly identified non-LC histology as the one having better prognosis. In our own experience LC carried an unfavourable prognosis while differentiation between SCC and non-SCC histology proved to be important. In a pooled RTOG studies analysis (Cox et al. 1999), histology was related to pattern of failure. ADC had greater risk for distant metastasis than SCC, although in our study (Jeremic et al. 2011) LC fared even worse. Also, it was shown by the RTOG authors that ADC progressed at the primary site more often than either SCC or LC carcinoma, which is only partially in agreement with our findings (Jeremic et al. 2011). Regardless of this, the RTOG study (Cox et al. 1999) clearly emphasized the importance of histology for treatment outcome and suggested separation of SCC from both ADC and LC carcinoma.

Of treatment-related factors, interfraction interval in hyperfractionated (Hfx) RT regimens was shown to be an independent prognosticator of treatment outcome (OS and LPFS) (Jeremic and Shibamoto 1996, Jeremic et al.2004). Contrary to our repeated findings, RTOG (Werner-Wasik et al. 1999) did not confirm any influence of interfraction interval on treatment outcome. However, this study suffered from serious shortcomings which we discussed earlier (Jeremic et al. 2004). First, definition of interfraction interval (mean of all daily intervals) was not optimal because a patient could be assigned an interval of 6 h when half of the treatments were given with 4 h and half with 8 h. Second, a number of CHT regimens were used, including concurrent and induction administration. Third, patients with stage II were included as well, and no separate analysis was provided for them. Fourth, no information on the influence of interval on endpoints other than oesophageal acute and late toxicity was provided. Fifth, only 3 pretreatment prognostic factors were correlated with 2 treatment-related factors (interval and CHT). Finally and most importantly, no information was provided on the influence of interval on local control, a vital part of this analysis, since interval might influence overall survival by influencing local control first. Concurrent CHT was proven to be an independent prognosticator of survival in several analyses. This is in contrast with findings by Ball et al. (2002) and Basaki et al. (2006), but is in agreement with the available data from RTOG and CALGB (Werner-Wasik et al. 1999; Socinsky et al. 2004) and findings from our previous studies (Jeremic et al. 1995, 1996). This has also been recently confirmed by the outcome of a meta-analysis that showed a significant advantage of concurrent RT-CHT over RT alone (Auperin et al. 2006). Only rarely published analyses included not only OS but two additional endpoints, namely LPFS and DMFS. Results of our most recent multivariate analysis (Jeremic et al. 2011) using LPFS as an endpoint mimicked those of OS, and confirmed our previous findings (Jeremic et al. 1995).

In patients not suitable for radical radiotherapy who were included in a randomised study of different palliative RT regimens, PS, weight loss and appetite loss were the most important prognostic factors for survival (Sundstrom et al. 2006). For example, 2-year survival was 22 % (no appetite loss) versus 3 % (appetite loss) in patients irradiated to 42 or 50 Gy.

4 Predictors of Response to Induction Therapy in Locally Advanced NSCLC

Although controversial, induction therapy followed by surgery in locally advanced NSCLC has been evaluated in many studies. The investigators aimed to define the most appropriate group for this approach, i.e. patients benefitting in terms of survival. Among the patients entering a course of induction CHT or RT-CHT, not all can complete the prescribed or planned procedure. Cerfolio et al. (2008) evaluated 402 patients with biopsy-proven, non-bulky N2 disease who underwent neoadjuvant RT-CHT and surgery. Among these patients 81 % completed their neoadjuvant therapy, 50 % returned for definitive pathologic restaging and 37 % underwent thoracotomy for attempted resection. Multivariate analysis found that only age younger than 70 years, more than one lymph node involvement and response to neoadjuvant therapy remained significant predictors of moving forward to the surgical arena after neoadjuvant therapy. The 5-year survival was 8 % for the 253 patients who did not return for restaging but was 47 % for the 149 patients who underwent thoracotomy ($p < 0.001$). The 5-year survival for selected subgroups of patients who underwent complete resection was 42 % for the 14 patients who had unsuspected residual N2 disease, 49 % for the 65 patients who had a partial response (PR), and 53 % for the 34 patients who had a complete response (CR).

Mediastinal downstaging after induction therapy is one of the most important and evaluated factors for long term survival (Albain et al. 1995; Betticher et al. 2006; Bueno et al. 2000; De Waele et al. 2006). Patients with persisting mediastinal involvement after induction therapy have a poor prognosis and will usually not benefit from surgical resection. Therefore accurate staging of the mediastinum is of utmost importance to determine the appropriate subgroup of patients for surgical resection after induction. Either minimally invasive techniques (transthoracic fine-needle aspiration biopsy—FNAB, transbronchial needle aspiration—TBNA, endobronchial ultrasound with FNAB—EBUS, endoscopic esophageal ultrasound with FNAB—EUS) or invasive techniques (re-mediastinoscopy, video assisted surgery—VATS) can be used for this approach and have a sensitivity between 70 and 80 %. All of these approaches require experience within the field. The non-invasive re-staging modalities with CT and PET have a rather low accuracy of 64 and 72 % (Annema et al. 2003; Herth et al. 2008; Kunst et al. 2007; De Waele et al. 2008, 2011; Marra et al. 2008; de Leyn et al. 2007). Betticher et al. (2003) for the Swiss Group for Clinical Cancer Research (SAKK) evaluated 90 potentially operable patients with stage IIIApN2 receiving 3 cycles of cisplatin plus docetaxel followed by surgical resection. Postoperative RT to 60 Gy was administered for positive resection margins or involvement of the uppermost mediastinal lymph node. Seventy-five patients (83 %) underwent resection. The overall response rate was 66 %, with 19 % pathological complete response (pCR). The median survival was 27.6 months and the 3-year survival was 33 %. Mediastinal nodal clearance and complete surgical resection were strong independent predictors of increased survival in a multivariate analysis.

A French group aimed to evaluate whether pCR in early stage NSCLC after platinum-based neoadjuvant CHT resulted in improved outcome, where pCR was defined by the absence of viable cancer cells in the resected surgical specimen. Among the 492 patients analyzed, 8.3 % achieved pCR and in the pCR group, 5-year overall survival was 80 % compared with 55.8 % in the non-pCR group ($p = 0.0007$). In multivariate analyses, pCR, SCC, weight loss less than or equal to 5 %, and stage-IB disease was found to be favorable prognostic factors of overall survival. Five-year DFS was 80.1 % in the pCR group compared to 44.8 % in the non-pCR group ($p < 0.0001$). SCC was the only independent predictor of pCR in the study population (Moulliet et al. 2012). All patients with pCR were clinically considered to be responders, either CR ($n = 5$) or PR ($n = 36$). These results confirm the previously reported findings, showing that cCR was predictive of pCR, and that CT assessments likely underestimate pCR rate (Milleron et al. 2005).

In a very recent retrospective analysis by Lococo et al. (2013) the long term results of the patients with pCR after induction therapy followed by surgery for locally advanced NSCLC were evaluated. Among the 195 patients treated with induction therapy, 137 were operated with radical intent. Among these, 27 % showed a pCR. Within this pCR group the overall 3- and 5-year long-term survival and disease-free survival rates were 67 and 64 %, and 68 and 71 %, respectively. Initial single N2 station involvement ($p = 0.010$), resection to a lesser extent than pneumonectomy ($p = 0.005$) and adjuvant therapy ($p = 0.005$) were found to be predictors of increased 5-year survival. Most of the recurrences in this cohort were distant.

One of the most important factors for the survival outcomes after surgery preceded by induction therapy is postoperative mortality. Several studies reported increased mortality after surgery with induction treatment, especially with concurrent RT-CHT, and with pneumonectomy. The Memorial Sloan Kettering Cancer Centre group updated their operative mortality and the factors associated with this from their surgical database of 549 patients. All received CHT, and 17 % also had radiation. The most common procedures were lobectomy (71 %) and pneumonectomy (13 %). Hospital mortality was 1.8 %, with only one death after right pneumonectomy. Multivariate analysis showed that predicted postoperative pulmonary function tests (predictive postoperative product, predicted postoperative diffusion capacity, and preoperative percentage of predicted postoperative diffusion capacity) were important indicators for postoperative morbidity and mortality (Barnett et al. 2011).

Perioperative mortality was assessed in a meta-analysis after neoadjuvant therapy and pneumonectomy for NSCLC. Based on 27 studies, 30- and 90-day perioperative mortalities were 7 and 12 % in the entire cohort. Cumulative mortalities were 11 and 5 % for right and left pneumonectomies. Both 30- and 90-day mortality remained greater in right than left pneumonectomy ($p = 0.02$). Among 11 studies providing both 30- and 90-day mortalities, mortality difference was 5 % ($p < 0.0001$) (Kim et al. 2012).

The predictive effect of nutritional parameters was investigated in a retrospective European study. Fifty-one patients with locally advanced NSCLC undergoing concurrent RT-CHT followed by surgery were evaluated. Postoperative complications occurred in 49 %. Weight loss $\geq$5 % during induction period was associated with shorter OS ($p = 0.03$), and especially overweight patients experiencing weight loss $\geq$5 % during the induction period had shorter OS and also PFS (van der Meij et al. 2011).

5 Predictors of Toxicity of Definitive Radiotherapy and Radiochemotherapy

5.1 Lung

Lung is one of the most sensitive tissues to ionizing radiation. Damage to normal lung tissue remains the most important limitation for effective treatment with RT or RT-CHT of this disease, apart from rapid progression. Recent decades brought many radiobiologically and/or technologically oriented RT dose intensification approaches. Moreover, concurrent RT-CHT became standard treatment in locally advanced NSCLC and limited disease (LD) SCLC. With these, toxicity was observed more frequently, both acute and late, leading sometimes to not only serious adverse events (grades 3–4), but also toxic deaths (grade 5). Therefore reducing RT or RT/CHT induced normal lung tissue damage is of critical importance in improving the therapeutic window and patients' quality of life. Acute lung injury starts from 1 to 3 months after RT and the most common symptom is severe dyspnea. Chronic lung damage which is usually irreversible evolves 6–24 months after irradiation. Prolonged follow-up is especially important as it enables better insight into events that may initially not be reported. In one such report, Miller et al. (2005) reported on an unexpected rate of bronchial stenosis using 1.6 Gy bid up to 70.8–86.4 Gy in NSCLC. Eight out of 103 (8 %) patients experienced clinically significant and symptomatic bronchial stenosis 2–48 months after RT, with a 1- and 4-year actuarial rate of 7 and 38 %, respectively. In stereotactic hypofractionated radiotherapy, the radiation tolerance of central structures including trachea and large vessels must also be considered. In general, radiographic abnormalities are seen more frequently than clinical symptoms which can be defined as haziness in the areas irradiated, a shift in the mediastinum and diaphragm of the irradiated area and pericardial and pleural fluid accumulation.

A number of clinical factors were investigated in order to determine their influence on the occurrence of bronchopulmonary and other toxicity in lung cancer patients treated with either RT alone or RT-CHT. Our previous multivariate analyses (Jeremic et al. 2004, 2012) in patients with stage III NSCLC treated with Hfx RT and concurrent low-dose CHT identified no clinical variable influencing acute grade $\geq$3 bronchopulmonary toxicity. Robnett et al. (2000), however, have found correlations with both female gender and KPS, while Rancati et al. (2003) and Claude et al. (2004) did not find that gender influenced bronchopulmonary toxicity. Brooks et al. (1986) and Claude et al. (2004) did not find correlations between toxicity and KPS. Except for Claude et al. (2004) who found adverse influence of age on the rate of symptomatic pneumonitis, other authors (Rancati et al. 2003; Brooks et al. 1986; Hernando et al. 2001; Quon et al. 1999) did not find such predictive influence. Regarding the use of CHT, Robnett et al. (2000), Lee et al. (1996), Inoue et al. (2001), and Hernando et al. (2001) did not find influence of CHT, while Brooks et al. (1986), Robert et al. (1999), Rancati et al. (2003), Yamada et al. (1998) and Byhardt et al. (1998) did so. Similarly to the latter, Singh et al. (2003) found adverse influence of concurrent CHT, and Werner-Wasik et al. (2000a, b) confirmed their finding in a multivariate analysis. In that study, even more profound negative influence of concurrent CHT was found when it was combined with Hfx RT. Moreno et al. (2007) could not identify any of the investigated clinical and therapeutic factors to be associated with bronchopulmonary toxicity, admittedly due to low incidence of these events. Similarly a Swedish group (De Petris et al. 2005) found no influence of age, gender, PS and stage on bronchopulmonary toxicity of concurrent RT-CHT. In other studies, total dose, fractionation and volume were occasionally identified as influencing bronchopulmonary toxicity. Interestingly, Roach et al. (1995) found somewhat favourable effect of Hfx RT on bronchopulmonary toxicity. Weight loss and concurrent CHT independently influenced occurrence of late grade $\geq$3 bronchopulmonary toxicity, contrasting our previous study which identified only stage as independent predictor of high-grade late bronchopulmonary toxicity (Jeremic et al. 2004).

Another set of measures of RT-induced lung toxicity include changes in pulmonary function tests (PFTs) such as Forced Expiratory Volume in 1 s (FEV_1), Forced Vital capacity (FVC), and carbon monoxide diffusion capacity (DL_{co}). A decline in PFTs was apparent at 6 months and continued well beyond 1 year (Miller et al. 2003), suggesting progressive RT-induced lung disease. In addition, others observed dose-dependent reduction in regional perfusion with prolonged follow-up post-RT, with most of this injury being manifest within 12 months post-RT (Woel et al. 2002).

Over many years various dosimetric parameters have been evaluated for RT-induced pulmonary toxicity. Of these, mean lung dose (MLD), the V_{dose} and Normal Tissue Complication probability (NTCP) are most commonly reported. MLDs of $\leq$15 Gy, 17.5–20 Gy, 22.5–25 Gy, and $\geq$27.5 Gy resulted in 0, 13, 21, and 43 % incidence of all grades of radiation pneumonitis (Oetzel et al. 1995). In a pooled analysis of 540 patients who received thoracic radiation by Kwa et al. (1998), the MLD was found to correlate with an increased risk of pneumonitis. A commonly recommended limit is to keep the MLD $\leq$ 20 Gy. The cut-off values of the percent volume of the total lung receiving a dose greater than e.g. 10 Gy (V10), 20 Gy (V20), 25 Gy (V25), 30 Gy (V30), 40 Gy (V40) or 50 Gy (V50) were reported by numerous authors, and such values were frequently found to be associated with radiation induced pneumonitis. Unfortunately, different endpoints (severity of pneumonitis) were used (Hernando et al. 2001; Claude et al. 2004; Armstrong et al. 1995; Graham et al. 1999) obscuring the picture. It is commonly recommended to limit V20 to $\leq$35 Gy ($\leq$20 Gy for preoperative RT-CHT). Correlations between calculated NTCP values and the risk of pneumonitis were documented in several studies. In one study (Martel et al. 1994), NTCP average values were 73 % in patients with pulmonary toxicity and 25 % in patients without it. Similarly, using Grade $\geq$2 pneumonitis as an endpoint, patients with and without it had NTCP values of 19.6 and 12.0 %, respectively (Hernando et al. 2001). In a study by Lee et al. (2003), the mean NTCP value for the ipsilateral lung was higher in the group with pneumonitis (66.0 %) versus the group without pneumonitis

(26.4 %). In other studies (Oetzel et al. 1995; Armstrong et al. 1995), various cut-off values of NTCP (≥12 and 30 %, respectively) were used, showing that values higher than the cut-off value in both studies led to higher incidence of pneumonitis than that observed with NTCP values lower than cut-off value. Due to inconsistent data existing in the literature of these dosimetric factors, some embarked on combining them with clinical and location-related factors into a single predictive model for radiation pneumonitis (Hope et al. 2004). Recently, Hope et al. (2006) showed that models most frequently selected included tumour position, maximum dose, and D35 (minimum dose to the 35 % volume receiving the highest doses) ($R = 0.28$). The most frequently selected two- or three-parameter models outperformed commonly used metrics, including V20 and MLD ($R = 0.18$). More recently, in a proposed nomogram Bradley et al. (2007) evaluated a number of possible predictors of pneumonitis. The final model incorporated two effects: greater risk due to irradiation of inferior parts of the lung, and greater risk for increasing normal lung mean dose. Similarly, a multi-institutional study (Kocak et al. 2007) suggested a model which included parameters such as MLD, RT dose to perfused lung and pre-RT lung function to form low versus high risk group of patients experiencing RT-induced toxicity. Though this study was unable to accurately segregate patients into these two risk groups on a prospective basis, considered retrospectively, the data were consistent with prior studies suggesting that dosimetric and functional parameters are predictive of RT-induced pneumonitis.

Biochemical detection markers have also been investigated upon their predictive role in RT-related pneumonitis. Interleukin (IL)-1α and IL-6 (Chen et al. 2001, 2002), Soluble Intracellular Adhesion Molecule (SICAM)-1 (Ishii and Kitamura 1999), Serum mucin-like glycoprotein antigen Kl-6 (Goto et al. 2001), pulmonary surfactant protein D (Sasaki et al. 2001) as well as Transforming Growth Factor (TGF)-β1 (Anscher et al. 1998; Vujaskovic and Groen 2000; Barthelemy-Brichant et al. 2004; De Jaeger et al. 2004; Novakova-Jiresova et al. 2004) have all been scrutinized with regard to early prediction of RT-pneumonitis. Conflicting results have been achieved with all of these, indicating need for further refinement of such approaches. Of interest is that Hart et al. (2005) undertook cytokine profiling for prediction of symptomatic RT-induced lung injury using a panel of 17 proinflammatory cytokines to find that only patients with lower levels of plasma IL-8 before RT might be at increased risk for developing such injury. Of additional interest is that Chen et al. (2005) used a prospective protocol which enabled them to show that in direct comparison IL-6 globally outperformed IL-1α in predicting radiation pneumonitis, having both higher positive predictive and negative predictive values. While these could theoretically be used to identify RT-pneumonitis in early stages, their overall effect would be doubtful in case they do not result in RT dose reduction. It should be clearly stated that dosimetric parameters of RT in general show a low predictive value of 69–80 %. Depending on the studied molecule, the negative predictive value of biomarkers was approximately 50 %. Obviously, additional work needs to be done in refining these approaches and integrating various predictors of RT-induced lung toxicity into a decision-making process in patients with lung cancer.

5.2 Heart, Oesophagus and Bone

In contrast to breast cancer, where incidental heart irradiation has received considerable attention, this issue is less well studied in lung cancer, presumably due to the lower likelihood of long-term survival. In addition, lung and oesophageal toxicity might influence outcomes after quite short follow-up, leading to treatment interruption and/or hospitalization in case of severe dysphagia. Heart doses should be minimized whenever possible, e.g. mean dose ≤26 Gy and V30 ≤45 %. However, it is not fully understood which substructures are most important and how reduced heart and lung function interfere with each other. Lung cancer, dysphagia is a common complication of lung radiotherapy when target volumes are close to the oesophagus, radiation tolerance. A nomogram predicting this side effect has been developed and validated (Dehing-Oberije et al. 2010). Predictive factors included age, gender, PS, mean oesophageal dose, maximum oesophageal dose and overall treatment time. Simpler recommendations were focused on V50 ≤ 40 %, V70 ≤ 20 % and Dmax ≤75 Gy. Bone injury following stereotactic radiotherapy (3 fractions) might develop several months after treatment (Taremi et al. 2012). On multivariate analysis, age, female gender and dose to 0.5 cc of the ribs (D0.5) were significant predictors for increased fracture risk. The authors developed a nomogram, which requires validation in larger datasets. Other data suggest that chest wall volumes of 5 and 15 cc receiving 40 Gy predicted a 10 and 30 % risk of toxicities, merely pain, respectively (Andolino et al. 2011). Stephans et al. (2012) recommended restricting V30 to ≤30 cc and V60 to ≤3 cc. Body mass index might also impact on lung cancer, chest wall toxicity risk. More details on normal tissue reactions and constraints for stereotactic radiotherapy were summarized by Lo et al. (2012).

6 Prognostic Factors in SCLC

Regarding patient-related parameters, gender was documented as an important prognostic factor for treatment outcome, with the combination of female sex and younger age (<60 years) carrying improved response rates, median survival, and 2-year survival rate. This observation was independent of any other relevant prognostic variable and has been known for decades (Osterlind and Anderson 1986; Spiegelman et al. 1989; Albain et al. 1990; Wolf et al. 1991; Buccheri and Ferrigno 1994). It was repeatedly confirmed in more recent trials, using different types of CHT (Paesmans et al. 2000; Singh et al. 2005), but many groups caution against basing treatment decision on these factors alone. Similarly to NSCLC, both KPS and the Eastern Cooperative Oncology Group Performance Status (ECOG PS) have been extensively used, with suggestion that ECOG PS might be easier to apply and better to discriminate the patients' prognosis (Buccheri et al. 1996). Irrespective of these findings, the majority of authors found that performance status was a significant prognostic factor (Osterlind and Anderson 1986; Spiegelman et al. 1989; Albain et al. 1990; Rawson and Peto 1990; Buccheri and Ferrigno 1994; Paesmans et al. 2000). In addition, weight loss has been identified as important prognostic factor also in SCLC (Stanley 1980; Tamura et al. 1998; Bremnes et al. 2003).

Of tumour-related factors, the most powerful prognostic factor in most of the published series using the IASLC definition (Sheperd et al. 2007; Micke et al. 2002; Paesmans et al. 2000; Jorgensen et al. 1996) is stage. When discriminating between LD SCLC and extensive disease (ED) SCLC, according to a rather old staging classification, it has been continuously shown that the median survival is around 20–30 months in the former, in contrast to about 10 months in latter group of patients (Jeremic et al. 1997a, b, 1999a, b; Yip and Harper 2000; Takada et al. 2002), and this has a major implication on treatment decisions. Besides that, a number of other prognostic factors related to the extent of tumour and the number or locations of metastatic sites have been evaluated (superior vena cava syndrome, pleural effusion, nodal involvement, involvement of different organs like liver, brain, or bone) (Albain et al. 1990; Würschmidt et al. 1995; Tamura et al. 1998; Bremnes et al. 2003). Mediastinal involvement and the infiltration of several organs might impair the prognosis of the patient, as has been demonstrated regarding long-term survival by Tai et al. (2003). However, the data are not consistent and therefore, these factors are not generally used as a basis for treatment decisions. SCLC can carry a mixture of different tumour cells in up to 20 % of cases, large-cell carcinoma being the most commonly combined cell type. This caused IASLC pathology committee to adopt three new subtypes of SCLC: small cell, mixed large and small cell, and combined small cell carcinomas (Hirsch et al. 1988). Unfortunately, several subsequent studies could not document a different clinical outcome for these three subgroups. As a consequence, actual WHO classification abandoned the idea of different subgroups (Brambilla et al. 2001). Nevertheless, the high percentage of patients with various combinations of SCLC and NSCLC might explain the divergent response to CHT, and support the idea of salvage resection for locally confined poor-responding cancer (Sheperd et al. 1991). No histological factors have been identified as predictive of prognosis in SCLC (Fissler-Eckhoff 2010).

Besides the tumour extent, serological factors (tumour markers), produced by tumour cells and released into the bloodstream, have been evaluated in a number of different studies. Due to their low tumour-specificity only a few of them have certain prognostic value: neuron specific enolase (NSE) and cytokeratin-19-fragments (Cyfra 21-1). NSE has been tested in several large trials, and a significant correlation was found between elevated NSE levels and poor prognosis in multivariate analyses, making it one of the most powerful prognostic factors (Bremnes et al. 2003; Jorgensen et al. 1996). Using NSE together with PS of the patient and tumour extent in a simple algorithm produces a clearly defined prognostic classification that can be used for treatment decisions (Jorgensen et al. 1996). Cyfra 21-1 has been the most commonly studied cytokeratin, and besides extensive disease and increased levels of lactate dehydrogenase (LDH) and NSE, levels >3.6 ng/ml significantly indicated a poor outcome of the patient (Pujol et al. 2003). Among the additionally tested serological markers only the serum carcinoembryonic antigen (CEA) has attracted scientific attention due to some positive studies, whereas chromogranin A (CgA), pro-gastrin releasing peptide (ProGRP) and creatinine kinase-BB (CPK-BB) have not yet been confirmed as important predictors in this disease (Ferrigno et al. 1994; Lamy et al. 2000; Sunaga et al. 1999).

A series of potential prognostic factors were evaluated through laboratory tests in SCLC: LDH, hemoglobin (Hb), albumin, alkaline phosphatase (AP), sodium, calcium, creatinine, bicarbonates, bilirubin, erythrocytes, leucocytes, neutrophilia, and thrombocytes. Elevated LDH seems to be the strongest haematological prognosticator with high accuracy predicting poor outcome. It seems to be even more important than some tumour markers (NSE), and is recommended by different groups as the most valid marker (and the cheapest one) for SCLC as a stratification criteria for clinical trials (Quoix et al. 2000; Rawson and Peto 1990; Osterlind and Anderson 1986). Of all the other factors mentioned before, the results are more or less inhomogeneous: low serum albumin concentration, normal sodium and uric acid levels, decreased plasmatic level of haemoglobin, leucocytosis, increased alkaline phosphatase (AP) and serum bicarbonate were only positive in some of the trials in which they were evaluated, and cannot be integrated in clinical routine decision making (Bremnes et al. 2003; Quoix et al. 2000; Rawson and Peto 1990; Osterlind and Anderson 1986). In principle, an elevated LDH should be seen as a risk factor for poor survival and an indicator of a larger tumour burden, at least demanding for a complete assessment of tumour stage. Based on the work of the Subcommittee for the Management of Lung cancer in the UK on almost 4000 patients, performance status, disease stage, and AP, sodium, aspartate aminotransferase and LDH should be measured in all future trials to assist comparisons between the clinical trials (Rawson and Peto 1990). Together with performance status and tumour stage, sodium, AP, and LDH have been combined as the Manchester Prognostic Score, and later modified by a Japanese group into a new three tiered classification (Kawahara et al. 1999). This model can differentiate 1-year survival rates of more than 50 % in the best versus 0 % in the worst group, or median survival rates of 16.0 versus 6.6 months, respectively. These classifications can be used to design clinical trials and to tailor individual treatment as well.

Of treatment-related factors, the response to treatment has been found to highly significantly influence the survival of patients treated with CHT and RT-CHT. Complete responders had a better survival than partial responders, who had a superior outcome than non-responders (Lebeau et al. 1995; Ray et al. 1998; Paesmans et al. 2000). Addition of RT to CHT was proven to significantly improve survival in two meta-analyses (Pignon et al. 1992; Warde and Payne 1992). In several randomized trials evaluating the timing of administration of RT and CHT it has also been documented that early concurrent RT-CHT improves the outcome of patients with LD SCLC compared to late RT-CHT, and that altered fractionation of irradiation might further enhance the results (Warde and Payne 1992; Murray et al. 1993; Jeremic et al. 1997a, b; Work et al. 1997; Lebeau et al. 1999; Turrisi et al. 1999; Takada et al. 2002). In retrospective trials the importance of total RT dose has been pronounced (Tai et al. 2003), and two randomized trials comparing higher doses of conventional RT with either Hfx or accelerated (Acc) RT schedules are still ongoing, and the answer to this important question is, therefore, lacking. While the place and role of RT is well established in LD SCLC, recent data point to the direction of using thoracic RT in selected cases of ED SCLC, frequently termed "limited extensive" SCLC. A pioneering study (Jeremic et al. 1999a, b) showed that thoracic RT leads to an improvement in survival through an improvement in local tumour control in patients experiencing complete response at distant sites and either complete response or partial response intrathoracically after induction platinum-etoposide CHT. Studies coming from different parts of the world (Zhu et al. 2011; Yee et al. 2012) corroborated this observation, which is currently being tested prospectively in Europe and the US. Finally, prophylactic cranial irradiation (PCI) added to RT-CHT in both LD SCLC (Auperin et al. 1999) and ED SCLC (Slotman et al. 2007) significantly improves overall survival due to an improved CNS control.

7 Conclusions

Identification of prognostic and predictive factors remains an important aspect in the treatment decision-making process in lung cancer. Various prognostic factors that theoretically could influence outcomes after RT or RT-CHT in both NSCLC and SCLC were evaluated and only a few were consistently shown to independently influence outcomes. This is also true when using induction (neoadjuvant) therapy before surgery in locally advanced NSCLC. Of a number of patient-, tumour- or treatment-related predictors of treatment-related toxicity dosimetric ones are most commonly used. More studies investigating these important aspects of optimization of the use of RT or RT-CHT in lung cancer patients are urgently needed.

References

Albain KS, Crowley JJ, Leblanc M, Livingston RB (1990) Determinants of improved outcome in small-cell lung cancer: an analysis of the 2,580-patient Southwest Oncology Group data base. J Clin Oncol 8:1563–1574

Albain KS, Rusch VW, Crowley JJ et al (1995) Concurrent cisplatin/etoposide plus chest radiotherapy followed by surgery for stages IIIA (N2) and IIIB non-small-cell lung cancer: mature results of Southwest Oncology Group phase II study 8805. J Clin Oncol 13:1880–1892

Alberg AJ, Ford JG, Samet JM (2007) American College of Chest Physicians. Epidemiology of lung cancer: ACCP evidence-based clinical practice guidelines (2nd edition). Chest 132:29S–55S

Andolino DL, Forquer JA, Henderson MA et al (2011) Chest wall toxicity after stereotactic body radiotherapy for malignant lesions of the lung and liver. Int J Radiat Oncol Biol Phys 80:692–697

Andratschke N, Zimmermann F, Boehm E et al (2011) Stereotactic radiotherapy of histologically proven inoperable stage I non-small cell lung cancer: patterns of failure. Radiother Oncol 101:245–249

Annema JT, Veselic M, Versteegh MI et al (2003) Mediastinal restaging: EUS-FNA offers a new perspective. Lung Cancer 42:311–318

Anscher MS, Kong FM, Andrews K et al (1998) Plasma transforming growth factor $\beta 1$ as a predictor of radiation pneumonitis. Int J Radiat Oncol Biol Phys 41:1029–1035

Armstrong JG, Zelefsky MJ, Leibel SA et al (1995) Strategy for dose escalation using 3-dimensional conformal radiation therapy for lung cancer. Ann Oncol 6:693–697

Auperin A, Arriagada R, Pignon JP et al (1999) Prophylactic cranial irradiation for patients with small-cell lung cancer in complete remission. Prophylactic cranial irradiation overview collaborative group. N Engl J Med 341:476–484

Auperin A, Le Pechoux C, Pignon JP et al (2006) Concomitant radiochemotherapy based on platin compounds in patients with locally advanced non-small cell lung cancer (NSCLC): a meta-analysis of individual data from 1764 patients. Ann Oncol 17:473–483

Ball D, Smith J, Wirth A (2002) Failure of T stage to predict survival in patients with non-small-cell lung cancer treated with radiotherapy with or without concomitant chemotherapy. Int J Radiat Oncol Biol Phys 54:1007–1013

Barnett SA, Rusch VW, Zheng J et al (2011) Contemporary results of surgical resection of non-small cell lung cancer after induction therapy: a review of 549 consecutive cases. J Thorac Oncol 6:1530–1536

Barthelemy-Brichant N, Bosquee L, Cataldo D et al (2004) Increased IL-6 and TGF- $\beta 1$ concentrations in bronchoalveolar lavage fluid associated with thoracic radiotherapy. Int J Radiat Oncol Biol Phys 58:758–767

Basaki K, Abe Y, Aoki M et al (2006) Prognostic factors for survival in stage III non-small-cell lung cancer treated with definitive radiation therapy: impact of tumor volume. Int J Radiat Oncol Biol Phys 64:449–454

Betticher DC, Schmitz SH, Totsch M et al (2003) Mediastinal lymph node clearance after docetaxel-cisplatin neoadjuvant chemotherapy is prognostic of survival in patients with stage IIIA pN2 non-small-cell lung cancer: a multicenter phase II trial. J Clin Oncol 21:1752–1759

Betticher DC, Hsu Schmitz SF, Tötsch M et al (2006) Prognostic factors affecting long-term outcomes in patients with resected stage IIIA pN2 non-small-cell lung cancer: 5-year follow-up of a phase II study. Br J Cancer 94:1099–1106

Bradley JD, Hope A, El Naqa I (2007) A nomogram to predict radiation pneumonitis, derived from a combined analysis of RTOG 9311 and institutional data. Int J Radiat Oncol Biol Phys 69:985–992

Brambilla E, Travis WD, Colby TV et al (2001) The new World Health Organization classification of lung tumours. Eur Respir J 18:1059–1068

Bremnes RM, Sundstrom S, Aasebo U et al (2003) The value of prognostic factors in small cell lung cancer: results from a randomized multicenter study with minimum 5 year follow-up. Lung Cancer 39:303–313

Brooks BJ Jr, Seifter EJ, Walsh TE et al (1986) Pulmonary toxicity with combined modality therapy for limited stage small-cell lung cancer. J Clin Oncol 4:200–209

Brundage MD, Feldman-Stewart D, Cosby R et al (2001) Phase I study of a decision aid for patients with locally advanced non-small cell lung cancer. J Clin Oncol 19:1326–1335

Brundage MD, Davies D, Mackillop WJ (2002) Prognostic factors in non-small cell lung cancer: a decade of progress. Chest 122: 1037–1057

Buccheri G, Ferrigno D (1994) Prognostic factors in lung cancer: tables and comments. Eur Respir J 7:1350–1364

Buccheri G, Ferrigno D, Tamburini M (1996) Karnofsky and ECOG performance status scoring in lung cancer: a prospective, longitudinal study of 536 patients from a single institution. Eur J Cancer 32A:1135–1141

Bueno R, Richards WG, Swanson SJ, et al (2000) Nodal stage after induction therapy for stage IIIA lung cancer determines patient survival. Ann Thorac Surg 70:1826–1831

Byhardt RW, Scott C, Sause WT et al (1998) Response, toxicity, failure patterns, and survival in five Radiation Therapy Oncology Group (RTOG) trials of sequential and/or concurrent chemotherapy and radiotherapy for locally advanced non-small-cell carcinoma of the lung. Int J Radiat Oncol Biol Phys 42:469–478

Cerfolio RJ, Maniscalco L, Bryant AS (2008) The treatment of patients with stage IIIA non-small cell lung cancer from N2 disease: who returns to the surgical arena and who survives. Ann Thorac Surg 86:912–920

Chen Y, Rubin P, Williams J et al (2001) Circulating IL-6 as a predictor of radiation pneumonitis. Int J Radiat Oncol Biol Phys 49:641–648

Chen Y, Williams J, Ding I et al (2002) Radiation pneumonitis and early circulatory cytokine markers. Semin Radiat Oncol 12:26–33

Chen Y, Hyrien O, Williams J et al (2005) Interleukin (IL)-1A and IL-6: applications to the predictive diagnostic testing of radiation pneumonitis. Int J Radiat Oncol Biol Phys 62:260–266

Chen M, Hayman JA, Ten Haken RK et al (2006) Long-term results of high-dose conformal radiotherapy for patients with medically inoperable T1–3N0 non-small-cell lung cancer: is low incidence of regional failure due to incidental nodal irradiation? Int J Radiat Oncol Biol Phys 64:120–126

Cheung PC, Mackillop WJ, Dixon P et al (2000) Involved-field radiotherapy alone for early-stage non-small-cell lung cancer. Int J Radiat Oncol Biol Phys 48:703–710

Claude L, Perol D, Ginestet C et al (2004) A prospective study on radiation pneumonitis following conformal radiation therapy in non-small-cell lung cancer: clinical and dosimetric factors analysis. Radiother Oncol 71:175–181

Cooper JF, Pearson FG, Todd TR, et al (1985) Radiotherapy alone for patients with operable carcinoma of the lung. Chest 87:289–292

Cox JD, Scott CB, Byhardt RW et al (1999) Addition of chemotherapy to radiation therapy alters failure patterns by cell type within non-small cell carcinoma of lung (NSCLC): analysis of Radiation Therapy Oncology Group (RTOG) trials. Int J Radiat Oncol Biol Phys 43:505–509

Curran WJ Jr, Scott CB, Horton J et al (1993) Recursive partitioning analysis of prognostic factors in three Radiation Therapy Oncology Group malignant glioma trials. J Natl Cancer Inst 85:704–710

De Jaeger K, Seppenwoolde Y, Kampinga HH et al (2004) Significance of plasma transforming growth factor β levels in radiotherapy for non-small-cell lung cancer. Int J Radiat Oncol Biol Phys 58:1378–1387

De Leyn P, Lardinois D, Van Schil PE et al (2007) ESTS guidelines for preoperative lymph node staging for non-small cell lung cancer. Eur J Cardiothorac Surg 32:1–8

De Petris L, Lax I, Sirzén F, Friesland S (2005) Role of gross tumor volume on outcome and of dose parameters on toxicity of patients undergoing chemoradiotherapy for locally advanced non-small cell lung cancer. Med Oncol 22:375–381

De Waele M, Hendriks J, Lauwers P et al (2006) Nodal status at repeat mediastinoscopy determines survival in non-small cell lung cancer with mediastinal nodal involvement, treated by induction therapy. Eur J Cardiothorac Surg 29:240–243

De Waele M, Serra-Mitjans M, Hendriks J et al (2008) Accuracy and survival of repeat mediastinoscopy (reMS) after induction therapy for non-small cell lung cancer in a combined series of 104 patients. Eur J Cardiothorac Surg 33:824–828

De Waele M, Hendriks J, Lauwers P et al (2011) Restaging the mediastinum in non-small cell lung cancer after induction therapy: non-invasive versus invasive procedures. Acta Chir Belg 111:161–164

Dehing-Oberije C, De Ruysscher D, Petit S et al (2010) Development, external validation and clinical usefulness of a practical prediction model for radiation-induced dysphagia in lung cancer patients. Radiother Oncol 97:455–461

Dosoretz DE, Katin MJ, Blitzer PH et al (1992) Radiation therapy in the management of medically inoperable carcinoma of the lung: results and implications for future treatment strategies. Int J Radiat Oncol Biol Phys 25:3–9

Dosoretz DE, Galmarini D, Rubenstein JH et al (1993) Local control in medically inoperable lung cancer: an analysis of its importance in outcome and factors determining the probability of tumour eradication. Int J Radiat Oncol Biol Phys 27:507–516

Edge SB, Byrd DR, Compton CC et al (2009) American Joint Committee on Cancer, American Cancer Society. AJCC cancer staging manual, 7th edn. Springer, Berlin

Edmonson JH, Lagakos SW, Selawry OS et al (1976) Cyclophosphamide, and CCNU in the treatment of inoperable small cell carcinoma and adenocarcinoma of the lung. Cancer Treat Rep 60:925–932

Emami B, Mirkovic N, Scott C et al (2003) The impact of regional nodal radiotherapy (dose/volume) on regional progression and survival in unresectable non-small cell lung cancer: an analysis of RTOG data. Lung Cancer 41:207–214

Fakiris AJ, McGarry RC, Yiannoutsos CT et al (2009) Stereotactic body radiation therapy for early-stage non-small-cell lung carcinoma: four-year results of a prospective phase II study. Int J Radiat Oncol Biol Phys 75:677–682

Fang LC, Komaki R, Allen P et al (2006) Comparison of outcomes for patients with medically inoperable stage I non-small-cell lung cancer treated with two-dimensional versus three-dimensional radiotherapy. Int J Radiat Oncol Biol Phys 66:108–116

Feinstein AR (1972) Clinical biostatistics XIV: the purposes of prognostic stratification. Clin Pharmacol Ther 13:285–297

Ferrigno D, Buccheri D, Biggi A (1994) Serum tumour markers in lung cancer: history, biology and clinical applications. Eur Respir J 7:186–197

Firat S, Byhardt RW, Gore E for the Radiation Therapy Oncology Group (2002a) Comorbidity and Karnofsky performance score are independent prognostic factors in stage III non-small-cell lung cancer: an institutional analysis of patients treated on four RTOG studies. Int J Radiat Oncol Biol Phys 54:357–364

Firat S, Bousamra M, Gore E, Byhardt RW (2002b) Comorbidity and KPS are independent prognostic factors in stage I non-small-cell lung cancer. Int J Radiat Oncol Biol Phys 52:1047–1057

Fissler-Eckhoff A (2010) Prognostic factors in histopatholgy of lung cancer. In: Heide J, Schmittel A, Kaiser D, Hinkelbein W (eds) Controversies in the treatment of lung cancer. Frontier radiation therapy oncology, vol 42. Karger, Basel, pp 1–14

Furuta M, Hayakawa K, Katano S et al (1996) Radiation therapy for stage I-II non-small cell lung cancer in patients aged 75 years and older. Jpn J Clin Oncol 26:95–98

Gauden SJ, Tripcony L (2001) The curative treatment by radiation therapy alone of stage I non-small cell lung cancer in a geriatric population. Lung Cancer 32:71–79

Gauden S, Ramsay J, Tripcony L (1995) The curative treatment by radiotherapy alone of stage I non-small cell carcinoma of the lung. Chest 108:1278–1282

Glatstein E, Makuch RW (1984) Illusion and reality: practical pitfalls in interpreting clinical trials. J Clin Oncol 2:488–497

Goldstraw P, Crowley J, Chansky K et al (2007) The IASLC lung cancer staging project: proposals for the revision of the TNM stage groupings in the forthcoming (seventh) edition of the TNM classification of malignant tumours. J Thorac Oncol 2:706–714

Goto K, Kodama T, Sekine I et al (2001) Serum levels of Kl-6 are useful biomarkers for severe radiation pneumonitis. Lung Cancer 34:141–148

Graham PH, Gebski VJ, Langlands AO (1995) Radical radiotherapy for early nonsmall cell lung cancer. Int J Radiat Oncol Biol Phys 31:261–266

Graham MV, Purdy JA, Emami B et al (1999) Clinical dose-volume histogram analysis for pneumonitis after 3D treatment for non-small cell lung cancer (NSCLC). Int J Radiat Oncol Biol Phys 45:323–329

Haffty BG, Goldberg NB, Gerstley J et al (1988) Results of radical radiation therapy in clinical Stage I, technically operable non-small cell lung cancer. Int J Radiat Oncol Biol Phys 15:69–73

Hart JP, Broadwater G, Rabbani Z et al (2005) Cytokine profiling for prediction of symptomatic radiation-induced lung injury. Int J Radiat Oncol Biol Phys 63:1448–1454

Hayakawa K, Mitsuhashi N, Nakajima N et al (1992) Radiation therapy for stage III epidermoid carcinoma of the lung. Lung Cancer 8:213–224

Hayakawa K, Mitsuhashi N, Saito Y et al (1996) Definite radiation therapy for medically inoperable patients with stage I and II non-small cell lung cancer. Radiat Oncol Invest 4:165–170

Hayakawa K, Mitsuhashi N, Saito Y et al (1999) Limited field irradiation for medically inoperable patients with peripheral stage I non-small cell lung cancer. Lung Cancer 26:137–142

Hernando ML, Marks LB, Bentel GC et al (2001) Radiation-induced pulmonary toxicity: a dose-volume histogram analysis in 201 patients with lung cancer. Int J Radiat Oncol Biol Phys 51:650–659

Herth FJ, Annema JT, Eberhardt R et al (2008) Endobronchial ultrasound with transbronchial needle aspiration for restaging the mediastinum in lung cancer. J Clin Oncol 26:3346–3350

Hirsch FR, Matthews MJ, Aisner S et al (1988) Histopathologic classification of small cell lung cancer. Changing concepts and terminology. Cancer 62:973–977

Hope AJ, el Naqa I, Bradley JD et al (2004) Radiation pneumonitis/fibrosis risk based on dosimetric, clinical, and location-related factors. Int J Radiat Oncol Biol Phys 6:S204

Hope AJ, Lindsay PE, El Naqa I et al (2006) Modeling radiation pneumonitis risk with clinical, dosimetric, and spatial parameters. Int J Radiat Oncol Biol Phys 65:112–124

Inoue A, Kunitoh H, Sekine, et al (2001) Radiation pneumonitis in lung cancer patients: a retrospective study of risk factors and the long-term prognosis. Int J Radiat Oncol Biol Phys 49:649–655

Ishii Y, Kitamura S (1999) Soluble intercellular adhesion molecule-1 as an early detection marker for radiation pneumonitis. Eur Respir J 13:733–738

Ishikawa H, Nakayama Y, Kitamoto Y et al (2006) Effect of histologic type on recurrence pattern in radiation therapy for medically inoperable patients with stage I non-small-cell lung cancer. Lung Cancer 184:347–353

Jeremic B, Shibamoto Y (1996) Effect of interfraction interval in hyperfractionated radiotherapy with or without concurrent chemotherapy for stage III nonsmall cell lung cancer. Int J Radiat Oncol Biol Phys 34:303–308

Jeremic B, Shibamoto Y, Acimovic L et al (1995) Pre-treatment prognostic factors in patients with stage III non-small cell lung cancer treated with hyperfractionated radiation therapy with or without concurrent chemotherapy. Lung Cancer 13:21–30

Jeremic B, Shibamoto Y, Acimovic LJ et al (1996) Hyperfractionated radiation therapy with or without concurrent low-dose daily carboplatin/etoposide for stage III non-small-cell lung cancer: a randomized study. J Clin Oncol 14:1065–1070

Jeremic B, Shibamoto Y, Acimovic LJ et al (1997a) Hyperfractionated radiotherapy alone for clinical stage I nonsmall cell lung cancer. Int J Radiat Oncol Biol Phys 38:521–525

Jeremic B, Shibamoto Y, Acimovic L, Milisavljevic S (1997b) Initial versus delayed accelerated hyperfractionated radiation therapy and concurrent chemotherapy in limited small cell lung cancer. J Clin Oncol 15:893–900

Jeremic B, Shibamoto Y, Nikolic N et al (1999a) The role of radiation therapy in the combined modality treatment of patients with extensive disease small-cell lung cancer (ED SCLC): a randomized study. J Clin Oncol 17:2092–2099

Jeremic B, Shibamoto Y, Acimovic LJ et al (1999b) Hyperfractionated radiotherapy for clinical stage II nonsmall cell lung cancer. Radiother Oncol 51:141–145

Jeremic B, Classen J, Bamberg M (2002) Radiation therapy alone in technically operable, medically inoperable early stage (I/II) non-small-cell lung cancer. Int J Radiat Oncol Biol Phys 54:119–130

Jeremic B, Milicic M, Dagovic A et al (2004) Interfraction interval in patients with stage III non-small cell lung cancer treated with hyperfractionated radiation therapy with or without concurrent chemotherapy. Final results in 536 patients. Am J Clin Oncol 27:616–625

Jeremic B, Milicic B, Acimovic L et al (2005) Concurrent hyperfractionated radiotherapy and low-dose daily carboplatin/paclitaxel in patients with early stage (I/II) non-small cell lung cancer (NSCLC). Long -term results of a phase II study. J Clin Oncol 23:6873–6880

Jeremic B, Milicic B, Milisavljevic S (2012) Toxicity of concurrent hyperfractionated radiation therapy and chemotherapy in locally advanced (stage III) non-small cell lung cancer (NSCLC). Single institution experience in 600 patients. Clin Transl Oncol 14:613–618

Jeremić B, Milicic B, Dagović A et al (2006) Pretreatment prognostic factors in patients with early stage (I/II) nonsmall cell lung cancer treated with hyperfractionated radiation therapy alone. Int J Radiat Oncol Biol Phys 65:1112–1119

Jeremić B, Miličić B, Milisavljevic S (2011) Clinical prognostic factors in patients with locally advanced (stage III) nonsmall cell lung cancer treated with hyperfractionated radiation therapy with and without concurrent chemotherapy: single-institution experience in 600 patients. Cancer 117:2995–3003

Jorgensen LG, Osterlind K, Genollá J et al (1996) Serum neuron-specific enolase (S-NSE) and the prognosis in small cell lung cancer (SCLC): a combined multivariate analysis. Br J Cancer 74:463–467

Kaskowitz L, Graham MV, Emami B et al (1993) Radiation therapy alone for stage I non-small cell lung cancer. Int J Radiat Oncol Biol Phys 27:517–523

Kawahara M, Fukuoka M, Saijko N et al (1999) Prognostic factors and prognostic staging system for small cell lung cancer. Jpn J Clin Oncol 27:158–165

Kim AW, Boffa DJ, Wang Z et al (2012) An analysis, systematic review, and meta-analysis of the perioperative mortality after neoadjuvant therapy and pneumonectomy for non-small cell lung cancer. J Thorac Cardiovasc Surg 143:55–63

Kl Miller, Zhou S-M, Barrier RC et al (2003) Long-term changes in pulmonary function tests after definitive radiotherapy for lung cancer. Int J Radiat Oncol Biol Phys 56:611–615

Kocak Z, Borst GR, Zeng J et al (2007) Prospective assessment of dosimetric/psychiologic-based models for predicting radiation pneumonitis. Int J Radiat Oncol Biol Phys 67:178–186

Komaki R, Scott CB, Byhardt RW et al (1998) Failure patterns by prognostic group determined by recursive partitioning analysis (RPA) of 1547 patients on four Radiation Therapy Oncology Group (RTOG) studies in inoperable nonsmall-cell lung cancer (NSCLC). Int J Radiat Oncol Biol Phys 42:263–267

Kunst PW, Lee P, Paul MA et al (2007) Restaging of mediastinal nodes with transbronchial needle aspiration after induction chemoradiation for locally advanced non-small cell lung cancer. J Thorac Oncol 2:912–915

Kupelian PA, Komaki R, Allen P (1996) Prognostic factors in the treatment of node-negative nonsmall cell lung carcinoma with radiotherapy alone. Int J Radiat Oncol Biol Phys 36:607–613

Lagerwaard FJ, Senan S, van Meerbeeck JP, Graveland WJ (2002) Has 3-D conformal radiotherapy (3D-CRT) improved local tumour control for stage I non-small cell lung cancer? Radiother Oncol 63:151–157

Lamy P, Grenier J, Kramar A, Pujol J (2000) Pro-gastrinreleasing peptide, neuron specific enolase and chromogranin A as serum markers of small cell lung cancer. Lung Cancer 29:197–203

Langer C, Hsu C, Curran D et al (2001) Do elderly patients with locally advanced non-small cell lung cancer benefit from combined modality therapy? A secondary analysis of RTOG 94–10. Int J Radiat Oncol Biol Phys 51:20–21

Lebeau B, Chastang C, Schuller MP et al (1995) Chimiothérapie des cancers ronchiques. Importance prognostique d'une résponse complète (1,280 patients). La Presse Médicale 24:217–221

Lebeau B, Urban T, Brechot JM et al (1999) A randomized clinical trial comparing concurrent and alternating thoracic irradiation for patients with limited small-cell lung cancer. Cancer 86:1480–1487

Lee JS, Scott C, Komaki R et al (1996) Concurrent chemoradiation therapy with oral etoposide and cisplatin for locally advanced inoperable non-small cell lung cancer: radiation Therapy Oncology Group protocol 91–06. J Clin Oncol 14:1055–1064

Lee SW, Choi EK, Lee JS et al (2003) Phase II study of three-dimensional conformal radiotherapy and concurrent mitomycin-C, vinblastin and cisplatin chemotherapy for stage III locally advanced, unresectable, non-small-cell lung cancer. Int J Radiat Oncol Biol Phys 56:996–1004

Lo SS, Sahgal A, Ma L, et al (2012) Normal tissue constraints. In: Lo SS, Teh BS, Lu JJ, Schefter TE (eds) Stereotactic body radiation therapy. Springer, Heidelberg

Lococo F, Cesario A, Margaritora S et al (2013) Long-term results in patients with pathological complete response after induction radiochemotherapy followed by surgery for locally advanced non-small-cell lung cancer. Eur J Cardiothorac Surg 43:e71–e81

Machtay M, Seiferheld W, Komaki R et al (1999) Is prolonged survival possible for patients with supraclavicular node metastasis in non-small cell lung cancer treated with chemoradiotherapy?: analysis of the Radiation Therapy Oncology Group experience. Int J Radiat Oncol Biol Phys 44:847–853

Mackillop MJ (2001) The importance of prognosis in cancer medicine. In: Gospodarowicz MK, Henson DE, Hutter RBP et al (eds) Prognostic factors in cancer. Wiley, New York

Marra A, Hillejan L, Fechner S, Stamatis G (2008) Remediastinoscopy in restaging of lung cancer after induction therapy. J Thorac Cardiovasc Surg 135:843–849

Martel MK, Ten Haken RK, Hazuka MB et al (1994) Dose-volume histogram and 3-D treatment planning evaluation of patients with pneumonitis. Int J Radiat Oncol Biol Phys 28:575–581

Matsuo Y, Shibuya K, Nagata Y et al (2011) Prognostic factors in stereotactic body radiotherapy for non-small-cell lung cancer. Int J Radiat Oncol Biol Phys 79:1104–1111

Micke P, Faldum A, Metz T et al (2002) Staging small cell lung cancer: Veterans Administration Lung Study Group versus International Association for the study of lung cancer–what limits limited disease? Lung Cancer 37:271–276

Miller K, Shafman T, Anscher M et al (2005) Bronchial stenosis: an underreported complication of high dose external beam radiotherapy for lung cancer? Int J Radiat Oncol Biol Phys 61:64–70

Milleron B, Westeel V, Quoix E et al (2005) French Thoracic Cooperative Group. Complete response following preoperative chemotherapy for resectable non-small cell lung cancer: accuracy of clinical assessment using the French trial database. Chest 128:1442–1447

Moreno M, Aristu J, Ramos LI et al (2007) Predictive factors for radiation-induced pulmonary toxicity after three-dimensional conformal chemoradiation in locally advanced non-small-cell lung cancer. Clin Transl Oncol 9:596–602

Morita K, Fuwa N, Suzuki Y et al (1997) Radical radiotherapy for medically inoperable non-small cell lung cancer in clinical stage I: retrospective analysis of 149 patients. Radiother Oncol 42:31–36

Morrison R, Delley TJ, Cleland WP (1963) The treatment of carcinoma of the bronchus. A clinical trial to compare surgery and supervoltage radiotherapy. Lancet 1:683–684

Mouillet G, Monnet E, Milleron B et al (2012) Pathologic complete response to preoperative chemotherapy predicts cure in early-stage non-small-cell lung cancer: combined analysis of two IFCT randomized trials. J Thorac Oncol 7:841–849

Murray N, Coy Patel J, Hodson I et al (1993) Importance of timing for thoracic irradiation in the combined modality treatment of limited stage small cell lung cancer. J Clin Oncol 11:336–344

Noordijk EM, Poest Clement Evd, Hermans J et al (1988) Radiotherapy as an alternative to surgery in elderly patients with respectable lung cancer. Radiother Oncol 13:83–89
Novakova-Jiresova A, Van Gameren MM, Coppes R et al (2004) Transforming growth factor-beta plasma dynamics and post-irradiation lung injury in lung cancer patients. Radiother Oncol 71:183–189
Oetzel D, Schraube P, Hensley F (1995) Estimation of pneumonitis risk in three-dimensional treatment planning using dose-volume histogram analysis. Int J Radiat Oncol Biol Phys 33:455–460
Ono R, Egawa S, Suemasu K et al (1991) Radiotherapy in inoperable stage I lung cancer. Jpn J Clin Oncol 21:125–128
Osterlind K, Anderson PK (1986) Prognostic factors in small cell lung cancer: a multivariate model base on 778 patients treated with chemotherapy with or without irradiation. Cancer 46:4189–4194
Paesmans M, Sculier JP, Lecomte J et al (2000) Prognostic factors for patients with small cell lung cancer. Cancer 89:523–533
Pfister DG, Johnson DH, Azzolli CG et al (2004) American Society of Clinical Oncology treatment of unresectable non-small-cell lung cancer guideline. J Clin Oncol 22:330–353
Pignon JP, Arriagada R, Ihde DC et al (1992) A meta-analysis of thoracic radiotherapy for smallcell lung cancer. N Engl J Med 327:1618–1624
Pujol JL, Quantin X, Jacot W et al (2003) Neuroendocrine and cytokeratin serum markers as prognostic determinants of small cell lung cancer. Lung Cancer 39:131–138
Quoix E, Purohit A, Faller-Beau M et al (2000) Comparative prognostic value of lactate dehydrogenase and neuron-specific enolase in small-cell lung cancer patients treated with platinum-based chemotherapy. Lung Cancer 30:127–134
Quon H, Shepherd FA, Payne DG et al (1999) The influence of age on the delivery, tolerance, and efficacy of thoracic irradiation in the combined modality treatment of limited stage small cell lung cancer. Int J Radiat Oncol Biol Phys 43:39–45
Rancati T, Ceresoli GL, Gagliardi G et al (2003) Factors predicting radiation pneumonitis in lung cancer patients: a retrospective study. Radiother Oncol 67:275–283
Rawson NSB, Peto J (1990) An overview of prognostic factors in small cell lung cancer. A report from the subcommittee for the management of lung cancer of the United Kingdom coordinating committee on cancer research. Br J Cancer 61:597–604
Ray R, Quantin X, Grenier J, Pujol JL (1998) Predictive factors of tumor response and prognostic factors of survival during lung cancer chemotherapy. Cancer Detect Prev 22:293–304
Roach M III, Gandara DR, Yuo HS et al (1995) Radiation pneumonitis following combined modality therapy for lung cancer: analysis of prognostic factors. J Clin Oncol 13:2606–2612
Robert F, Childs HA, Spencer SA et al (1999) Phase I/IIa study of concurrent paclitaxel and cisplatin with radiation therapy in locally advanced non-small cell lung cancer: analysis of early and late pulmonary morbidity. Semin Radiat Oncol 9:136–147
Robnett TJ, Machtay M, Vines EF et al (2000) Factors predicting severe radiation pneumonitis in patients receiving definitive chemoradiation for lung cancer. Int J Radiat Oncol Biol Phys 48:89–94
Rosenthal SA, Curran WJ Jr, Herbert SH et al (1992) Clinical stage II non-small cell lung cancer treated with radiation therapy alone. The significance of clinically staged ipsilateral hilar adenopathy (N1 disease). Cancer 70:3410–3417
Sandler HM, Curran WJ Jr, Turrisi AT III (1990) The influence of tumor size and pre-treatment staging on outcome following radiation therapy alone for stage I non-small cell lung cancer. Int J Radiat Oncol Biol Phys 19:9–13
Sasaki R, Oejima T, Matsumoto A et al (2001) Clinical significance of serum pulmonary surfactant proteins A and D for the early detection of radiation pneumonitis. Int J Radiat Oncol Biol Phys 50:301–307
Sheperd FA, Ginsberg R, Patterson GA et al (1991) Surgical treatment for limited small-cell lung cancer. J Cardiovasc Surg 101:385–393
Shepherd FA, Crowley J, Van Houtte P, Postmus PE, Carney D, Chansky K, Shaikh Z, Goldstraw P (2007) International Association for the Study of Lung Cancer International Staging Committee and Participating Institutions. The International Association for the Study of Lung Cancer staging project: proposals regarding the clinical staging of small cell lung cancer in the forthcoming (seventh) edition of the tumor, node, metastasis classification for lung cancer. J Thorac Oncol 2:1067–1077
Sibley GS, Jamieson TA, Marks LB et al (1998) Radiotherapy alone for medically inoperable stage I non-small-cell lung cancer: The Duke experience. Int J Radiat Oncol Biol Phys 40:149–154
Siegel R, Naishadham D, Jemal A (2012) Cancer statistics, 2012. CA Cancer J Clin 62:10–29
Simon R (1984) Importance of prognostic factors in cancer clinical trials. Cancer Treat Rep 68:185–192
Singh AK, Lockett MA, Bradley JD (2003) Predictors of radiation induced esophageal toxicity in patients with non-small-cell lung cancer treated with three- dimensional conformal radiotherapy. Int J Radiat Oncol Biol Phys 55:337–341
Singh S, Parulekar W, Murray N (2005) Influence of sex on toxicity and treatment outcome in small-cell lung cancer. J Clin Oncol 23:850–856
Sl Kwa, Lebesque JV, Theuws JC et al (1998) Radiation poneumonitis as a function of mean lung dose: ana analysis of pooled data of 540 patients. Int J Radiat Oncol Biol Phys 42:1–9
Slotman BJ, Karim AB (1994) Curative radiotherapy for technically operable stage I nonsmall cell lung cancer. Int J Radiat Oncol Biol Phys 29:33–37
Slotman BJ, Antonisse IE, Njo KH (1996) Limited field irradiation in early stage (T1–2 N0) non-small cell lung cancer. Radiother Oncol 41:41–44
Slotman B, Faivre-Finn C, Kramer G et al (2007) EORTC Radiation oncology group lung cancer group prophylactic cranial irradiation in extensive small-cell lung cancer. N Engl J Med 357:664–672
Socinski MA, Zhang C, Herndon JE II et al (2004) Combined modality trials of the cancer and leukemia group B in stage III non-small-cell lung cancer: analysis of factors influencing survival and toxicity. Ann Oncol 15:1033–1041
Spiegelman D, Maurer LH, Ware JH et al (1989) Prognostic factors in small-cell carcinoma of the lung: an analysis of 1,521 patients. J Clin Oncol 7:344–354
Stanley KE (1980) Prognostic factors for survival in patients with inoperable lung cancer. J Natl Cancer Inst 65:25–32
Stephans KL, Djemil T, Tendulkar RD et al (2012) Prediction of chest wall Toxicity from lung stereotactic body radiotherapy (SBRT). Int J Radiat Oncol Biol Phys 82:974–980
Straif K, Benbrahim-Tallaa L, Baan R et al (2009) A review of human carcinogens–part C: metals, arsenic, dusts, and fibres. Lancet Oncol 10:453–454
Sunaga N, Tsuchiya S, Minato K et al (1999) Serum progastrin-releasing peptide is a useful marker for treatment monitoring and survival in small-cell lung cancer. Oncology 57:143–148
Sundstrom S, Bremnes RM, Brunsvig P et al (2006) Palliative thoracic radiotherapy in locally advanced non-small cell lung cancer: can quality of life assessments help in selection of patients for short or long course radiotherapy? J Thorac Oncol 1:816–824
Tai P, Tonita J, Yu E, Skarsgard D (2003) Twenty-year follow up study of long-term survival of limited-stage small-cell lung cancer and overview of prognostic and treatment factors. Int J Radiat Oncol Biol Phys 56:626–633

Takada M, Fukuoka M, Kawahara M et al (2002) Phase III study of concurrent versus sequential thoracic radiotherapy in combination with cisplatin and etoposide for limited-stage small-cell lung cancer: results of the Japan clinical oncology group study 9104. J Clin Oncol 20:3054–3060
Tamura M, Ueoka H, Kiura K et al (1998) Prognostic factors of small-cell lung cancer in Okayama lung cancer study group trials. Acta Med Okayama 52:105–111
Taremi M, Hope A, Lindsay P et al (2012) Predictors of radiotherapy induced bone injury (RIBI) after stereotactic lung radiotherapy. Radiat Oncol 7:159
Turrisi AT, Kim K, Blum R et al (1999) Twice-daily compared with one-daily thoracic radiotherapy in limited small cell lung cancer treated concurrently with cisplatin and etoposide. N Engl J Med 340:265–271
van der Meij BS, Phernambucq EC, Fieten GM et al (2011) Nutrition during trimodality treatment in stage III non-small cell lung cancer: not only important for underweight patients. J Thorac Oncol 6:1563–1568
Vujaskovic Z, Groen HJ (2000) TGF-beta, radiation-induced pulmonary injury and lung cancer. Int J Radiat Biol 76:511–516
Warde P, Payne D (1992) Does thoracic irradiation improve survival and local control in limited-stage small-cell carcinoma of the lung? A meta-analysis. J Clin Oncol 10:890–895
Watine J (1998) Further comments on a practical prognostic index for inoperable non-small-cell lung cancer: a clinical biologist's point of view. J Cancer Res Clin Oncol 124:581–583
Werner-Wasik M, Scott C, Graham ML et al (1999) Interfraction interval does not affect survival of patients with non-small cell lung cancer treated with chemotherapy and/or hyperfractionated radiotherapy: a multivariate analysis of 1076 RTOG patients. Int J Radiat Oncol Biol Phys 44:327–331
Werner-Wasik M, Scott C, Cox JD et al (2000a) Recursive portioning analysis of 1999 Radiation Therapy Oncology Group (RTOG) patients with locally-advanced non-small-cell lung cancer (LA-NSCLC): identification of five groups with different survival. Int J Radiat Oncol Biol Phys 48:1475–1482
Werner-Wasik M, Pequignot E, Leeper D et al (2000b) Predictors of severe esophagitis include use of concurrent chemotherapy, but not the length of irradiated esophagus: a multivariate analysis of patients with lung cancer with nonoperative therapy. Int J Radiat Oncol Biol Phys 48:689–696
Woel RT, Munley MT, Hollis D et al (2002) The time course of radiation therapy-induced reductions in regional perfusion: a prospective study with >5 years of follow-up. Int J Radiat Oncol Biol Phys 52:58–67
Wolf M, Holle R, Hans K et al (1991) Analysis of prognostic factors in 766 patients with small cell lung cancer (SCLC): the role of sex as a predictor for survival. Br J Cancer 63:986–992
Work E, Nielson OS, Bentzen SM et al (1997) Randomized study of initial versus late chest irradiation combined with chemotherapy in limited-stage small-cell lung cancer. J Clin Oncol 15:3030–3037
Würschmidt F, Bünemann H, Heilmann HP (1995) Small cell lung cancer with and without vena cava syndrome: a multivariate analysis of prognostic factors in 408 cases. Int J Radiat Oncol Biol Phys 33:77–82
Yamada M, Kudoh S, Hirata K et al (1998) Risk factors of pneumonitis following chemoradiotherapy for lung cancer. Eur J Cancer 34:71–75
Yamada K, Soejima T, Ota Y et al (2003) Radiotherapy for medically inoperable non-small cell lung cancer at clinical stage I and II. Tumori 89:75–79
Yee D, Butts C, Reiman A et al (2012) Clinical trial of post-chemotherapy consolidation thoracic radiotherapy for extensive-stage small cell lung cancer. Radiother Oncol 102:234–238
Yip D, Harper PG (2000) Predictive and prognostic factors in small cell lung cancer: current status. Lung Cancer 28:173–185
Zhang HX, Yin WB, Zhang LJ et al (1989) Curative radiotherapy of early operable non-small cell lung cancer. Radiother Oncol 14:89–94
Zhao L, West BT, Hayman JA et al (2007) High radiation dose may reduce negative effect of large gross tumor volume in patients with medically inoperable early-stage non-small-cell lung cancer. Int J Radiat Oncol Biol Phys 68:103–110
Zhu H, Zhou Z, Wang Y et al (2011) Thoracic radiation therapy improves the overall survival of patients with extensive-stage small cell lung cancer with distant metastasis. Cancer 117:5423–5431

Esophageal Cancer

Robert L. Eil, F. E. M. Voncken, J. Torres-Roca, and Charles R. Thomas Jr.

Contents

R. L. Eil
Department of Surgery,
Oregon Health & Science University,
3181 SW Sam Jackson Park Road,
Portland, OR 97239, USA

F. E. M. Voncken
Department of Radiotherapy,
The Netherlands Cancer Institute-Antoni
van Leeuwenhoek Hospital, Plesmanlaan 121,
1066 CX, Amsterdam, Netherlands

J. Torres-Roca
Department of Radiation Oncology,
H Lee Moffitt Cancer Center,
12902 USF Magnolia Dr,
Tampa, FL 33612, USA

C. R. Thomas Jr. (✉)
Department Radiation Medicine,
Oregon Health & Science University,
3181 SW Sam Jackson Park Road,
Portland, OR 97239, USA
e-mail: thomasch@ohsu.edu

Abstract

Despite ongoing advances, the vast majority of those afflicted with esophageal cancer go on to die of their disease. While some respond notably to chemoradiotherapy, others-with seemingly similar disease characteristics based on existing clinical assays-have a limited or absent response. The current climate is suitable for the development of predictive tools and novel methods of evaluation to aid in individualised patient treatment planning. In the preoperative setting our clinical staging and varied imaging modalities, although imperfect are used to determine which patients will likely receive from chemoradiotherapy. No permutation of the data currently available can predict, with a satisfactory accuracy, whether an individual patient will have a substantial response to neoadjuvant treatment with minimal morbidity. Potentially, the addition of molecular assays in tandem with standardization of radiologic data will allow the development of increasingly powerful tools to predict the likelihood of response to treatment without complication for an individual patient.

1 Introduction

Esophageal cancer is a significant worldwide health problem, of which the incidence in the USA and Western Europe is rapidly increasing (Holmes and Vaughan 2007;

C. Nieder and L. E. Gaspar (eds.), *Decision Tools for Radiation Oncology*, Medical Radiology. Radiation Oncology,
DOI: 10.1007/174_2013_919, © Springer-Verlag Berlin Heidelberg 2013
Published Online: 19 October 2013

Siegel et al. 2012). Patients frequently present with advanced stage disease, poor performance status, and have a poor prognosis. Over recent years, the addition of neoadjuvant chemoradiotherapy (CRT) to surgery has improved 5-year survival probability from 34 % for patients treated with surgery alone to 47 % for patients treated with chemoradiotherapy and surgery (van Hagen et al. 2012).

However, responses to neoadjuvant treatment vary, with heterogeneous responses for patients with similar clinical stage. If neoadjuvant treatment produces a pathologically complete response (pCR), outcomes are better: patients with a pCR can expect a 5-year survival rate of 48 vs. 18 % for non-responding patients (Berger et al. 2005).

Without the benefit of knowing the pathologic stage, it is difficult to select patients who will benefit from this aggressive treatment. So far, three characteristics on which prediction can be based have been identified: clinical factors, biomarkers, and imaging modalities. While these last two are promising, at this current time no combination of available clinical data is reliable enough to indicate which patients are going to have a robust response to CRT and benefit from esophagectomy, and which should be treated with only selected modalities. Thus, traditional clinical factors such as tumor stage, age and performance status are still used to select the best therapy for a particular patient.

With regard to biomarkers, new strategies for subdividing esophageal cancer patients into prognostic groups may result in patients being selected for CRT or not on the basis of molecular assays, in addition to the 'traditional' methods of stage and imaging modalities. While these markers are promising, the exact clinical setting in which biomarkers will routinely be of utility in guiding treatment has yet to be defined.

The third characteristic, imaging, involves the use of modalities such as endoscopic ultrasound (EUS), computed tomography (CT), positron emission tomography (PET)-CT and magnetic resonance imaging (MRI). As a group, the information these assays provide continues to play an important role in staging and re-staging and thus in patient selection for CRT.

Combining these clinical data allows for our growing field of interest, where prognostic models and nomograms attempt to predict individual prognosis and response to CRT, with the potential to individualize treatment and isolate high-risk groups for novel treatments.

The above patient and tumor characteristics are the main basis upon which multidisciplinary treatment plans are made. In this chapter we review these decision tools and their implications for prognosis, treatment response and toxicity in the progressively individualized treatment of esophageal cancer.

2 Prognosis and Treatment Response

2.1 Disease Characteristics

Currently, no single clinical parameter can be used to predict which patients will achieve a pathological complete response (pCR) following CRT or survive their disease. However, there are several clinical and oncologic factors that have consistently proven to be significantly associated with outcome.

2.1.1 Patient Characteristics

Several patient-related factors are associated with survival and response to CRT. Factors as AJCC stage, male gender, performance status, location of the tumor, high lifetime alcohol consumption, forced expiratory volume in 1 s (FEV1), number of involved lymph nodes and cigarette smoking are independent predictors of survival (Thrift et al. 2012; Situ et al. 2012). Parameters as gender, tumor grade, baseline EUS T-stage and histology are related to a pCR (Ajani et al. 2012). Achievement of pCR or any tumor response corresponds with better overall survival (Berger et al. 2005).

2.1.2 Histologic Characteristics

Histology of the tumor is an important differentiating factor, as the response at treatment differs substantially between adenocarcinomas and squamous cell carcinomas (SCC) (Rizk et al. 2007; Heath et al. 2000; Urba et al. 2001; Burmeister et al. 2005). Squamous cell carcinomas have a much higher likelihood to achieve a pCR than adenocarcinomas: a pCR in adenocarcinomas occurs in 20–30 % whereas for SCC, pCR occurs in up to 50 % of the patients (van Hagen et al. 2012). Although in general, achievement of a pCR is commonly associated with improved survival (Berger et al. 2005), this does not apply to SCC patients, since a higher rate of pCR for SCC patients does not seem to translate into better overall outcomes. Additionally, it is worth noting that while patients that have a pCR do have better prognosis when compared to all other patients with remaining invasive disease, a significant number of patients will succumb to their disease, with almost indistinguishable OS when compared to patients with stage I (Rizk et al. 2007). If one desires to predict which patients can safely go on to esophageal salvage following CRT, novel prognostic assays and use of the currently available data is required.

Histologic grade is a predictor for a pCR, long-term outcome (Ajani et al. 2012), and is implemented in initial staging for differentiating prognostic groups. However, with increasing use of neoadjuvant therapy, this grading is solely based on endoscopic biopsy. With the accuracy of grade assessment on biopsy being only 73 %, it should be interpreted with caution (Dikken et al. 2012).

2.2 Staging Systems

Esophageal cancer staging has an important role in selecting patients for the appropriate treatment strategy and is related with long-term outcomes (Talsma et al. 2012). The TNM staging system of the American Joint Committee on Cancer (AJCC) and the International Union Against Cancer (UICC) for esophageal cancer is used universally and was recently revised. A major change between the 2002 (Union Internationale Contre le Cancer 2002) and the 2010 (Rice et al. 2010) editions were the development of separate stage groupings according to histology and a better description of the tumors located at the esophagogastric junction (EGJ) (Tables 1, 2, 3 and 4).

These tumors, at the esophagogastric junction (EGJ) and proximal 5 cm of the stomach that extend into the EGJ or esophagus, are staged as esophageal cancers (Table 5). While all other tumors with an epicenter in the stomach >5 cm from the EGJ, or those within 5 cm of the EGJ without extension into the esophagus are staged as gastric cancers. A sub classification of these junctional tumors can be made by the classification described by Siewert and Stein (1998) (Table 6).

A validation study of this 7th edition of the UICC-AJCC staging system was performed by Talsma et al., which showed for surgical esophageal cancer patients that the 7th edition of staging provided more accurate prognostic stratification for OS in comparison to the 6th edition (Talsma et al. 2012).

Table 1 TNM staging of esophageal squamous cell cancer (SCC) UICC-AJCC 7th edition (Rice et al. 2010)

Primary tumor (T)	
TX	Primary tumor cannot be assessed
T0	No evidence of primary tumor
Tis	High-grade dysplasia (HGD)
T1	Tumor invades lamina propria, muscularis mucosae, or submucosa
T1a	Tumor invades lamina propria or muscularis mucosae
T1b	Tumor invades submucosa
T2	Tumor invades muscularis propria
T3	Tumor invades adventitia
T4	Tumor invades adjacent structures
T4a	Resectable tumor invading pleura, pericardium, or diaphragm
T4b	Unresectable tumor invading other adjacent structures, such as aorta, vertebral body, trachea, etc.
Regional lymph nodes (N)	
NX	Regional lymph node(s) cannot be assessed
N0	No regional lymph node metastasis
N1	Metastasis in 1–2 regional lymph nodes
N2	Metastasis in 3–6 regional lymph nodes
N3	Metastasis in seven or more regional lymph nodes
Distant metastasis (M)	
M0	No distant metastasis
M1	Distant metastasis
Histologic grade (G)	
GX	Grade cannot be assessed—stage grouping as G1
G1	Well differentiated
G2	Moderately differentiated
G3	Poorly differentiated
G4	Undifferentiated—stage grouping as G3 squamous

2.3 Imaging

Imaging modalities as EUS, CT, PET-CT and MRI currently play an important role in staging and in patient selection before CRT. They may also be utilized for post CRT clinical re-staging (ycTNM) after induction treatment or response monitoring during treatment, however the results should be interpreted with caution in this setting (Ribeiro et al. 2006). During these different phases of the patient care some have attempted to identify a distinctive role for each modality.

2.3.1 EUS

2.3.1.1 Staging

Endoscopic ultrasound (EUS) uses a high frequency ultrasound transducer to obtain detailed images of the tumor mass and the relationship with the five-layered structure of the esophageal wall. EUS attempts to provide measurements of tumor thickness and is regularly used to estimate tumor extension in initial staging for esophageal cancer (Ribeiro et al. 2006). The discriminatory power for distinguishing between early stage tumors and those with deeper invasion may approach 80–90 %. Some have found this gross distinction prognostic in identifying those patients at risk for a positive circumferential resection margin (CRM), if treated with isolated surgery (Reid et al. 2012). However, its exact TNM accuracy is the least prognostic of available clinical information in predicting pre operative stage (Reid et al. 2012; van Vliet et al. 2008; Thosani et al. 2012).

While, EUS remains a frequently used clinical estimate of primary tumor staging, there are technical limitations to its ubiquitous use. Not all patients are capable of receiving a complete EUS due to esophageal stenosis. Additionally, the accuracy of EUS is operator dependent and is subject to a

Table 2 Prognostic groups by TNM stage/anatomic stage for squamous cell carcinoma UICC-AJCC 7th edition (Rice et al. 2010)

Anatomic stage/prognostic groups					
Squamous cell carcinoma					
Stage	T	N	M	Grade	Tumor location
0	Tis (HGD)	N0	M0	1, X	Any
IA	T1	N0	M0	1, X	Any
IB	T1	N0	M0	2–3	Any
	T2–3	N0	M0	1, X	Lower, X
IIA	T2–3	N0	M0	1, X	Upper, middle
	T2–3	N0	M0	2–3	Lower, X
IIB	T2–3	N0	M0	2–3	Upper, middle
	T1–2	N1	M0	Any	Any
IIIA	T1–2	N2	M0	Any	Any
	T3	N1	M0	Any	Any
	T4a	N0	M0	Any	Any
IIIB	T3	N2	M0	Any	Any
IIIC	T4a	N1–2	M0	Any	Any
	T4b	Any	M0	Any	Any
	Any	N3	M0	Any	Any
IV	Any	Any	M1	Any	Any

learning curve (Fockens et al. 1996). Ultimately, preoperative staging of lymph node status is challenging. A recently proposed tool from Gaur et al. (2010) for predicting pathologic lymph node involvement based on clinical information is discussed in further detail below in Nomograms and Predictive models section.

2.3.1.2 Re-staging

For response evaluation, EUS continues to be used as the primary diagnostic modality. However, the accuracy of EUS restaging varies significantly across several recent retrospective analyses (Ribeiro et al. 2006; Giovannini et al. 1997; Chak et al. 2000).

Different methods have been proposed for response assessment with EUS. The first method is to restage according to the TNM staging system (Fockens et al. 1996), second method is to measure the relative reduction in thickness of the tumor (Gaur et al. 2010; Giovannini et al. 1997) and a third method is to measure the relative tumor shrinkage at the maximum cross-sectional area (MCSA) (Gaur et al. 2010; Chak et al. 2000). However, with these different methods the accuracy is still poor and ranges from 17 to 59 % (Sloof 2006; Hirata et al. 1997; Zuccaro et al. 1999; Bowrey et al. 1999). Even when a EUS is combined with biopsy, the accuracy does not exceed 31 % to correctly predict a pCR (Sarkaria et al. 2009). Of patients that have a negative biopsy on restaging endoscopy (cCR) less than 30 % will have a pCR (Sarkaria et al. 2009).

Table 3 TNM staging of esophageal and esophagogastric junction (EGJ) adenocarcinoma UICC-AJCC 7th edition (Rice et al. 2010)

Primary tumor (T)	
TX	Primary tumor cannot be assessed
T0	No evidence of primary tumor
Tis	High-grade dysplasia (HGD)
T1	Tumor invades lamina propria, muscularis mucosae, or submucosa
T1a	Tumor invades lamina propria or muscularis mucosae
T1b	Tumor invades submucosa
T2	Tumor invades muscularis propria
T3	Tumor invades adventitia
T4	Tumor invades adjacent structures
T4a	Resectable tumor invading pleura, pericardium, or diaphragm
T4b	Unresectable tumor invading other adjacent structures, such as aorta, vertebral body, trachea, etc.
Regional lymph nodes (N)	
NX	Regional lymph node(s) cannot be assessed
N0	No regional lymph node metastasis
N1	Metastasis in 1–2 regional lymph nodes
N2	Metastasis in 3–6 regional lymph nodes
N3	Metastasis in seven or more regional lymph nodes
Distant metastasis (M)	
M0	No distant metastasis
M1	Distant metastasis
Histologic grade (*G*)	
GX	Grade cannot be assessed—stage grouping as G1
G1	Well differentiated
G2	Moderately differentiated
G3	Poorly differentiated
G4	Undifferentiated—stage grouping as G3 squamous

A possible explanation for this discrepancy between endoscopic staging and subsequent pathologic staging is that EUS may not be able to differentiate between post-treatment inflammation or fibrosis and residual tumor (Jamil et al. 2008).

2.3.2 CT

2.3.2.1 Staging

Computed tomography (CT) is usually one of the first steps in staging esophageal cancer patients and is used to evaluate the region of the primary tumor and evaluate for distant metastases. However, the accuracy for locoregional staging is limited. Accuracy for tumor staging has been reported with a range of 42 68 % (Lowe et al. 2005; Wu et al. 2003) and for regional lymph node metastases the pooled sensitivity and specificity is only 0.50 (95 % C.I. 0.41–0.6)

Table 4 Prognostic groups by TNM stage/anatomic stage for adenocarcinoma UICC-AJCC 7th edition (Rice et al. 2010)

Anatomic stage/prognostic groups				
Adenocarcinoma carcinoma				
Stage	T	N	M	Grade
0	Tis (HGD)	N0	M0	1, X
IA	T1	N0	M0	1–2, X
IB	T1	N0	M0	3
	T2	N0	M0	1–2, X
IIA	T2	N0	M0	3
IIB	T3	N0	M0	Any
	T1–2	N1	M0	Any
IIIA	T1–2	N2	M0	Any
	T3	N1	M0	Any
	T4a	N0	M0	Any
IIIB	T3	N2	M0	Any
IIIC	T4a	N1–2	M0	Any
	T4b	Any	M0	Any
	Any	N3	M0	Any
IV	Any	Any	M1	Any

Table 5 Primary site of esophageal cancer based on proximal edge of tumor according to the UICC-AJCC 7th edition (Rice et al. 2010)

Anatomic name	Esophageal location	Anatomic boundaries	Endoscopic distance from incisors
Cervical	Upper	Hypopharynx to sternal notch	15 to <20 cm
Thoracic	Upper	Sternal notch to azygos vein	20 to <25 cm
	Middle	Lower border of azygos vein to inferior pulmonary vein	25 to <30 cm
	Lower	Lower border of inferior pulmonary vein to esophagogastric junction	30 to <40 cm
Abdominal	Lower	Esophagogastric junction to 5 cm below esophagogastric junction	40–45 cm
	Esophagogastric junction/cardia	Esophagogastric junction to 5 cm below esophagogastric junction	40–45 cm

Table 6 Siewert classification (Siewert and Stein 1998)

Type	Description
Type I	Located between 5 and 1 cm proximal to the anatomical cardia. Adenocarcinoma of the distal esophagus that usually arises from an area with specialized intestinal metaplasia
Type II	Located between 1 cm proximal and 2 cm distal to the anatomical cardia. True carcinoma of the cardia arising from the cardiac epithelium or short segments with intestinal metaplasia
Type III	Located between 2 and 5 cm distal to the anatomical cardia. Subcardial gastric carcinoma that infiltrates the EGJ and distal esophagus from below

(van Vliet et al. 2008). Also, when used for screening for distant metastases CT-scans have difficulty recognizing small distant metastases, while a PET-CT is more sensitive (van Vliet et al. 2008).

2.3.2.2 Re-staging

CT scan is the most commonly used diagnostic modality in monitoring response of nonsurgical therapy for solid tumors. For esophageal cancer restaging, however, its role remains ambiguous. CT gives good visualization of the tumor bulk in majority of the patients. However, when tumor shrinkage is correlated to pathological response following neoadjuvant treatment some have found a clear correlation (Swisher et al. 2004; Voncken et al. 2012), while others failed (Griffith et al. 1999; Jones et al. 1999).

This difference could be due to an overestimation of edema, inflammation and fibrosis for residual tumor (Westerterp et al. 2005). While, CT remains one of many modalities in re-staging after induction treatment, primary tumor response should be interpreted with caution.

2.3.3 PET

FDG-PET is a nuclear imaging modality that evaluates tumor physiology and allows for a quantitative functional assessment of the primary via the standardized uptake value (SUV). Nearly all primary esophageal cancers have high levels of cellular metabolism, increased glycolysis, and an increased number of glucose transporters. In almost all cases, SCC primary tumors have a high uptake of FDG. In adenocarcinomas this FDG accumulation is more variable, with a minority (6 %) of the tumors being non-avid, usually the mucous containing and poorly differentiated tumor types or tumors too small to detect (<5 mm) by FDG-PET (Wagner et al. 2009; Stahl et al. 2003; Wong and Chambers 2008).

2.3.3.1 Staging

FDG-PET can provide information in initial staging, especially for finding regional nodal metastases and silent distant metastases, where it has a role in selecting patients that will benefit from neoadjuvant CRT. In addition, FDG-PET can contribute to localization, size measurement and GTV definition of the primary tumor and lymph nodes (Katsoulis et al. 2007).

2.3.3.2 Restaging

PET-CT provides several pieces of clinically relevant information in restaging after induction treatment. A PET-CT can detect occult metastases after induction treatment and thus saving patients from undergoing a non-curative esophagectomy. A PET-CT after induction treatment detects metastases in 8 % of patients with a consequent adjustment in therapeutic plan (Bruzzi et al. 2007).

An additional advantage of response monitoring with PET-CT is the prognostic value in the decrease, or lack there of, in SUV of the primary tumor. While a PET-directed therapy does have the potential to change clinical practice and improve outcomes, it cannot currently be considered a standard approach in isolation. Standardization of quantitative results across facilities continues to be a technical roadblock. Several methods have been proposed as standard procedure for metabolic response analysis using the standard uptake value (SUV) as a semi quantitative measure of FDG uptake. Proposed methods are: SUV pre-treatment, SUV after chemoradiation, percentage of decline of SUV, attainment of a metabolic complete response after chemoradiation and to show an early metabolic response 14 days after start of chemoradiation.

These different methods were analyzed in a systematic review of Omloo et al. evaluating 31 studies (Omloo et al. 2011). Fifteen of these studies tested the pretreatment FDG uptake as a predictive factor. On univariate analysis, SUV was a predictor of survival in 12 out of 15 studies and multivariate analysis showed only in two out of eight studies that SUV was an independent predictor of survival. SUV decrease after completion of neoadjuvant treatment was predictive in only two out of six studies. Finally, there were six studies looking at the SUV decrease and prognosis early during neoadjuvant therapy. SUV decrease was a predictor of response in all of these six studies and a predictor of survival in five of these six studies.

Comparative analysis across FDG-PET articles is challenging due the non-standardization of the image acquisition process and subsequent analytic thresholds. Since the methodology for image acquisition varies, the SUV threshold to predict prognosis varies significantly between analyses (from 3 to 10.5) and cutoff values for amount of SUV change differentiating responders from non-responders also varies depending on the publication (from −30 to −70 %) (Omloo et al. 2011). This illustrates the difficulty to translate these results to clinical practice, although the field of treatment stands to benefit from an adequately powered prospective trial evaluating the true relevance of early SUV decline during CRT. In conclusion, early SUV response assessment holds promise to potentially guide ongoing treatment, but the implementation and technical applicability have not yet developed to the extent required to find a clinical role for routine use.

2.3.4 MRI

The recent development of functional MRI imaging has opened a new window of opportunities for staging esophageal tumors, monitoring response to treatment and potentially even predicting biological behavior (Chang 2009; Riddell et al. 2007). Esophageal imaging with MRI has some technological challenges due to local cardiorespiratory motion artifact. However, with an accurately tuned sequence accurate images can be acquired.

For staging the esophageal tumor, EUS is the modality of first choice, however for 6 % of newly diagnosed patients, EUS is not possible due to a narrowing of the esophageal lumen and subsequent inability to pass the endoscope. CT is less accurate in differentiating depth of tumor invasion, thus for staging those patients, MRI could be an alternative (Riddell et al. 2007).

Staging the depth of tumor growth with MRI has an accuracy of about 60 % (Jamil et al. 2008), but with the MRI technique still under development, imaging reaches a higher level of precision, however this has not yet been correlated with accuracy of overall stage (Riddell et al. 2007). MRI cannot differentiate each layer of the esophageal wall, therefore an alternative T differentiation standard is described by Botet et al. (1991) and by Riddell et al. (2007) (Table 7).

Recently developed MRI techniques such as diffusion weighted imaging (DWI) and dynamic contrast-enhanced (DCE) MRI may provide a relative increased accuracy in clinical staging and response assessment of esophageal tumors.

In diffusion-weighted magnetic resonance imaging (DWI) each voxel reflects the amount of water diffusion at that location. This diffusion process can be quantified by measuring the apparent diffusion coefficients (ADCs) of a voxel. ADC measurements have been suggested for staging or as predictive markers. However, its role for staging looks not as promising as its role as a predictor (Sakurada et al. 2009; Aoyagi et al. 2011). Further investigation is warranted to determine the exact role of DWI.

Dynamic contrast enhanced (DCE-) MRI has the ability to show alterations of vascular integrity that result from pathologic angiogenesis. Esophageal cancer is associated with a higher vascularization and an increase in vascular density, compared with normal esophageal tissue. In DCE-MRI, after a bolus of gadolinium chelate is administered intravenously, flow signal and leak can be observed. Two parameters are of importance, the contrast reagent transfer

Table 7 Radiographic staging criteria as described by Botet et al. (1991) and Riddell et al. (2007)

	Staging according to Botet	MRI features defined by Riddell
T stage		
T1	Thickening less than 5 mm	No discernable tumor
T2	Thickening of the wall greater than 5 mm and less than 15 mm	Intermediate signal intensity within the high signal submucosa and muscularis propria (low signal). Low signal outer margin of muscularis propria clearly defined and remains intact
T3	Thickening of the wall greater than 15 mm with irregularity of the outer margin	Nodular irregularity of the outer margin of the muscularis propria. Intermediate signal intensity nodules extending from the esophageal wall into the peri-esophageal tissues
T4	Tumor invasion of adjacent structures such as the trachea, aortic pericardium, or vertebral body	Intermediate signal intensity tumor extending into adjacent structures. Loss of a high signal fat plane between intermediate signal intensity tumor and an adjacent structure
N stage		
N0	Lymph nodes less than 10 mm in diameter were considered benign nodes	Uniform high signal intensity returned from peri-esophageal tissues
N1	Lymph nodes greater than 10 mm in short axis diameter were considered abnormal	Nodular intermediate signal intensity nodules >2 mm in size within the peri-esophageal tissues

between plasma and interstitial space (Ktrans) and the volume fraction of the interstitial space (Ve). These parameters can help distinguishing normal tissue from tumor tissue. DCE-MRI could have a role in the staging phase as it distinguishes histologic subtypes (Oberholzer et al. 2008). But it also perceives tumor microvascular density changes during chemoradiotherapy and can be imaged by DCE-MRI signal (Chang et al. 2008). Therefore, for monitoring response following CRT it holds the most promise.

2.3.5 Molecular Markers/Signatures

2.3.5.1 Background

Concurrent chemoradiation with or without surgery is commonly utilized as primary management of patients with non-metastatic disease. However, there is significant heterogeneity of response, suggesting that there are subpopulations that derive differential treatment benefit from RT. For example, approximately 30 % of patients experience a complete pathological response (Berger et al. 2005; Donahue et al. 2009). A molecular diagnostic that can identify these patients could be utilized clinically to avoid surgery for these patients. In contrast for patients that are predicted to be less responsive to RT, their management could be impacted by either offering RT dose intensification and/or prioritization of surgery (without RT).

At its most basic, a molecular signature is a collection of features that attempt to explain a complex phenotype. While a single predictive molecular marker would be ideal, such an isolated predictor of response to therapy in esophageal cancer has not been documented. In lieu of such a discovery, the technique of combining multiple analytes provides an opportunity to develop a predictive molecular assay; there continue to be a relatively small number of molecular signatures that are routinely part of clinical practice.

2.3.5.2 Molecular Signature Development

Developing a molecular signature typically involves two steps. In the first step, features (genes, proteins, microRNAs etc.) are selected that define the phenotype of interest (i.e. responders to radiation therapy). Once the features are selected then an algorithm is generated to predict the phenotype in an unknown sample. A classic approach is to use samples in a dataset as a "training set" to identify the features and develop the signature. Once the signature is developed, its predictive accuracy is tested on a validation set, ideally independent of the training set. A significant problem in the field of molecular signatures has been their inherent dependence on the "training set" and thus a lack of robust validation analysis (Watanabe et al. 2006; Dalton and Friend 2006).

2.3.5.3 Radiation Therapy Molecular Signatures

The majority of molecular signatures in the literature have been developed to describe disease prognosis (independent of treatment), molecular subtypes and/or response prediction to chemotherapy. However, two independent groups have developed RT-specific signatures that have considerable clinical validation. Weichselbaum and colleagues developed an interferon-related gene signature for DNA damage, which was independently validated as a predictor of adjuvant chemotherapy efficacy and for local–regional control after RT in breast cancer (Weichselbaum et al. 2008). Separately, Eschrich and colleagues utilized a systems biology approach to identify a molecular signature of intrinsic tumor radiosensitivity (Eschrich et al. 2009a, b). Using ten specific genes they modeled a radiosensitivity index (RSI) that has been independently validated in multiple disease sites (rectal, esophagus, head and neck, breast) in over 1,000 patients. Of the two signatures, RSI has been validated in a small dataset of esophageal cancer patients (n = 12). The predicted RSI was significantly different in responders (R) vs. nonresponders (NR) in esophageal (RSI R vs. NR 0.37 vs. 0.50, p = 0.05). A low RSI value is consistent with a more radiosensitive tumor. The range of RSI values for 7 responders was 0.11–0.53 and for 5 nonresponders was 0.46–0.54. Therefore it is possible that this signature can be adjusted to support specific clinical decisions to improve clinical care for esophageal cancer patients.

2.3.5.4 Clinical Applications for an RT Molecular Signature in Esophageal Cancer

A challenge to the development of a clinically relevant radiosensitivity molecular signature stems from RT's broad applicability as a therapeutic agent in cancer. Since RT is used in different settings depending on disease site, the clinical utility of the signature would vary depending on the clinical application. A requirement for any signature that is to be applied routinely in the clinic is the development of a standardized and reliable process for tissue acquisition, processing, RNA isolation and gene expression measurement. Recently, the National Cancer Institute selected RSI for commercial development through the recently created Clinical Assay Development Program (CADP). The purpose of the project is the development of an analytically validated, commercial-grade diagnostic platform for RSI that will be ready for testing in clinical trials.

There remains significant opportunity to improve the clinical outcomes for esophageal cancer patients by identifying biological sub-populations that will derive differential treatment benefit from RT. Tailoring RT to fit a particular molecular RT profile will lead to the development of biology-based radiation oncology and result in better RT utilization.

3 Toxicity

The evolution of treatment for locally advanced esophageal cancer from single-modality surgery or radiotherapy to multimodality therapy has resulted in improved outcomes. Unfortunately, CRT comes with a potential increase in toxicity and resultant detriment to a patient's short-term quality of life (van Meerten et al. 2008).

The risks vs. benefits of the treatment are decisive in patient's decision to receive CRT. To make a well-considered decision, patients should be counseled before start of treatment about the potential toxicities. We give an overview of potential risks and toxicities for patients receiving multimodality treatment or single modality radiotherapy. We provide parameters, where available, that predict toxicity.

Among the many challenges with estimating toxicity risk based on the available publications, is that toxicity scoring systems are not uniform—making direct comparison impossible. The most frequently used scoring systems for toxicity are the Common Terminology Criteria for Adverse Events (CTCAE) (Trotti et al. 2003) of the National Cancer Institute (NCI) and the toxicity criteria from the Radiation Therapy Oncology Group (RTOG) system.

3.1 Esophagitis

The most common acute and late toxicity, excluding fatigue, for esophageal cancer patients treated with (chemo-) radiotherapy is, as expected, esophagitis.

3.1.1 Acute Esophagitis

Radiation induced acute esophagitis presents as dysphagia with resultant malnutrition and dehydration, requiring nutritional support (enteral or parenteral) in 17–35 % of the patients (Ahn et al. 2005).

The incidence of acute esophagitis (any grade) ranges from 19 to 79 % and grade $\geq$3 esophagitis is reported in 1–43 % of patients. This broad scale of the reported esophagitis depends, primarily, on the differences in toxicity reporting and definition. Other potential risk factors for esophagitis include dose schedules and treated volume of the esophagus. Finally, the incidence of esophagitis increases with the addition of chemotherapy to radiotherapy and may vary depending on the chemotherapy schedule given (Meluch et al. 2003; Urba et al. 2003; van Meerten et al. 2006; Cooper et al. 1999; Ajani et al. 2008).

3.1.2 Late Esophageal Toxicity

Late esophagitis can present as dysphagia, stricture, necrosis or fistula of the esophagus. The incidence rates of this late toxicity are mainly based on definitive chemoradiation studies. Late esophageal toxicity of any grade occurs in about 35 % of the patients and a grade $\geq$3 late esophageal toxicity has been seen in 8–21 % of the patients (Cooper et al. 1999).

The strongest predictor for late esophageal toxicity is the severity of acute esophagitis, as a result of consequential late effects. Other predicting parameters for esophageal toxicity are dosimetric.

3.1.3 Parameters Predicting Esophagitis

From lung cancer series we have learned several predicting parameters for acute and late esophageal toxicity. As described earlier, the strongest parameter is the severity of the acute toxicity, but other parameters are a combination of radiation dose and treated volume of the esophagus.

A number of dosimetric parameters have been developed in an effort to reduce the continuously distributed dose-volume histogram (DVH) to a few clinically relevant indices. These relevant indices include: the percent organ volume receiving at least a certain dose (V_{20Gy}, V_{30Gy}, V_{40Gy}); the surface area receiving at least a certain dose (SA_{20Gy}, SA_{30Gy}, SA_{40Gy}); the length of the esophagus included in the radiation field to a threshold dose ($LETT_{20Gy}$, $LETT_{30Gy}$, $LETT_{40Gy}$); the mean esophageal dose (MED), defined as the average dose to the esophagus; and the maximal dose, defined as the highest point-dose within the irradiated esophageal volume (Milano et al. 2007; Rose et al. 2009).

Rose et al. (2009) provided a clear review of 18 lung cancer studies reporting dosimetric parameters predicting esophagitis. They identified 83 unique dosimetric parameters, of which only 6 were evaluated in 5 or more studies that were significantly associated with radiation esophagitis: MED, V_{20Gy}, V_{30Gy}, V_{40Gy}, V_{45Gy} and V_{50Gy}. Correlation was found for acute radiation esophagitis with MED, V_{20Gy}, V_{30Gy}, V_{40Gy} and V_{45Gy}. Correlation with the combined endpoint of acute and chronic radiation esophagitis was found with MED and V_{50Gy}. Logistic models relating DVH parameters to clinically significant acute esophagitis were identified.

For esophageal cancer, dosimetric predictors for esophagitis have not been reviewed with this precision and one could argue that these dosimetric predictors for esophagitis could be similar for esophageal cancer patients as for lung cancer patients. However, the etiology of esophageal cancer is different from lung cancer and the esophagus of esophageal cancer patients has been subjected to other treatment modalities and received greater inflammatory insult than the esophagus of lung cancer patients. Therefore it is not certain if the relatively normal esophagus of lung cancer patients is proportionally as sensitive to radiation damage and may not respond similarly. It may not be appropriate to extrapolate these dosimetric parameters to esophageal cancer patients.

3.2 Pneumonitis

Radiation pneumonitis (RP) is a major adverse event after thoracic irradiation. While the majority of patients with RP present with mild symptoms such as a dry cough, RP can result in severe morbidity and potential mortality.

Incidences of radiation pneumonitis grade ≥ 2 have been reported as high as 20–22 % (Hsu et al. 2009; Nomura et al. 2012) for esophageal cancer patients treated with definitive chemoradiation.

3.2.1 Parameters Predicting Pneumonitis

Predictive factors for RP have extensively been reported for irradiated lung cancer patients (Vogelius and Bentzen 2012), but there are only a few reports of esophageal cancer available (Hsu et al. 2009; Nomura et al. 2012; Wang et al. 2008; Asakura et al. 2010; Tucker et al. 2006). Predictive parameters for RP in lung cancer patients include clinical factors such as older age, disease located in mid-lower lung (Vogelius and Bentzen 2012), and dosimetric parameters such as mean lung dose (MLD) (Kwa et al. 1998), the percent of lung volume receiving at least 20 Gy (V_{20Gy}), 13 Gy (V_{13Gy}), 10 Gy (V_{10Gy}) or 5 Gy (V_{5Gy}) (Palma et al. 2012).

For esophageal cancer patients, predictors for pulmonary complications were studied on much smaller study cohorts and mainly on studies involving neoadjuvant chemoradiation and surgery. Pulmonary complications in these studies include both radiation pneumonitis as pneumonia, atelectasis, pleural effusion and pulmonary embolism. Significant predictors for pulmonary complications were the clinical parameters: stage IV, induction chemotherapy before CRT (Wang et al. 2006) and impaired pulmonary function (FEV1) before surgery, as well as the dosimetric parameters of mean lung dose, effective dose, V_{10Gy} and absolute volume of lung receiving <5 Gy were significant predictors for pulmonary complications.

Radiation oncologists have to balance all dosimetric and patient specific predictors for pulmonary complications of radiotherapy before approval of the treatment plan.

3.3 Hematologic Toxicity

Hematologic toxicity is the most common side effect in patients treated with chemotherapy. The severity of these adverse events depends on the chemotherapy regimen and number of cycles given.

Generally, these hematologic toxicities consist of neutropenia, anemia, and thrombocytopenia. As expected, regimens that use lower doses and fewer cycles report lower toxicity rates (Urba et al. 2001; Minsky et al. 2002; David 2008).

The most common regimens used are 5-fluorouracil (5-FU) and cisplatin based, but other regimens including carboplatin combined with paclitaxel are increasingly employed, likely due to better patient tolerance (van Hagen et al. 2012). Still, their remains a great variety of chemotherapeutic regimens, prescribed doses and number of cycles used.

In the studies that subdivide hematologic toxicity, the most common toxicity reported is neutropenia and with incidences of 9–78 % (van Hagen et al. 2012; Urba et al. 2001) with the highest incidence of myelotoxicity reported for triple agent chemotherapy regimens.

3.4 Cardiac Toxicity

The most common manifestation of late radiation injury to the heart is pericardial effusion, which may present as acute pericarditis, chronic pericardial effusion, or remain asymptomatic. Although myocardial damage is less frequent, it can result in severe toxicities, such as myocardial infarction.

From long term survivors of Hodgkin lymphoma and left sided breast cancer we have learned that radiation induced cardiac pathology leads to significant morbidity and mortality. With the overall survival of esophageal cancer patients improving, along with increasing numbers of long-term survivors, late cardiac toxicity becomes a growing concern.

In a study of 101 patients treated with definitive chemoradiation for esophageal cancer 28 % developed pericardial effusion and V_{30Gy} was found to be the only significant predictor (Wei et al. 2008). Incidence of cardiopulmonary toxicity has been reported as high as 29 % in elderly compared to 3 % for younger patients (Morota et al. 2009).

Myocardial perfusion defects were detected in 54 % of the esophageal cancer patients treated with radiotherapy compared to 16 % of patients treated with surgery alone, 42 % had mild inferior wall ischemia compared to 4 % of the surgery only group. The perfusion defects were related to the area of the heart receiving $\geq$45 Gy (Gayed et al. 2006).

Other dosimetric predictors for late symptomatic cardiac toxicity besides V_{30Gy}, V_{45Gy} are mean heart dose (MHD) $\geq$ 40 Gy (Hashimoto et al. 2008) and thresholds for toxicity defined as $V_{20Gy} \geq 70$ %, $V_{30Gy} \geq 65$ % and $V_{40Gy} \geq 60$ % of the cardiac volume (Konski et al. 2012). Important risk factors for development of symptomatic cardiac toxicity is advanced age and female gender.

Validation of these predictors is necessary before these parameters can be implemented as constraints in treatment planning.

3.5 Quality of Life

It is increasingly recognized that health-related quality of life (HRQoL) is a central and increasingly quantified clinical outcome measure in oncology. Quality of life outcomes are important in new treatment regimens under evaluation or intensified regimens with small benefits in long-term outcomes. In a group of 202 patients comparing multimodality treatment with surgery alone there was a negative impact in HRQoL before surgery but postoperatively the HRQoL was similar to those who had surgery alone (Reynolds et al. 2006). This temporary negative effect of the HRQoL confirmed by the results of van Meerten et all, where the HRQoL scores were restored or even improved 1 year postoperatively (van Meerten et al. 2006). Chemoradiotherapy has a temporary negative effect on the quality of life.

In conclusion, the use of multimodality therapy of esophageal cancer results in a significant negative impact in the short-term quality of life. However, this is a temporarily effect and 1 year after surgery the HRQoL was restored and similar for patients treated with multimodality and surgery-alone.

4 Treatment Technique

Over the past several decades there has been a tremendous evolution of technological advances in radiotherapy treatment planning. Although two dimensional treatment planning was once the standard of care, the implementation of the computed tomography (CT) to treatment planning has made 3D conformal radiation therapy (3D-CRT) possible. With better anatomical visualization and target delineation, this technique created the first step to sparing normal tissue.

Recently, this 'classic' 3D-CRT evolved to intensity-modulated radiotherapy (IMRT) using multiple beams, allowing more concave dose distributions around the target volume and therewith avoiding normal structures. IMRT plans improve target conformity and spares organs at risks when compared with 3D-CRT.

Volumetric-arc-therapy (VMAT) is the novel form of IMRT where intensity modulated radiation is delivered during one or more gantry arcs, with continuous variable beam aperture, variable dose rates and gantry speed modulation. This has advantages in terms of simplicity of optimization and fast delivery. This fast delivery results in a shorter beam-on time. Subsequently, with a VMAT plan, as compared to IMRT plan, there is a reduction of the amount of monitor units given of 20–67 % (Vivekanandan et al. 2012; Yin et al. 2012; Van Benthuysen et al. 2011). VMAT further reduces the dose to the heart and lungs and slightly improves the dose coverage to the PTV.

4.1 Parameters to Evaluate Treatment Plans of Different Techniques

Irradiation of esophageal cancer comes with the risk of significant toxicity, with the organs at risk being the heart, lung, esophagus and spinal cord. The aim of the implementation of these novel techniques is to reduce the toxicities to these organs while retaining or improving target coverage.

4.2 Heart

VMAT and IMRT treatment plans reduce the heart dose compared to 3D-CRT. When the parameter V_{30Gy} of the heart is measured, a significant reduction from 55 to 31 % with VMAT vs. 3DCRT (Hashimoto et al. 2008) is seen, for IMRT vs. 3DCRT this is from 61 to 24.8 % (Konski et al. 2012) and a reduction of 33.5 % in favor of VMAT over IMRT (Wei et al. 2008). This dosimetric parameter V_{30Gy} is correlated to symptomatic cardiac disease (Vogelius and Bentzen 2012) and a reduction of the dose to the heart should lead to a reduction in late cardiac toxicity. Long-term studies are necessary to determine the contribution of this dose reduction to the incidence and severity of cardiac toxicity.

4.3 Lung

A similar reduction is also seen for lung doses, where there is a general reduction of the dosimetric parameters (V_{10Gy}, V_{20Gy}, V_{30Gy}) (David 2008; Wei et al. 2008) when comparing VMAT to IMRT. However, there is a slight increase of the mean lung dose (MLD) of 2 % and an increase up to 13 % of the V_{5Gy} in thoracic esophageal tumors (Wei et al. 2008). How this reduction of the V_{20Gy} and increase of V_{5Gy} and MLD will affect pulmonary toxicity remains unclear.

A retrospective review compared 676 patients treated with 3DCRT and IMRT. Treatment modality IMRT (vs. 3DCRT), in addition to known prognostic factors as stage and performance status, was associated with overall survival, locoregional control and noncancer-related death (Lin et al. 2012).

IMRT and VMAT plans result in better target dose coverage, reduces doses to the heart and high dose volumes to the lung and potentially leads to better outcomes. VMAT reduces the amount of monitor units given, reduces the high dose to heart or lung even further, but slightly increases the low radiation dose to body or lungs.

5 Nomograms and Prognostic/Predictive Models

5.1 Goals of Predictive Models in Esophageal Cancer

Clinical prediction tools used in the management of esophageal cancer aim to estimate the likelihood of specified outcomes, both dichotomous and time to event data, based on relevant clinical variables. Particularly for esophageal cancer—due to its baseline poor survival and the high morbidity of the required medical intervention, accurate and applicable estimates of treatment outcomes are essential for medical decision-making, patient counseling, and clinical trial design. Recent randomized and appropriate powered clinical data demonstrates the survival benefit of neoadjuvant chemoradiotherapy (CRT) followed by esophagectomy rather than isolated esophagectomy for specified patient populations (Berger et al. 2005). However, in this investigation, similarly, groups were stratified based on TNM staging and a heterogeneous pathologic response to CRT was observed. The survival benefit observed within the advanced stage patients is not uniformly shared, concentrated within those patients that have a pathologic response and may be entirely absent for those with no observable downstaging.

Estimates of the survival benefit derived from CRT for a particular patient given their demographic information and oncologic staging can be an aid for patient education while aiding in medical decision making and potentially improving outcomes by employing therapies predicted to be the most beneficial for each patient. It is likely that the variables included in relevant decision tools will include data beyond classical TNM staging and may ultimately involve molecular markers and novel post treatment re-staging data (molecular and genetic markers were covered already in this chapter and will not be discussed in this subsection).

Standard pathologic TNM staging from the surgical specimen following neoadjuvant CRT (ypTNM) continues to be more prognostic of survival than any restaging or pre operative data—despite a, currently unpredictable, variable downstaging effect. A neoadjuvant treatment strategy makes estimating the survival benefit of chemoradiotherapy based on surgical stage difficult given that the final pathologic stage may not be the same as the stage at diagnosis. Concurrently, current techniques for clinical TNM staging and restaging techniques are unreliable.

Tools beyond predicting response and survival benefit to neoadjuvant CRT are required to model the risk for an individual patient undergoing or abstaining from some portion of trimodal therapy. Accurately predicting an individual patient's risk of morbidity and mortality from each treatment, particularly esophagectomy, will be an important tool in recommending an individualized treatment plan.

While nomograms are available for many of the aspects of esophageal cancer treatment mentioned above, careful examination of the data used, the covariates analyzed, and the patients included is required to avoid inappropriate application of a prediction tool to a specific patient. The general technical considerations of nomogram creation, propensity weighting, regression analysis, and data interpretation are covered separately in "Statistics of Survival Prediction and Nomogram Development" of this text and will not specifically be addressed here.

a

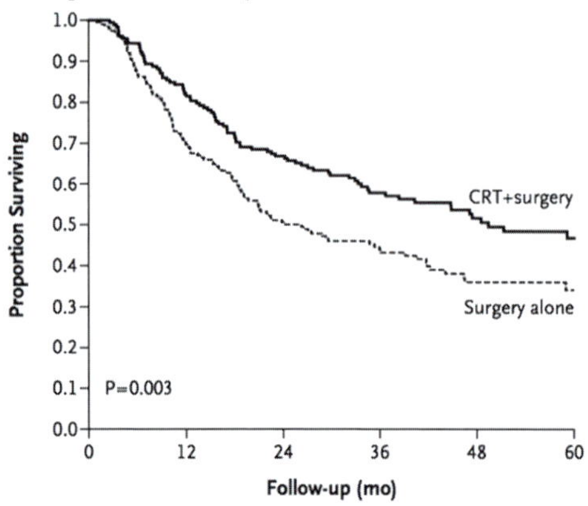

No. at Risk	0	12	24	36	48	60
CRT+surgery	178	145	119	75	49	28
Surgery alone	188	131	94	62	33	17
Total	366	276	213	137	82	45

b

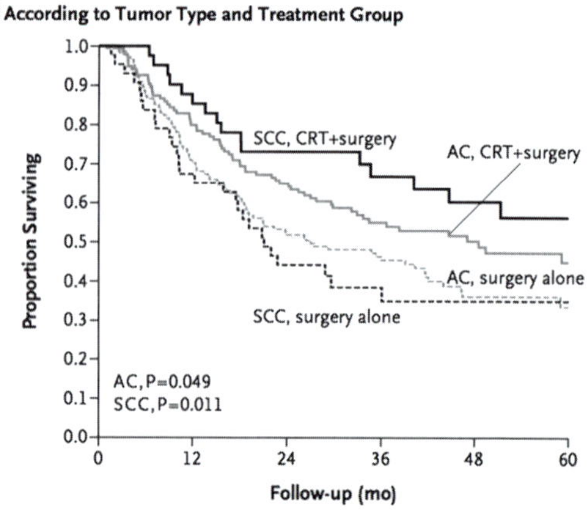

No. at Risk	0	12	24	36	48	60
AC, CRT+surgery	134	107	87	53	34	18
AC, surgery alone	141	99	73	50	25	10
SCC, CRT+surgery	41	35	30	21	15	8
SCC, surgery alone	43	29	19	11	8	4
Total	359	270	209	135	82	40

Fig. 1 Kaplan–Meier plots of estimated overall 5-year survival. **a** Scohows a Kaplan–Meier plot of the estimated overall 5-year survival among patients with esophageal or esophagogastric-junction cancer who underwent neo-adjuvant chemoradiotherapy (CRT) followed by surgery (178 patients) or surgery alone (188), acrding to an intention-to-treat analysis. **b** Shows a Kaplan–Meier plot of the estimated overall 5-year survival among the 134 patients with adenocarcinoma (AC) treated with neoadjuvant chemoradiotherapy followed by surgery and the 141 treated with surgery alone, and the 41 patients with squamous-cell carcinoma (SCC) treated with chemoradiotherapy followed by surgery and the 43 treated with surgery alone, according to an intention-to-treat analysis. Other tumor types were excluded from this analysis. Adapted from van Hagen et al. (2012)

5.2 Predicting Benefit from Neoadjuvant Chemoradiotherapy

Accurately predicting the benefit for a specific patient and evaluating the response to neoadjuvant treatment continues to a challenge and potential point of controversy. Although already discussed in this chapter, it is appropriate to again address the recent evidence supporting neoadjuvant CRT in subpopulations of those affected with esophageal cancer. A recently published, appropriately powered, randomized controlled trial from van Hagen et al. (van Hagen et al. 2012) evaluating patients with disease beyond T1N0 and up to T3N1 based on clinical staging, demonstrated an overall statistically significant survival benefit, seen below in Fig. 1a (all patients) and 1b (stratified by histology). Overall, patients receiving trimodality therapy had a median survival of 49.4 vs. 24.0 months in the surgery only group ($p = 0.003$).

Traditional Kaplan–Meier survival analysis demonstrates that their selected population will have an overall survival benefit from neoadjuvant CRT. When performing subgroup survival analysis, this benefit remained statistically significant both for adenocarcinoma (AC) and for squamous cell (SCC) histology.

However, the survival benefit of chemoradiotherapy is likely not distributed evenly across all patients. Those patients who have a pathologic complete response (pCR), with no residual tumor identifiable in the surgical specimen, or even those with partial response following neoadjuvant CRT have a better prognosis than those that have no appreciable or minimal response to CRT. Identification of a molecular or histologic marker predictive of response to CRT, similar to the RSI discussed above, would provide useful adjunctive clinical information. Several institutions have attempted to predict clinical surrogates for benefit from CRT (Ajani et al. 2012). However, ypTNM remains a useful prognosticator of outcome and was recently employed in the construction of a predictive web based tool (Eil et al. 2013).

While the prognostic power of the ypTNM has been validated previously (Holmes and Vaughan 2007) the exact benefit of neoadjuvant CRT on patients by their documented ypTNM has not been examined. Eil et al. (2013) proposed a survival prediction tool applicable to resected patients with or without neoadjuvant CRT based on a SEER-Medicare database of 824 patients. The multivariate regression coefficients and OR are shown below in Table 8. A web browser based nomogram was built from this model to create individual estimates of survival and is available at http://skynet.ohsu.edu/nomograms/.

The beta coefficients and odd ratios predicted from the regression model are represented in Table 8. The predicted survival benefit from neoadjuvant CRT persisted for advanced stage disease present after treatment (Eil et al. 2013). For example, based upon the model, a 70 year old male with adenocarcinoma and 12 lymph nodes harvested

Table 8 SEER—medicare predictive log logistic multivariate regression model parameters

Covariate	Beta coefficient	P	OR	95 % CI
(Intercept)	6.4560	0.0096		
Age	−0.0310	0.4026	1.1	0.9–1.18
Age′	−0.3009	0.0680	1.7	0.9–2.8
Age″	0.8060	0.0218	0.3	0.01–0.8
Sex = female	0.3055	0.0002	0.6	0.5–0.8
Tstage = 2	−0.3188	0.0097	1.7	1.13–2.6
Tstage = 3	−0.8054	<0.0001	3.9	2.6–5.7
Tstage = 4	−1.1091	<0.0001	6.4	3.5–11.8
Tx = CRT	−0.8059	<0.0001	3.8	2.5–5.9
Histology = squamous	−0.2701	0.0003	1.6	1.23–2.0
Nodes = 1	−0.7019	<0.0001	3.2	2.2–4.7
Nodes = 2	−0.9804	<0.0001	5.2	3.3–8.1
Nodes = 3	−1.2394	<0.0001	8.0	3.6–17.4
TotalLN	0.0286	<0.0001		
Tstage = 2 × tx = CRT	0.5523	0.0011		
Tstage = 3 × tx = CRT	0.6674	<0.0001		
Tstage = 4 × tx = CRT	1.2559	<0.0001		
Tx = CRT × nodes = 1	0.9149	<0.0001		
Tx = CRT × nodes = 2	0.3996	0.0262		
Tx = CRT × nodes = 3	0.4749	0.1284		
Tx = CRT × totalLN	−0.0167	0.0243		
Log (scale)	−0.5176	<0.0001		
Log (scale)	−0.5176	<0.0001		

Log logistic multivariate regression model beta coefficients. The associated odds ratio (OR) and 95 % CI are also provided. Note: age modeled using restricted cubic spline function with four knots, requiring three independent coefficients: Age, Age′, and Age″. Interaction terms indicate how the influence of adjuvant chemo-therapy or CRT varies by T and N stages and total LN (Eil et al. 2013)

with ypT4N2 stage having received neoadjuvant CRT would have a predicted 3 year OS of 29 vs. 12 % without CRT. A similar patient with ypT2N1 disease is predicted to have a 3 year OS of 64 % with neoadjuvant CRT vs. 45 % with isolated esophagectomy (Eil et al. 2013).

This analytic tool, being based on pathologic stage, is most applicable in the post-operative setting—when the ypTNM stage is available for postoperative counseling, comparison, and treatment planning. Additionally, such risk modeling is helpful in the design of research protocols for identifying homogenous high risk groups. One would expect the model to underestimate of the benefit of neoadjuvant therapy due to its expected downstaging effect on ypTNM as compared to cTNM. The ultimate goal of a predictive decision aid for designing an individualized treatment course would include early identification, or even prediction, of responders and non-responders—leading to avoidance of ineffective and dangerous application of both chemoradiotherapy and surgery.

With the above predictive tool, one can estimate the benefit of neoadjuvant CRT based on the final pathologic stage. However, this definitive information is not available when considering whether to administer neoadjuvant treatment. Pre-treatment knowledge, or at least likelihood of nodal status would aid in guiding treatment—as patients N1 or greater benefit significantly from neoadjuvant treatment (Eil et al. 2013). In 2010, with a training sample of 164 patients resected with curative intent at M.D. Anderson Cancer Center and excluding those that received neoadjuvant therapy Gaur and colleagues developed a tool for predicting nodal involvement based on preoperative clinical characteristics (Gaur et al. 2010). The nomogram was validated externally, showing a concordance index (CI) of 0.77. Their predictive tool, represented in Fig. 2 below, was adapted into a traditional point system with the strongest clinical indicator being valued at 100 points and other variables being weighed against this as described by Jasonos et al. (2008).

In reviewing their point scale weighting, the most heavily weighted variable was tumor length, which the authors chose to dichotomize at 2 cm. Clinical evaluation of nodal status (cN), or EUS, was not significantly associated

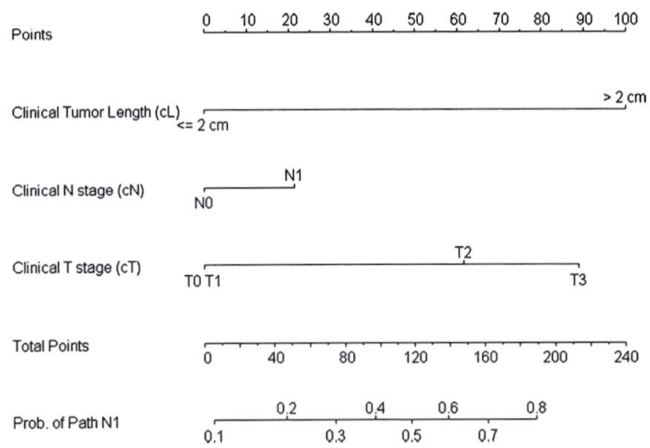

Fig. 2 Nomogram to predict pathologic lymph node involvement (path N1) using clinical measurements for M. D. Anderson training set. The nomogram consists of six rows. Row 1 (points row) is the point assignment for each variable. Rows 2–4 correspond to the variables included in the model. For an individual patient, each variable in rows 2–4 is assigned a point value, which is determined by drawing a vertical line from the appropriate position on the variable row to the points row. The assigned points for all three variables are added, and the total is marked in row 5 (total points). Then, the risk of path N1 is calculated by drawing a vertical line from the appropriate position on the total-points row to the final row (predicted path N1 probability). Point scale nomogram adapted from Gaur et al. (2010)

with pathologic nodal status on multivariate analysis, with an OR of 1.5 (0.5–5.5; p = 0.5). This predictive tool estimates that a cT2N0 patient with a tumor that measures <2 cm has only a 27 % chance of having N1 disease, while a cT2N0 patient with a tumor >2 cm has a 72 % of having N1 disease. This is troubling data given the inherent clinical confidence most place in EUS data, as well as the need for certainty in predicting nodal status—which many weight heavily when determining whether to offer neoadjuvant therapy. Additionally, the lowest risk oncologic features as measured by Gaur's nomogram, a T2 patient maintains a 27 % risk of having nodal disease. Many would consider this a high enough likelihood to consider CRT, given the documented benefit. More precise predictive tools are required to narrow the spectrum of patients considered for trimodal treatment.

5.3 Predicting Pathologic Complete Response After Neoadjuvant Chemoradiotherapy

The ability to confidently predict which patients with an apparent clinical CR (cCR) will have a pCR would provide an opportunity to further stratify which patients may not obtain a survival benefit from esophagectomy following chemoradiotherapy. However, a pCR does not guarantee disease free survival. Many patients with a documented pCR have documented disease recurrence and ultimately succumb to their disease. However, the prognosis is significantly improved and the likelihood of a local failure is greatly reduced for patients with no residual disease when compared to all other patients with residual disease (Chirieac et al. 2005; Donahue et al. 2009; Brucher et al. 2006). Those patients that respond with a pCR, approximately 30 % of those undergoing neoadjuvant CRT, demonstrate a 55 % 5 year survival vs. 34 % for all patients treated with neoadjuvant CRT followed by surgery. The prognostic power of the pathologic response has been reproducible, with some advocating for its addition to the traditional TNM stage (Swisher et al. 2005). Of those who achieve a preoperative cCR, a small minority have a true pCR. Some are found to have a partial response, and others have no demonstrable response to neoadjuvant CRT in comparison to estimated pretreatment TNM (cTNM). However, based on the SEER-Medicare based nomogram discussed above, even patients with advanced ypTNM stage benefitted from neoadjuvant CRT (Eil et al. 2013). Given the reliable prognostic power of response to CRT, the accuracy of the clinical stage found prior to neoadjuvant treatment is critical to ultimately determining which strategy will result in the greatest survival benefit.

Several series have demonstrated post neoadjuvant CRT restaging techniques to be concerningly inaccurate. Post treatment biopsies have an accuracy approaching 30 % and are not prognostic of outcome. Post treatment endoscopic biopsy reveals no residual malignancy in approximately 80 % of patients, while the incidence of pCR is 25–30 %.

Regarding the accuracy of EUS ycTNM, Kalha and colleagues performed a retrospective review of 83 patients from MD Anderson revealed that EUS restaging correctly identified the T stage in only 29 % of patients (Kalha et al. 2004). The sensitivity for detecting nodal disease was only 51 %. Of the 22 patients who responded to the neoadjuvant chemoradiotherapy with a complete pathologic response, 19 were restaged by EUS as having residual disease. Given the above findings, some have endeavored to find modes of post treatment evaluation other than clinical restaging to estimate the patient's state of disease and response to treatment.

Of the diagnostic modalities currently available, the change in PET standard uptake value (SUV) before and after treatment has proven to be the most reliable indicator of response (Ajani et al. 2012). In the setting of these diagnostic limitations, at the end of 2012 a predictive nomogram with an end point of pCR based on clinical parameters following CRT was released based on the institutional database of MD Anderson. The strongest predictor of pCR was the SUV after treatment. Unfortunately, PET scanning calibration is not standardized across institutions. In the face of these limitations, they produced a model with a bias-corrected area under the curve (AUC) of 0.7 (95 % CI = 0.64–0.73). Figure 3 represents their point scale nomogram.

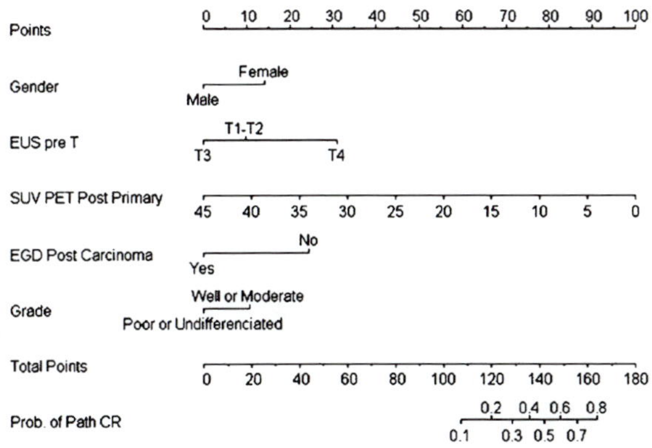

Fig. 3 The nomogram consists of eight rows. Row 1 (points row) is the point assignment for each variable. Rows 2–6 correspond to the variables included in the model. For an individual patient, each variable is assigned a point value, which is determined by drawing a vertical line from the appropriate position on the variable row to the points row. The demonstrates that combining variables can increase the probability of predicting pathCR to as high as 80 % if a patient scores >160 points. Among the most influential factors for attaining the highest scores for predicting pathCR were lower postchemoradiation SUVmax and the absence of cancer cells on postchemoradiation biopsy specimens. Point scale nomogram adapted from Ajani et al. (2012)

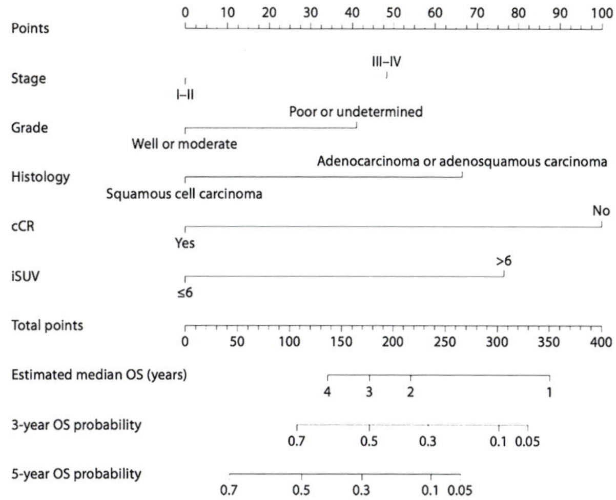

Fig. 4 Row 1 (points row) is the point assignment for each variable. Rows 2–6 correspond to the variables included in the model. For an individual patient, each variable is assigned a point value, which is determined by drawing a vertical line from the appropriate position on the variable row to the points row. Point scale nomogram adapted from Suzuki et al. (2012)

While these predictive tools hold promise for improving individualized treatment regimens, their discriminatory power is not yet such that one could depend upon it for embarking upon an esophageal preservation strategy for a specific patient. Molecular markers and oncogenetics hold promise to increase our predictive power in the future. This topic is discussed elsewhere in this chapter and will not be addressed in this section.

5.4 Predicting Survival for Patients Receiving Definitive Chemoradiotherapy

A tool predicting survival for patients unfit, unwilling, or of too advanced stage for surgery may not intuitively be of value—what decision is there to make when the planned treatment is already determined? However, when one considers the purpose of a nomogram and brings the information provided by such a tool into the larger clinical arena, it could advance all of the goals of a clinical prediction tool: aid in medical decision making, provide straightforward information for patients, supply baseline outcomes to aid in research protocol design, and potentially a baseline to compare against similar patients who did undergo CRT followed by surgery.

In contemplating the benefit of an esophageal preservation strategy for some patients based on their cCR and other appropriate variables, a predictive survival tool for those that have received definitive CRT would be immediately useful. Using their institutional clinical database including 257 patients undergoing definitive CRT Suzuki et al. (2012) produced a nomogram predicting benefit from definitive CRT. Similarly to Ajani et al., discussed above, for predicting pCR, PET SUV was a significant predictor of outcome. However, here post treatment endoscopic biopsy was the strongest predictor of OS following treatment, as no pathologic staging data was available. Their final CI was 0.7 for predicting OS. Given the baseline complex medical history, making many of them inappropriate for operative intervention, OS analysis may be confounded by deaths due to non-oncologic etiologies (Fig. 4).

5.5 Predicting Perioperative Mortality

As part of a comprehensive strategy to correctly predict which patients will benefit from treatment, one must ultimately incorporate the potential mortality from treatment itself. Several nomograms for prediction of complications following esophagectomy have been published and are discussed below. As a general assertion one can say that these nomograms have been difficult to apply outside of their home institution due to the multifactorial etiology of the end outcomes, differing patient populations, operative techniques, and post operative management.

In 2006 Steyerberg et al. (2008) reported a predictive model for mortality following esophagectomy based on SEER-Medicare data from 1991 to 1996 and validated on several other cohorts. Perhaps due to the complex multifactorial nature of post operative outcomes, the Medicare database, and the low incidence of perioperative mortality the predictive power was low—a CI of 0.58 when externally validated.

Table 9 Score chart to estimate 30-day mortality after cancer-directed surgery for esophageal cancer

Characteristic	Score
Age, years	
50	−1
65	0
80	1
Comorbidity	
Pulmonary	1
Cardiovascular	1
Diabetes	1
Hepatic	1
Renal	1
Neoadjuvant therapy	
Radiotherapy	1.5
Chemoradiotherapy	1
Hospital volume, No. of esophagectomy/year	
Low (≤1)	0
Intermediate (1.1–2.5)	−0.5
High (≥2.6)	−1.5
Very high (±50)	−2

Sum score is obtained by adding scores. Intermediate scores for age can be approximated by linear interpolation. For example, age 72 corresponds to a score of +0.5. The formula to calculate the predicted probability of surgical mortality is P (mortality) −1/[1 + exp (2.41 − 0.32 × score)]. Cancer. Adapted from Steyerberg et al. (2008)

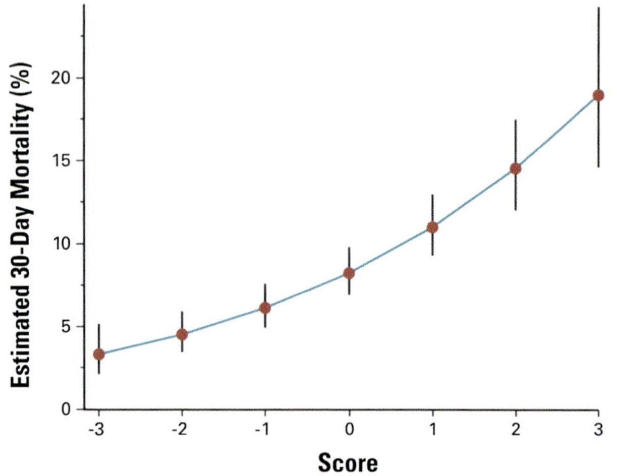

Fig. 6 Estimated surgical mortality in relation to the sum cumulative score that can be obtained from Table 9. The 95 % CIs are based on analysis of four cohorts, containing 3,592 patients undergoing surgery for esophageal cancer using the aforementioned scale and formula. Adapted from Steyerberg et al. (2008)

Table 9 below shows the variables considered in their nomogram with Fig. 5 graphically demonstrating the estimated 30-day perioperative mortality.

While the above model is not independently adequate for medical decision-making in its current state with a CI of 0.58, it provides a template for a more precise prediction tool. A more accurate, perhaps institution specific, prediction tool for perioperative mortality may be of use. Such a

Fig. 5 Adapted from Steyerberg et al. Score chart to estimate 30-day mortality after cancer-directed surgery for esophageal cancer

Characteristic	Score
Age, years	
50	−1
65	0
80	1
Comorbidity	
Pulmonary	1
Cardiovascular	1
Diabetes	1
Hepatic	1
Renal	1
Neoadjuvant therapy	
Radiotherapy	1.5
Chemoradiotherapy	1
Hospital volume; No. of esophagectomy/year	
Low (≤ 1)	0
Intermediate (1.1-2.5)	−0.5
High (≥ 2.6)	−1.5
Very high (± 50)	−2

tool could be of use in counseling high-risk patients with advanced stage to avoid esophagectomy based on a high estimate of postoperative mortality. Additionally, a peri-operative mortality risk prediction tool may be used in conjunction with those predicting survival after cCR from chemoradiotherapy—identifying those patients most appropriate for esophageal salvage (Fig. 6).

6 Summary

While esophageal cancer continues to claim the lives of a significant number of those that it affects, aggressive trimodal treatment strategies within a targeted population has resulted in progressive increases in survival. However, neoadjuvant CRT followed by esophagectomy has the potential to provide significant survival benefit to patients whose tumor biology is responsive to CRT, despite advanced disease. However, the oncologic response to treatment is heterogenous across and within clinically stratified treatment groups. Accurately identifying those patients that will benefit from aggressive treatment, and sparing non-responders the risks associated with trimodality treatment will depend on novel utilization of existing prognostic tools and the development of additional assays.

References

Ahn SJ, Kahn D, Zhou S et al (2005) Dosimetric and clinical predictors for radiation-induced esophageal injury. Int J Radiat Oncol Biol Phys 61(2):335–347

Ajani JA, Winter K, Komaki R et al (2008) Phase II randomized trial of two nonoperative regimens of induction chemotherapy followed by chemoradiation in patients with localized carcinoma of the esophagus: RTOG 0113. J Clin Oncol 26(28):4551–4556

Ajani JA, Correa AM, Hofstetter WL et al (2012) Clinical parameters model for predicting pathologic complete response following preoperative chemoradiation in patients with esophageal cancer. Ann Oncol 23(10):2638–2642

Aoyagi T, Shuto K, Okazumi S, Shimada H, Kazama T, Matsubara H (2011) Apparent diffusion coefficient values measured by diffusion-weighted imaging predict chemoradiotherapeutic effect for advanced esophageal cancer. Dig Surg 28(4):252–257

Asakura H, Hashimoto T, Zenda S et al (2010) Analysis of dose-volume histogram parameters for radiation pneumonitis after definitive concurrent chemoradiotherapy for esophageal cancer. Radiother Oncol 95(2):240–244

Berger AC, Farma J, Scott WJ et al (2005) Complete response to neoadjuvant chemoradiotherapy in esophageal carcinoma is associated with significantly improved survival. J Clin Oncol 23(19):4330–4337

Botet JF, Lightdale CJ, Zauber AG, Gerdes H, Urmacher C, Brennan MF (1991) Preoperative staging of esophageal cancer: comparison of endoscopic US and dynamic CT. Radiology 181(2):419–425

Bowrey DJ, Clark GW, Roberts SA et al (1999) Serial endoscopic ultrasound in the assessment of response to chemoradiotherapy for carcinoma of the esophagus. J Gastrointest Surg 3(5):462–467

Brucher BL, Becker K, Lordick F, Fink U, Sarbia M, Stein H, Busch R, Zimmerman F, Molls M, Hofler H, Siewart JR (2006) The clinical impact of histopathologic response assessment by residual tumor cell quantification in esopahgeal squamous cell carcinomas. Cancer 106(10):2119–2126

Bruzzi JF, Swisher SG, Truong MT et al (2007) Detection of interval distant metastases: clinical utility of integrated CT-PET imaging in patients with esophageal carcinoma after neoadjuvant therapy. Cancer 109(1):125–134

Burmeister BH, Smithers BM, Gebski V et al (2005) Surgery alone versus chemoradiotherapy followed by surgery for resectable cancer of the oesophagus: a randomised controlled phase III trial. Lancet Oncol 6(9):659–668

Chak A, Canto MI, Cooper GS et al (2000) Endosonographic assessment of multimodality therapy predicts survival of esophageal carcinoma patients. Cancer 88(8):1788–1795

Chang EY (2009) Esophageal cancer: principles and practice. Demos Medical Publisher, New York

Chang EY, Li X, Jerosch-Herold M et al (2008) The evaluation of esophageal adenocarcinoma using dynamic contrast-enhanced magnetic resonance imaging. J Gastrointest Surg 12(1):166–175

Chirieac LR, Swisher SG, Ajani JA, Komaki RR, Correa AM, Morris JS, Roth JA, Rashid A, Hamilton SR, Wu TT (2005) Posttherapy pathologic stage predicts survival in patients with esophageal carcinoma receiving preoperative chemoradiation. Cancer 103:1347–1355

Cooper JS, Guo MD, Herskovic A et al (1999) Chemoradiotherapy of locally advanced esophageal cancer: long-term follow-up of a prospective randomized trial (RTOG 85-01). Radiation Therapy Oncology Group. JAMA 281(17):1623–1627

Dalton WS, Friend SH (2006) Cancer biomarkers—An invitation to the table. Science 312:1165–1168

David IH (2008) Esophageal cancer chemotherapy: recent advances. Gastrointest Cancer Res 2:85–92

Dikken JL, Coit DG, Klimstra DS et al (2012) Prospective impact of tumor grade assessment in biopsies on tumor stage and prognostic grouping in gastroesophageal adenocarcinoma: relevance of the seventh edition American joint committee on cancer staging manual revision. Cancer 118(2):349–357

Donahue JM, Nichols FC, Li Z, Schomas DA, Allen MS, Cassivi SD, Jatoi A, Miller RC, Wigle DA, Shen R, Deschamps C (2009a) Complete pathologic response after neoadjuvant chemoradiotherapy for esophageal cancer is associated with enchanced survival. Ann Thoracic Surg 87(2):392–399

Donahue JM, Nichols FC, Li Z, Schomas DA, Allen MS, Cassivi SD, Jatoi A, Miller RC, Wigle DA, Shen R, Deschamps C (2009b) Complete pathologic response after neoadjuvant chemoradiotherapy for esophageal cancer is associated with enchanced survival. Ann Thoracic Surg 87(2):392–399

Eil R, Diggs BS, Wang SJ, Dolan J, Hunter JG, Thomas CR (2013) Nomogram for predicting the benefit of neoadjuvant chemoradiotherapy for esophageal cancer – A SEER – medicare analysis. Presented: ASCO Annual Meeting, 31 May to 4 June 2013, Chicago

Eschrich S, Zhang H et al (2009a) Systems biology modeling of the radiation sensitivty network: a biomarker discovery platform. Int J Radiat Oncol Biol Phys 75(2):497–505

Eschrich S, Pramana J et al (2009b) A gene expression model of intrinsic tumor radiosensitivity: prediction of response and prognosis after chemoradiation. Int J Radiat Oncol Biol Phys 75(2):489–496

Fockens P, Van den Brande JH, van Dullemen HM, van Lanschot JJ, Tytgat GN (1996) Endosonographic T-staging of esophageal carcinoma: a learning curve. Gastrointest Endosc 44(1):58–62

Gaur P, Sepesi B, Hofstetter WL, Correa AM, Bhutani MS, Vaporciyan AA, Watson TJ, Swisher SG (2010) A clinical nomogram predicting pathologic lymph node involvement in esophageal cancer patients. Ann Surg 252(4):611–617

Gayed IW, Liu HH, Yusuf SW et al (2006) The prevalence of myocardial ischemia after concurrent chemoradiation therapy as detected by gated myocardial perfusion imaging in patients with esophageal cancer. J Nucl Med 47(11):1756–1762

Giovannini M, Seitz JF, Thomas P et al (1997) Endoscopic ultrasonography for assessment of the response to combined radiation therapy and chemotherapy in patients with esophageal cancer. Endoscopy 29(1):4–9

Griffith JF, Chan AC, Chow LT et al (1999) Assessing chemotherapy response of squamous cell oesophageal carcinoma with spiral CT. Br J Radiol 72(859):678–684

Hashimoto T, Asakura H, Zenda S et al (2008) Cardiac toxicities after concurrent chemoradiotherapy for esophageal cancer- dose volume histogram. Int J Radiat Oncol Biol Phys 72(1):S130

Heath EI, Burtness BA, Heitmiller RF et al (2000) Phase II evaluation of preoperative chemoradiation and postoperative adjuvant chemotherapy for squamous cell and adenocarcinoma of the esophagus. J Clin Oncol 18(4):868–876

Hirata N, Kawamoto K, Ueyama T, Masuda K, Utsunomiya T, Kuwano H (1997) Using endosonography to assess the effects of neoadjuvant therapy in patients with advanced esophageal cancer. AJR Am J Roentgenol 169(2):485–491

Holmes RS, Vaughan TL (2007) Epidemiology and pathogenesis of esophageal cancer. Semin Radiat Oncol 17(1):2–9

Hsu FM, Lee YC, Lee JM et al (2009) Association of clinical and dosimetric factors with postoperative pulmonary complications in esophageal cancer patients receiving intensity-modulated radiation therapy and concurrent chemotherapy followed by thoracic esophagectomy. Ann Surg Oncol 16(6):1669–1677

Jamil LH, Gill KR, Wallace MB (2008) Staging and restaging of advanced esophageal cancer. Curr Opin Gastroenterol 24(4):530–534

Jasonos A, Schrag D, Raj G, Panageas K (2008) How to build and interpret a nomogram for cancer prognosis. J Clin Oncol 26:1364–1370

Jones DR, Parker LA Jr, Detterbeck FC, Egan TM (1999) Inadequacy of computed tomography in assessing patients with esophageal carcinoma after induction chemoradiotherapy. Cancer 85(5):1026–1032

Kalha I, Kaw M, Fukami N, Patel M, Singh S, Gagneja H, Cohen D, Morris J (2004) The accuracy of endoscopic ultrasound for restaging esophageal carcinoma after chemoradiation therapy. Cancer 101(5):940–947

Katsoulis IE, Wong WL, Mattheou AK, Damani N, Chambers J, Livingstone JI (2007) Fluorine-18 fluorodeoxyglucose positron emission tomography in the preoperative staging of thoracic oesophageal and gastro-oesophageal junction cancer: a prospective study. Int J Surg 5(6):399–403

Konski A, Li T, Christensen M et al (2012) Symptomatic cardiac toxicity is predicted by dosimetric and patient factors rather than changes in 18F-FDG PET determination of myocardial activity after chemoradiotherapy for esophageal cancer. Radiother Oncol 104(1):72–77

Kwa SL, Lebesque JV, Theuws JC et al (1998) Radiation pneumonitis as a function of mean lung dose: an analysis of pooled data of 540 patients. Int J Radiat Oncol Biol Phys 42(1):1–9

Lin SH, Wang L, Myles B et al (2012) Propensity score-based comparison of long-term outcomes with 3-dimensional conformal radiotherapy vs intensity-modulated radiotherapy for esophageal cancer. Int J Radiat Oncol Biol Phys 84(5):1078–1085

Lowe VJ, Booya F, Fletcher JG et al (2005) Comparison of positron emission tomography, computed tomography, and endoscopic ultrasound in the initial staging of patients with esophageal cancer. Mol Imaging Biol 7(6):422–430

Meluch AA, Greco FA, Gray JR et al (2003) Preoperative therapy with concurrent paclitaxel/carboplatin/infusional 5-FU and radiation therapy in locoregional esophageal cancer: final results of a Minnie Pearl cancer research network phase II trial. Cancer J 9(4):251–260

Milano MT, Constine LS, Okunieff P (2007) Normal tissue tolerance dose metrics for radiation therapy of major organs. Semin Radiat Oncol 17(2):131–140

Minsky B, Pajak T, Ginsberg R, Pisansky T, Martenson J, Komaki R, Okawara G, Rosenthal S, Kelsen D (2002) INT 0123 (radiation therapy oncology group 94–05) phase III trial of combined mortality therapy for esophageal cancer: high-dose versus standard-dose radiation therapy. JCO 20:1167–1174

Morota M, Gomi K, Kozuka T et al (2009) Late toxicity after definitive concurrent chemoradiotherapy for thoracic esophageal carcinoma. Int J Radiat Oncol Biol Phys 75(1):122–128

Nomura M, Kodaira T, Furutani K, Tachibana H, Tomita N, Goto Y (2012) Predictive factors for radiation pneumonitis in oesophageal cancer patients treated with chemoradiotherapy without prophylactic nodal irradiation. Br J Radiol 85(1014):813–818

Oberholzer K, Pohlmann A, Schreiber W et al (2008) Assessment of tumor microcirculation with dynamic contrast-enhanced MRI in patients with esophageal cancer: initial experience. J Magn Reson Imaging 27(6):1296–1301

Omloo JM, van Heijl M, Hoekstra OS, van Berge Henegouwen MI, van Lanschot JJ, Sloof GW (2011) FDG-PET parameters as prognostic factor in esophageal cancer patients: a review. Ann Surg Oncol 18(12):3338–3352

Palma DA, Senan S, Tsujino K, et al (2012) Predicting radiation pneumonitis after chemoradiation therapy for lung cancer: an international individual patient data meta-analysis. *Int J Radiat Oncol Biol Phys* 85(2):444–450

Reid TD, Chan DS, Roberts SA, Crosby TD, Williams GT, Lewis WG (2012) Prognostic significance of circumferential resection margin involvement following oesophagectomy for cancer and the predictive role of endoluminal ultrasonography. Br J Cancer 107(12):1925–1931

Reynolds JV, McLaughlin R, Moore J, Rowley S, Ravi N, Byrne PJ (2006) Prospective evaluation of quality of life in patients with localized oesophageal cancer treated by multimodality therapy or surgery alone. Br J Surg 93(9):1084–1090

Ribeiro A, Franceschi D, Parra J et al (2006) Endoscopic ultrasound restaging after neoadjuvant chemotherapy in esophageal cancer. Am J Gastroenterol 101:1216–1221

Rice TW, Blackstone EH, Rusch VW (2010) 7th edition of the AJCC cancer staging manual: esophagus and esophagogastric junction. Ann Surg Oncol 17(7):1721–1724

Riddell AM, Allum WH, Thompson JN, Wotherspoon AC, Richardson C, Brown G (2007) The appearances of oesophageal carcinoma demonstrated on high-resolution, T2-weighted MRI, with histopathological correlation. Eur Radiol 17(2):391–399

Rizk NP, Seshan VE, Bains MS et al (2007a) Prognostic factors after combined modality treatment of squamous cell carcinoma of the esophagus. J Thorac Oncol 2(12):1117–1123

Rizk NP, Venkatraman E, Bains MS et al (2007b) American joint committee on cancer staging system does not accurately predict survival in patients receiving multimodality therapy for esophageal adenocarcinoma. J Clin Oncol 25(5):507–512

Rose J, Rodrigues G, Yaremko B, Lock M, D'Souza D (2009) Systematic review of dose-volume parameters in the prediction of esophagitis in thoracic radiotherapy. Radiother Oncol 91(3):282–287

Sakurada A, Takahara T, Kwee TC et al (2009) Diagnostic performance of diffusion-weighted magnetic resonance imaging in esophageal cancer. Eur Radiol 19(6):1461–1469

Sarkaria IS, Rizk NP, Bains MS et al (2009) Post-treatment endoscopic biopsy is a poor-predictor of pathologic response in patients undergoing chemoradiation therapy for esophageal cancer. Ann Surg 249(5):764–767

Siegel R, DeSantis C, Virgo K et al (2012) Cancer treatment and survivorship statistics. CA Cancer J Clin 62(4):220–241

Siewert JR, Stein HJ (1998) Classification of adenocarcinoma of the oesophagogastric junction. Br J Surg 85(11):1457–1459

Situ D, Wei W, Lin P, et al (2012) Do tumor grade and location affect survival in esophageal squamous cell carcinoma? Survival analysis of 302 cases of pT3N0M0 esophageal squamous cell carcinoma. *Ann Surg Oncol* 20:580–585

Sloof GW (2006) Response monitoring of neoadjuvant therapy using CT, EUS, and FDG-PET. Best Pract Res Clin Gastroenterol 20(5):941–957

Stahl A, Ott K, Weber WA et al (2003) FDG PET imaging of locally advanced gastric carcinomas: correlation with endoscopic and histopathological findings. Eur J Nucl Med Mol Imaging 30(2): 288–295

Streyerberg EW, Neville BA, Koppert LB, Lemmens VE, Tilanus HW, Coebergh JW, Weeks JC, Earle CC (2008) Surgical mortality in patients with esophageal cancer: development and validation of a simple risk score. JCO 24:4277–4283

Suzuki A, Xiao L, Hayashi Y, Blum M, Welsh J, Lin S, Lee J, Bhutani M, Weston B, Maru D, Rice D, Swisher S, Hostetter W, Erasmus J, Ajani JA (2012) Nomograms for prognostication of outcome in patients with esophageal and gastroesophageal carcinoma underoing definitive chemoradiotherapy. Oncology 82:108–113

Swisher SG, Maish M, Erasmus JJ, et al (2004) Utility of PET, CT, and EUS to identify pathologic responders in esophageal cancer. Ann Thorac Surg 78(4):1152–1160; discussion 1152–1160

Swisher S, Hofstetter W, Wu T, Correa AM, Ajani JA, Komaki RR, Chirieac L, Hunt K, Liao Z, Phan A, Rice D, Vaporciyan AA, Walsh G, Roth J (2005) Proposed revision of the esophgeal cancer staging sytem to accommodate pathologic following preoperative chemoradiation. Ann Surg 241(5):810–820

Talsma K, van Hagen P, Grotenhuis BA et al (2012) Comparison of the 6th and 7th editions of the UICC-AJCC TNM classification for esophageal cancer. Ann Surg Oncol 19(7):2142–2148

Thosani N, Singh H, Kapadia A et al (2012) Diagnostic accuracy of EUS in differentiating mucosal versus submucosal invasion of superficial esophageal cancers: a systematic review and meta-analysis. Gastrointest Endosc 75(2):242–253

Thrift AP, Nagle CM, Fahey PP et al (2012) The influence of prediagnostic demographic and lifestyle factors on esophageal squamous cell carcinoma survival. Int J Cancer 131(5):E759–E768

Trotti A, Colevas AD, Setser A et al (2003) CTCAE v3.0: development of a comprehensive grading system for the adverse effects of cancer treatment. Semin Radiat Oncol 13(3):176–181

Tucker SL, Liu HH, Wang S et al (2006) Dose-volume modeling of the risk of postoperative pulmonary complications among esophageal cancer patients treated with concurrent chemoradiotherapy followed by surgery. Int J Radiat Oncol Biol Phys 66(3):754–761

Union Internationale Contre le Cancer (2002) TNM classification of malignant tumours, 6th edn. Wiley-Liss, New York

Urba SG, Orringer MB, Turrisi A, Iannettoni M, Forastiere A, Strawderman M (2001) Randomized trial of preoperative chemoradiation versus surgery alone in patients with locoregional esophageal carcinoma. J Clin Oncol 19(2):305–313

Urba SG, Orringer MB, Ianettonni M, Hayman JA, Satoru H (2003) Concurrent cisplatin, paclitaxel, and radiotherapy as preoperative treatment for patients with locoregional esophageal carcinoma. Cancer 98(10):2177–2183

Van Benthuysen L, Hales L, Podgorsak MB (2011) Volumetric modulated arc therapy vs. IMRT for the treatment of distal esophageal cancer. Med Dosim 36(4):404–409

van Hagen P, Hulshof MC, van Lanschot JJ et al (2012) Preoperative chemoradiotherapy for esophageal or junctional cancer. N Engl J Med 366(22):2074–2084

van Meerten E, Muller K, Tilanus HW et al (2006) Neoadjuvant concurrent chemoradiation with weekly paclitaxel and carboplatin for patients with oesophageal cancer: a phase II study. Br J Cancer 94(10):1389–1394

van Meerten E, van der Gaast A, Looman CW, Tilanus HW, Muller K, Essink-Bot ML (2008) Quality of life during neoadjuvant treatment and after surgery for resectable esophageal carcinoma. Int J Radiat Oncol Biol Phys 71(1):160–166

van Vliet EP, Heijenbrok-Kal MH, Hunink MG, Kuipers EJ, Siersema PD (2008) Staging investigations for oesophageal cancer: a meta-analysis. Br J Cancer 98(3):547–557

Vivekanandan N, Sriram P, Kumar SA, Bhuvaneswari N, Saranya K (2012) Volumetric modulated arc radiotherapy for esophageal cancer. Med Dosim Spring 37(1):108–113

Vogelius IR, Bentzen SM (2012) A literature-based meta-analysis of clinical risk factors for development of radiation induced pneumonitis. Acta Oncol 51(8):975–983

Voncken FE, Jiang H, Kim J, et al (2012) Degree of tumor shrinkage following neoadjuvant chemoradiotherapy: a potential predictor for complete pathological response in esophageal cancer? Dis Esophagus. doi: 10.1111/j.1442-2050.2012.01445.x

Wagner TD, Javie M, Yang G (2009) Esophageal cancer: principles and practice. Demos Medical Publisher, New York

Wang SL, Liao Z, Vaporciyan AA et al (2006) Investigation of clinical and dosimetric factors associated with postoperative pulmonary complications in esophageal cancer patients treated with concurrent chemoradiotherapy followed by surgery. Int J Radiat Oncol Biol Phys 64(3):692–699

Wang S, Liao Z, Wei X et al (2008) Association between systemic chemotherapy before chemoradiation and increased risk of treatment-related pneumonitis in esophageal cancer patients treated with definitive chemoradiotherapy. J Thorac Oncol 3(3):277–282

Watanabe T, Komuro Y, Kiyomatsu T, Kanazawa T, Kazama Y, Tanaka J, Tanaka T, Yamamoto Y, Shirane M, Muto T, Nagawa H (2006) Prediction of sensitivity of rectal cancer cells in response to preoperative radio- therapy by DNA microarray analysis of gene expression profiles. Cancer Res 66:3370–3374

Wei X, Liu HH, Tucker SL et al (2008) Risk factors for pericardial effusion in inoperable esophageal cancer patients treated with definitive chemoradiation therapy. Int J Radiat Oncol Biol Phys 70(3):707–714

Weichselbaum RR, Ishwaranc H et al (2008) An interferon-related gene signature for DNA damage resistance is a predictive marker for chemotherapy and radiation for breast cancer. PNAS 105:18490–18495

Westerterp M, van Westreenen HL, Reitsma JB et al (2005) Esophageal cancer: CT, endoscopic US, and FDG PET for assessment of response to neoadjuvant therapy–systematic review. Radiology 236(3):841–851

Wong WL, Chambers RJ (2008) Role of PET/PET CT in the staging and restaging of thoracic oesophageal cancer and gastro-oesophageal cancer: a literature review. Abdom Imaging 33(2):183–190

Wu LF, Wang BZ, Feng JL et al (2003) Preoperative TN staging of esophageal cancer: comparison of miniprobe ultrasonography, spiral CT and MRI. World J Gastroenterol 9(2):219–224

Yin L, Wu H, Gong J et al (2012) Volumetric-modulated arc therapy vs. c-IMRT in esophageal cancer: a treatment planning comparison. World J Gastroenterol 18(37):5266–5275

Zuccaro G Jr, Rice TW, Goldblum J et al (1999) Endoscopic ultrasound cannot determine suitability for esophagectomy after aggressive chemoradiotherapy for esophageal cancer. Am J Gastroenterol 94(4):906–912

Gastric Cancer

Trevor Leong

Contents

Abstract

The use of radiotherapy for treatment of gastric cancer has become commonplace over the past 10 years following reporting of the US Intergroup Trial 0116. However, gastric irradiation has proved to be very challenging for radiation oncologists. Aside from the technical difficulties associated with radiotherapy, there are also many clinical challenges faced by clinicians when deciding optimal treatment for patients with gastric cancer. With increasing use of perioperative chemotherapy and more extensive surgical resection, the indications for radiotherapy have become less well defined. Radiation oncologists are also wary of the acute and potential late toxicities associated with abdominal irradiation. This chapter will describe the challenges faced by radiation oncologists when treating gastric cancer and summarise the available evidence regarding prognostic and predictive factors for survival, response and toxicity after radiotherapy.

1 Introduction

The use of radiotherapy for treatment of gastric cancer has only become commonplace over the past 10 years following reporting of the Gastric Surgical Adjuvant Trial (INT0116) that demonstrated a major survival advantage to the use of postoperative adjuvant chemoradiotherapy (Macdonald et al. 2001). This trial randomly assigned 556 patients following surgery to either observation or adjuvant therapy with 4 monthly cycles of bolus 5-fluorouracil (5-FU) and leucovorin combined with 45 Gy of external beam radiotherapy. With a median follow-up period of 5 years, the 3 year survival rate was 50 % in the chemoradiotherapy group versus 41 % in the surgery alone group ($p = 0.005$). The Intergroup trial highlighted the fact that many radiation oncologists are not familiar with the complex techniques of radiotherapy planning and delivery for gastric cancer. An

T. Leong (✉)
Division of Radiation Oncology,
Peter MacCallum Cancer Centre, Locked Bag 1,
A'Beckett Street, Melbourne, VIC 8006, Australia
e-mail: Trevor.Leong@petermac.org

C. Nieder and L. E. Gaspar (eds.), *Decision Tools for Radiation Oncology*, Medical Radiology. Radiation Oncology,
DOI: 10.1007/174_2013_829,
Published Online: 5 April 2013

evaluation of the radiotherapy treatment planning issues related to implementation of the adjuvant program in this study demonstrated that 35 % of the patients reviewed for initial compliance had major or minor deviations in protocol radiation therapy at the time of initial pretreatment review (Smalley et al. 2002). Until recently, many clinical trial protocols for treatment of gastric cancer (including INT0116) employed 2D treatment planning and parallel-opposed anteroposterior-posteroanterior (AP-PA) field arrangements, resulting in large radiotherapy target volumes. However, many radiation oncologists are reluctant to treat such large abdominal volumes with anterior and posterior fields due to concerns about normal tissue toxicity, particularly in relation to the kidneys, liver and spinal cord. Current modern techniques of radiation delivery including 3-dimensional conformal radiotherapy (3D-CRT) and intensity-modulated radiotherapy (IMRT) employ multiple radiation fields that conform more accurately to the high-risk volume and produce superior dose distributions with the potential to reduce normal tissue toxicity. However, despite the use of CT-based target volume delineation and conformal radiation techniques, many radiation oncologists continue to experience difficulties with gastric irradiation. In a recently reported multi-institutional national study that employed CT planning and 3D-conformal techniques, 35 % of treatment plans contained protocol violations relating to target volume delineation despite the provision of detailed protocol guidelines including a contouring atlas (Leong et al. 2011).

Aside from the technical challenges of gastric irradiation, there are also many clinical challenges faced by practicing radiation oncologists when deciding optimal treatment for patients with gastric cancer. The decision making process has been made more difficult by recent developments in treatment including the use of alternative neo/adjuvant strategies. Although postoperative chemoradiotherapy has been adopted as standard of care in some parts of the world, it is still uncommonly used in other parts. This relates mainly to criticism of INT0116 with regard to surgical quality as 54 % of patients underwent less than a D1 lymph node dissection despite the recommendation for a D2 dissection. However, there are also concerns amongst medical and radiation oncologists regarding the outdated chemoradiation regimen that was employed and the toxicity associated with the treatment. The combined modality regimen in this program was associated with grade 3 and grade 4 toxicity in 41 and 32 % of cases, respectively. The recently published MRC MAGIC trial provides a new option for the treatment of resectable gastric cancer (Cunningham et al. 2006). This trial randomly assigned 503 patients with resectable gastric cancer to either perioperative chemotherapy (3 preoperative and 3 postoperative cycles of epirubicin, cisplatin, 5-FU [ECF]) and surgery or surgery alone. With a median follow-up of 4 years, the 5 year survival rate was 36 % in the perioperative chemotherapy group versus 23 % in the surgery alone group ($p = 0.0009$). The MAGIC study has expanded the range of treatment options available for resectable gastric cancer. For patients seen preoperatively, a regimen of perioperative ECF represents an alternative standard of care for adjuvant therapy. Therefore, in Western countries there are 2 standards of care for patients with resectable gastric cancer, and since the publication of the INT0116 and MAGIC studies, clinicians have been faced with the dilemma of which strategy to employ. Perioperative chemotherapy is used mainly in the United Kingdom and parts of Europe, while postoperative chemoradiation is used mainly in North America.

As with other GI tumour sites, there is increasing interest in the use of preoperative chemoradiotherapy for gastric cancer, which has several distinct advantages compared to postoperative treatment. One of the main advantages is the potential for tumour downstaging with an increase in the complete R0 resection rate. Preoperative therapy is also much better tolerated than postoperative therapy, thereby ensuring that all patients receive the intended treatment. Both of these advantages were clearly demonstrated in the MAGIC study. Preoperative treatment also allows the radiation oncologist to delineate radiotherapy target volumes with greater ease and accuracy because the stomach is intact and the precise location of the primary tumour is known. The strategy of preoperative chemoradiotherapy has been reported in several phase II studies. Ajani et al. reported the results of a multi-institutional phase II study of 34 patients treated with 2 cycles of 5-FU/folinic acid/cisplatin followed by chemoradiation (45 Gy with concurrent continuous infusional 5-FU) and then surgery (Ajani et al. 2004). The R0 resection rate was 70 % and the pathological complete response (pCR) rate was 30 %. The median survival time was 34 months, which is similar to postoperative chemoradiotherapy reported in INT0116. In the RTOG 99-04 phase II study, there were 49 patients who were treated with 2 cycles of 5-FU/folinic acid/cisplatin prior to chemoradiation (45 Gy with concurrent continuous infusional 5-FU/paclitaxel) and subsequent surgery (Ajani et al. 2006). The R0 resection rate was 77 % and the pCR rate was 26 %. Importantly, both studies reported acceptable toxicity and no increase in postoperative morbidity. Preoperative radiotherapy alone has been investigated in a phase III trial from Beijing in which 370 patients with gastric cancer were randomised to radiotherapy (40 Gy in 20 fractions) and surgery, or surgery alone (Zhang et al. 1998). The ten-year survival rates were 20 % for preoperative radiotherapy and 13 % for surgery alone (p = 0.009). The R0 resection rate was higher for patients undergoing preoperative radiotherapy (80 versus 62 %), and the pCR rate for this group was 11 %. Morbidity and mortality rates were not increased in patients receiving preoperative treatment. Although preoperative chemoradiation is still an investigational approach, which is being tested in the ongoing *TOPGEAR* randomised phase III trial (Leong et al. 2012), there is an increasing number of reports in the medical literature describing this approach.

Because gastric irradiation is a relatively new treatment strategy, there is little in the published literature regarding prognostic and predictive factors for survival, response and toxicity after radiotherapy. Nevertheless, this chapter will describe the challenges faced by radiation oncologists when treating gastric cancer and summarise the available evidence that may be used in the decision making process.

2 Prognostic Factors for Survival in Resectable Gastric Cancer. Which Patients Need Radiotherapy?

2.1 AJCC Staging System

With increasing use of perioperative chemotherapy and more extensive surgical resection, the indications for adjuvant radiotherapy have become less well defined. Patients were eligible for the INT0116 study if either, (1) The primary tumour penetrated the muscularis propria or extended to adjacent organs; or (2) The regional lymphatics were involved (T3,4 and/or N1,2 according to the 1988 staging criteria of the American Joint Commission on Cancer [AJCC]). This was based on pattern-of-failure data from the Minnesota Re-operative Series documenting that approximately 60 % of those with positive lymph nodes or extension of the primary tumour through the serosa relapse in the tumour bed, regional lymph nodes, stump, or anastomosis (Gunderson and Sosin 1982). Pathological tumour stage is still the main criterion for determining the need for postoperative chemoradiation. AJCC stage is used as a surrogate measure for predicting individual patient risk after surgery. Since the INT0116 trial, the AJCC staging system has undergone four revisions leading to the current 7th edition in 2010 Table 1. The aim of each revision was to improve the prognostic value of the staging system by adding subgroups to existing stage groupings and introducing new predictive parameters, while keeping the staging system simple and intuitive. Dikken et al. have recently evaluated the changes in the 7th edition AJCC staging system compared to the 6th edition with regard to complexity and predictive accuracy (Dikken et al. 2012). Differences between the 2 staging systems were evaluated using a combined data set of 2,196 patients from Memorial Sloan-Kettering Cancer Centre (MSKCC) and the Dutch Gastric Cancer Trial who underwent an R0 resection for gastric cancer. Within this patient cohort, 16 % received preoperative chemotherapy, 16 % received postoperative chemotherapy and 5 % received postoperative radiotherapy. The concordance index for each staging system was calculated to examine its accuracy for predicting stage-specific survival. Concordance index for a staging system measures how closely the ranking of patient stage correlates with the ranking of actual patient outcome (100 % = absolute concordance). The new staging system was found to be more complex with 9 stage groups compared to 7 in the previous edition. Redefinition of nodal staging into N1, N2 and N3 groups has resulted in a more even distribution with improved predictive accuracy of N classification. However, the predictive accuracy of the AJCC 7th edition was significantly worse than that of the AJCC 6th edition (concordance index 0.697 versus 0.711; $P < 0.01$). Although subdivision of AJCC 6th edition stage II into 7th edition stage IIA, IIB and IIIA has produced 3 significantly different prognostic groups, the subdivision of 6th edition stage IIIA into 7th edition stage IIIA and IIIB has produced 2 groups with virtually identical stage-specific survival. The authors concluded that for individual patient outcome, no improvements were detected from the 6th to the 7th edition staging systems.

2.2 Nomograms

Selecting patients for adjuvant therapy based solely on AJCC stage is not entirely accurate. The AJCC stage groupings stratify disease-specific survival after an R0 resection into risk groups based on the depth of tumour invasion and the number of positive lymph nodes. All patients grouped within a particular AJCC stage group are assumed to have the same prognosis and are therefore treated in the same way. However, for individual patients, risk can vary substantially within a particular stage group depending on other prognostic factors. Tools for individual patient prognostication have been developed that outperform the AJCC classification in prognostic accuracy. In 2003, Kattan et al. from MSKCC developed a postoperative nomogram for predicting disease-specific survival after an R0 resection for gastric cancer (Kattan et al. 2003) (Fig. 1). Rather than stratifying patients into risk groups, nomograms are tools that combine all proven prognostic factors to

Table 1 AJCC TNM classification of gastric cancer

Stage	Description
Primary tumor (T)	
TX	Primary tumor cannot be assessed
TO	No evidence of primary tumor
Tis	Carcinoma in situ: intraepithelial tumor without invasion of the lamina propria
T1a	Tumor invades lamina propria or muscularis mucosae
T1b	Tumor invades submucosa
T2	Tumor invades muscularis propria[a]
T3	Tumor penetrates subserosal connective tissue without invasion of visceral peritoneum[b] or adjacent structures (including spleen, transverse colon, liver, diaphragm, pancreas, abdominal wall, adrenal gland, kidney, small intestine, and retroperitoneum)
T4a	Tumor invades serosa (visceral peritoneum)
T4b	Tumor invades adjacent structures
Regional lymph nodes (N)	
NX	Regional lymph nodes cannot be assessed
N0	No regional lymph node metastasis (pN0 denotes negative finding in all examined lymph nodes, regardless of the total number removed and examined)
N1	Metastasis in 1–2 regional lymph nodes
N2	Metastasis in 3–6 regional lymph nodes
N3a	Metastasis in 7–15 regional lymph nodes
N3b	Metastasis in ≥16 regional lymph nodes
Distant metastasis (M)	
M0	No distant metastasis
M1	Distant metastasis (including seeding of the peritoneum and positive peritoneal cytology)

[a] Penetration to the muscularis propria with extension into the gastrocolic or gastrohepatic ligaments, or into the greater or lesser omentum, without perforation of the visceral peritoneum covering these structures is categorized as T3; perforation of the visceral peritoneum covering the gastric ligaments or the omentum is categorized as T4

[b] Intramural extension to the duodenum or esophagus is classifi ed by the depth of the greatest invasion in any of these sites including stomach

Source Edge et al. (2009)

predict individual patient risk. The MSKCC nomogram utilised data from 1,039 patients who had undergone R0 resections. Nomogram predictor variables included age, sex, primary tumour site, Lauren histology, number of positive lymph nodes, number of negative lymph nodes, and depth of invasion. The concordance index for the model was 0.80. The concordance index provides the probability that for two randomly selected patients in which one patient has an event before the other, the patient who had the event first has a poorer predicted outcome from the nomogram (for concordance, higher is better). When compared with the predictive ability of AJCC stage, the nomogram discrimination was superior (concordance index 0.80 versus 0.77; $P < 0.001$). The authors noted heterogeneity within several of the AJCC stage groups with a range of nomogram-predicted probabilities within each group.

In the last 10 years, D2 lymph node dissection has become more commonly practiced worldwide despite the fact that published randomised trials have not demonstrated improved survival with more extensive nodal dissections (Bonenkamp et al. 1999; Cuschieri et al. 1999). One of the main criticisms of the INT0116 trial has been the lack of quality assurance relating to surgical technique. It has been claimed that the benefits of chemoradiation are only due to the compensation of poor surgery, and that these benefits would not be seen if a D2 dissection had been performed. D2 nodal dissection has been the standard of care in Eastern countries for many decades and the survival rates for Eastern patients with gastric cancer are consistently higher than those for Western patients (MacDonald 2011; Strong et al. 2010). A nomogram predicting 5- and 10 year overall survival after D2 gastrectomy in Eastern patients has recently been reported (Han et al. 2012). Han et al. analysed data from 7,954 patients who underwent D2 gastrectomy at Seoul National University Hospital (SNUH) in Korea. The nomogram was constructed and validated by randomly assigning two-thirds of the patients to the training set ($n = 5{,}300$) and one-third to the validation set ($n = 2{,}654$). Nomogram predictor variables included age, sex, primary tumour location, depth of invasion, number of metastatic lymph nodes, and number of examined lymph nodes. The nomogram was validated firstly using the SNUH validation set and then an additional

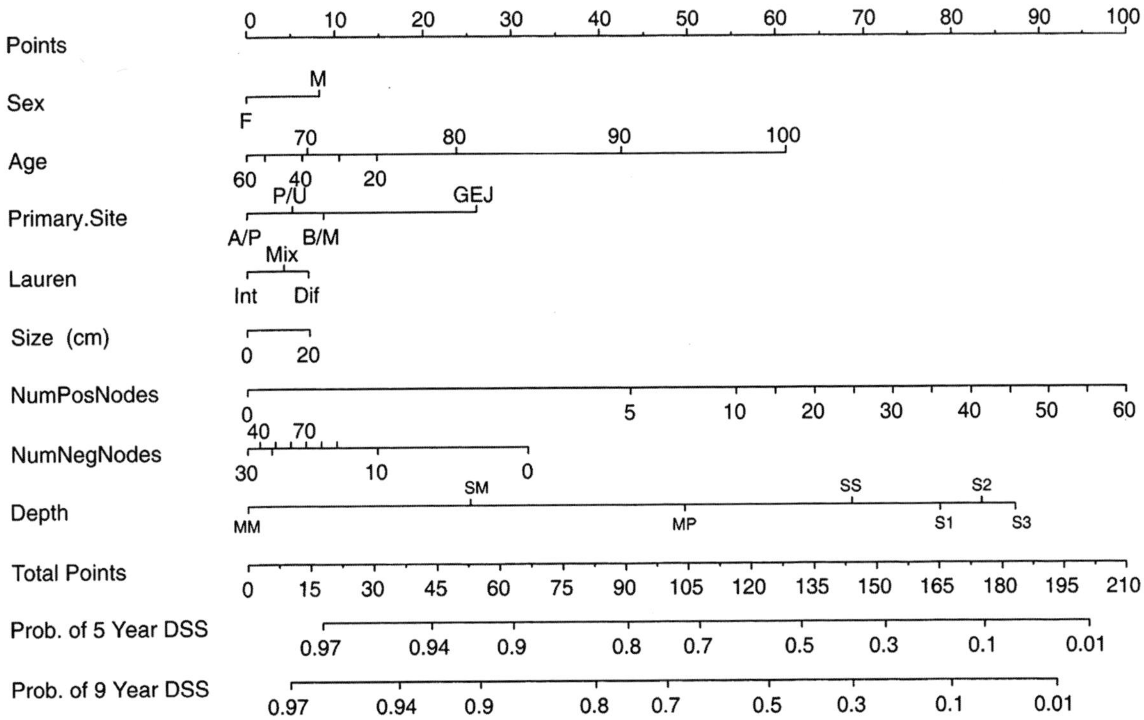

Instructions for Physician: Locate the patient's sex on the **Sex** axis. Draw a line straight upwards to the **Points** axis to determine how many points towards gastric cancer-specific death the patient receives for his or her sex. Repeat this process for the other axes, each time drawing straight upward to the **Points** axis. Sum the points achieved for each predictor and locate this sum on the **Total Points** axis. Draw a line straight down to the disease-specific survival axes to find the patient's probability of surviving gastric cancer assuming he or she does not die of another cause first.

Fig. 1 Memorial Sloan-Kettering Cancer Center nomogram for disease-specific survival (DSS). Number of positive nodes (*NumPosNodes*); number of negative nodes (*NumNegNodes*) probability (*Prob.*); antrum or pyloric (*A/P*), body or middle one-third (*B/M*), gastroesophageal junction (*GEJ*); proximal or upper one-third (*P/U*); intestinal (*int*); mixed (*mix*); diffuse (*Dif*); mucosa (*MM*); propria muscularis (*MP*); suspected serosal invasion (*S1*); definite serosal invasion (*S2*); adjacent organ involvement (*S3*); submucosa (*SM*); and subserosa (*SS*). Reprinted with permission © (2003) American Society of Clinical Oncology. All rights reserved. Kattan et al. (2003)

external validation was performed using a data set (n = 2,500) from the Cancer Institute Ariake Hospital (CIAH) in Tokyo, Japan. In the SNUH validation set, the actual survival corresponded closely with the predicted survival, and the nomogram exhibited superior discrimination power compared with the current 7th edition of the AJCC staging system for gastric cancer (concordance index 0.78 versus 0.69; $P < 0.001$). Similar to the MSKCC nomogram, a wide range of predicted survivals could be identified within each AJCC stage group. In the CIAH validation set, the concordance index was 0.79 and the predicted survival was within a 10 % margin of nomogram prediction.

The use of a nomogram can improve prognostic accuracy when trying to predict outcome after surgery in an individual patient. The information derived can be used to decide whether adjuvant treatment is required if the predicted risk of treatment failure exceeds some predefined threshold. For generalised use of a nomogram by other institutions or other countries, it is important to minimise the effect of differences in surgical technique and pathologic examination. Details regarding D2 gastrectomy and the minimum number of nodes examined are not provided in the report by Kattan. Nevertheless, the MSKCC nomogram has been externally validated for accuracy in several Western patient cohorts (Koc et al. 2009; Novotny et al. 2006; Peeters et al. 2005). In the SNUH data set, all patients underwent a D2 gastrectomy and patients were excluded if the number of examined lymph nodes was less than 16. However, although this nomogram may be useful in Korea and Japan where D2 gastrectomy is routinely performed, it has not been validated using a Western patient cohort. The universal applicability of these nomograms across both Eastern and Western populations remains a question for several reasons. Firstly, the treatment paradigms for adjuvant therapy are different in the East and West. In Eastern countries, adjuvant therapy consists almost exclusively of postoperative chemotherapy, and there is very little use of radiotherapy or preoperative treatment (Bang et al. 2012; Sakuramoto et al. 2007). Secondly, there are clear differences in the epidemiology and clinical presentation of gastric cancer in the East compared with the West (Bunt et al. 1995; Guggenheim and Shah 2012; Verdecchia et al. 2003). Some studies also suggest that Eastern patients may have better survival rates, stage-for-stage compared with Western patients, even after controlling for the extent of surgical resection (Strong et al. 2010).

2.3 Combining Postoperative Chemoradiation with Preoperative Chemotherapy

One dilemma faced by clinicians is how to manage patients who commence treatment with preoperative ECF but show no evidence of tumour downstaging at surgery. Should these patients continue with postoperative ECF according to the MAGIC regimen, or should they change to postoperative chemoradiation? This question is being addressed in the ongoing *CRITICS* trial that is being conducted in the Netherlands and Scandinavia. *CRITICS* is a randomised trial of preoperative epirubicin, cisplatin and capecitabine [ECX] followed by either surgery and additional ECX (i.e., MAGIC), or by surgery and postoperative chemoradiation (i.e., INT0116). The question being addressed by this trial is whether postoperative chemoradiation improves survival and/or locoregional control compared to postoperative chemotherapy alone in patients that receive preoperative chemotherapy followed by surgery. Currently, in the absence of any randomised data to guide treatment decisions, it is not unreasonable to offer postoperative chemoradiation to those patients who have not demonstrated any evidence of downstaging with preoperative chemotherapy (i.e., those with pathological T3-4 tumours or node positive tumours). It is known from the INT0116 trial that postoperative chemoradiation is effective in these patients, while the contribution of postoperative chemotherapy as given in the MAGIC trial is controversial given that only 42 % of patients completed the postoperative chemotherapy (Macdonald et al. 2001).

2.4 Molecular Biomarkers

The development of new molecular biomarkers can be used to identify subgroups of tumours with different biological and clinical behavior. Several molecular techniques have been utilized to identify potential predictors of lymph node status in patients with gastric cancer including altered DNA copy number and expression of specific genes, genome wide mRNA expression analysis, and gene expression profiling (Buffart et al. 2009; Li et al. 2008; Marchet et al. 2007; Teramoto et al. 2005; Wu et al. 2008; Zheng et al. 2006). However, none of the identified markers have shown clinical utility and the gold standard to predict prognosis after surgery remains TNM staging.

3 Prognostic and Predictive Markers Associated with Chemoradiotherapy

3.1 Clinico-Pathological Features

3.1.1 Postoperative Chemoradiotherapy

There is very little information in the published literature reporting prognostic factors for survival after chemoradiation for gastric cancer. The 5 year survival estimates for patients treated on INT0116 show decreasing survival with increasing T-stage and number of positive lymph nodes (MacDonald 2011). Patients with T1-2 tumours had 56 % 5 year survival compared to 38 % for patients with T3 tumours. The 5 year survival estimates for patients with N0, N1-3, and N > 4 nodal disease were 60, 50 and 30 % respectively. In a recent update of the INT0116 trial, Smalley et al. performed exploratory subset analyses of treatment effect for the following variables; sex, race, T-stage, N-stage, D level of resection, primary tumour location, and histology (Smalley et al. 2012). These analyses showed that postoperative chemoradiation was beneficial in all subsets with the exception of patients with diffuse histology who exhibited minimal non-significant treatment effect. The authors were unable to explain this finding and caution that it may be a random observation of an unplanned subset analysis.

Several studies have shown lymph node status to be an important prognostic factor for survival following adjuvant chemoradiation. Quero et al. have recently reported a series of 52 patients who underwent gastrectomy and postoperative chemoradiotherapy for gastric cancer (Quero et al. 2012). The proportion of patients who had D1 and D2 lymph node dissection was 71 and 15 % respectively. This study reported pathologic nodal status to be predictive of disease-free survival. Patients with $\leq$6 positive lymph nodes had a 5-year disease-free survival rate of 57 % compared to 32 % for patients with 7–15 positive nodes and 18 % for patients with >15 positive nodes ($p = 0.02$). Osti et al. reported a series of 55 patients with gastric cancer who underwent D2 gastrectomy followed by postoperative chemoradiotherapy (Osti et al. 2012). In this study, lymph node ratio (LNR: defined as the ratio of the number of metastatic nodes to the number of removed nodes) $\geq$4 and N3 nodal stage were significant prognostic factors for overall survival and relapse. In addition, stage III–IV disease was also identified as being a significant prognostic factor for survival. Chang and co-workers treated a series of 120 patients with gastric cancer over a 10 year period using the INT0116 regimen (Chang et al. 2011). Fifty-two percent of patients underwent conventional radiotherapy planning and were treated with simple AP-PA techniques, while 48 % underwent CT planning. This study showed that stage of disease, and particularly nodal stage was an important prognostic factor for survival. Interestingly, the authors also reported that CT planning was a favourable predictor of survival as compared with conventional planning. Kassam et al. from the Princess Margaret Hospital reported a series of 82 patients with resected gastric cancer who were treated with postoperative chemoradiotherapy (Kassam et al. 2006). Only 6.1 % of patients underwent a D2 lymph node dissection, while 48 % underwent less than a D1 dissection. In this series, tumour and nodal stage significantly influenced relapse-free and overall survival. Three year relapse-free survival was 74 % for patients with T1/2 tumours compared to 36 % for patients with T3/4 tumours ($p = 0.008$). Three year overall survival was 85 % for T1/2 tumours versus 53 % for T3/4 tumours ($p = 0.02$). Patients with N0/1 tumours had a 3-year relapse-free survival of 63 % compared to 0 % for patients with N2/3 tumours ($p < 0.001$). Three year overall survival was 80 % for N0/1 tumours versus 0 % for N2/3 tumours ($p < 0.001$). Zhu et al. have recently reported the results of a randomised, multicentre trial from China that compared IMRT plus concurrent chemotherapy with chemotherapy alone in 380 gastric cancer patients treated with D2 gastrectomy (Zhu et al. 2012). IMRT was associated with an increase in the median duration of relapse-free survival (50 months for IMRT versus 32 months for chemotherapy alone; $p = 0.029$), although there was no significant difference in overall survival. An analysis of prognostic factors showed that lymph node metastasis and TNM stage were both independent prognostic factors. This study provides the first phase III evidence of benefit for postoperative chemoradiation in patients undergoing D2 gastrectomy.

Verheij et al. have recently assessed the performance of the MSKCC gastric nomogram in a cohort of 139 patients who received postoperative chemoradiation after an R0 resection for gastric cancer (Verheij et al. 2012). As previously described, this nomogram was developed from a data set of patients who had undergone R0 resections without any adjuvant therapy. The concordance index of the nomogram was 0.64 for patients who received postoperative chemoradiation, which was lower than the concordance index for patients who received no adjuvant therapy (0.80). The observed survival of patients receiving postoperative chemoradiation was approximately 20 % higher than that predicted by the nomogram. The authors concluded that the MSKCC nomogram significantly underpredicted the survival of this patient group, confirming the survival benefit conferred by postoperative chemoradiation. This study highlights the need to update current postoperative nomograms with incorporation of patient cohorts receiving adjuvant therapy.

3.1.2 Preoperative Chemoradiotherapy

Several investigators have reported prognostic factors for survival after preoperative chemoradiotherapy for gastric cancer. In the RTOG 99-04 phase II study of preoperative chemoradiotherapy, Ajani et al. reported that 82 % of patients with a pCR following preoperative chemoradiotherapy were alive compared with 69 % of patients with less than pCR (Ajani et al. 2006). A similar correlation between pCR and overall survival in gastric cancer patients treated with preoperative chemoradiation has been reported by other groups (Ajani et al. 2004; Reed et al. 2008). Rostom et al. reported a study of 41 patients with operable gastric cancer who were treated with 2 cycles of induction chemotherapy (fluorouracil, docetaxel, and cisplatin) followed by 45 Gy of radiation with concurrent fluorouracil and docetaxel, and then surgery (Rostom et al. 2012). The pCR rate was 24 % and the 3 year overall survival rate was 47.3 %. In this study, overall survival was significantly correlated with pathological response, R0 resection, dissected pathologically positive lymph nodes, and post-surgery T-stage. Investigators from the MD Anderson Cancer Center investigated the role of surgical pathology stage following preoperative chemoradiation as a prognosticator of overall survival (Rohatgi et al. 2006). The patient cohort for this study comprised 74 patients enrolled on 2 prospectively conducted, preoperative chemoradiation trials. All patients were staged with endoscopic ultrasound (EUS) and laparoscopy and were treated with induction chemotherapy followed by chemoradiation to 45 Gy, and then surgery. This analysis did not show any correlation between baseline clinical stage as determined by EUS and overall survival. However, there was a significant correlation between postsurgical T, N, and overall stages with overall survival. Of all the factors assessed, the pathologic AJCC stage was the strongest predictor of overall survival. Patients with stages 0-II tumours survived significantly longer than patients with stages III-IV tumours (median time not reached vs 12 months respectively; $p = 0.001$). In addition, patients who achieved a pCR survived significantly longer than those who did not (median time not reached versus 53 months; $p = 0.004$). The authors concluded that when preoperative chemoradiation is employed, the surgical pathology stage is a better prognosticator of overall survival than the baseline clinical stage. In a separate study utilising the same patient cohort, the same investigators have shown that clinical stage after preoperative chemoradiation is also a better predictor of patient outcome than baseline clinical stage (Patel et al. 2007). Amongst the 74 patients who received preoperative chemoradiation, 35 underwent repeat preoperative staging with EUS. For these patients, the correlation between baseline EUS stage and overall survival was not statistically significant. However, there was a significant correlation between pre-surgical EUS stage and overall survival. Patients with pre-surgical stages I-II tumours survived significantly longer than patients with pre-surgical stages III-IV tumours (median time not reached versus 15.2 months respectively; $p = 0.01$).

3.2 Molecular Biomarkers

Although there are many reports describing molecular biomarkers associated with response to chemotherapy in gastric cancer (Mutze et al. 2011; Robb and Mariette 2012; Van Cutsem et al. 2012; Wang et al. 2012), there is very little published data relating to molecular biomarkers associated with the use of chemoradiotherapy. This reflects the relatively short period of time that radiotherapy has been used as part of curative treatment for gastric cancer. Lee et al. investigated the impact of E2F-1 expression on the clinical outcome of gastric cancer patients treated with surgery and adjuvant chemoradiation (Lee et al. 2008). E2F-1 is a transcription factor that can act either as an oncogene or a tumour suppressor gene depending on the primary tumour type, and it controls the transcription of several genes involved in DNA synthesis (Bell and Ryan 2004; La Thangue 2003; Wu et al. 2001). The patient cohort for this study comprised 467 patients from a single centre in Korea who all underwent D2 gastrectomy followed by adjuvant chemoradiation using the INT0116 regimen (45 Gy of radiation plus 5-FU and leucovorin). Immunohistochemical studies using tissue microarrays showed that E2F-1 immunopositivity predicted more favourable survival as compared with E2F-1 immunonegativity [$p = 0.050$, hazard ratio = 0.702, 95 % confidence interval 0.487–1.013]. However, AJCC stage was still the most powerful prognostic factor in this series. Soyuer et al. investigated the prognostic significance of CD9 expression in 49 patients with locally advanced gastric cancer treated with surgery and adjuvant chemoradiation (Soyuer et al. 2010). CD9 is a tetraspanin transmembrane protein that plays an important role in inhibiting cell motility in several tumour cell lines, including gastric cancer. Immunohistochemical evaluation showed CD9 positivity to be a significant prognostic factor for disease-free and overall survival. Ongoing and future clinical trials will continue the search to identify molecular biomarkers of response and survival, but currently there are no reliable prognostic markers to identify gastric cancer patients who may benefit from adjuvant chemoradiotherapy.

4 Toxicity of Chemoradiotherapy for Gastric Cancer

4.1 Acute and Late Toxicities

A major concern amongst radiation oncologists when contemplating gastric irradiation is toxicity. Radiotherapy to the abdomen can result in significant acute toxicity related to hepatic and gastrointestinal mucosal exposure. In addition, gastric irradiation may also affect critical normal tissues such as the kidneys, liver, lungs, and heart, resulting in late toxicities. The combined modality regimen employed in INT0116 was associated with considerable acute toxicity, with grade 3 and grade 4 toxicity occurring in 41 and 32 % of cases, respectively (Macdonald et al. 2001). Only 64 % of patients completed treatment as planned and 17 % of patients were unable to complete radiotherapy due to treatment related toxicity. The main toxicities associated with this treatment were haematologic and gastrointestinal. Major grade 3/4 haematologic toxicity occurred in 54 % of patients while major grade 3/4 gastrointestinal toxicity occurred in 33 % of patients. There have been no reports of late treatment-related toxicities with long-term follow-up, although 21 patients in the chemoradiation arm developed second malignancies compared to 8 in the observation arm (Smalley et al. 2012). Other investigators have also reported high toxicity rates when using the INT0116 regimen. In the study by Chang et al. of 120 patients treated with the INT0116 regimen, the reported rate of grade 3 or greater acute toxicity was 66 %, while the rate of grade 4 toxicity was 22 % (all due to neutropenia) (Chang et al. 2011). Grade 3 gastrointestinal toxicity occurred in 8 % of patients while grade 3/4 haematologic toxicity occurred in 61 % of patients. The authors reported that anaemia and gastritis were the most commonly occurring late complications of treatment. Twelve patients developed gastritis that was confirmed by gastroscopy and was either grade 1 or 2. Three patients developed anastomotic strictures, 2 patients developed malabsorption, and 1 patient developed a bowel obstruction. Grade 1 renal impairment was observed in 3 patients and was manifested clinically as mildly elevated serum creatinine or proteinuria. Interestingly, ultrasound and CT performed on these 3 patients demonstrated atrophic left kidneys that were attributed to radiation. Kundel et al. have recently evaluated the tolerability of the INT0116 regimen in 166 patients treated over a 7 year period (Kundel et al. 2011). Treatment compliance was relatively poor with only 54 % of patients completing the entire chemoradiation regimen (87 % completed radiotherapy and 57 % completed chemotherapy). In all cases, treatment discontinuation was due to treatment related toxicity. Acute toxicity was considerable with 46 % of patients experiencing grade ≥3 toxicity. Grade ≥3 haematologic toxicity occurred in 32 % of patients with the most common being neutropenia and leukopenia (grade ≥3 in 30 and 25 % respectively). Febrile neutropenia was reported in 15 % of patients. Grade ≥3 non-haematologic toxicity occurred in 25 % of patients with the most common being nausea, vomiting and diarrhoea (10 % for each toxicity). Three patients (1.8 %) died from treatment related toxicity and 48 patients (29 %) were hospitalised for toxicity. Late radiation toxicity was not reported for this study.

It should be noted that the majority of patients in the above studies were treated according to the original INT0116 protocol i.e., bolus 5-FU/leucovorin chemotherapy combined with radiotherapy delivered using AP-PA fields. In the decade that has elapsed since publication of the INT0116 trial, several alternative chemoradiation regimens for gastric cancer have been reported that combine more current systemic treatment with modern techniques of radiotherapy delivery. The aim of any new regimen is to enhance the therapeutic ratio by improving efficacy and reducing toxicity. We recently reported the results of a prospective, multi-centre study that evaluated a regimen of ECF chemotherapy combined with chemoradiation (Leong et al. 2011). In this study, 54 patients received adjuvant treatment consisting of 1 cycle of ECF chemotherapy, followed by radiotherapy (45 Gy) with concurrent continuous infusional 5-FU, and then 2 further cycles of ECF. All patients were treated using multiple-field 3D conformal techniques (Leong et al. 2005). The proportion of patients completing cycles 1, 2, and 3 of ECF chemotherapy were 100, 81, and 67 % respectively. Ninety-four percent of patients completed radiotherapy as planned. Grade 3/4 neutropenia occurred in 66 % of patients with 7.4 % developing febrile neutropenia. Grade 3/4 gastrointestinal toxicity occurred in 28 % of patients. At a median follow-up period of 36 months, the 3 year overall survival rate was 61.6 %. While overall treatment compliance in this study was similar to that observed in INT0116 where 64 % of patients completed treatment as planned, the radiotherapy compliance was higher than in INT0116 where 17 % of patients were unable to complete radiotherapy due to treatment related toxicity. The higher radiotherapy completion rate observed in our study compared to INT0116 may be due in part to the conformal radiotherapy techniques that were employed compared to the AP-PA field arrangements used in INT0116. Intergroup trial CALGB 80101 is the follow-on study to INT0116, and it has recently been reported in abstract form (Fuchs et al. 2011). This randomised phase III trial compared the INT0116 regimen with an ECF-based regimen, which is almost identical to the one used in our study. An analysis of the toxicity profiles favors the ECF arm. The rates of diarrhoea, mucositis, dehydration and grade 4 neutropenia in the ECF arm were approximately half that in the control arm (15 versus 7 %; 15 versus 7 %; 9 versus 4 %; 33 versus 19 %). Overall grade 4 toxicity was 40 % in the control arm vs 26 % in the ECF arm ($p < 0.001$). However, there was no difference in overall survival between the 2 arms (5 year overall survival 44 % for ECF arm versus 41 % for control arm; $p = 0.80$).

4.2 Predictive Factors for Toxicity After Gastric Irradiation

There are no reports in the published literature describing factors that predict for acute toxicity after gastric irradiation. Radiation oncologists need to be cognizant of the toxicity profile associated with this treatment, and carefully select patients for adjuvant therapy after considering factors such as age, performance status, comorbidity and nutritional status. Patients also require appropriate ancillary care including nutritional support, anti-emetics and regular blood counts to ensure that the prescribed treatment is completed with minimal toxicity.

4.2.1 Renal Toxicity

Aside from the acute toxicity of treatment, radiation oncologists are particularly wary of the potential late complications of gastric irradiation. Perhaps the most critical organs in this regard are the kidneys, owing to their relatively lower tolerance compared to other normal tissue structures. Risk estimates for radiation-associated kidney injury are currently based on dosimetric factors derived from dose volume histogram (DVH) analysis. Unfortunately, our current understanding of kidney dose response is still rudimentary. Partial-kidney irradiation risk estimates are still based on very basic dose-volume models, which fail to take into account the spatial distribution of both radiation dose and existing kidney function. There is a paucity of information in the medical literature regarding partial kidney tolerance after modern chemoradiation for gastrointestinal malignancies. Most of the published studies have been in lymphoma and seminoma where the radiation doses are lower and the volumes of kidney irradiated are smaller compared with those for gastric cancer. Jansen et al. reported the results of a prospective study investigating late renal toxicity following postoperative chemoradiation for gastric cancer (Jansen et al. 2007). In this study, renal function was monitored in 44 patients using Tc^{99m}-thiatide renography performed before and at regular intervals after postoperative chemoradiation. The left-to-right ratio in activity was used as an index of the division of renal function between the 2 kidneys. The study demonstrated a progressive decline in relative left kidney function of approximately 11 % after 6 months ($p = 0.012$) and 52 %

after 18 months ($p < 0.001$). The V_{20} (percentage volume receiving 20 Gy) for the left kidney and the mean left kidney dose were found to be associated with decreased kidney function. One patient who was followed up for more than 18 months developed clinically symptomatic renovascular hypertension. May et al. analysed the clinical and dosimetric factors associated with changes in renal function in 63 patients who received abdominal irradiation for gastrointestinal malignancies (May et al. 2010). Changes in renal function were assessed using creatinine clearance measured before radiotherapy and at 6 month intervals after radiotherapy. Median follow-up was 17.5 months and median radiation dose was 50.4 Gy. This study demonstrated a progressive decline in renal function over time with creatinine clearance decreasing 21.37 % (SD 21.77) from 98.46 mL/min (SD 36.95) before radiotherapy to 74.20 mL/min (SD 25.74) one year after radiotherapy ($p < 0.0001$). Multivariate analysis showed pre-radiotherapy creatinine clearance, V_{10} (percentage of bilateral renal volume receiving 10 Gy), and mean kidney dose to be significantly associated with the development of grade ≥ 2 renal complications at 1 year after chemoradiation ($p = 0.0025$, 0.0170, and 0.0095, respectively). Because the kidney partial tolerance to radiotherapy is largely unknown, it is difficult to make firm recommendations about dose constraints for renal irradiation. The recently published QUANTEC paper on radiation-associated kidney injury provides the best summary of studies that have been reported to date (Dawson et al. 2010). In this paper, the authors have produced a composite schematic of combined kidney DVH of data from these studies, which provides some broad guidelines for clinicians (Fig. 2). One of the major difficulties encountered with gastric irradiation is how to balance the dose constraints for the liver with those of the kidneys. Whether or not the dose constraints for all organs can be met, will depend in part, on the tolerance doses imposed for each organ. In the majority of cases, gastric irradiation is associated with relatively high radiation doses to either, or both kidneys, so any dose constraints that are imposed need to be realistically achievable. It should also be remembered that use of nephrotoxic chemotherapy with abdominal radiotherapy can reduce renal tolerance and compound renal toxicity (Stewart et al. 1989; Tarbell et al. 1988).

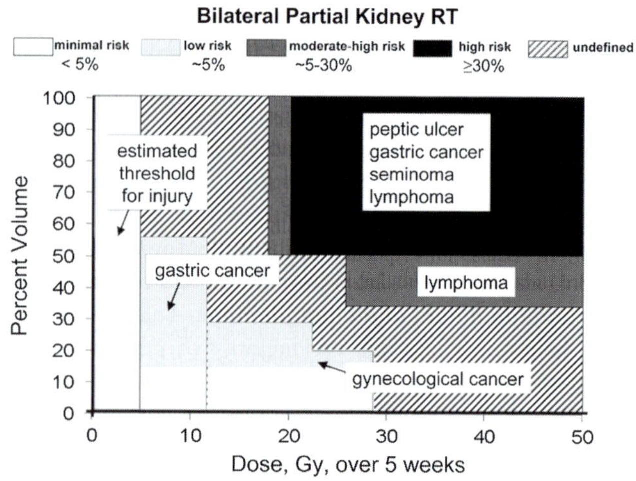

Fig. 2 Composite schematic of combined kidney DVH of data from published studies, represented as regions associated with minimal (<5 %), low (~5 %), moderate-to-high (~5–30 %), high (≥30 %), or undocumented estimated toxicity risks. Clinical experience that yielded risk estimates for each region also indicated. Actual risks associated with using each region on its own or regions in combination are plan-specific and associated with substantial uncertainty. Reprinted with permission. © (2010) Elsevier Ltd. All rights reserved. Dawson et al. (2010)

4.2.2 Liver Toxicity

In contrast to radiation-associated kidney injury, the data relating to radiation-induced liver disease (RILD) has been reasonably well studied and analysed. One of the largest reported series of patients treated with partial liver irradiation comes from the University of Michigan (Dawson et al. 2001, 2002). These studies have demonstrated that small portions of the liver can be irradiated to a very high dose. Estimates of the liver doses associated with a 5 % risk of RILD for uniform irradiation of one-third, two-thirds, and the whole liver were 90, 47, and 31 Gy, respectively. Mean liver dose was also associated with RILD, with no cases reported in patients with a mean liver dose of less than 31 Gy. The recently published QUANTEC paper on radiation-associated liver injury has proposed guidelines for normal liver dose constraints; for a 5 % or less risk of RILD, the mean normal liver dose (liver minus gross tumour volume) should be <32 Gy in 2 Gy fractions (Pan et al. 2010). There are several factors that may render patients more susceptible to RILD including pre-existing liver dysfunction, hepatitis B carrier status, concurrent chemotherapy, and portal vein tumour thrombosis (Cheng et al. 2004; Dawson et al. 2002; Kim et al. 2007; Liang et al. 2006).

4.3 Strategies Aimed at Reducing Toxicity

4.3.1 IMRT

There are several treatment strategies that may potentially reduce acute and long-term sequelae of chemoradiation while maintaining adequate coverage of the target volume. IMRT can potentially reduce toxicity by decreasing radiation exposure to adjacent critical normal tissues. Previously reported studies have shown that compared to 3D-CRT, IMRT for postoperative treatment of gastric cancer can reduce radiation dose to the kidneys, spinal cord and liver (Alani et al. 2009; Dahele et al. 2010; Minn et al. 2010).

The majority of these studies have been dosimetric comparisons with only a few reporting clinical outcomes. Chakravarty et al. reported their experience using IMRT as preoperative treatment for localized gastric cancer (Chakravarty et al. 2012). In this series from the MD Anderson Cancer Center, 25 patients were treated with induction chemotherapy followed by preoperative IMRT with concurrent chemotherapy, and then surgical resection. Following preoperative treatment, the R0 resection rate was 80 % and the pCR rate was 20 %. These rates are similar to those reported in previous studies of preoperative chemoradiation for gastric cancer using 3D-CRT (Ajani et al. 2004, 2006). Interestingly, the rates of grade 3 acute toxicity, hospitalisation, and feeding tube use did not appear to be lower in patients treated with IMRT when compared to those in a group of 50 patients treated at the same institution with preoperative 3D-CRT (56 versus 54 %; 24 versus 28 %; 76 versus 78 % respectively). The authors postulate that acute toxicity in these patients is likely due to irradiation of the gastric mucosa, which will be the same regardless of the radiation technique employed. Grade 3 acute toxicities included dehydration (40 %), nausea (32 %), anorexia (20 %), fatigue (8 %), dysphagia (4 %), and odynophagia (4 %). There were no reports of grade 4 or higher toxicity. Although IMRT did not appear to reduce the rates of acute toxicity in this study, it did lead to dosimetric sparing of the liver and kidneys. Minn et al. compared the clinical outcomes and toxicity in patients treated with postoperative chemoradiation for gastric cancer using IMRT versus 3D-CRT (Minn et al. 2010). In this study of 57 patients, 31 were treated with IMRT and 26 with 3D-CRT. Similar to the MD Anderson series, grade $\geq$2 acute gastrointestinal toxicity was found to be similar between the 3D-CRT and IMRT patients (61.5 versus 61.2 %, respectively). However, 3 patients in the 3D-CRT group required a treatment break due to toxicity, whereas no patient in the IMRT group required a treatment break. IMRT led to improved sparing of the liver (V_{30} 16.1 % for IMRT versus 28 % for 3D-CRT) as well as the kidneys (median V_{20} 18 % for IMRT versus 22 % for 3D-CRT). With a median follow-up of 1.3 years, grade 3 late toxicity was experienced by 3 patients in the 3D-CRT group, all of whom developed small bowel obstruction. For the IMRT group, grade 3 toxicity was experienced by 1 patient who developed a stricture requiring surgery. This study also suggested that IMRT may potentially preserve kidney function over 3D-CRT. The median 'pre-irradiation serum creatinine to most recent post-irradiation creatinine' was unchanged in the IMRT group (0.80 mg/dL) but increased in the 3D-CRT group from 0.80 mg/dL to 1.0 mg/dL ($p = 0.02$).

4.3.2 Preoperative Chemoradiation

Preoperative radiotherapy can also potentially reduce target volumes and dose to normal tissues compared to postoperative radiotherapy. Tillman et al. compared normal tissue radiation doses using preoperative versus postoperative radiotherapy for locally advanced gastroesophageal junction and proximal gastric cancers (Tillman et al. 2008). In this dosimetric comparison, hypothetical preoperative treatment plans were generated for 5 patients who had undergone postoperative radiotherapy with curative intent. The preoperative treatment plans were then compared to the postoperative plans used to treat the patient with respect to prespecified dose volume parameters. The study showed that target volumes were smaller using preoperative radiotherapy by an average of 23 %. This was mainly due to the fact that with preoperative treatment, there is no requirement to cover anastomotic sites that are often located high in the chest following surgery for gastroesophageal junction tumours. For the same reason, the resultant composite lung doses were reduced in the preoperative plans by 50–79 %. In all patients, the V_{20} for the lungs was reduced from a mean of 16 to 2.9 %. Likewise, the V_{30} for the heart was also reduced in all preoperative plans (15.8 versus 35.4 %). In contrast, the radiation doses to the kidneys, liver and spinal cord were similar with both approaches.

5 Conclusion

In contrast to most other tumour sites, the use of radiotherapy in the curative treatment of gastric cancer is a relatively new treatment strategy. As such, there is a paucity of information in the published literature regarding prognostic and predictive factors for response, survival and toxicity after radiotherapy. The majority of published studies have been small, single institution series and have not been validated in larger patient cohorts or randomised phase III trials. Clinicians must currently rely on traditional clinicopathological factors such as TNM staging to guide clinical decision making. Nevertheless, considerable efforts are being directed towards gastric cancer research with large phase III chemoradiation trials such as *CRITICS* and *TOPGEAR* due for completion in the next few years. These trials incorporate well designed correlative science studies that will hopefully identify molecular biomarkers of response and survival, thereby allowing a more personalised approach to patient management.

References

Ajani JA, Mansfield PF, Janjan N, Morris J, Pisters PW, Lynch PM, Feig B, Myerson R, Nivers R, Cohen DS, Gunderson LL (2004) Multi-institutional trial of preoperative chemoradiotherapy in patients with potentially resectable gastric carcinoma. J Clin Oncol 22(14):2774–2780

Ajani JA, Winter K, Okawara GS, Donohue JH, Pisters PW, Crane CH, Greskovich JF, Anne PR, Bradley JD, Willett C, Rich TA (2006) Phase II trial of preoperative chemoradiation in patients with localized gastric adenocarcinoma (RTOG 9904): quality of combined modality therapy and pathologic response. J Clin Oncol 24(24):3953–3958

Alani S, Soyfer V, Strauss N, Schifter D, Corn BW (2009) Limited advantages of intensity-modulated radiotherapy over 3D conformal radiation therapy in the adjuvant management of gastric cancer. Int J Radiat Oncol Biol Phys 74(2):562–566. doi:10.1016/j.ijrobp.2008.09.061

Bang YJ, Kim YW, Yang HK, Chung HC, Park YK, Lee KH, Lee KW, Kim YH, Noh SI, Cho JY, Mok YJ, Ji J, Yeh TS, Button P, Sirzen F, Noh SH (2012) Adjuvant capecitabine and oxaliplatin for gastric cancer after D2 gastrectomy (CLASSIC): a phase 3 open-label, randomised controlled trial. Lancet 379(9813):315–321. doi:10.1016/S0140-6736(11)61873-4

Bell LA, Ryan KM (2004) Life and death decisions by E2F-1. Cell Death Differ 11(2):137–142. doi:10.1038/sj.cdd.4401324

Bonenkamp JJ, Hermans J, Sasako M, van de Velde CJ (1999) Extended lymph-node dissection for gastric cancer. Dutch gastric cancer group. N Engl J Med 340(12):908–914

Buffart TE, van Grieken NC, Tijssen M, Coffa J, Ylstra B, Grabsch HI, van de Velde CJ, Carvalho B, Meijer GA (2009) High resolution analysis of DNA copy-number aberrations of chromosomes 8, 13, and 20 in gastric cancers. Virchows Archiv Int J pathol 455(3):213–223. doi:10.1007/s00428-009-0814-y

Bunt AM, Hermans J, Smit VT, van de Velde CJ, Fleuren GJ, Bruijn JA (1995) Surgical/pathologic-stage migration confounds comparisons of gastric cancer survival rates between Japan and Western countries. J Clin Oncol 13(1):19–25

Chakravarty T, Crane CH, Ajani JA, Mansfield PF, Briere TM, Beddar AS, Mok H, Reed VK, Krishnan S, Delclos ME, Das P (2012) Intensity-modulated radiation therapy with concurrent chemotherapy as preoperative treatment for localized gastric adenocarcinoma. Int J Radiat Oncol Biol Phys 83(2):581–586. doi:10.1016/j.ijrobp.2011.07.035

Chang AT, Ng WT, Law AL, Ku KM, Lee MC, Lee AW (2011) Adjuvant chemoradiation for resected gastric cancer: a 10 year experience. Gastric Cancer 14(1):63–71. doi:10.1007/s10120-011-0011-y

Cheng JC, Wu JK, Lee PC, Liu HS, Jian JJ, Lin YM, Sung JL, Jan GJ (2004) Biologic susceptibility of hepatocellular carcinoma patients treated with radiotherapy to radiation-induced liver disease. Int J Radiat Oncol Biol Phys 60(5):1502–1509. doi:10.1016/j.ijrobp.2004.05.048

Cunningham D, Allum WH, Stenning SP, Thompson JN, van de Velde CJ, Nicolson M, Scarffe JH, Lofts FJ, Falk SJ, Iveson TJ, Smith DB, Langley RE, Verma M, Weeden S, Chua YJ, Participants MT (2006) Perioperative chemotherapy versus surgery alone for resectable gastroesophageal cancer. N Engl J Med 355(1):11–20

Cuschieri A, Weeden S, Fielding J, Bancewicz J, Craven J, Joypaul V, Sydes M, Fayers P (1999) Patient survival after D1 and D2 resections for gastric cancer: long-term results of the MRC randomized surgical trial. Surgical co-operative group. Br J Cancer 79(9–10):1522–1530

Dahele M, Skinner M, Schultz B, Cardoso M, Bell C, Ung YC (2010) Adjuvant radiotherapy for gastric cancer: A dosimetric comparison of 3-dimensional conformal radiotherapy, tomotherapy and conventional intensity modulated radiotherapy treatment plans. Med Dosim 35(2):115–121. doi:10.1016/j.meddos.2009.03.003

Dawson LA, Kavanagh BD, Paulino AC, Das SK, Miften M, Li XA, Pan C, Ten Haken RK, Schultheiss TE (2010) Radiation-associated kidney injury. Int J Radiat Oncol Biol Phys 76(3):S108–S115. doi:10.1016/j.ijrobp.2009.02.089

Dawson LA, Normolle D, Balter JM, McGinn CJ, Lawrence TS, Ten Haken RK (2002) Analysis of radiation-induced liver disease using the Lyman NTCP model. Int J Radiat Oncol Biol Phys 53(4):810–821

Dawson LA, Ten Haken RK, Lawrence TS (2001) Partial irradiation of the liver. Semin Radiat Oncol 11(3):240–246

Dikken JL, van de Velde CJ, Gonen M, Verheij M, Brennan MF, Coit DG (2012) The new American joint committee on cancer/international union against cancer staging system for adenocarcinoma of the stomach: increased complexity without clear improvement in predictive accuracy. Ann Surg Oncol 19(8):2443–2451. doi:10.1245/s10434-012-2403-6

Edge SB, Byrd DR, Compton CC et al (2009) American Joint Committee on Cancer, American Cancer Society. AJCC cancer staging manual, 7th edn. Springer, Berlin Heidelberg New York

Fuchs CS, Tepper JE, Niedzwiecki D, Hollis D, Mamon HJ, Swanson R, Haller DG, Dragovich T, Alberts SR, Bjarnason GA, Willett CG, Enzinger PC, Goldberg RM, Venook AP, Mayer RJ (2011) Postoperative adjuvant chemoradiation for gastric or gastroesophageal junction (GEJ) adenocarcinoma using epirubicin, cisplatin, and infusional (CI) 5-FU (ECF) before and after CI 5-FU and radiotherapy (CRT) compared with bolus 5-FU/LV before and after CRT: intergroup trial CALGB 80101. J Clin Oncol 29(15):4003

Guggenheim DE, Shah MA (2012) Gastric cancer epidemiology and risk factors. J Surg Oncol. doi:10.1002/jso.23262

Gunderson LL, Sosin H (1982) Adenocarcinoma of the stomach: areas of failure in a re-operation series (second or symptomatic look) clinicopathologic correlation and implications for adjuvant therapy. Int J Radiat Oncol Biol Phys 8(1):1–11

Han DS, Suh YS, Kong SH, Lee HJ, Choi Y, Aikou S, Sano T, Park BJ, Kim WH, Yang HK (2012) Nomogram predicting long-term survival after D2 gastrectomy for gastric cancer. J Clin Oncol 30(31):3834–3840. doi:10.1200/JCO.2012.41.8343

Jansen EP, Saunders MP, Boot H, Oppedijk V, Dubbelman R, Porritt B, Cats A, Stroom J, Valdes Olmos R, Bartelink H, Verheij M (2007) Prospective study on late renal toxicity following postoperative chemoradiotherapy in gastric cancer. Int J Radiat Oncol Biol Phys 67(3):781–785. doi:10.1016/j.ijrobp.2006.09.012

Kassam Z, Lockwood G, O'Brien C, Brierley J, Swallow C, Oza A, Siu L, Knox JJ, Wong R, Cummings B, Kim J, Moore M, Ringash J (2006) Conformal radiotherapy in the adjuvant treatment of gastric cancer: review of 82 cases. Int J Radiat Oncol Biol Phys 65(3):713–719. doi:10.1016/j.ijrobp.2006.01.001

Kattan MW, Karpeh MS, Mazumdar M, Brennan MF (2003) Postoperative nomogram for disease-specific survival after an R0 resection for gastric carcinoma. J Clin Oncol 21(19):3647–3650. doi:10.1200/JCO.2003.01.240

Kim TH, Kim DY, Park JW, Kim SH, Choi JI, Kim HB, Lee WJ, Park SJ, Hong EK, Kim CM (2007) Dose-volumetric parameters predicting radiation-induced hepatic toxicity in unresectable hepatocellular carcinoma patients treated with three-dimensional conformal radiotherapy. Int J Radiat Oncol Biol Phys 67(1):225–231. doi:10.1016/j.ijrobp.2006.08.015

Koc M, Dizen H, Ozalp N, Keskek M, Karakose N, Tez M (2009) External validation of a US-derived nomogram that predicts individual survival after gastric cancer resection. Langenbeck's Arch Surg 394(4):755–756. doi:10.1007/s00423-008-0426-z

Kundel Y, Purim O, Idelevich E, Lavrenkov K, Man S, Kovel S, Karminsky N, Pfeffer RM, Nisenbaum B, Fenig E, Sulkes A, Brenner B (2011) Postoperative chemoradiation for resected gastric cancer–is the Macdonald regimen tolerable? a retrospective multi-institutional study. Radiat Oncol 6:127. doi:10.1186/1748-717X-6-127

La Thangue NB (2003) The yin and yang of E2F–1: balancing life and death. Nature Cell Biol 5(7):587–589. doi:10.1038/ncb0703-587

Lee J, Park CK, Park JO, Lim T, Park YS, Lim HY, Lee I, Sohn TS, Noh JH, Heo JS, Kim S, Lim do H, Kim KM, Kang WK (2008) Impact of E2F–1 expression on clinical outcome of gastric adenocarcinoma patients with adjuvant chemoradiation therapy. Clin Cancer Res 14(1):82–88. doi:10.1158/1078-0432.CCR-07-0612

Leong T, Joon DL, Willis D, Jayamoham J, Spry N, Harvey J, Di Iulio J, Milner A, Mann GB, Michael M (2011) Adjuvant chemoradiation for gastric cancer using epirubicin, cisplatin, and 5-fluorouracil before and after three-dimensional conformal radiotherapy with concurrent infusional 5-fluorouracil: a multicenter study of the Trans-Tasman Radiation Oncology Group. Int J Radiat Oncol Biol Phys 79(3):690–695. doi:10.1016/j.ijrobp.2009.11.042

Leong T, Smithers M, Michael M, Gebski V, Boussioutas A, Miller D, Zalcberg JR, Wong R, Haustermans K (2012) TOPGEAR: An international randomized phase III trial of preoperative chemoradiotherapy versus preoperative chemotherapy for resectable gastric cancer (AGITG/TROG/EORTC/NCIC CTG). J Clin Oncol 30(15) (May 20 Supplement):TPS4141

Leong T, Willis D, Joon DL, Condron S, Hui A, Ngan SY (2005) 3D Conformal radiotherapy for gastric cancer-results of a comparative planning study. Radiother Oncol 74(3):301–306

Li SG, Ye ZY, Zhao ZS, Tao HQ, Wang YY, Niu CY (2008) Correlation of integrin beta3 mRNA and vascular endothelial growth factor protein expression profiles with the clinicopathological features and prognosis of gastric carcinoma. World J Gastroenterol 14(3):421–427

Liang SX, Zhu XD, Xu ZY, Zhu J, Zhao JD, Lu HJ, Yang YL, Chen L, Wang AY, Fu XL, Jiang GL (2006) Radiation-induced liver disease in three-dimensional conformal radiation therapy for primary liver carcinoma: the risk factors and hepatic radiation tolerance. Int J Radiat Oncol Biol Phys 65(2):426–434. doi:10.1016/j.ijrobp.2005.12.031

MacDonald JS (2011) Gastric Cancer: Nagoya is not New York. J Clin Oncol 29(33):4348–4350

Macdonald JS, Smalley SR, Benedetti J, Hundahl SA, Estes NC, Stemmermann GN, Haller DG, Ajani JA, Gunderson LL, Jessup JM, Martenson JA (2001) Chemoradiotherapy after surgery compared with surgery alone for adenocarcinoma of the stomach or gastroesophageal junction. N Engl J Med 345(10):725–730

Marchet A, Mocellin S, Belluco C, Ambrosi A, DeMarchi F, Mammano E, Digito M, Leon A, D'Arrigo A, Lise M, Nitti D (2007) Gene expression profile of primary gastric cancer: towards the prediction of lymph node status. Ann Surg Oncol 14(3):1058–1064. doi:10.1245/s10434-006-9090-0

May KS, Khushalani NI, Chandrasekhar R, Wilding GE, Iyer RV, Ma WW, Flaherty L, Russo RC, Fakih M, Kuvshinoff BW, Gibbs JF, Javle MM, Yang GY (2010) Analysis of clinical and dosimetric factors associated with change in renal function in patients with gastrointestinal malignancies after chemoradiation to the abdomen. Int J Radiat Oncol Biol Phys 76(4):1193–1198. doi:10.1016/j.ijrobp.2009.03.002

Minn AY, Hsu A, La T, Kunz P, Fisher GA, Ford JM, Norton JA, Visser B, Goodman KA, Koong AC, Chang DT (2010) Comparison of intensity-modulated radiotherapy and 3-dimensional conformal radiotherapy as adjuvant therapy for gastric cancer. Cancer 116(16):3943–3952. doi:10.1002/cncr.25246

Mutze K, Langer R, Schumacher F, Becker K, Ott K, Novotny A, Hapfelmeier A, Hofler H, Keller G (2011) DNA methyltransferase 1 as a predictive biomarker and potential therapeutic target for chemotherapy in gastric cancer. Eur J Cancer 47(12):1817–1825. doi:10.1016/j.ejca.2011.02.024

Novotny AR, Schuhmacher C, Busch R, Kattan MW, Brennan MF, Siewert JR (2006) Predicting individual survival after gastric cancer resection: validation of a US-derived nomogram at a single high-volume center in Europe. Ann Surg 243(1):74–81

Osti MF, Agolli L, Bracci S, Monaco F, Tubin S, Minniti G, De Sanctis V, Enrici RM (2012) Adjuvant chemoradiation with 5-fluorouracil or capecitabine in patients with gastric cancer after D2 nodal dissection. Anticancer Res 32(4):1397–1402

Pan CC, Kavanagh BD, Dawson LA, Li XA, Das SK, Miften M, Ten Haken RK (2010) Radiation-associated liver injury. Int J Radiat Oncol Biol Phys 76(3 Suppl):S94–S100. doi:10.1016/j.ijrobp.2009.06.092

Patel PR, Mansfield PF, Crane CH, Wu TT, Lee JH, Lynch PM, Morris J, Pisters PW, Feig B, Sunder PK, Izzo JG, Ajani JA (2007) Clinical stage after preoperative chemoradiation is a better predictor of patient outcome than the baseline stage for localized gastric cancer. Cancer 110(5):989–995. doi:10.1002/cncr.22870

Peeters KC, Kattan MW, Hartgrink HH, Kranenbarg EK, Karpeh MS, Brennan MF, van de Velde CJ (2005) Validation of a nomogram for predicting disease-specific survival after an R0 resection for gastric carcinoma. Cancer 103(4):702–707. doi:10.1002/cncr.20783

Quero L, Bouchbika Z, Kouto H, Baruch-Hennequin V, Gornet JM, Munoz N, Cojean-Zelek I, Houdart R, Panis Y, Valleur P, Aparicio T, Maylin C, Hennequin C (2012) Postoperative chemotherapy followed by conformal concomitant chemoradiotherapy in high-risk gastric cancer. Int J Radiat Oncol Biol Phys 83(2):574–580. doi:10.1016/j.ijrobp.2011.07.031

Reed VK, Krishnan S, Mansfield PF, Bhosale PR, Kim M, Das P, Janjan NA, Delclos ME, Lowy AM, Feig BW, Pisters PW, Ajani JA, Crane CH (2008) Incidence, natural history, and patterns of locoregional recurrence in gastric cancer patients treated with preoperative chemoradiotherapy. Int J Radiat Oncol Biol Phys 71(3):741–747. doi:10.1016/j.ijrobp.2007.10.030

Robb WB, Mariette C (2012) Predicting the response to chemotherapy in gastric adenocarcinoma: who benefits from neoadjuvant chemotherapy? Recent Res Cancer Res 196:241–268. doi:10.1007/978-3-642-31629-6_17

Rohatgi PR, Mansfield PF, Crane CH, Wu TT, Sunder PK, Ross WA, Morris JS, Pisters PW, Feig BW, Gunderson LL, Ajani JA (2006) Surgical pathology stage by American Joint Commission on cancer criteria predicts patient survival after preoperative chemoradiation for localized gastric carcinoma. Cancer 107(7):1475–1482. doi:10.1002/cncr.22180

Rostom Y, Zaghloul H, Khedr G, El-Shazly W, Abd-Allah D (2012) Docetaxel-based preoperative chemoradiation in localized gastric cancer: impact of pathological complete response on patient outcome. J Gastrointest Cancer. doi:10.1007/s12029-012-9449-3

Sakuramoto S, Sasako M, Yamaguchi T, Kinoshita T, Fujii M, Nashimoto A, Furukawa H, Nakajima T, Ohashi Y, Imamura H, Higashino M, Yamamura Y, Kurita A, Arai K (2007) Adjuvant chemotherapy for gastric cancer with S-1, an oral fluoropyrimidine. New Engl J Med 357(18):1810–1820. doi:10.1056/NEJMoa072252

Smalley SR, Benedetti JK, Haller DG, Hundahl SA, Estes NC, Ajani JA, Gunderson LL, Goldman B, Martenson JA, Jessup JM, Stemmermann GN, Blanke CD, Macdonald JS (2012) Updated analysis of SWOG-directed intergroup study 0116: a phase III trial of adjuvant radiochemotherapy versus observation after curative

gastric cancer resection. J Clin Oncol 30(19):2327–2333. doi:10.1200/JCO.2011.36.7136
Smalley SR, Gunderson L, Tepper J, Martenson JA, Minsky B, Willett C, Rich T (2002) Gastric surgical adjuvant radiotherapy consensus report: rationale and treatment implementation. Int J Radiat Oncol Biol Phys 52(2):283–293
Soyuer S, Soyuer I, Unal D, Ucar K, Yildiz OG, Orhan O (2010) Prognostic significance of CD9 expression in locally advanced gastric cancer treated with surgery and adjuvant chemoradiotherapy. Pathol Res Pract 206(9):607–610. doi:10.1016/j.prp.2010.04.004
Stewart FA, Oussoren Y, Bartelink H (1989) The influence of cisplatin on the response of mouse kidneys to multifraction irradiation. Radiother Oncol 15(1):93–102
Strong VE, Song KY, Park CH, Jacks LM, Gonen M, Shah M, Coit DG, Brennan MF (2010) Comparison of gastric cancer survival following R0 resection in the United States and Korea using an internationally validated nomogram. Ann Surg 251(4):640–646. doi:10.1097/SLA.0b013e3181d3d29b
Tarbell NJ, Guinan EC, Niemeyer C, Mauch P, Sallan SE, Weinstein HJ (1988) Late onset of renal dysfunction in survivors of bone marrow transplantation. Int J Radiat Oncol Biol Phys 15(1):99–104
Teramoto K, Tada M, Tamoto E, Abe M, Kawakami A, Komuro K, Matsunaga A, Shindoh G, Takada M, Murakawa K, Kanai M, Kobayashi N, Fujiwara Y, Nishimura N, Shirata K, Takahishi T, Ishizu A, Ikeda H, Hamada J, Kondo S, Katoh H, Moriuchi T, Yoshiki T (2005) Prediction of lymphatic invasion/lymph node metastasis, recurrence, and survival in patients with gastric cancer by cDNA array-based expression profiling. J Surg Res 124(2):225–236. doi:10.1016/j.jss.2004.10.003
Tillman GF, Pawlicki T, Koong AC, Goodman KA (2008) Preoperative versus postoperative radiotherapy for locally advanced gastroesophageal junction and proximal gastric cancers: a comparison of normal tissue radiation doses. Dis Esophagus 21(5):437–444. doi:10.1111/j.1442-2050.2007.00794.x
Van Cutsem E, de Haas S, Kang YK, Ohtsu A, Tebbutt NC, Ming XuJ, Peng Yong W, Langer B, Delmar P, Scherer SJ, Shah MA (2012) Bevacizumab in combination with chemotherapy as first-line therapy in advanced gastric cancer: a biomarker evaluation from the AVAGAST randomized phase III trial. J Clin Oncol 30(17):2119–2127. doi:10.1200/JCO.2011.39.9824
Verdecchia A, Mariotto A, Gatta G, Bustamante-Teixeira MT, Ajiki W (2003) Comparison of stomach cancer incidence and survival in four continents. Eur J Cancer 39(11):1603–1609
Verheij M, Dikken J, Coit D, Baser R, Gonen M, Goodman K, Brennan M, Jansen E, Boot H, van de Velde C (2012) Performance of a nomogram predicting disease-specific survival after an R0 resection for gastric cancer in patients receiving postoperative chemoradiation therapy. Int J Radiat Oncol Biol Phys 84(3):S194
Wang S, Wu X, Chen Y, Zhang J, Ding J, Zhou Y, He S, Tan Y, Qiang F, Bai J, Zeng J, Gong Z, Li A, Li G, Roe OD, Zhou J (2012) Prognostic and predictive role of JWA and XRCC1 expressions in gastric cancer. Clin Cancer Res 18(10):2987–2996. doi:10.1158/1078-0432.CCR-11-2863
Wu L, Timmers C, Maiti B, Saavedra HI, Sang L, Chong GT, Nuckolls F, Giangrande P, Wright FA, Field SJ, Greenberg ME, Orkin S, Nevins JR, Robinson ML, Leone G (2001) The E2F1-3 transcription factors are essential for cellular proliferation. Nature 414(6862):457–462. doi:10.1038/35106593
Wu Y, Guo E, Yu J, Xie Q (2008) High DcR3 expression predicts stage pN2-3 in gastric cancer. Am J Clin Oncol 31(1):79–83. doi:10.1097/COC.0b013e3180ca77ad
Zhang ZX, Gu XZ, Yin WB, Huang GJ, Zhang DW, Zhang RG (1998) Randomized clinical trial on the combination of preoperative irradiation and surgery in the treatment of adenocarcinoma of gastric cardia (AGC)–report on 370 patients. Int J Radiat Oncol Biol Phys 42(5):929–934
Zheng H, Takahashi H, Murai Y, Cui Z, Nomoto K, Niwa H, Tsuneyama K, Takano Y (2006) Expressions of MMP-2, MMP-9 and VEGF are closely linked to growth, invasion, metastasis and angiogenesis of gastric carcinoma. Anticancer Res 26(5A):3579–3583
Zhu WG, Xua DF, Pu J, Zong CD, Li T, Tao GZ, Ji FZ, Zhou XL, Han JH, Wang CS, Yu CH, Yi JG, Su XL, Ding JX (2012) A randomized, controlled, multicenter study comparing intensity-modulated radiotherapy plus concurrent chemotherapy with chemotherapy alone in gastric cancer patients with D2 resection. Radiother Oncol 104(3):361–366. doi:10.1016/j.radonc.2012.08.024

Pancreatic Cancer

Carsten Nieder and Thomas B. Brunner

Contents

Abstract

Treatment of pancreatic cancer is challenging. Both delayed diagnosis, locoregional disease extension, likelihood of local relapse and distant metastases contribute to disappointing outcome. Many patients are not amenable to curative surgical resection. Controversy exists around role and concepts of neoadjuvant and adjuvant chemo- and chemoradiation in common ductal adenocarcinoma scenarios, regarding both resectable and borderline resectable disease. Palliative treatment including chemoradiation and stereotactic body radiotherapy continues to evolve. The focus of this chapter is prognostic and predictive models for patients with ductal adenocarcinoma.

1 Introduction

When the use of chemoradiation for localized pancreatic cancer is considered, it is important to appreciate several disease characteristics that differ greatly from those of most other malignancies. In patients who cannot undergo curative resection the median survival is usually 12 months or less, with eventual progression of local and distant disease occurring commonly after chemoradiation or chemotherapy, and modest improvement in median survival to be expected. Even if the primary tumor is completely resected, disease-specific mortality is typically in the order of 80 % due to the problems of local disease recurrence and distant metastases. Most pancreatic cancer patients have some combination of host-related factors, such as advanced age, poor performance status, and medical comorbidity, or tumor related factors, such as anorexia and exocrine insufficiency, that often make them relatively poor candidates for aggressive therapy. A recent study evaluated all cases diagnosed between 2007 and 2009 in the Region of Southern Denmark (population: 1,200,000). Six-hundred-eighteen cases were registered,

C. Nieder (✉)
Oncology and Palliative Medicine, Nordland Hospital, 8092 Bodø, Norway
e-mail: carsten.nieder@nlsh.no

T. B. Brunner
Radiation Oncology, University Hospital Freiburg, 79106 Freiburg, Germany

C. Nieder and L. E. Gaspar (eds.), *Decision Tools for Radiation Oncology*, Medical Radiology. Radiation Oncology,
DOI: 10.1007/174_2013_870, © Springer-Verlag Berlin Heidelberg 2013
Published Online: 6 July 2013

25 of which did not have adenocarcinoma (Bjerregaard et al. 2013). Patients were divided in 3 clinical groups based on initial therapy; group 1: resection (n = 64), group 2: chemotherapy or chemo-radiotherapy (n = 191), group 3: no tumor directed therapy (n = 324). Median survival in the three groups was 25.7, 8.1 and 1.1 months respectively.

Decision making in pancreatic cancer is complex and requires dedicated multidisciplinary teams. Since outcome is so poor with standard therapies in localized pancreatic cancer, these patients are appropriate for clinical trials incorporating novel chemotherapeutic and molecularly targeted agents (Brunner and Scott-Brown 2010). While improved local tumor control with more effective radiosensitization could have a modest impact on median survival in patients with locally advanced and resectable pancreatic cancer, significant improvement in median survival duration will require the development of more effective systemic regimens that address the dominant distant failure pattern. It is hoped that current efforts will lead to gradual improvements in outcome for patients with pancreatic cancer. In this chapter, prognostic and predictive models are discussed with an emphasis on recent clinical trials that included sufficiently large patient cohorts.

2 Diagnosis, Staging, and Initial Management of Pancreatic Cancer

The initial goals in the evaluation and treatment of symptomatic patients are to determine resectability, establish a histologic diagnosis, and reestablish biliary tract outflow. Accurate clinical staging is critical in the multidisciplinary management of pancreatic cancer. Abdominal computed tomography (CT) is the most common diagnostic imaging technique used to reliably confirm and determine the stage of suspected pancreatic malignancies. In many centers, endoscopic ultrasonographically guided fine-needle biopsy of the pancreas is the procedure of choice for the diagnosis of pancreatic malignancies. Accurate determination of resectability is the most important aspect of clinical staging (Callery et al. 2009). Surgical resectability is based on involvement of the superior mesenteric vessels and the celiac artery and its branches. The American Joint Committee on Cancer (AJCC) staging system for exocrine pancreatic duct cancer is shown in Table 1. Basically, three criteria are necessary for resectability: (1) localized disease, (2) lack of involvement of the celiac axis or superior mesenteric artery, and (3) patency of the superior mesenteric/portal venous confluence. Inaccurate clinical determination of surgical resectability leads to incomplete resections which are not curative and do not prolong median survival (Neoptolemos et al. 2001).

Table 1 AJCC TNM classification of carcinoma of exocrine pancreas

Stage	Descriptions		
Primary Tumor (T)			
TX	Primary tumor cannot be assessed		
T0	No evidence of primary tumor		
Tis	Carcinoma in situ		
T1	Tumor limited to the pancreas, 2 cm or less in greatest dimension (resectable primary tumor)		
T2	Tumor limited to the pancreas, more than 2 cm in greatest dimension (resectable primary tumor)		
T3	Tumor extends beyond the pancreas but without involvement of the celiac axis or superior mesenteric artery (potentially resectable primary tumor)		
T4	Tumor involves the celiac axis or the superior mesenteric artery (unresectable primary tumor)		
Regional Lymph Nodes (N)			
NX	Regional lymph nodes cannot be assessed		
N0	No regional lymph node metastasis		
N1	Regional lymph node metastasis. Regional lymph node sampling from nodes around common hepatic artery, celiac artery, splenic hilum, infrapyloric nodes are required during Whipple's procedure in pathological staging. Ideally, >10 lymph nodes should be sampled during surgery		
Distant Metastasis (M)			
MX	Distant metastasis cannot be assessed		
M0	No distant metastasis		
M1	Distant metastasis (including seeding of the peritoneum and positive peritoneal cytology)		
Stage Grouping			
T1	T2	T3	T4
N0 IA	IB	IIA	III
N1 11B	IIB	IIB	III
MI IV	IV	IV	IV

Source Edge et al (2010)

3 Multidisciplinary Management of Resectable Tumors

Multiple studies have demonstrated that clinicopathologic factors such as tumor size, histologic differentiation, margin status, and nodal involvement are statistically significant prognostic variables (Corsini et al. 2008; Miller et al. 2009). The pancreatic nomogram , originally developed in the Memorial Sloan-Kettering Cancer Center (MSKCC) in the USA, combines clinicopathological and operative data to predict disease-specific survival at 1, 2 and 3 years from initial resection. It was based on prospectively collected data from 555 pancreatic resections for adenocarcinoma (Brennan et al. 2004). Factors include age, gender, weight loss, T stage, number of positive and negative nodes, differentiation, margins and others. An external patient cohort from a retrospective pancreatic adenocarcinoma database at the Academic Medical Centre in Amsterdam was used to test the validity of the nomogram (De Castro et al. 2009). The cohort included 263 consecutive patients who had surgery between 1985 and 2004. The 1-, 2- and 3-year disease-specific survival rates were 61, 30 and 16 % respectively. The nomogram concordance index was 0.61. The calibration analysis of the model showed that the predicted survival did not significantly deviate from the actual survival. Thus, this model may aid in counseling patients.

Historically, chemoradiation has been shown to reduce the probability of local tumor recurrence (Anonymous 1987). Chemoradiation accomplishes this by eradicating microscopic residual disease remaining in the tumor bed after complete tumor resection or through the reduction in regional lymph node recurrence (Belka et al. 2006). In the case of pancreatic cancer, the retroperitoneal margin is nearly always close and often positive, and isolated lymph node recurrences are rare. Therefore, at least in theory, locoregional therapy in pancreatic cancer can be optimized with complete gross tumor resection and treatment of microscopic disease at the retroperitoneal margin with chemoradiation. Unfortunately, however, multiinstitutional trials have reported strikingly high rates of local tumor recurrence. Local tumor recurrence (or more likely) persistence was identified as a component of the first site of failure in 39 % of patients enrolled on the GITSG trial (Anonymous 1987), 53 % of patients enrolled on the EORTC trial (Klinkenbijl et al. 1999), and 62 % of patients enrolled on the ESPAC-1 trial (Neoptolemos et al. 2004). Moreover, several trials questioned whether chemoradiation truly improves survival more than adjuvant chemotherapy. Schmidt et al. reported a randomized phase III trial of adjuvant chemoradiation plus interferon alfa-2b versus fluorouracil (5-FU) and folinic acid (FA) for patients with resected pancreatic adenocarcinoma (Schmidt et al. 2012). Between 2004 and 2007, 132 R0/R1 resected patients received either 5-FU, cisplatin, and interferon alfa-2b plus radiotherapy followed by two cycles of 5-FU (arm A, n = 64) or six cycles of 5-FU monotherapy (arm B, n = 68). Median survival for all randomly assigned patients was 26.5 months in arm A and 28.5 months in arm B. The hazard ratio was 1.04, p = 0.99. A randomized phase II intergroup study explored the feasibility and tolerability of a gemcitabine-based regimen after R0 resection of pancreatic head cancer (Van Laethem et al. 2010). Patients (n = 90) were randomly assigned to receive either four cycles of gemcitabine (control arm) or gemcitabine for two cycles followed by weekly gemcitabine with concurrent radiation (50.4 Gy; CRT arm). Treatment was completed per protocol by 87 and 73 % in the control and CRT arms, respectively, and grade 4 toxicity was 0 and 5 %, respectively. In the CRT arm, three patients experienced grade 3-related late toxicity. Median DFS was 12 months in the CRT arm and 11 months in the control arm. Median OS was 24 months in both arms. First local recurrence was less frequent in the CRT arm (11 % vs. 24 %).

As compared to Europe, adjuvant chemoradiation is more commonly used in the United States (Kimple et al. 2012; Van Laethem et al. 2012). For adjuvant therapy, the Radiation Therapy Oncology Group (RTOG) has defined in a consensus panel guidelines for the delineation of the clinical target volume (CTV) in pancreatic head cancer (Goodman et al. 2012). In addition to the preoperative tumor volume and the pancreaticojejunostomy these guidelines define the following elective nodal volumes: celiac artery, superior mesenteric artery, portal vein and aorta. One of their landmark clinical trials was RTOG 9704 (Willett et al. 2003; Regine et al. 2011). After resection of pancreatic adenocarcinoma, patients were randomized to pre- and post-chemoradiation 5-FU versus pre- and post-chemoradiation gemcitabine. CRT was provided at 50.4 Gy with continuously provided 5-FU. Four hundred fifty-one patients were eligible. Univariate analysis showed no difference in overall survival (OS). Pancreatic head tumor patients (n = 388) had a median survival and 5-year OS of 20.5 months and 22 % with gemcitabine versus 17.1 months and 18 % with 5-FU. On multivariate analysis, patients on the gemcitabine arm with pancreatic head tumors experienced a trend toward improved OS (p = 0.08). The sequencing of 5-FU CRT with gemcitabine as done in this trial was not associated with a statistically significant improvement in OS. Despite local recurrence being approximately half of that reported in previous adjuvant trials, distant disease relapse still occurred in more than 70 % of patients. These findings served as the basis for the ongoing EORTC/U.S. Intergroup RTOG 0848 phase III adjuvant trial evaluating the impact of CRT after completion of a full course of gemcitabine. RTOG 9704 data were also used to determine the influence of lymph node factors (number of positive nodes (NPN), total nodes examined (TNE), and lymph node ratio (LNR ratio of NPN to TNE)) on OS and disease-free survival (DFS). Both TNE, NPN, and LNR were associated with OS and DFS (Showalter et al. 2011). A previous multivariate analysis of RTOG 9704 demonstrated two significant factors that predicted OS: nodal involvement (hazard ratio 1.5) and CA 19-9 level >90 (hazard ratio 3.3) (Berger et al. 2008). CA 19-9 is a stratification factor for the current RTOG adjuvant pancreas trial (0848) (Table 2).

A different North American study was reported by Moghanaki et al. (2011). Between 1984 and 2006, this group retrospectively analyzed 91 patients with pancreatic cancer treated with pancreaticoduodenectomy or total pancreatectomy followed by adjuvant 5-FU-based chemoradiation at

Table 2 Major prognostic factors in pancreatic adenocarcinoma

Resectable stages	Locally advanced, non-metastatic disease
Tumor size	Performance status
Tumor location (head versus other)	Age
Nodal involvement	CA 19-9 level
Histologic differentiation	Uncertainty regarding distant metastases (stage Mx)
CA 19-9 level	PET-CT related features such as SUVmax and tumor volume
Better prognosis is also expected in patients with younger age, less weight loss and female gender	

the University of Pennsylvania. The prognostic significance of demographic factors, stage, year of surgery, tumor location, grade, resection status, and number of positive lymph nodes on overall survival were examined. With a median follow-up of 6.5 years, the overall median survival was 2.3 years, and the 5-year overall survival was 29 %. In multivariate analysis, completeness of resection ($p<0.001$), fewer number of positive lymph nodes (0 vs. 1–2 vs. 3 or more) ($p = 0.004$), and age ≤60 years ($p = 0.006$) were all independently associated with improved overall survival. Some centers have used intraoperative radiotherapy (IORT) with or without external beam radiotherapy (EBRT) and chemotherapy (Pisters et al. 1998; Jingu et al. 2012). However, the focus of this chapter is not on technical aspects of radiotherapy.

4 Down-Staging Patients with Locally Advanced Disease

There is a widespread perception that some unresectable pancreatic tumors can be converted to resectable ones with the use of chemotherapy or chemoradiation. The interpretation of published studies is limited by inconsistent and subjective definitions of resectability and by variable, in part inadequate preoperative radiologic assessments of resectability. Probably the most variable factor in determining resectability and thus interpreting whether a tumor has been converted to resectable from unresectable is the meaning of vascular involvement (Katz et al. 2013). Although most surgeons would agree that tumor encasement of either the celiac artery or the superior mesenteric artery constitutes unresectable disease, opinions vary with regard to more limited arterial involvement. It is probably in this group of patients that, theoretically, active cytotoxic therapy could lead to down-staging (Golcher et al. 2008). These cases are sometimes referred to as "marginally resectable" or borderline resectable . In a recent study, patients were deemed borderline resectable if they had severe unilateral superior mesenteric vein or portal vein impingement, tumor abutment of the superior mesenteric artery, gastroduodenal artery encasement up to the origin from the hepatic artery, or colon invasion (Kim et al. 2013). Sixty-eight evaluable patients received treatment at 4 centers. Treatment consisted of two 28-day cycles of gemcitabine (1,000 mg/m^2 on days 1, 8, and 15) and oxaliplatin (85 mg/m^2 on days 1 and 15) with radiotherapy during cycle 1 (30 Gy in 2-Gy fractions). Patients were evaluated for surgery after cycle 2. Patients who underwent resection received 2 cycles of adjuvant chemotherapy. The only characteristic associated significantly with R0 resection was CA 19-9 response. Comparing any increase ($n = 15$) with a 0–50 % decrease ($n = 13$) and a >50 % decrease ($n = 27$) demonstrated that a decrease in CA 19-9 was associated with R0 resection ($p = 0.02$). Resection (R0 vs R1/R2 vs none), baseline quality of life, female gender, tumor in the pancreatic body or tail (compared with the pancreatic head), and lower CA 19-9 levels at baseline were associated with improved survival (all $p < 0.05$). In the patients who underwent surgical resection ($n = 43$), longer surgery time ($p = 0.03$) and increased blood loss during surgery ($p = 0.02$) were associated with poorer survival, and marginal associations were observed with surgical procedure (Whipple was inferior to distal-subtotal pancreatectomy; $p = 0.057$) and histologic treatment effect ($p = 0.068$).

In Heidelberg, Germany, a total of 215 patients with locally advanced pancreatic cancer were treated with chemoradiation at a single institution (Habermehl et al. 2012). Radiotherapy was delivered with a median dose of 52.2 Gy in single fractions of 1.8 Gy. Chemotherapy was applied concomitantly as gemcitabine at a dose of 300 mg/m^2 weekly, followed by adjuvant cycles of full-dose gemcitabine (1,000 mg/m^2). After neoadjuvant treatment restaging was done to evaluate secondary resectability. After chemoradiation a total of 26 % of all patients with primary unresectable disease were offered secondary resection. Tumor-free resection margins could be achieved in 39 % (R0-resection). Patients with complete resection after CRT showed a significantly increased median overall survival with 22.1 compared to 11.9 months in non-resected patients. In most cases the first site of disease progression was systemic with hepatic (52 %) and peritoneal (36 %) metastases. A different study population from the United States was comprised of 240 consecutive patients who received neoadjuvant chemoradiation and surgery, and was compared with 60 patients who had no neoadjuvant therapy between 1999 and 2007 (Estrella et al. 2012). Among the 240 treated patients, the 1-year and 3-year DFS rates were 52 and 32 %, with a median DFS of 15.1 months. The 1-year and 3-year OS rates were 95 and 47 %, with a median

OS of 33.5 months. By univariate analysis, DFS was associated with age, post-therapy tumor stage (ypT), lymph node status (ypN), number of positive lymph nodes, and AJCC stage, whereas OS was associated with intraoperative blood loss, margin status, ypT, ypN, number of positive lymph nodes, and AJCC stage. By multivariate analysis, DFS was independently associated with age, number of positive lymph nodes, and AJCC stage, and OS was independently associated with differentiation, margin status, number of positive lymph nodes, and AJCC stage. In addition, the treated patients had better OS and lower frequency of lymph node metastasis than those who had no neoadjuvant therapy. In a series of 132 North American patients (Breslin et al. 2001), survival duration was superior for women ($p = 0.04$) and for patients with no evidence of lymph node metastasis ($p = 0.03$). There was no difference in survival duration associated with patient age, dose of preoperative radiation therapy, the delivery of intraoperative radiotherapy, or the histologic grade of chemoradiation treatment effect.

Currently, stereotactic body radiotherapy (SBRT) is also being explored in comparable patient groups (Polistina et al. 2010; Chuong et al. 2013). Approximately one-third of initially staged non-resectable tumor patients would be expected to have resectable tumors following neoadjuvant therapy, with comparable survival as initially resectable tumor patients (Gillen et al. 2010). A recent meta-analysis included 19 studies, which involved 2,148 patients (Laurence et al. 2011). Only cohort studies were included. The meta-analysis found that patients with unrespectable pancreatic cancer who underwent neoadjuvant chemoradiotherapy achieved similar survival outcomes to patients with resectable disease, even though only 40 % were ultimately resected. Neoadjuvant chemoradiotherapy was not associated with statistically significant increase in the rate of pancreatic fistula formation or total complications, although there was an increase in the risk of peri-operative death.

White et al. performed a study to evaluate the applicability of an already mentioned nomogram, which was developed for patients undergoing resection without preoperative chemoradiation and which incorporates several post-resection pathological factors (Brennan et al. 2004), to a population of patients who received preoperative CRT prior to resection (White et al. 2006). From 1994 to 2004, 82 patients with biopsy-proven, radiographically localized adenocarcinoma of the pancreatic head underwent preop CRT followed by pancreaticoduodenectomy (PD); 50 concurrent patients underwent PD without preoperative CRT. Mean nomogram-predicted disease-specific survival rates were compared with observed rates from the time of resection. Despite having more locally advanced tumors on initial staging (21 vs. 8 %; $p<0.05$), patients who received preoperative CRT had smaller resected tumors (mean 2.3 vs. 3.1 cm; $p<0.01$), were less likely to have T3 tumors (54 vs. 80 %, $p<0.01$), were less likely to have positive lymph nodes (29 vs. 58 %, $p< 0.01$), and had fewer positive lymph nodes (mean 0.4 vs. 1.9, $p<0.01$), all factors that imply treatment effect and favorably impact on nomogram-predicted outcome. Observed DSS was similar to predicted DSS in both groups. The similarity in observed and predicted DSS following resection in patients who received preoperative CRT suggested that the effects (whether treatment, selection, or no effect) were reflected by the nomogram. The ability of the nomogram to evaluate the effects of preoperative CRT on survival was limited by the potential effects of preoperative CRT on factors within the nomogram.

5 Chemoradiation in Locally Advanced Disease (LAPC)

Locally advanced pancreatic cancer is generally incurable and all therapies have significant limitations. In reality, patients probably benefit modestly from both systemic therapy and chemoradiation; these approaches are complementary and should both be considered in patients with locally advanced disease (Huguet et al. 2007). Acute toxicity can be reduced if the radiation fields are confined to the gross primary tumor and clinically enlarged lymph nodes, regardless of the radiosensitizing chemotherapy that is used (Jackson et al. 2010). Treating uninvolved regional lymph nodes requires larger amounts of gastric and duodenal mucosa to be treated which can lead to higher rates of gastrointestinal toxicity and is not likely to improve median survival.

In GITSG studies of 5-FU–based chemoradiation therapy in patients with locally advanced pancreatic adenocarcinoma (Anonymous 1979; Moertel et al. 1981) patients were randomly assigned to receive 40 Gy of radiation plus 5-FU, 60 Gy plus 5-FU, or 60 Gy without chemotherapy. Radiation therapy was delivered as a split course, with 20 Gy given over 2 weeks followed by a 2-week rest. 5-FU was delivered IV at a bolus dose of 500 mg/m^2/day for the first 3 days of each 20-Gy cycle and given weekly (500 mg/m^2) following the completion of chemoradiation therapy. The median survival was 10 months in each of the chemoradiation groups and 6 months for the group that received 60 Gy without 5-FU. In contrast to the results from the GITSG, an ECOG study suggested no benefit to chemoradiation therapy over 5-FU alone (Klaassen et al. 1985). The ECOG study randomly assigned patients with locally advanced or incompletely resected pancreatic adenocarcinoma to receive chemoradiation therapy (40 Gy and 600 mg/m^2/day 5-FU for 3 days) or 5-FU alone (600 mg/

m^2/week). The chemoradiation therapy group received weekly bolus administration of 5-FU following chemoradiation therapy until there was evidence of disease progression. The median survival was 8.3 months in the group that received chemoradiation therapy and 8.2 months in the group that received 5-FU alone. It was evident both in the GITSG studies and in the ECOG trial that patients with locally advanced, unresectable pancreatic cancer who are symptomatic to the point of not being fully ambulatory do not benefit from anticancer therapy. More recent trials of chemoradiation for locally advanced pancreatic cancer have investigated continuous-infusion 5-FU in combination with EBRT. Capecitabine appears to have similar efficacy to intravenously administered 5-FU and is an appropriate substitute for infusional or bolus 5-FU when used with radiotherapy. In a phase I trial, 800 mg/m^2 was the recommended dose when capecitabine was given on days of radiation only (Saif et al. 2005).

The introduction of gemcitabine was a step forward in the treatment of pancreatic cancer. Its value as a systemic agent and the recognition of its radiosensitizing properties stimulated the study of combinations of gemcitabine with EBRT for patients with localized pancreatic cancer (Blackstock et al. 1999; McGinn et al. 2001; Pipas et al. 2001; Wolff et al. 2001; Murphy et al. 2007; Girard et al. 2010; Brunner et al. 2011; Cardenes et al. 2011). Several strategies have been investigated including seven-weekly injections of gemcitabine with short course EBRT (30 Gy), twice-weekly gemcitabine with 50.4 Gy of EBRT, weekly gemcitabine with 50.4 Gy of EBRT, and full dose weekly gemcitabine with escalating doses of radiation. Most of these studies suggested gastrointestinal toxicity as a dose-limiting factor, but hematologic toxicity has also been observed. Several multiinstitutional studies have been completed evaluating gemcitabine-based chemoradiation. In a small study performed in Taiwan, 34 patients with locally advanced pancreatic cancer were randomized to receive 5-FU based chemoradiation (500 mg/m^2 daily for 3 days, every 14 days with radiation to a total dose of 50.4–61.2 Gy) or gemcitabine and radiation (600 mg/m^2 weekly with equivalent doses of radiation) (Li et al. 2003). The objective response rate to gemcitabine and radiation was 50 % and only 13 % for 5-FU chemoradiation. In addition, median survival was substantially better using gemcitabine compared with 5-FU (14.5 months vs. 6.7 months, $p = 0.027$). These efficacy results must be interpreted with caution because of the limited accrual (34 patients) and the poor results in the control group. A phase II study conducted in patients with locally advanced pancreatic cancer by the Cancer and Leukemia Group B evaluated gemcitabine given at 40 mg/m^2 twice weekly. In that study, there were 35 and 50 % grade 3 or 4 gastrointestinal and hematologic toxicities, respectively, and the median survival was only 8.5 months (Blackstock et al. 2001) Not surprisingly, the Cancer and Leukemia Group B abandoned this approach in locally advanced pancreatic cancer. Both of these studies used regional nodal fields that likely contributed to the significant gastrointestinal toxicity. In contrast, the approach that was developed at the University of Michigan delivered high doses of gemcitabine (1,000 mg/m^2) and a slightly lower radiotherapy dose (36 Gy in 15 fractions over 3 weeks), with conformal radiation fields encompassing the gross tumor volume alone. At that institution, the irradiation of a smaller volume of normal tissue was reported to be well tolerated (McGinn et al. 2001). Investigators have since embarked on further studies evaluating the same regimen. As reported in 2008, 41 patients enrolled at six institutions (Small et al. 2008). Among the 39 treated patients, the most common toxicities were grade 3 neutropenia (13 %), grade 3 nausea (10 %) and grade 3 vomiting (10 %). Thirteen (81 %) of 16 patients initially judged resectable, three (33 %) of nine borderline-resectable patients, and one (7 %) of 14 unresectable patients underwent resection after therapy. One-year survival rates were 73 % for all patients, 94 % for resectable patients, 76 % for borderline-resectable patients, and 47 % for unresectable patients. The authors concluded that full-dose gemcitabine with concurrent radiotherapy was well tolerated and active. Later it was shown that intensity-modulated radiotherapy (IMRT) to a total dose of 55 Gy can be given together with full-dose gemcitabine (Ben-Josef et al. 2012). However, the issue of radiation dose escalation in LAPC is controversial. In patients with limited survival expectation a favorable balance between toxicity, treatment time, resource utilization and survival outcome is crucial (Murphy et al. 2012).

A small randomized ECOG trial was reported in 2011 (Loehrer et al. 2011). Patients with localized unresectable adenocarcinoma of the pancreas were randomly assigned to receive gemcitabine alone (at 1,000 mg/m^2/week for weeks 1–6, followed by 1 week rest, then for 3 of 4 weeks) or gemcitabine (600 mg/m^2/week for weeks 1–5, then 4 weeks later 1,000 mg/m^2 for 3 of 4 weeks) plus radiotherapy (starting on day 1, 1.8 Gy per fraction, total dose 50.4 Gy). Of 74 patients entered, patients in the radiation arm had greater incidence of grades 4 and 5 toxicities (41 % vs. 9 %), but grades 3 and 4 toxicities combined were similar (77 % vs. 79 %). No statistical differences were seen in quality of life measurements at 6, 15 to 16, and 36 weeks. The primary end point was survival, which was 9.2 months and 11.1 months for arms A and B, respectively ($p = 0.017$). In conclusion, there was moderately improved overall survival with the addition of radiation therapy to gemcitabine. A different concept studied in France failed to improve survival (Chauffert et al. 2008). This randomized study ($n = 119$) compared chemoradiation (60 Gy, 2 Gy/fraction;

concomitant 5-FU, 300 mg/m^2/day, days 1–5 for 6 weeks; cisplatin, 20 mg/m^2/day, days 1–5 during weeks 1 and 5) and gemcitabine (1,000 mg/m^2 weekly for 7 weeks). Maintenance gemcitabine (1,000 mg/m^2 weekly, 3 of 4 weeks) was given in both arms until disease progression or toxicity. Actually, gemcitabine treatment was superior to chemoradiation. Regarding radiotherapy technical considerations in the management of LAPC the recent American-French consensus recommendations provide important guidance (Huguet et al. 2012).

The RTOG has published a phase II trial evaluating capecitabine-based chemoradiation (825 mg/m^2 twice daily) with bevacizumab (RTOG 0411) followed by systemic therapy with concurrent gemcitabine and bevacizumab (Crane et al. 2009). Eighty-two patients were treated. The addition of bevacizumab to chemoradiotherapy followed by bevacizumab and gemcitabine resulted in a similar median survival (11.9 months) to previous RTOG studies in patients with locally advanced pancreatic cancer. The purpose of the randomized phase II study RTOG 0020 was to evaluate the addition of weekly low- dose gemcitabine with concurrent paclitaxel/RT and to evaluate the efficacy and safety of the farnesyl transferase inhibitor R115777 following chemoradiation (Rich et al. 2012). Patients in Arm 1 received gemcitabine, 75 mg/m^2/week, and paclitaxel, 40 mg/m^2/week, for 6 weeks, with 50.4 Gy radiation. Patients in Arm 2 received an identical chemoradiation regimen but then received maintenance R115777 until disease progression or unacceptable toxicity. One hundred ninety-five patients were entered into this study, and 184 were analyzable. The median survival time was 11.5 months and 8.9 months for the chemoradiation and chemoradiation plus R115777 arms, respectively. A different phase II trial was designed to assess the efficacy and safety of cetuximab, gemcitabine, and oxaliplatin followed by cetuximab, capecitabine, and radiation therapy in LAPC (Crane et al. 2011). Sixty-nine patients received gemcitabine and oxaliplatin every 2 weeks for four doses, followed by radiation (50.4 Gy to the gross tumor only) with concurrent capecitabine (825 mg/m^2 twice daily). Cetuximab (500 mg/m^2) was started on day 1 of chemotherapy and was continued every 2 weeks during chemotherapy and chemoradiotherapy. Diagnostic cytology specimens were immunostained for Smad4(Dpc4) expression. Median overall survival time was 19.2 months. Acneiform rash correlated with improved survival ($p = 0.001$), but initial CA19-9, borderline resectable initial stage, and surgical resection ($n = 7$) did not. The 1-year and 2-year radiographic local progression rates were 23 and 61 %, respectively. Smad4(Dpc4) expression correlated with a local rather than a distant dominant pattern of disease progression ($p = 0.016$). Prospective validation of Smad4(Dpc4) expression in cytology specimens as a predictive biomarker is necessary before this parameter can be recommended for widespread use.

Recently, final results of a large randomized phase III trial among patients with LAPC and the first to test gene transfer against this malignancy were reported (Herman et al. 2013). The study compound, TNFerade biologic is a novel means of delivering tumor necrosis factor alpha to tumor cells by gene transfer. In all, 304 patients were randomly assigned 2:1 to standard of care plus TNFerade (SOC + TNFerade) versus standard of care alone (SOC). SOC consisted of 50.4 Gy in 28 fractions with concurrent fluorouracil (200 mg/m^2 per day continuous infusion). TNFerade was injected intratumorally before the first fraction of radiotherapy each week by using either a percutaneous transabdominal or an endoscopic ultrasound approach. Four weeks after chemoradiotherapy, patients began gemcitabine (1,000 mg/m^2) with or without erlotinib until progression or toxicity. The analysis included 187 patients randomly assigned to SOC + TNFerade and 90 to SOC. Median survival was 10 months for patients in both the SOC + TNFerade and SOC arms (hazard ratio 0.90; $p = 0.26$). Median progression-free survival was 6.8 months for SOC + TNFerade versus 7.0 months for SOC. Multivariate analysis identified five baseline characteristics prognostic for survival: age, M stage (M0 *v* Mx), prior cancer history, prior cancer treatment, and baseline CA19-9 (Table 2). Some authors have also reported that patients with decreasing level of CA 19-9 (marker dynamics after treatment) fared better than non-responders (Micke et al. 2005).

As mentioned in the sections dealing with resectable pancreatic tumors, SBRT including frameless image-guided approaches with individualized fractionation regimens is currently being evaluated for different patient groups, also those with unresectable disease, recurrent disease or previously irradiated (Koong et al. 2004; Chang et al. 2009). Initial results suggest that combination with gemcitabine appears feasible (Gurka et al. 2013). In the study by Didolkar et al. pain relief was noted in the majority of patients lasting for 18–24 weeks ($n = 85$, Didolkar et al. 2010). Most of the patients died of distant disease progression while their primary tumor was controlled. Overall median survival from diagnosis was 18.6 months and from SBRT it was 8.7 months. Another study suggested that freedom from local progression depends on tumor volume (cut-off 15 ml) and SBRT dose above 22 Gy (most patients received single fraction SBRT; Rwigema et al. 2011). Parameters correlating with duodenal toxicity after single fraction SBRT have been developed by the Stanford University group (Murphy et al. 2010). They included V(10)-V(25) and D(max) as well as Lyman NTCP model. This group also reported on prognostic value of PET-CT derived parameters in 55 patients and found that maximum standardized uptake value (SUVmax) was prognostic in multivariate analysis

(Schellenberg et al. 2010). 18Fluorodeoxyglucose (FDG) was used as PET tracer. A different small study suggested that FDG-PET-CT-defined gross tumor volume size might predict outcomes of LAPC patients treated with definitive chemoradiation (Parlak et al. 2012). A third small study with 20 patients suggested that FDG-PET may be used to decide whether or not patients could have complete surgical resection after chemoradiation (Choi et al. 2010). Larger studies are necessary to elucidate the role of PET-CT in patients assigned to radiotherapy.

One of the larger analyses of prognostic factors was performed by the Eastern Cooperative Oncology Group (ECOG) (Cohen et al. 2005). In that study, 114 patients were randomized to receive 59.4 Gy EBRT in 1.8-Gy fractions alone or in combination with 5-FU and mitomycin-C. Of multiple patient characteristics evaluated, only performance status (PS) was a significant predictor of both disease-free survival and overall survival ($p = 0.006$). The median survival time of PS 0–1 patients was 9.2 months, compared to 7.1 months for PS 2 patients. Authors from Denmark described the results in 178 LAPC patients treated from 2001 to 2010 and developed a prognostic model for both survival and the possibility of a subsequent resection (Bjerregaard et al. 2012). CRT consisted of 50 Gy in 27 fractions combined with tegafur-uracil(UFT)/folinic acid(FA). The median survival from diagnosis was 11.5 months. A Cox regression model for survival demonstrated resection (hazard ratio 0.12) and pre-CRT gemcitabine-based therapy (HR 0.57) as being associated with a favorable outcome. A logistic regression model showed stage III disease (odds ratio 0.16) and abnormal hemoglobin (OR 0.26) as being associated with lower odds of resection.

Systematic toxicity analyses are limited. The MD Anderson Cancer Center group evaluated medical records and treatment plans of 106 patients with LAPC who were treated with chemoradiation between 2005 and 2010 (Kelly et al. 2013). All patients received neoadjuvant and concurrent chemotherapy. Seventy-eight patients were treated with conventional radiation to 50.4 Gy in 28 fractions; 28 patients received dose-escalated radiation therapy (range, 57.5–75.4 Gy in 28–39 fractions). Treatment-related toxicity was graded according to Common Terminology Criteria for Adverse Events, version 4.0. Twenty patients had treatment-related duodenal toxicity events, such as duodenal inflammation, ulceration, and bleeding. Four patients had grade 1 events, 8 had grade 2, 6 had grade 3, 1 had grade 4, and 1 had grade 5. On univariate analysis, a toxicity grade ≥ 2 was associated with tumor location, low platelet count, an absolute volume (ccm) receiving a dose of at least 55 Gy > 1 ccm, and a maximum point dose >60 Gy. Of these factors, only V(55 Gy) = 1 ccm was associated with duodenal toxicity on multivariate analysis (hazard ratio 6.7; $p = 0.002$). The spinal cord dose is typically limited to 50 Gy. The mean dose to the entire liver should be kept below 32 Gy. The mean dose to bilateral entire kidneys should be limited to 18 Gy or less.

6 Conclusion

Improving the treatment of pancreatic cancer is a challenge. Variations in practice pattern are considerable, reflecting the limited number of high quality randomized trials performed in this disease. Major prognostic factors include tumor size and location, nodal involvement, distant metastases, histologic differentiation, CA 19-9 level, age, performance status and weight loss. Predictive factors for treatment response and toxicity are emerging, related for example to biomarkers, PET imaging characteristics and dosimetric factors. However, confirmatory analyses are needed before general recommendations can be made. The technical potential to deliver radiation to the upper abdomen in an unprecedentedly precise and normal tissue sparing manner has never been better than in the current era. With gradual improvements in systemic treatment beyond gemcitabine monotherapy, which impact micrometastatic disease as one competing cause of failure and eventually death, future trials have to determine whether or not improved local control can be achieved and how much this factor influences survival.

References

Anonymous (1979) A multi-institutional comparative trial of radiation therapy alone and in combination with 5-fluorouracil for locally unresectable pancreatic carcinoma. The Gastrointestinal Tumor Study Group. Ann Surg 189:205–208

Anonymous (1987) Further evidence of effective adjuvant combined radiation and chemotherapy following curative resection of pancreatic cancer. Gastrointestinal Tumor Study Group. Cancer 59:2006–2010

Belka C, Nieder C, Molls M (2006) Biological basis of combined radio- and chemotherapy. In: Brown JM, Mehta MP, Nieder C (eds) Multimodal concepts for integration of cytotoxic drugs and radiation therapy Springer Heidelberg. New York, Berlin, pp 3–18

Ben-Josef E, Schipper M et al (2012) A phase I/II trial of intensity modulated radiation (IMRT) dose escalation with concurrent fixed-dose rate gemcitabine (FDR-G) in patients with unresectable pancreatic cancer. Int J Radiat Oncol Biol Phys 84:1166–1171

Berger AC, Garcia M Jr et al (2008) Postresection CA 19–9 predicts overall survival in patients with pancreatic cancer treated with adjuvant chemoradiation: a prospective validation by RTOG 9704. J Clin Oncol 26:5918–5922

Bjerregaard JK, Mortensen MB et al (2012) Prognostic factors for survival and resection in patients with initial nonresectable locally advanced pancreatic cancer treated with chemoradiotherapy. Int J Radiat Oncol Biol Phys 83:909–915

Bjerregaard JK, Mortensen MB et al (2013) Characteristics, therapy and outcome in an unselected and prospectively registered cohort of pancreatic cancer patients. Eur J Cancer 49:98–105

Blackstock A, Tempero M et al (2001) Cancer and Leukemia Group B (CALGB) 89805: phase II chemoradiation trial using gemcitabine in patients with localoregional adenocarcinoma of the pancreas. Int J Radiat Oncol Biol Phys 51:31 abst #49

Blackstock AW, Bernard SA et al (1999) Phase I trial of twice-weekly gemcitabine and concurrent radiation in patients with advanced pancreatic cancer. J Clin Oncol 17:2208–2212

Brennan MF, Kattan MW et al (2004) Prognostic nomogram for patients undergoing resection for adenocarcinoma of the pancreas. Ann Surg 240:293–298

Breslin TM, Hess KR et al (2001) Neoadjuvant chemoradiotherapy for adenocarcinoma of the pancreas: treatment variables and survival duration. Ann Surg Oncol 8:123–132

Brunner TB, Scott-Brown M (2010) The role of radiotherapy in multimodal treatment of pancreatic carcinoma. Radiat Oncol 5:64

Brunner TB, Sauer R et al (2011) Gemcitabine/cisplatin versus 5-fluorouracil/mitomycin C chemoradiotherapy in locally advanced pancreatic cancer: a retrospective analysis of 93 patients. Radiat Oncol 6:88

Callery MP, Chang KJ et al (2009) Pretreatment assessment of resectable and borderline resectable pancreatic cancer: expert consensus statement. Ann Surg Oncol 16:1727–1733

Cardenes HR, Moore AM et al (2011) A phase II study of gemcitabine in combination with radiation therapy in patients with localized, unresectable, pancreatic cancer: a Hoosier Oncology Group study. Am J Clin Oncol 34:460–465

Chang DT, Schellenberg D et al (2009) Stereotactic radiotherapy for unresectable adenocarcinoma of the pancreas. Cancer 115: 665–672

Chauffert B, Mornex F et al (2008) Phase III trial comparing intensive induction chemoradiotherapy (60 Gy, infusional 5-FU and intermittent cisplatin) followed by maintenance gemcitabine with gemcitabine alone for locally advanced unresectable pancreatic cancer. Definitive results of the 2000-01 FFCD/SFRO study. Ann Oncol 19:1592–1599

Choi M, Heilbrun LK et al (2010) Using 18F-fluorodeoxyglucose positron emission tomography to monitor clinical outcomes in patients treated with neoadjuvant chemo-radiotherapy for locally advanced pancreatic cancer. Am J Clin Oncol 33:257–261

Chuong MD, Springett GM et al (2013) Stereotactic body radiation therapy for locally advanced and borderline resectable pancreatic cancer is effective and well tolerated. Int J Radiat Oncol Biol Phys 86:516–522

Cohen SJ, Dobelbower R Jr et al (2005) A randomized phase III study of radiotherapy alone or with 5-fluorouracil and mitomycin-C in patients with locally advanced adenocarcinoma of the pancreas: Eastern Cooperative Oncology Group study E8282. Int J Radiat Oncol Biol Phys 62:1345–1350

Corsini MM, Miller RC et al (2008) Adjuvant radiotherapy and chemotherapy for pancreatic carcinoma: the Mayo Clinic experience (1975–2005). J Clin Oncol 26:3511–3516

Crane CH, Winter K et al (2009) Phase II study of bevacizumab with concurrent capecitabine and radiation followed by maintenance gemcitabine and bevacizumab for locally advanced pancreatic cancer: Radiation Therapy Oncology Group RTOG 0411. J Clin Oncol 27:4096–4102

Crane CH, Varadhachary GR et al (2011) Phase II trial of cetuximab, gemcitabine, and oxaliplatin followed by chemoradiation with cetuximab for locally advanced (T4) pancreatic adenocarcinoma: correlation of Smad4(Dpc4) immunostaining with pattern of disease progression. J Clin Oncol 29:3037–3043

de Castro SM, Biere SS et al (2009) Validation of a nomogram for predicting survival after resection for adenocarcinoma of the pancreas. Br J Surg 96:417–423

Didolkar MS, Coleman CW et al (2010) Image-guided stereotactic radiosurgery for locally advanced pancreatic adenocarcinoma results of first 85 patients. J Gastrointest Surg 14:1547–1559

Edge SB, Byrd DR et al (2010). American joint committee on cancer, American Cancer Society. AJCC Cancer Staging Manual. 7th edn. Berlin, Springer

Estrella JS, Rashid A et al (2012) Post-therapy pathologic stage and survival in patients with pancreatic ductal adenocarcinoma treated with neoadjuvant chemoradiation. Cancer 118:268–277

Gillen S, Schuster T et al (2010) Preoperative/neoadjuvant therapy in pancreatic cancer: a systematic review and meta-analysis of response and resection percentages. PLoS Med 7:e1000267

Girard N, Mornex F et al (2010) Estimating optimal dose of twice-weekly gemcitabine for concurrent chemoradiotherapy in unresectable pancreatic carcinoma: mature results of GEMRT-01 Phase I trial. Int J Radiat Oncol Biol Phys 77:1426–1432

Golcher H, Brunner T et al (2008) Preoperative chemoradiation in adenocarcinoma of the pancreas. A single centre experience advocating a new treatment strategy. Eur J Surg Oncol 34:756–764

Goodman KA, Regine WF et al (2012) Radiation therapy oncology group consensus panel guidelines for the delineation of the clinical target volume in the postoperative treatment of pancreatic head cancer. Int J Radiat Oncol Biol Phys 83:901–908

Gurka MK, Collins SP et al (2013) Stereotactic body radiation therapy with concurrent full-dose gemcitabine for locally advanced pancreatic cancer: a pilot trial demonstrating safety. Radiat Oncol 8:44

Habermehl D, Kessel K et al (2012) Neoadjuvant chemoradiation with gemcitabine for locally advanced pancreatic cancer. Radiat Oncol 7:28

Herman JM, Wild AT et al (2013) Randomized phase III multi-institutional study of TNFerade biologic with fluorouracil and radiotherapy for locally advanced pancreatic cancer: final results. J Clin Oncol 31:886–894

Huguet F, André T et al (2007) Impact of chemoradiotherapy after disease control with chemotherapy in locally advanced pancreatic adenocarcinoma in GERCOR phase II and III studies. J Clin Oncol 25:326–331

Huguet F, Goodman KA et al (2012) Radiotherapy technical considerations in the management of locally advanced pancreatic cancer: American-French consensus recommendations. Int J Radiat Oncol Biol Phys 83:1355–1364

Jackson AS, Jain P et al (2010) Efficacy and tolerability of limited field radiotherapy with concurrent capecitabine in locally advanced pancreatic cancer. Clin Oncol (R Coll Radiol) 22:570–577

Jingu K, Tanabe T et al (2012) Intraoperative radiotherapy for pancreatic cancer: 30-year experience in a single institution in Japan. Int J Radiat Oncol Biol Phys 83:e507–e511

Katz MH, Marsh R et al (2013). Borderline resectable pancreatic cancer: Need for standardization and methods for optimal clinical trial design. Ann Surg Oncol 2013 Feb 23

Kelly P, Das P et al (2013) Duodenal toxicity after fractionated chemoradiation for unresectable pancreatic cancer. Int J Radiat Oncol Biol Phys 85:e143–e149

Kim EJ, Ben-Josef E et al (2013). A multi-institutional phase 2 study of neoadjuvant gemcitabine and oxaliplatin with radiation therapy in patients with pancreatic cancer. Cancer 2013 May 29

Kimple RJ, Russo S et al (2012) The role of chemoradiation for patients with resectable or potentially resectable pancreatic cancer. Expert Rev Anticancer Ther 12:469–480

Klaassen DJ, MacIntyre JM et al (1985) Treatment of locally unresectable cancer of the stomach and pancreas: a randomized comparison of 5-fluorouracil alone with radiation plus concurrent and maintenance 5-fluorouracil–an Eastern Cooperative Oncology Group study. J Clin Oncol 3:373–378

Klinkenbijl JH, Jeekel J et al (1999) Adjuvant radiotherapy and 5-fluorouracil after curative resection of cancer of the pancreas and periampullary region: phase III trial of the EORTC gastrointestinal tract cancer cooperative group. Ann Surg 230: 776–82; discussion 782–4
Koong AC, Le QT et al (2004) Phase I study of stereotactic radiosurgery in patients with locally advanced pancreatic cancer. Int J Radiat Oncol Biol Phys 58:1017–1021
Laurence JM, Tran PD et al (2011) A systematic review and meta-analysis of survival and surgical outcomes following neoadjuvant chemoradiotherapy for pancreatic cancer. J Gastrointest Surg 15:2059–2069
Li C-P, Chao Y et al (2003) Concurrent chemoradiotherapy treatment of locally advanced pancreatic cancer: Gemcitabine versus 5-fluorouracil, a randomized controlled study. Int J Radiat Oncol Biol Phys 57:98–104
Loehrer PJ Sr, Feng Y et al (2011) Gemcitabine alone versus gemcitabine plus radiotherapy in patients with locally advanced pancreatic cancer: an Eastern Cooperative Oncology Group trial. J Clin Oncol 29:4105–4112
McGinn CJ, Zalupski MM et al (2001) Phase I trial of radiation dose escalation with concurrent weekly full-dose gemcitabine in patients with advanced pancreatic cancer. J Clin Oncol 19:4202–4208
Micke O, Hesselmann S et al (2005) Results and follow-up of locally advanced cancer of the exocrine pancreas treated with radiochemotherapy. Anticancer Res 25:1523–1530
Miller RC, Iott MJ, Corsini MM (2009) Review of adjuvant radiochemotherapy for resected pancreatic cancer and results from Mayo Clinic for the 5th JUCTS symposium. Int J Radiat Oncol Biol Phys 75:364–368
Moertel CG, Frytak S et al (1981) Therapy of locally unresectable pancreatic carcinoma: a randomized comparison of high dose (6000 rads) radiation alone, moderate dose radiation (4000 rads + 5-fluorouracil), and high dose radiation + 5-fluorouracil: The Gastrointestinal Tumor Study Group. Cancer 48:1705–1710
Moghanaki D, Mick R et al (2011) Resection status, age and nodal involvement determine survival among patients receiving adjuvant chemoradiotherapy in pancreatic adenocarcinoma. JOP 12:438–444
Murphy JD, Adusumilli S et al (2007) Full-dose gemcitabine and concurrent radiotherapy for unresectable pancreatic cancer. Int J Radiat Oncol Biol Phys 68:801–808
Murphy JD, Christman-Skieller C et al (2010) A dosimetric model of duodenal toxicity after stereotactic body radiotherapy for pancreatic cancer. Int J Radiat Oncol Biol Phys 78:1420–1426
Murphy JD, Chang DT et al (2012) Cost-effectiveness of modern radiotherapy techniques in locally advanced pancreatic cancer. Cancer 118:1119–1129
Neoptolemos JP, Stocken DD et al (2001) Influence of resection margins on survival for patients with pancreatic cancer treated by adjuvant chemoradiation and/or chemotherapy in the ESPAC-1 randomized controlled trial. Ann Surg 234:758–768
Neoptolemos JP, Stocken DD et al (2004) A randomized trial of chemoradiotherapy and chemotherapy after resection of pancreatic cancer. New Engl J Med 350:1200–1210
Parlak C, Topkan E et al (2012) Prognostic value of gross tumor volume delineated by FDG-PET-CT based radiotherapy treatment planning in patients with locally advanced pancreatic cancer treated with chemoradiotherapy. Radiat Oncol 7:37
Pipas JM, Mitchell SE et al (2001) Phase I study of twice-weekly gemcitabine and concomitant external-beam radiotherapy in patients with adenocarcinoma of the pancreas. Int J Radiat Oncol Biol Phys 50:1317–1322
Pisters PW, Abbruzzese JL et al (1998) Rapid-fractionation preoperative chemoradiation, pancreaticoduodenectomy, and intraoperative radiation therapy for resectable pancreatic adenocarcinoma. J Clin Oncol 16:3843–3850
Polistina F, Costantin G et al (2010) Unresectable locally advanced pancreatic cancer: a multimodal treatment using neoadjuvant chemoradiotherapy (gemcitabine plus stereotactic radiosurgery) and subsequent surgical exploration. Ann Surg Oncol 17:2092–2101
Regine WF, Winter KA et al (2011) Fluorouracil-based chemoradiation with either gemcitabine or fluorouracil chemotherapy after resection of pancreatic adenocarcinoma: 5-year analysis of the U.S. Intergroup/RTOG 9704 phase III trial. Ann Surg Oncol 18:1319–1326
Rich TA, Winter K et al (2012) Weekly paclitaxel, gemcitabine, and external irradiation followed by randomized farnesyl transferase inhibitor R115777 for locally advanced pancreatic cancer. Onco Targets Ther 5:161–170
Rwigema JC, Parikh SD et al (2011) Stereotactic body radiotherapy in the treatment of advanced adenocarcinoma of the pancreas. Am J Clin Oncol 34:63–69
Saif MW, Eloubeidi MA et al (2005) Phase I study of capecitabine with concomitant radiotherapy for patients with locally advanced pancreatic cancer: Expression analysis of genes related to outcome. J Clin Oncol 23:8679–8687
Schellenberg D, Quon A et al (2010) 18Fluorodeoxyglucose PET is prognostic of progression-free and overall survival in locally advanced pancreas cancer treated with stereotactic radiotherapy. Int J Radiat Oncol Biol Phys 77:1420–1425
Schmidt J, Abel U et al (2012) Open-label, multicenter, randomized phase III trial of adjuvant chemoradiation plus interferon Alfa-2b versus fluorouracil and folinic acid for patients with resected pancreatic adenocarcinoma. J Clin Oncol 30:4077–4083
Showalter TN, Winter KA et al (2011) The influence of total nodes examined, number of positive nodes, and lymph node ratio on survival after surgical resection and adjuvant chemoradiation for pancreatic cancer: a secondary analysis of RTOG 9704. Int J Radiat Oncol Biol Phys 81:1328–1335
Small W Jr, Berlin J et al (2008) Full-dose gemcitabine with concurrent radiation therapy in patients with nonmetastatic pancreatic cancer: a multicenter phase II trial. J Clin Oncol 26:942–947
Van Laethem JL, Hammel P et al (2010) Adjuvant gemcitabine alone versus gemcitabine-based chemoradiotherapy after curative resection for pancreatic cancer: a randomized EORTC-40013-22012/FFCD-9203/GERCOR phase II study. J Clin Oncol 28:4450–4456
Van Laethem JL, Verslype C et al (2012) New strategies and designs in pancreatic cancer research: consensus guidelines report from a European expert panel. Ann Oncol 23:570–576
White RR, Kattan MW et al (2006) Evaluation of preoperative therapy for pancreatic cancer using a prognostic nomogram. Ann Surg Oncol 13:1485–1492
Willett CG, Safran H et al (2003) Clinical research in pancreatic cancer: The Radiation Therapy Oncology Group trials. Int J Radiat Oncol Biol Phys 56:31–37
Wolff RA, Evans DB et al (2001) Phase I trial of gemcitabine combined with radiation for the treatment of locally advanced pancreatic adenocarcinoma. Clin Cancer Res 7:2246–2253

Liver Cancer and Metastases

Christine F. Lauro and Tracey E. Schefter

Contents

C. F. Lauro · T. E. Schefter (✉)
Department of Radiation Oncology,
University of Colorado Denver,
Anschutz Medical Campus,
Mail Stop F706, 1665 Aurora Court,
Suite 1032, Aurora, CO 80045, USA
e-mail: tracey.schefter@ucdenver.edu

Abstract

The treatment of hepatocellular carcinoma and liver metastases pose unique considerations to the radiation oncologist. The increasing incidence of hepatocellular carcinoma in North America mandates the refinement of prevention strategies, identification of high-risk individuals, and further development of prognostic and predictive scoring systems for locally ablative therapies. Given the advances in systemic therapy for patients with colorectal malignancies, as well as for other primaries, there is a subset of patients who can experience a prolonged disease-free interval or are potentially curable from the ablation of metastatic liver lesions. More refined methods for identifying these patients using clinical and pathologic factors are currently under investigation. With the advent of conformal radiotherapy and stereotactic radiotherapy, there is a low risk of hepatic toxicity for patients with normal hepatic function. Caution should be exercised when treating patients with underlying hepatic compromise.

Abbreviations

HCC	Hepatocellular carcinoma
RILD	Radiation-induced veno-occlusive liver disease
SBRT	Stereotactic body radiation therapy
CP	Child-Pugh

1 Introduction

Primary hepatic malignancies are a global health issue. Primary liver cancer is the third most common cause of cancer death worldwide (Parkin and Ferlay et al. 2001). The most common histology of primary liver cancer is hepatocellular carcinoma, although cholangiocarcinoma and less commonly sarcoma and hepatoblastoma are other

C. Nieder and L. E. Gaspar (eds.), *Decision Tools for Radiation Oncology*, Medical Radiology. Radiation Oncology,
DOI: 10.1007/174_2013_835, © Springer-Verlag Berlin Heidelberg 2013
Published Online: 26 March 2013

pathologic variants (Cance and Stewart et al. 2000). The incidence of hepatocellular carcinoma is geographically dependent and parallels the incidence of hepatitis B and C viruses, as at least 80 % of primary liver malignancies are attributable to these infections (Bosch and Ribes et al. 2004). Given that the most common variant of primary liver cancer is hepatocellular carcinoma, we will focus our discussion on this histologic variant.

Metastatic disease to the liver is the most common hepatic malignancy (Memon and Lewandowski et al. 2011). It is a particularly common scenario for patients with colorectal primaries, as it has been estimated that 25 % of patients present with liver metastases at diagnosis, and an additional 50 % will experience hepatic metastatic disease progression within 5 years (Bengmark and Hafstrom 1969). The majority of these patients will die as a result of their hepatic metastatic disease (Foster 1984). Although the older paradigm for treatment of patients with metastatic colorectal cancer was generally palliative and/or supportive in nature, recent advances in chemotherapy have improved the survival of these patients, with median survivals of 2 and more years (Chang and Swaminath et al. 2011). Surgical series have documented that long-term survival can be obtained in a favorable subset of patients with hepatic metastases (Aloia and Vauthey et al. 2006; Simmonds and Primrose et al. 2006; Taniai and Yoshida et al. 2006; Tomizawa and Ohwada et al. 2006; Wei and Grant et al. 2006). However, approximately 80–90 % of colorectal patients with metastatic liver disease are not surgical candidates (Alberts and Horvath et al. 2005; Van Cutsem and Adam et al. 2006; Muratore and Bouzari et al. 2007; Daowood and Mahadevan et al. 2009), and it is estimated that only 10–30 % of these patients can be downstaged to a resectable state by the use of chemotherapy (Kemeny 2006). Therefore, there is a large population of patients with potentially curable disease that could benefit from non-operative, ablative therapeutic interventions. We will focus our discussion on the prognostic classification schemes and treatment-specific factors for liver metastases. This chapter focuses on metastatic liver disease and hepatocellular carcinoma, discussing clinical and treatment-related factors that determine clinical outcomes and radiological factors that facilitate radiation planning. Furthermore, since toxicity, particularly radiation-induced liver disease, is a major concern in the application of radiotherapy to the liver, this will be reviewed.

2 Primary Liver Cancer

2.1 Clinical Factors

The incidence of hepatocellular carcinoma is heavily influenced by regional rates of hepatitis infection. Hepatitis B infection accounts for the majority of hepatocellular carcinoma diagnoses in Southeast Asia and sub-Saharan Africa, whereas the preponderance of cases in Japan, Europe, and North America are due to hepatitis C.

In the United States, the cumulative lifetime risk of hepatocellular carcinoma is 0.88 % in men and 0.42 % in women (Ries and Kosary et al. 2004). In the year 2010, 24,120 new cases of liver and biliary cancers were diagnosed, resulting in 18,910 deaths, with a 3:1 male to female predominance (Jemal and Siegel et al. 2010). The incidence of hepatocellular carcinoma in the United States is rising, as reflected by a 30 % increase in death rate from 1991 to 2006 (Jemal and Siegel et al. 2010). This trend is largely attributable to hepatitis C infection, and it is estimated that 4 million Americans are infected with this virus (Spradling and Rupp et al. 2012). Although the incidence of hepatitis C infection has decreased in the last several decades, the two to four decade latency period between viral infection and the development of hepatocellular carcinoma is thought to be responsible for the rising incidence of hepatocellular carcinoma in the United States.

Chronic inflammation of the liver is the predominant mechanism of developing hepatocellular carcinoma. Hepatitis B and C as well as alcoholic cirrhosis are risk factors for the development of hepatocellular carcinoma. Individuals chronically infected with either hepatitis B or C appear to have a 100-fold increased risk for the development of hepatocellular carcinoma as compared with non-infected individuals (Beasley and Hwang et al. 1981; Heintges and Wands 1997). Coinfection with both hepatitis B and C appears to have a synergistic effect (Chen and Yu et al. 1997). While alcohol-induced cirrhosis clearly has been associated with the development of hepatocellular carcinoma (Hassan and Hwang et al. 2002), population-based studies have been confounded by coinfection with hepatitis.

The bulk of efforts striving to reduce the prevalence of hepatocellular carcinoma have focused upon the reduction of hepatitis B and C transmission. A vaccine for hepatitis B has been commercially available since 1982. Due to the genetic diversity of the hepatitis C virus, a vaccine has not yet been developed. Efforts to reduce this blood-borne pathogen include needle exchange programs, blood transfusion screening assays, universal precautions for health care providers, and treatment with interferon alpha for individuals known to be infected with hepatitis C (Benvegnu and Alberti 1996).

Other non-viral causes of hepatocellular carcinoma include alcoholic cirrhosis and/or excessive alcohol intake, nonalcoholic steatohepatitis (NASH), environmental exposure to alfatoxin, as well as rare inherited metabolic disorders including hereditary hemochromatosis, porphyria cutanea tarda, alpha 1-antitrypsin deficiency, Wilson's disease, and Stage IV primary biliary cirrhosis (Fattovich and

Table 1 Assessment of Hepatic Cirrhosis: The Child-Pugh Score

Score	Bilirubin (mg/dL)	Albumin (g/dL)	Prothrombin time (sec)	Hepatic Encephalopathy (grade)	Ascites
1	<2	>3.5	<4	None	None
2	2–3	2.8–3.5	4–6	1–2	Mild (detectable)
3	>3	<2.8	>6	3–4	Severe (tense)
Child class: A, 5–6; B, 7–9; C, > 9					

Child-Pugh classification of hepatic function is based on the international normalized ratio (INR), bilirubin and albumin serum levels, as well as the degree of ascites and encephalopathy

Stroffolini et al. 2004). It has been estimated that approximately 15–50 % of patients diagnosed with hepatocellular carcinoma do not have the classic risk features of viral hepatitis and/or heavy alcohol use (El-Seraq 2004).

Identification of patients at high risk for the development of hepatocellular carcinoma has the potential to identify individuals with early stage, and thereby potentially curable, disease. The NCCN identifies high-risk individuals as those diagnosed with viral, autoimmune, or alcoholic cirrhosis, NASH, or non-cirrhotic hepatitis B carriers. These patients are recommended to undergo serum alpha-fetoprotein and/or hepatic ultrasound evaluation every 6–12 months (Benson and Abrams et al. 2009). This recommendation is supported by a randomized controlled trial conducted in China, in which 18,816 patients with either a diagnosis of hepatitis B infection or chronic hepatitis were enrolled to undergo either clinical observation or surveillance with serum alpha-fetoprotein evaluation and ultrasound at 6 month intervals. There was a 37 % reduction in hepatocellular carcinoma mortality among those randomized to the screening arm, although <60 % of these patients complied with the screening protocol (Zhang and Tang et al. 2004).

Upon a histologic confirmation of hepatocellular carcinoma, a multidisciplinary evaluation is indicated, which includes a complete history and physical examination, hepatitis panel, and serum evaluation of hepatic function, including bilirubin, transaminases, alkaline phosphatase, PT or INR, albumin, BUN, creatinine, CBC, platelets, and AFP. Chest imaging should be performed, with bone scan as indicated. The Child-Pugh classification is a commonly utilized tool for assessment of hepatic function, which is based on the degree of ascites and encephalopathy as well as bilirubin, albumin, and international normalized ratio (INR) levels (Table 1).

Commonly used staging systems for hepatocellular carcinoma include the American Joint Committee on Cancer (AJCC) TNM staging system (Table 2), as well as the Barcelona Clinic Liver Cancer (BCLC) classification (Fig. 1). A criticism of the BCLC is that patients with portal invasion, node positive, and/or metastasis positive disease are collectively grouped, and focal therapies are not recommended for this heterogeneous cohort of patients. Other staging systems including the Okuda staging system (Okuda and Obata et al. 1985) and Cancer of the Liver Italian Program (CLIP) scoring system (Kanematsu and Hoshi et al. 1999), which are clinical staging systems best suited for patients with poor liver reserve and advanced disease. The presence of portal vein thrombosis alone has been shown to portend a poor prognosis, with a median survival of 3 months without treatment for these patients (Wang and Zhang et al. 2008).

2.2 Treatment-Specific Factors

The majority of patients with hepatocellular carcinoma are asymptomatic, and symptomatology from primary liver cancer portends a poor prognosis. Treatment options for hepatocellular carcinoma are dependent upon underlying liver function. Less than 30 % of patients present with potentially resectable, and thereby potentially curably disease (Bruix and Sherman 2005). Five-year survival for this favorable cohort of patients ranges between 40 and 70 %. Approximately, 20 % of patients are diagnosed with end stage, symptomatic disease. Treatment strategies for these patients are palliative in nature, and median survival is less than 3 months. The remainder of patients, approximately 50 %, are diagnosed with inoperable, locally advanced disease (Llovet and Bruix et al. 2003), and therapeutic modalities may include chemotherapy, percutaneous ablation, embolization, conformal radiotherapy, and/or SBRT.

2.2.1 Liver Transplantation in the Management of Hepatocellular Carcinoma

Liver transplantation is the gold standard treatment for hepatocellular carcinoma, as both the cirrhotic liver and primary disease are eradicated. The United Network for Organ Sharing (UNOS) uses the Milan criteria to identify patients who are suitable for transplant, which stipulates that one tumor should be ≤5 cm, or up to 3 tumors could measure up to 3 cm each, without extrahepatic spread or macrovascular invasion. For patients with these favorable features, the 4-year survival rate was reported to be 85 %, and the recurrence-free survival was 92 % (Mazzaferro and Doci et al. 1996).

Table 2 TNM Classification for Liver Tumors from the American Joint Committee on Cancer (AJCC) 7th edition (2010)

Primary Tumor (T)			
TX	Primary tumor cannot be assessed		
T0	No evidence of primary tumor		
T1	Solitary tumor without vascular invasion		
T2	Solitary tumor with vascular invasion or multiple tumors none more than 5 cm		
T3a	Multiple tumors more than 5 cm		
T3b	Single tumor or multiple tumors of any size involving a major branch of the portal vein or hepatic vein		
T4	Tumor(s) with direct invasion of adjacent organs other than the gallbladder or with perforation of visceral peritoneum		
Regional Lymph Nodes (N)			
NX	Regional lymph nodes cannot be assessed		
N0	No regional lymph node metastasis		
N1	Regional lymph node metastasis		
Distance Metastasis (M)			
M0	No distant metastasis		
M1	Distant metastasis		
Anatomic stage/Prognostic groups			
Stage I	T1	N0	M0
Stage II	T2	N0	M0
Stage IIIA	T3a	N0	M0
Stage IIIB	T3b	N0	M0
Stage IIIC	T4	N0	M0
Stage IVA	Any T	N1	M0
Stage IVB	Any T	Any N	M1

The original and primary source for this information is the AJCC Cancer Staging Manual, Seventh edition (2010) published by Springer Science and Business Media LLC (SBM)

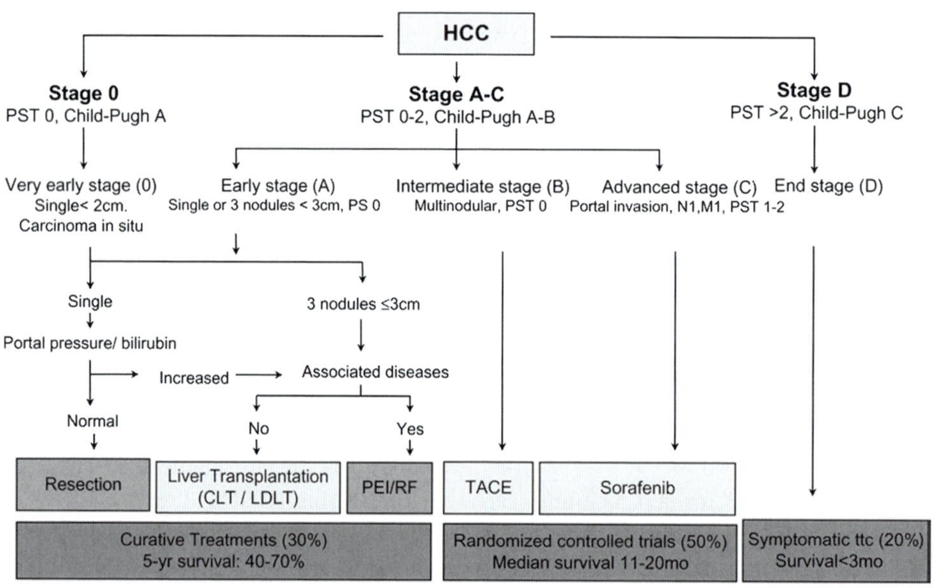

Fig. 1 Barcelona Clinic Liver Cancer (*BCLC*) classification for hepatocellular carcinoma (*HCC*). Llovet and Di Bisceglie et al. (2008) Barcelona Clinic Liver Cancer (*BCLC*) classification for hepatocellular carcinoma (*HCC*) including incidence, estimated survival, and management options. *PST*, performance status based on Eastern Cooperative Oncology Group score; *N* nodal stage; *M* metastases stage; *CLD* cadaver liver transplantation; *LDLT* living donor liver transplantation; *RF* radiofrequency ablation; *PEI* percutaneous ethanol injection; *TACE* transarterial chemoembolization (Llovet and Di Bisceglie et al. 2008)

Liver transplantation is limited by organ availability, and approximately 20 % of patients who have been listed on the liver transplant list have subsequently withdrawn due to tumor progression. Therefore, an interest in "bridge" therapies has emerged to maintain patient eligibility for liver transplant. Traditional bridge therapies have included radiofrequency ablation (Lu et al. 2005), chemoembolization (Heckman and Devera et al. 2008), and radioembolization with yttrium-90 microspheres (Kulik and van Holsbeeck et al. 2006). Hepatic resection as a bridge to transplant yielded higher operative mortality, increased recurrence, and poorer outcome than patients receiving primary liver transplantation in a prospective, single institution French experience, and has subsequently been abandoned as a bridge therapy (Adam and Azoulay et al. 2003).

More recently, SBRT has emerged as a viable bridge to transplant strategy. The Baylor experience reported a 5-year overall survival rate of 100 % for 10 patients with hepatocellular carcinoma who received bridge therapy in the form of SBRT to a median dose of 51 Gy in 3 Gy fractions prior to orthotopic transplant (O'Connor and Davis et al. 2012). The University of Rochester experience, which treated 11 evaluable lesions in 10 patients to a median dose of 50 Gy in 5-Gy fractions, reported no grade $\geq$ 3 toxicities and no radiation-induced liver disease. All patients were alive at a median follow-up of 19.6 months (Katz and Chawla et al. 2012). Finally, a prospective phase I-II trial conducted at indiana university treated 14 hepatocellular carcinoma patients with a Child-Pugh Class B score of <8 were treated to a total dose of 40 Gy in 5 fractions. Local control at 12 months was 87.5 % (Cardenes and Lasley et al. 2012). Three grade 4 toxicities were observed, which included hyperbilirubinemia, hypokalemia, and thrombocytopenia.

2.2.2 Surgical Resection in the Management of Hepatocellular Carcinoma

Hepatic resection is a potentially curative option for patients with early stage disease. Prediction of post-operative hepatic reserve is an essential component of the preoperative evaluation of these patients. To assess for the adequacy of the future liver remnant, the Child-Pugh classification has historically been employed (Table 1). In North America, the current evaluation for resection typically includes the determination of the presence of portal hypertension, as quantified by hepatic vein catheterization (Bruix and Castells et al. 1996). Other methods to clinically assess for portal hypertension include the presence of splenomegaly and/or thrombocytosis. The literature is mixed regarding the exact margin required for adequate removal of the tumor, although 1–2 cm is generally recommended.

2.2.3 Percutaneous Ablation in the Management of Hepatocellular Carcinoma

Percutaneous ablation is a local therapy whereby substances (alcohol or acetic acid) are injected into a focal liver lesion, or the temperature is changed (via radiofrequency ablation, microwave, laser, or cryotherapy). Ethanol and radiofrequency ablation are the two most commonly reported ablative techniques. In a retrospective analysis of five randomized trials, it appears that radiofrequency was superior to ethanol ablation in terms of overall survival and local control for small HCC (Chen and Li et al. 2006). Radiofrequency ablation was directly compared to hepatic resection in a randomized trial of 230 patients conducted in China. Hepatic resection was found to be significantly superior to radiofrequency ablation, with an overall survival rate of 75.6 % versus 54.8 %, and recurrence-free survival of 51.3 % versus 28.7 %, respectively (Huang and Yan et al. 2010). The NCCN currently endorses ablation as a local treatment modality for patients with a small burden (tumors $\leq$ 3 cm) of unresectable disease (Benson and Abrams et al. 2009). Lesions not suitable to ablation include lesions near the dome, as they are less well visualized with ultrasound, and lesions near large blood vessels, due to concerns of heat sink from nearby circulation.

2.2.4 Endovascular Therapies in the Management of Hepatocellular Carcinoma

Endovascular therapies for the treatment of hepatocellular carcinoma include radioembolization and chemoembolization. These techniques exploit the differential perfusion of hepatic malignancies and parenchyma, given that tumor cells derive their blood supply from the hepatic artery, whereas normal hepatocytes rely on the hepatic vein. In this way, cancerous cells are preferentially targeted with relative sparing of normal hepatocytes. Radioembolization is a catheter-based, liver-directed therapy that involves the hepatic intra-arterial injection of isotopes, typically yttrium-90, bound to resin microspheres. While the major mechanism of radioembolization is due to radiation, embolization also attempts to induce ischemic necrosis of the tumor. In contrast, transcatheter arterial chemoembolization attempts to both increase the local concentration of chemotherapeutic agents and induce ischemic necrosis of the tumor. In hepatocellular carcinoma, chemoembolization and radioembolization have been used to delay disease progression, bridge to potential liver transplantation, or palliate symptoms.

Multiple randomized trials comparing transcatheter arterial chemoembolization versus best supportive care for patients with unresectable hepatocellular carcinoma and without severe liver disease found no advantage to transarterial chemoembolization versus conservative therapy (Pelletier 1990; Hepatocellulaire 1995), although a meta-analysis of 7 randomized, controlled trials found a significant 2-year overall survival benefit of chemoembolization versus control (Adam and Azoulay et al. 2003). The NCCN endorses chemoembolization as a treatment option for patients with unresectable hepatocellular carcinoma without main portal vein thrombosis, as ischemic hepatitis is a known complication of this procedure (Benson and Abrams et al. 2009).

A recent comparative analysis study of patients with unresectable hepatocellular carcinoma without portal vein thrombosis compared 122 patients who received chemoembolization and 123 who received radioembolization (Salem and Lewandowski et al. 2011). The acute side effects of abdominal pain and transaminitis were significantly more frequent in the chemoembolization cohort. Time to progression was statistically improved from 8.4 to 13.3 months, favoring patients who underwent radioembolization as opposed to chemoembolization. Various older, retrospective studies have concluded that radioembolization and chemoembolization are equivalent locoregional therapies with similar effectiveness and safety profiles (Poon and Lau et al. 2007; Shannon and Williams 2008).

The most commonly used radioisotope for radioembolization is yttrium-90 (^{90}Y), which is a pure beta-emitter with a half-life of 64.2 h. In a recent, prospective report of long-term outcomes of patients receiving ^{90}Y, overall time to progression was 7.9 months (Poon and Lau et al. 2007). Patients with Child-Pugh A disease, with or without portal vein thrombosis, enjoyed the longest survival. Survival times significantly differed between patients with Child-Pugh A and B disease, at 17.2 months and 8.8 months, respectively. Patients with Child-Pugh B disease who had portal vein thrombosis fared the poorest, with a median survival of 5.6 months. Baseline patient characteristics, including age and performance status, as well as serum indicators of hepatic function predicted for survival.

2.2.5 External Beam Radiotherapy in the Management of Hepatocellular Carcinoma

Prior to the development of conformal radiotherapy, the utilization of radiotherapy in the management of hepatocellular carcinoma was limited by toxicity, given that the whole liver was necessarily encompassed in the radiation portal. Radiation-induced veno-occlusive liver disease (classic RILD) was the dose-limiting complication, which was pathologically first described by Reed and Cox in the early 1960s (Reed 1966).

The advent of conformal radiotherapy permitted delin eation of target lesions, thereby enabling partial volumes of the liver to be spared from radiotherapy. Furthermore, the dose-volume relationship between liver irradiation and RILD became better elucidated. In 2002, a Normal Tissue Complication Probability (NTCP) model was described which estimated a 50 % complication risk of RILD for whole-organ irradiation of 39.8 Gy for patients with primary hepatobiliary cancer. (Dawson and Normolle et al. 2002).

One of largest experiences of conformal radiotherapy in the treatment of hepatocellular carcinoma is derived from the Seong experience in Korea, which is a retrospective series of 298 patients with hepatocellular carcinoma. The majority (81.9 %) of patients were treated with conformal radiotherapy to a total dose of $\geq$45 Gy. On multivariate analysis, a BED of >53.1 Gy was shown to be a significant factor for better prognosis (Seong and Lee et al. 2009).

In the United States, the University of Michigan conducted a series of trials with conventionally fractionated, conformal partial liver radiotherapy which was delivered in doses up to 90 Gy in 1.5-Gy fractions on a twice-daily schedule with concurrent intra-arterial hepatic fluorodeoxyuridine (Robertson and Walker et al. 1997; McGinn and Ensminger et al. 1998; Dawson and McGinn et al. 2000; Ben-Josef and Normolle et al. 2005). For the 35 patients enrolled in these trials with hepatocellular carcinoma, an objective response was obtained in 56 % of patients, and median survival was 15.2 months. There was a statistically significant effect for dose, as patients who received a total dose of $\geq$75 Gy enjoyed improved progression free survival than patients who received lesser total radiotherapy doses (Ben-Josef and Normolle et al. 2005). A summary of trials of conformal radiotherapy is provided in Table 3. Typically, local control has been reported between 54 and 81 %, and 1-year overall survival ranges between 43 and 65 %.

2.2.6 Stereotactic Body Radiotherapy in the Management of Hepatocellular Carcinoma

Stereotactic body radiation therapy (SBRT) has emerged as powerful, non-invasive ablative technique with the capacity for local tumor eradication in the absence of surgery. The experience of SBRT for hepatocellular carcinoma is relatively small, given the new application of SBRT in the treatment of this entity. Several trials have reported their experiences with hepatocellular carcinoma and SBRT, with total doses typically between 36 and 60 Gy delivered in 3–6 fractions (Table 4) (Liang and Zhu et al. 2006; Mendez-Romero and Wunderink et al. 2006; Tse and Hawkins et al. 2008; Cardenes and Price et al. 2010; Goyal and Einstein 2010; Kwon and Bae et al. 2010; Louis and Dewas et al. 2010; Seo and Kim et al. 2010). In contrast to patients with metastatic liver tumors, the majority of patients with hepatocellular carcinoma have cirrhotic livers, so estimation of post-treatment hepatic function is increasingly important. Further details regarding the toxicity of SBRT in

Table 3 Trials of conformal, conventionally fractionated radiotherapy for Hepatocellular Carcinoma

Study	Patients	CP Class A (%)	Total dose (dose per fraction)	1-year local control	1-year overall survival
Liu and Li et al. 2004 (Liu and Li et al. 2004)	44	86	40–60 Gy, fractional dose unreported	61 %	61
Ben-Josef and Normolle et al. 2005 (Ben-Josef and Normolle et al. 2005)	35	100	40–90 Gy in 1.5 Gy fx BID	81 %	57
Liang and Zhu et al. 2005 (Liang and Zhu et al. 2005)	128	84	36–68 Gy, majority 4- to 6-Gy fx	69 % at 3 months	65
Kim and Kim et al. 2006 (Kim and Kim et al. 2006)	70	88	44–54 Gy in 2- to 3-Gy fx	54 %	43
Mornex and Girard et al. 2006 (Mornex and Girard et al. 2006)	27	59	36–66 Gy in 2-Gy fx	78 %	NA
Seong and Lee et al. 2009 (Seong and Lee et al. 2009)	398	77	25–60 Gy, majority 1.8- to 5-Gy fx	NA	45

Abbreviations: *BID* twice daily; *CP* Child-Pugh; *fx* fractions

Table 4 Studies of stereotactic body radiotherapy for Hepatocellular Carcinoma

Study	Patients	CP Class A (%)	Total dose (fractions)	1-year local control (%)	1-year overall survival (%)
Mendez-Romero and Wunderink et al. 2006 (Mendez-Romero and Wunderink et al. 2006)	8	75	37.5 Gy (3 fractions) for < 4 cm 25 Gy (5 fractions) or 30 Gy (3 fractions) for ≥ 4 cm	75	75
Tse and Hawkins et al. 2008 (Tse and Hawkins et al. 2008)	31	100	24–54 Gy (6 fractions)	65	48
Cardenes and Price et al. 2010 (Cardenes and Price et al. 2010)	17 (25 tumors)	35	36–48 Gy (3 fractions) for CPA 36–42 Gy (3 fractions) or 40 Gy (5 fractions) for CPB	100	75
Goyal and Einstein et al. 2010 (Goyal and Einstein et al. 2010)	6	NA	24–45 Gy (1–3 fractions)	100	67
Seo and Kim et al. 2010 (Seo and Kim et al. 2010)	38	89	33–57 Gy (3–4 fractions)	79	68
Kwon and Bae et al. 2010 (Kwon and Bae et al. 2010)	42	90	30–39 Gy (3 fractions)	72	93
Louis and Dewas et al. 2010 (Louis and Dewas et al. 2010)	25	88	45 Gy (3 fractions)	95	79
Stenmark and Liu et al. 2011 (Stenmark and Liu et al. 2011, January 20–22)	31	69	Majority 50 Gy (5 fractions) or 60 Gy (3 fractions)	88	81

Abbreviations: *CPA* Child-Pugh Class A; *CPB* Child-Pugh Class B

hepatocellular carcinoma are reviewed later in the "Toxicity" section.

One of the largest prospective trials of SBRT in hepatocellular carcinoma was conducted at the Princess Margaret Hospital. In this phase 1 trial, 31 patients with unresectable hepatocellular carcinoma with Child-Pugh A liver function were treated with 6 fraction SBRT. The total SBRT dose was dependent upon NTCP calculations that estimated the risk of RILD from 5 to 20 % based on the University of Michigan experience. The median tumor dose was 36 Gy (range 24–54 Gy). A median overall survival of 11.7 months was observed for patients with hepatocellular carcinoma. There was a 24 % rate of Grade 3 transaminitis, and no acute Grade 4–5 toxicities. There was one late Grade 5 toxicity resulting from a GI bleed (Tse and Hawkins et al. 2008).

2.2.7 Chemotherapy in the Management of Hepatocellular Carcinoma

Sorafenib is an oral multikinase inhibitor of vascular endothelial growth factor and platelet-derived growth factor receptors. The SHARP (Sorafenib Hepatocellular Carcinoma Assessment Randomized Protocol) trial was a large phase 3, randomized, placebo-controlled trial that evaluated sorafenib in patients with advanced hepatocellular carcinoma (Llovet and Ricci et al. 2007). Patients receiving sorafenib experienced a 3 month improvement in median survival than those randomized to placebo (10.7 months vs 7.9 months, $P < 0.001$). Time to radiographic progression was also significantly improved with the addition of sorafenib by approximately 3 months. Similar in design to the SHARP trial, the Asia–Pacific trial found a statistically significant improvement in overall survival (6.5 months vs 4.2 months) as well as median time to progression (2.8 months vs 1.4 months) for patients treated with sorafenib versus placebo (Cheng and Kang et al. 2009). The NCCN designates sorafenib as the only treatment option with a category 1 designation for Child-Pugh Class A patients with unresectable disease (Benson and Abrams et al. 2009).

3 Metastatic Liver Disease

3.1 Clinical Factors

The spectrum of metastatic disease to the liver is broad, ranging from a single metastatic lesion to innumerable hepatic metastases. Traditionally, the presence of liver metastases denoted an incurable state, and interventions were largely restricted to systemic therapy and/or palliative in nature. However, surgical series of metastasectomy have challenged this assumption, with recent studies documenting 5-year survival rates from 42 to 71 % for patients with solitary hepatic metastases (Aloia and Vauthey et al. 2006; Simmonds and Primrose et al. 2006; Taniai and Yoshida et al. 2006; Tomizawa and Ohwada et al. 2006; Wei and Grant et al. 2006). From these observations, the concept of 'oligometastases' denoted that, for patients with limited volume and sites of metastatic disease, localized cancer therapies have the potential to be curative in nature (Weichselbaum and Hellman 2011).

The identification of patients with hepatic metastases who have disease that is potentially amenable to curative, locoregional therapies has been investigated in a retrospective manner by surgical series. There is evidence that patients presenting synchronously with a primary colon cancer and liver metastases may have a more disseminated disease state and corresponding shorter disease-free interval than for patients developing metachronous metastases (Tsai and Su et al. 2007). Fong et al. examined the clinical and pathologic findings of 1,001 consecutive patients at a single institution undergoing partial liver resection for metastatic colorectal disease. Five-year survival for all patients was 37 %, and the 10-year survival was 22 %. Findings that portended a poor long-term survival on multivariate analysis included positive surgical margins, extrahepatic disease, node positive primary, disease-free interval of <12 months, >1 hepatic metastasis, largest hepatic tumor >5 cm, and CEA > 200 mg/mL (Fong and Fortner et al. 1999). A clinical risk score corresponding to tumor recurrence at 1, 2, 3, 4, and 5 years was developed from these findings (Table 5).

Table 5 Clinical risk score for tumor recurrence

	Survival (%)					
Score	1 year	2 year	3 year	4 year	5 year	Median (mo)
0	93	79	72	60	60	74
1	91	76	66	54	44	51
2	89	73	60	51	40	47
3	86	67	42	25	20	33
4	70	45	38	29	25	20
5	71	45	27	14	14	22

Each of the following risk factors are one point: Node-positive primary, disease-free interval <12 months, >1 tumor, size >5 cm, CEA > 200 ng/ml (Fong and Fortner et al. 1999)

Similarly, Pawlik et al. conducted a multicenter, retrospective analysis of 557 patients undergoing hepatic resection. At a median follow-up of 29 months, the median survival for patients with a positive surgical margin was significantly inferior to patients with negative margins, with a median survival of 49 months for the former group, and the median survival was not reached for the latter group. Width of the negative surgical margin did not appear to predict for survival (Pawlik and Scoggins et al. 2005).

3.2 Treatment-Specific Factors

3.2.1 Fractionated Radiotherapy in the Management of Metastatic Liver Disease

The use of radiotherapy in the management of metastatic liver disease has classically been limited by toxicity. In the 1970s and 1980s, numerous studies suggested that low-dose whole-liver radiotherapy (generally 21–30 Gy in 2- to 3-Gy fractions) conferred an improvement in pain control in up to 90 % of patients, without an overall survival benefit (Prasad and Hendrickson et al. 1977; Sherman and Order 1978; Borgelt and Gelber et al. 1981). Median survival was poor in these studies, as demonstrated by an 11 week median survival observed in RTOG 76-05 (Borgelt and Gelber et al. 1981). Studies which sought to augment the efficacy of low-dose whole-liver radiotherapy with various methods, including hyperfractionation, misonidazole radiosensitization, and radiolabelled antibodies, did not suggest significant benefit as compared with whole-liver radiotherapy alone (Liebel and Massullo et al. 1987; Stillwagon and Guse et al. 1989; Abrams and Pajak et al. 1998).

The advent of 3-dimensional, conformal radiotherapy enabled the delivery of partial liver radiotherapy, permitting tumor dose escalation without the inherent dose limitations of whole-liver radiotherapy. The University of Michigan published the results of a phase I-II trial in 1995, which escalated the dose of conformal radiotherapy from 48 to 72.6 Gy in 1.5- to 1.65-Gy fractions with concurrent intra-arterial hepatic flurordeoxyuridine (Robertson and Walker et al. 1995). Fifty percent of patients achieved an objective response (11 of 22 patients), with the remainder of patients experiencing stable disease. The median survival was 20 months, which compared favorably to older, whole-liver series. In another study, 45 patients with colorectal liver metastases were treated with either low-dose whole-liver radiotherapy to a total dose of 8–31 Gy in 2- to 3-Gy fractions, versus low-dose whole-liver radiotherapy followed by tumor boost to 33–60 Gy (Mohiuddin and Ahmad et al. 1996). Median survival was improved from 4 to 14 months with the addition of the boost.

3.2.2 Stereotactic Body Radiotherapy in the Management of Liver Metastases

Stereotactic body radiotherapy (SBRT) is a hypofractionated radiation technique that utilizes both increased target conformality and steep dose gradients outside the planning target volume to deliver an ablative tumor dose (Schefter and Kavanagh 2011). Several clinical developments are necessary for the delivery of SBRT: (1) secure patient immobilization; (2) accurate repositioning from simulation to treatment delivery; (3) multiple arcing small aperture fields; (4) assessment of organ motion; (5) stereotactic registration of the target; and (6) ablative dose fractionation (Timmerman and Kavanagh et al. 2007). An early application of SBRT was in the treatment of medically inoperable, early stage lung cancer. A phase II North American study evaluated 55 patients who received 54 Gy in 3 Gy fractions to a non-small cell lung primary (Timmerman and Galvin et al. 2010). The documented 3-year survival rate of 55.8 % and local tumor control rate of 97.6 % compared favorably to the outcomes of conventionally fractionated management, with a low rate of treatment toxicity. From the findings of this phase II trial and the work of others, SBRT is now an NCCN recognized management approach for medically inoperable primary lung cancer (Ettinger and Bepler 2010).

Early reports of the use of SBRT in the treatment of liver lesions emanated from Stockholm in the 1990s (Blomgren and Lax et al. 1995; Lax and Blomgren et al. 1998). Subsequently, several phase I-II trials have investigated the use of SBRT in liver lesions (Table 6) (Herfarth and Debus et al. 2001; Hoyer and Roed et al. 2006; Mendez-Romero and Wunderink et al. 2006; Lee and Kim et al. 2009; Rusthoven and Kavanagh et al. 2009; Goodman and Wiegner et al. 2010; Rule and Timmerman et al. 2011). Typically, eligible patients had one to five hepatic metastases, all <5 cm in diameter. While the majority of the metastases were secondary to colorectal primaries, metastatic lesions from other gastrointestinal cancers, renal cell carcinoma, breast cancer, bladder cancer, and ovarian cancer were treated. It has been postulated that the best candidates for SBRT are similar to those most suitable for metastasectomy, in that they have controlled primary tumors, a limited burden of metastatic disease, metachronous appearance of primary and metastatic disease, younger age, and higher performance status (Timmerman and Bizekis et al. 2009).

The results of the phase I/II series describing liver SBRT have championed its use as a safe, ablative nonsurgical technique. One of the earliest series was reported by Herfarth and Debus et al. in 2001, where 60 liver lesions (56 metastases, 4 primary tumors) in 36 patients were treated with doses escalated from 14 to 26 Gy in a single fraction. The actuarial local control rate after 18 months was 81 % (Herfarth and Debus et al. 2001). Every patient experienced post-treatment, CT findings of a sharply demarcated hypodense area surrounding the target, at a median time of 1.8 months following SBRT (Herfarth and Hof et al. 2003).

A multi-institutional phase I/II study from the University of Colorado treated patients with one to three hepatic lesions with individual tumor diameters <6 cm with three fraction SBRT (Schefter and Kavanagh et al. 2005; Rusthoven and Kavanagh et al. 2009). During phase I, the total dose was safely escalated from 36 to 60 Gy, and the phase II dose was 60 Gy. Actuarial in-field local control rates at one and 2 years post-treatment were 95 % and 92 %, respectively. Toxicities were minimal, as demonstrated by a 2 % rate of grade $\geq$ 3 toxicity (one patient experienced a grade 3 soft tissue toxicity). In a phase I trial at the University of Texas Southwestern, patients were treated in three dose-escalation cohorts: 30 Gy in 3 fractions, 50 Gy in 5 fractions, and 60 Gy in 5 fractions (Rule and Timmerman et al. 2011). A critical non-tumorous hepatic volume of 700 mL was spared from doses >21 Gy. There was a statistically significant difference in local control between the 60- and 30- Gy cohorts, with a 2 year local control rate of 100 and 56 %, respectively. There were no toxicities grade 3 or greater reported.

Table 6 Outcomes of phase I/II studies of SBRT for liver metastases

Study	Patients	No. of tumors by type: metastasis/primary	Total dose (fractions)	Local control	Time
Herfarth and Debus et al. 2001	37	56/4	14–26 Gy (1 fraction)	67 %	18 Months
Phase I/II				81 % with ≥20 Gy	
(Herfarth and Debus et al. 2001)					
Mendez-Romero and Wunderink et al. 2006	25	34/11	37.5 Gy (3 fractions)	82 %	24 Months
Phase I/II					
(Mendez-Romero and Wunderink et al. 2006)					
Hoyer and Roed et al. 2006	44	NR	45 Gy (3 Fractions)	79 %	24 Months
Phase II					
(Hoyer and Roed et al. 2006)					
Lee and Kim et al. 2009	68	141/0	Variable NTCP-based	71 %	12 Months
Phase I					
(Lee and Kim et al. 2009)			Median 42 Gy (6 fractions)		
Rusthoven and Kavanagh et al. 2009	47	63/0	36–60 Gy (3 fractions)	92 %	24 Months
Phase I/II					
(Rusthoven and Kavanagh et al. 2009)					
Goodman and Wiegner et al. 2010	26	33/7	18–30 Gy (1 fraction)	77 %	12 Months
Phase I					
(Goodman and Wiegner et al. 2010)					
Rule and Timmerman et al. 2011	27	37/0	30 Gy (3 fractions)	56 %	24 Months
				89 %	
Phase I			50 Gy (5 fractions)	100 %	
(Rule and Timmerman et al. 2011)			60 Gy (5 fractions)		

In a multi-institutional study, 65 patients with 102 colorectal metastases treated with one to six fraction SBRT were retrospectively analyzed (Chang and Swaminath et al. 2011). On multivariate analysis by lesion, total dose, dose per fraction, and BED all correlated significantly with local control. Conversely, patient characteristics including age and number of prior chemotherapy regimens were not associated with local control. A tumor control probability model estimated that the dose required for >90 % local control was 46- to 52-Gy in 3 fractions. There was a trend correlating local tumor control with overall survival, suggesting that hepatic tumor control is a significant clinical objective.

3.2.3 Radiofrequency Ablation in the Management of Liver Metastases

Radiofrequency ablation is a procedure that utilizes an alternating electrical current to generate thermal ablation of interstitial tissue via an open, laparoscopic, or percutaneous approach. The experience of radiofrequency ablation (RFA) in the management of liver metastases has been limited to retrospective studies (Gleisner and Choti et al. 2008; de Jong and Pulitano et al. 2009; Hur and Ko et al. 2009; (Reuter and Scoggins et al. 2009). Toxicity of RFA appears to be modest, with a major complication rate ranging between 0 and 2 % (Wong and Mangu et al. 2010). There is wide range of reported outcomes in these studies, with 5-year survival ranging between 14 and 55 %, and local control rates reported as 3.6–60 % (Wong and Mangu et al. 2010). The predominance of the literature suggests that RFA yields inferior local recurrence and overall survival outcomes as compared with surgical resection (Abdalla 2009; de Jong and Pulitano et al. 2009). The 2009 ASCO clinical evidence review and 2012 Cochrane Database Systemic Review concluded that, given the lack of randomized trials, there is insufficient evidence to form the basis of clinical recommendations for the use of RFA (Wong and Mangu et al. 2010; Cirocchi and Trastulli et al. 2012).

3.2.4 Radioembolization in the Management of Liver Metastases

As described previously, radioembolization is a catheter-based, liver-directed therapy that involves the hepatic intra-arterial injection of isotopes, typically yttrium-90, bound to resin microspheres. The data regarding radioembolization has reported little toxicity, although the experience is limited to small trials with highly selected patients. A recent multi-center phase III study of 46 patients compared intravenous fluorouracil with or without radioembolization for patients with unresectable, chemotherapy-refractory liver-limited metastatic colorectal cancer. The results suggested a significant improvement in terms of median time to tumor progression of 2.1 and 4.5 months, favoring the radioembolization arm, without a statistically significant difference in grade 3 or 4 toxicities (Hendlisz and Van den Eynde et al. 2010).

4 Radiation Planning Techniques

There are several issues unique to the treatment planning for liver metastases and primary liver cancer. Given the proximity of critical adjacent normal structures and the potential for radiation-induced liver injury to the normal hepatic parenchyma, it is critical to accurately define the tumor and reproducibly localize the lesion(s) on a daily basis.

Hepatic lesions are difficult to discriminate from normal hepatic parenchyma in noncontrast, computed tomography (CT) imaging. The addition of intravenous, timed contrast can permit improved visualization of both primary and metastatic liver lesions. Primary hepatocellular carcinoma more avidly enhances than normal hepatic parenchyma during the arterial phase (acquired after a 20- to 30-second delay) and washes out during the venous (50–60 second) or late delayed (>180 second) phases of imaging (Bruix and Sherman 2011). In contrast, metastatic lesions are better visualized with addition of intravenous contrast timed for the venous phase. Furthermore, the additional imaging modalities of magnetic resonance imaging (MRI) and positron emission tomography (PET) can assist in the discrimination of hepatic lesions. As these studies must be registered to the planning CT scan, it is advisable to perform these ancillary studies in the same immobilization device to facilitate registration (Brock 2011).

Breathing motion and daily changes of the liver position may be substantial. Motion management strategies include abdominal compression and breath-hold techniques. Imaging techniques for motion assessment include repeat 3-dimensional imaging between two extreme states of the breath cycle, or four-dimensional assessment of the respiratory cycle.

Daily localization of the liver lesion is critical to permit for dose escalation and sparing of the normal hepatic parenchyma. Various imaging modalities are utilized for treatment delivery, including two-dimensional images, ultrasound, kV and MV volumetric guidance, and IGRT. Image-guided radiotherapy (IGRT) may facilitate tumor dose escalation via reduction of PTV margins and improved precision of radiotherapy. The placement of fiducial markers is utilized to assist with IGRT, and is associated with little toxicity (Kothary and Heit et al. 2009).

5 Toxicity

Prior to the development of conformal radiotherapy, the utilization of radiotherapy in the management of metastatic and primary liver lesions was limited by toxicity. Toxicity to the liver is dependent upon the volume of liver irradiated, radiation dose, functional reserve of the liver, and other medical comorbidities.

The two most challenging complications after hepatic irradiation are radiation-induced liver disease and chest wall toxicities. These will be the topic of further discussion.

5.1 Radiation-Induced Liver Disease

Radiation-induced veno-occlusive liver disease (RILD) was historically the dose-limiting complication, which was pathologically described by Reed (1966). These pathologic findings are responsible for both "classic" and "nonclassic" RILD. In "classic" RILD, which typically occurs within 4 months after completion of radiotherapy, patients present with fatigue, weight gain, increased abdominal girth, hepatomegaly, anicteric ascites, and an isolated elevation in alkaline phosphatase without accompanying transaminitis (Lawrence and Robertson et al. 1995). In contrast, "non-classic" RILD is usually experienced by patients with underlying cirrhosis. This clinical scenario is characterized by jaundice and/or significant transaminitis within 3 months post completion of hepatic radiotherapy (Cheng and Wu et al. 2002; Liang and Zhu et al. 2006; Xu and Liang et al. 2006).

In 1965, Ingold first described the relationship between total liver dose and RILD (Ingold and Kaplan et al. 1965). RILD occurred in 1 out of 8 patients who received a total liver dose of 30–35 Gy, as compared with 12 of 27 who received doses in excess of 36 Gy. This observation was confirmed in RTOG 84-05, which was a phase I-II study which escalated the whole-liver dose from 27 Gy to 33 Gy in 1.5-Gy fractions with twice-daily scheduling (Russell and Wasserman et al. 1993). No patients experienced RILD at a total dose of 30 Gy, as compared with 10 % of patients who received 33 Gy. In the Emami paper, the probability of a

Table 7 Quantitative Assessment of Normal Tissue Effects in the Clinic (QUANTEC) recommendations for dose constraints for external beam radiotherapy to the liver

	Liver metastases	Primary liver cancer	Descriptor
Whole-liver RT	≤30 Gy, 2 Gy/fx	≤28 Gy, 2 Gy/fx	Whole-organ prescription dose
	21 Gy/7 fx	21 Gy/7 fx	
Partial liver RT, conventional fractionation	<32 Gy	<28 Gy	Mean normal liver dose for tumor dose ≤2 Gy/fraction
SBRT, 3–6 fractions	<15 Gy/3 fx	<13 Gy/3 fx	Mean normal liver dose
	<20 Gy/6 fx	<18 Gy/6 fx	
		CPB < 6 Gy, in 4–6 Gy/fx	
SBRT, 3–5 fractions	≥700 mL of normal liver receives ≤15 Gy		Critical volume model

Abbreviations: *CPB* Child-Pugh Class B; *fx* fractions; *RT* radiotherapy; *SBRT* stereotactic body radiotherapy

5 % complication within 5 years from treatment (TD5/5) for the whole liver was defined as 30 Gy in 2-Gy fractions (Emami and Brown et al. 1991).

The liver is an organ organized in radiobiologically parallel architecture, with numerous, repetitive functional subunits. A significant portion of the liver can be ablated without resultant hepatic dysfunction, if a portion of the normal liver is spared from a mean dose. Furthermore, the organ is capable of regeneration, which may provide long-term recovery from radiotherapy. This notion is supported by surgical series, which have demonstrated that as much as 80 % of the noncirrhotic liver can be removed without triggering liver failure (Penna 2002; Shah and Coates et al. 2007).

Studies investigating the use of SBRT for hepatic metastases have reported low rates of RILD, presumably because this cohort of patients are without underlying hepatic dysfunction. The University of Colorado prospective phase I/II trial demonstrated the safety of escalating doses for hepatic metastases to 60 Gy in 3 fractions (Schefter and Kavanagh et al. 2005; Rusthoven and Kavanagh et al. 2009). In this study, a "critical volume" model mandated that at least 700 mL of normal liver receive <15 Gy of total dose. Support for these constraints were extrapolated from the surgical literature where, as previously noted, as much as 80 % of normal liver could be resected without precipitating liver failure (Penna 2002; Shah and Coates et al. 2007). Assuming an average liver size of 2,000 mL, the deliberate sparing of 700 mL would ensure at least 35 % uncompromised liver volume. In this series, no grade 3 or higher hepatotoxicity was noted. No prospective dose-escalation trials have reached maximum tolerated doses (MTD) (Herfarth and Debus et al. 2001; Rusthoven and Kavanagh et al. 2009; Goodman and Wiegner et al. 2010; Rule and Timmerman et al. 2011) and reports have consistently demonstrated that patients with adequate baseline liver function can tolerate SBRT with minimal hepatotoxicity.

In contrast, investigators the Princess Margaret Hospital utilized a conceptually different approach to normal liver constraints for SBRT to hepatic metastases. The Lyman normal tissue complication probability model dictated the 6-fraction SBRT total dose. In this way, individualized radiation doses were designated to maintain the nominal risk of RILD for three estimated risk levels (5, 10, and 20 %). The median SBRT dose was 41.8 Gy in 6 fractions. Two patients experienced grade 3 transaminitis. No RILD was observed, suggesting that the Lyman normal tissue complication probability model likely overestimates the risk of hepatic injury. One patient experienced a grade 4 duodenal bleed and grade 5 malignant small bowel obstruction. This patient received maximum doses to 5 cc of the stomach and duodenum of 31.1 Gy and 33.1 Gy, respectively.

In contrast to patients with hepatic metastases, patients with hepatocellular carcinoma typically have compromised underlying liver function. Therefore, dose constraints for both conventionally fractionated treatment and SBRT must account for post-treatment liver reserve. In the study of SBRT for hepatocellular carcinoma reported by Son et al., 36 patients were treated with SBRT for unresectable hepatocellular carcinoma to doses of 30–39 Gy in 3 fractions (Son and Choi et al. 2010). Grade 2 or higher hepatic toxicity was noted in 33 % of patients, and 11 % of patients developed progression of Child-Pugh class. On multivariate analysis, the only parameter associated with the progression of Child-Pugh class was the total liver volume receiving a dose <18 Gy. The investigators proposed that the total liver volume receiving <18 Gy should be >800 cc to reduce the risk of hepatic function deterioration.

The Quantitative Assessment of Normal Tissue Effects in the Clinic (QUANTEC) recommendations reflect the differential dose considerations for patients with liver metastases as opposed to primary liver cancer, and are summarized in Table 7.

Treatment of radiation-induced liver injury is largely supportive, as no pharmacologic therapies are currently approved for the treatment of RILD. Treatment typically involves diuresis for fluid retention, analgesics for discomfort, paracentesis for ascites, and correction of coagulopathy (Guha and Kavanagh 2011). Animal studies have suggested that glutathione or a combination of selenium and vitamin E may offer hepatic radioprotection (DeLeve 1998; Gençel and Naziroglu et al. 2010).

5.2 Chest Wall Toxicity

Chest wall pain and rib fracture are other reported toxicities of liver and lung SBRT. A commonly used metric for quantification of chest wall dose is the volume receiving >30 Gy (V30)(Dunlap and Cai et al. 2010; Bongers and Haasbeek et al. 2011; Creach and El Naqa et al. 2012). Creach et al. identified that a V30 threshold of 0.7 % and V40 threshold of 0.19 % correlate with a 15 % risk of chest wall pain (Creach and El Naqa et al. 2012). Woody et al. created a predictive model of chest wall pain using a modified equivalent uniform dose model created from four distinct SBRT fractionation schemes (Woody and Videtic et al. 2012).

References

Abdalla E (2009) Commentary: radiofrequency ablation for colorectal liver metastases: do not blame the biology when it is the technology. Am J Surg 197:737–739

Abrams R, Pajak T et al (1998) Survival results among patients with alpha-fetoprotein-positive, unresectable hepatocellular carcinoma: analysis of three sequential treatments of the RTOG and Johns Hopkins Oncology Center. Cancer J Sci Am 4:178–184

Adam R, Azoulay D et al (2003) Liver resection as a bridge to transplantation for hepatocellular carcinoma on cirrhosis: a reasonable strategy? Ann Surg 238:508–519

Alberts S, Horvath W et al (2005) Oxaliplatin, flurouracil, and leucovorin for patients with unresectable liver-only metastases from colorectal cancer: a North Central Cancer Treatment Group phase II study. J Clin Oncol 23:9243–9249

Aloia T, Vauthey J et al (2006) Solitary colorectal liver metastasis: resection determines outcome. Arch Surg 141:460–467

Beasley R, Hwang L et al (1981) Hepatocellular carcinoma and hepatitis B virus. A prospective study of 22 707 men in Taiwan. Lancet 2:1129–1133

Ben-Josef E, Normolle D et al (2005) Phase II trial of high-dose conformal radiation therapy with concurrent hepatic artery floxuridine for unresectable intrahepatic malignancies. J Clin Oncol 23:8739–8747

Bengmark S, Hafstrom L (1969) The natural history of primary and secondary tumors of the liver. I. The prognosis for patients with hepatic metastases from colonic and rectal carcinoma by laparatomy. Cancer 23:198–202

Benson A, Abrams T et al (2009) NCCN clinical practice guidelines in oncology: hepatobiliary cancers. J Natl Compr Canc Netw 7:350–391

Benvegnu L, Alberti A (1996) Risk factors and prevention of hepatocellular carcinoma in HCV infection. Dig Dis Sci 41:S49–S55

Blomgren H, Lax I et al (1995) Stereotactic high dose fraction radiation therapy of extracranial tumors using an accelerator. Acta Oncol 34:861–870

Bongers E, Haasbeek C et al (2011) Incidence and risk factors for chest wall toxicity after risk-adapted stereotactic radiotherapy for early-stage lung cancer. J Thorac Oncol 6:252–257

Borgelt B, Gelber R et al (1981) The palliation of hepatic metastases: results of the Radiation Therapy Oncology Group pilot study. J Radiat Oncol Biol Phys 7:587–591

Bosch F, Ribes J et al (2004) Primary liver cancer: Worldwide incidence and trends. Gastroenterology 127:S5–S16

Brock K (2011) Imaging and image-guided radiation therapy in liver cancer. Semin Radiat Oncol 21:247–255

Bruix J, Castells A et al (1996) Surgical resection of hepatocellular carcinoma in cirrhotic patients: prognostic value of preoperative portal pressure. Gastroenterology 111:1018–1022

Bruix J, Sherman M (2011) Management of hepatocellular carcinoma: an update. Hepatology 53:1020–1022

Bruix J, Sherman M (2005) Management of hepatocellular carcinoma. Hepatology 42:1208–1236

Cance W, Stewart A et al (2000) The National Cancer Data Base Report on treatment patterns for hepatocellular carcinomas: improved survival of surgically resected patients, 1985–1996. Cancer 88:912–920

Cardenes H, Price T et al (2010) Phase I feasibility trial of stereotactic body radiation therapy for primary hepatocellular carcinoma. Clin Transl Oncol 12:218–225

Cardenes, H., Lasley, F. et al. (2012). Stereotactic body radiotherapy (SBRT) in patients with hepatocellular carcinoma with Child-Pugh class B. J Clin Oncol 30(suppl; abstr) e14683

Chang D, Swaminath A et al (2011) Stereotactic body radiotherapy for colorectal liver metastases. Cancer 117:4060–4069

Chen C, Yu M et al (1997) Epidemiological characteristics and risk factors of hepatocellular carcinoma. J Gastroenterol Hepatol 12:S294–S308

Chen M, Li J et al (2006) A prospective randomized trial comparing percutaneous local ablative therapy and partial hepatectomy for small hepatocellular carcinoma. Ann Surg 243:321–328

Cheng A, Kang Y et al (2009) Efficacy and safety of sorafenib in patients in the Asia-Pacific region with advanced hepatocellular carcinoma: A phase III randomized, double-blind, placebo-controlled trial. Lancet Oncol 10:25–34

Cheng J, Wu J et al (2002) Radiation-induced liver disease after three-dimensional conformal radiotherapy for patients with hepatocellular carcinoma: dosimetric analysis and implication. Int J Radiat Oncol Biol Phys 54:156–162

Cirocchi, R., Trastulli, S. et al. (2012). Radiofrequency ablation in the treatment of liver metastases from colorectal cancer. Cochrane Datab Syst Rev 6 CD006317

Creach K, El Naqa I et al (2012) Dosimetric predictors of chest wall pain after lung stereotactic body radiotherapy. Radiother Oncol 104:23–27

Daowood O, Mahadevan A et al (2009) Stereotactic body radiation therapy for liver metastases. Eur J Cancer 45:2947–2959

Dawson L, McGinn C et al (2000) Escalated focal liver radiation and concurrent hepatic artery fluorodeoxyuridine for unresectable intrahepatic malignancies. J Clin Oncol 18:2210–2218

Dawson L, Normolle D et al (2002) Analysis of radiation-induced liver disease using the Lyman NTCP model. Int J Radiat Oncol Biol Phys 53:810–821 de Jong M, Pulitano C et al (2009) Rates and patterns of recurrence following curative intent surgery for colorectal liver metastasis: an international multi-institutional analysis of 1669 patients. Ann Surg 250:440–448

DeLeve L (1998) Glutathione defense in non-parenchymal cells. Semin Liver Dis 18:403–413

Dunlap N, Cai J et al (2010) Chest wall volume receiving >=30 Gy predicts risk of severe pain and/or rib fracture after lung stereotactic body radiotherapy. Int J Radiat Oncol Biol Phys 76:796–801

El-Seraq H (2004) Hepatocellular carcinoma: recent trends in the United States. Gastroenterology 127:S27–S34

Emami B, Brown L et al (1991) Tolerance of normal tissue to therapeutic irradiation. Int J Radiat Oncol Biol Phys 21:109–122

Ettinger D, Bepler A (2010) Non-small cell lung cancer. J Natl Compr Canc Netw 8:740–801

Fattovich G, Stroffolini T et al (2004) Hepatocellular carcinoma in cirrhosis: incidence and risk factors. Gastroenterology 127:S35–S50

Fong Y, Fortner J et al (1999) Clinical score for predicting recurrence after hepatic resection for metastatic colorectal cancer: analysis of 1001 consecutive cases. Ann Surg 230:309–318

Foster J (1984) Treatment of metastatic disease of the liver: a skeptic's view. Semin Liver Dis 4:170–179

Gençel O, Naziroglu M et al (2010) Selenium and vitamin E modulates radiation-induced liver toxicity in pregnant and non-pregnant rat: effects of colemanite and hematite shielding. Biol Trace Element Res 135:253–263

Gleisner A, Choti M et al (2008) Colorectal liver metastases: recurrence and survival following hepatic resection, radiofrequency ablation, and combined resection-frequency ablation. Arch Surg 143:1204–1212

Goodman K, Wiegner E et al (2010) Dose-escalation study of single-fraction stereotactic body radiotherapy for liver malignancies. Int J Radiat Oncol Biol Phys 78:486–493

Goyal K, Einstein D et al (2010) Cyberknife stereotactic body radiation therapy for nonresectable tumors of the liver: preliminary results. HPB Surg 309780

Guha C, Kavanagh B (2011) Hepatic radiation toxicity: avoidance and amelioration. Semin Radiat Oncol 21:256–263

Hassan M, Hwang LY et al (2002) Risk factors for hepatocellular carcinoma: synergism of alcohol with viral hepatitis and diabetes mellitus. Hepatology 36:1206–1213

Heckman J, Devera M et al (2008) Bridging locoregional therapy for hepatocellular carcinoma prior to liver transplantation. Ann Surg Oncol 15:3169–3177

Heintges T, Wands J (1997) Hepatitis C virus: epidemiology and transmission. Hepatology 26:521–526

Hendlisz A, van den Eynde M et al (2010) Phase III trial comparing protracted intravenous fluorouracil infusion alone or with yttrium-90 resin microspheres radioembolization for liver-limited metastatic colorectal cancer refractory to standard chemotherapy. J Clin Oncol 28:3687–3694

Hepatocellulaire GdEedTdC (1995) A comparison of lipiodol chemoemboliation and conservation treatment for unresectable hepatocellular carcinoma. N Engl J Med 332:1256–1261

Herfarth K, Debus J et al (2001) Stereotactic single-dose radiation therapy of liver tumors: results of a phase I/II trial. J Clin Oncol 19:164–170

Herfarth K, Hof H et al (2003) Assessment of focal liver reaction by multiphasic CT after stereotactic single-dose radiotherapy of liver tumors. Int J Radiat Oncol Biol Phys 57:444–451

Hoyer M, Roed H et al (2006) Phase II study on stereotactic body radiotherapy of colorectal metastases. Acta Oncol 45:823–830

Huang J, Yan L et al (2010) A randomized trial comparing radiofrequency ablation and surgical resection for HCC conforming to the Milan criteria. Ann Surg 252:903–912

Hur H, Ko Y et al (2009) Comparative study of resection and radiofrequency ablation in the treatment of solitary colorectal liver metastases. Am J Surg 197:728–736

Ingold J, Kaplan R et al (1965) Radiation hepatitis. AJR Am J Roentgenol 93:200–208

Jemal A, Siegel R et al (2010) Cancer statistics. CA Cancer J Clin 60:277–300

Kanematsu M, Hoshi H et al (1999) Small hepatic nodules in cirrhosis: ultrasonographic, CT, and MR imaging findings. Abdom Imaging 24:47–55

Katz A, Chawla S et al (2012) Stereotactic hypofractionated radiation therapy as a bridge to transplantation for hepatocellular carcinoma: clinical outcome and pathologic correlation. Int J Radiat Oncol Biol Phys 83:895–900

Kemeny N (2006) Management of liver metastases from colorectal cancer. Oncology 20:1161–1176

Kim T, Kim D et al (2006) Three-dimensional conformal radiotherapy of unresectable hepatocellular carcinoma patients for whom transcatheter arterial chemoembolization was ineffective or unsuitable. Am J Clin Oncol 29:568–575

Kothary N, Heit J et al (2009) Safety and efficacy of percutaneous fiducial marker implantation for image-guided radiation therapy. J Vasc Intervent Radiol 20:235–239

Kulik L, van Holsbeeck A et al (2006) Yttrium-90 microspheres (TheraSphere) treatment of unresectable hepatocellular carcinoma: downstaging to resection, RFA and bridge to transplantation. J Surg Oncol 94:572–586

Kwon J, Bae S et al (2010) Long-term effect of stereotactic body radiation therapy for primary hepatocellular carcinoma ineligible for local ablation therapy or surgical resection. Stereotactic radiotherapy for liver cancer. BMC Cancer 10:475

Lawrence TS, Robertson JM et al (1995) Hepatic toxicity resulting from cancer treatment. Int J Radiat Oncol Biol Phys 31:1237–1248

Lax I, Blomgren D et al (1998) Extracranial stereotactic radiosurgery of localized targets. J Radiosurg 1:135–148

Lee M, Kim J et al (2009) Phase I study of individualized stereotactic body radiotherapy of liver metastases. J Clin Oncol 27:1585–1591

Liang SX, Zhu XD et al (2005) Hypofractionated three-dimensional conformal radiation therapy for primary liver carcinoma. Cancer 103:2181–2188

Liang SX, Zhu XD et al (2006) Radiation-induced liver disease in three-dimensional conformal radiation therapy for primary liver carcinoma: the risk factors and hepatic radiation tolerance. Int J Radiat Oncol Biol Phys 65:426–434

Liebel S, Massullo P et al (1987) A comparison of misonidazole sensitized radiation therapy to radiation therapy alone for the palliation of hepatic metastases: results of a Radiation Therapy Oncology Group randomized prospective trial. Int J Radiat Oncol Biol Phys 13:1057–1064

Liu MT, Li SH et al (2004) Three-dimensional conformal radiation therapy for unresectable hepatocellular carcinoma patients who had failed with or were unsuited for transcatheter arterial chemoembolization. Japan J Clin Oncol 34:532–539

Llovet JM, Bruix BA et al (2003) Hepatocellular carcinoma. Lancet 362:1907–1917

Llovet JM, Di Bisceglie AM et al (2008) Design and endpoints of clinical trials in hepatocellular carcinoma. J Natl Cancer Inst 100:698–711

Llovet J, Ricci S, Mazzaferro V et al (2007) Sharp investigators sorafenib improves survival in advanced hepatocellular carcinoma (hcc): results of a phase III randomized placebo-controlled tria! J Clin Oncol LBA1

Louis C, Dewas S et al (2010) Stereotactic radiotherapy of hepatocellular carcinoma: preliminary results. Technol Cancer Res Treat 9:479–487

Lu DS, Yu N, Raman S (2005) Percutaneous radiofrequency ablation of hepatocellular carcinoma as a bridge to liver transplantation. Hepatology 41:1130–1137

Mazzaferro V, Doci RE et al (1996) Liver transplantation for the treatment of small hepatocellular carcinomas in patients with cirrhosis. N Engl J Med 334:693–699

McGinn CJ, Ensminger T et al (1998) Treatment of intrahepatic cancers with radiation doses based on a normal tissue complication probability model. J Clin Oncol 16:2246–2252

Memon K, Lewandowski RJ et al (2011) Radioembolization for primary and metastatic liver cancer. Semin Radiat Oncol 21:294–302

Mendez-Romero A, Wunderink W et al (2006) Stereotactic body radiation therapy for primary and metastatic liver tumors: a single institution phase I-II study. Acta Oncol 45:831–837

Mohiuddin M, Ahmad CE et al (1996) Combined liver radiation and chemotherapy for palliation of hepatic metastases from colorectal cancer. J Clin Oncol 14:722–728

Mornex F, Girard N et al (2006) Feasibility and efficacy of high-dose three-dimensional-conformal radiotherapy in cirrhotic patients with small-size hepatocellular carcinoma non-eligible for curative therapies—mature results of the French Phase II RTF-1 trial. Int J Radiat Oncol Biol Phys 66:1152–1158

Muratore A, Bouzari ZD et al (2007) Asymptomatic colorectal cancer with un-resectable liver metastases: immediate colorectal resection or up-front systemic chemotherapy? Ann Surg Oncol 14:766–770

O'Connor JK, Davis TJ et al (2012) Long-term outcomes of stereotactic body radiation therapy in the treatment of hepatocellular cancer as a bridge to transplantation. Liver Transpl 18:949–954

Okuda K, Obata OT et al (1985) Natural history of hepatocellular carcinoma and prognosis in relation to treatment. Study of 850 patients. Cancer 56:918–928

Parkin DM, Ferlay BF et al (2001) Estimating the world cancer burder: GLOBOCAN 2000. Int J Cancer 94:153–156

Pawlik T, Scoggins C et al (2005) Effect of surgical margin status on survival and site of recurrence after hepatic resection for colorectal metastases. Ann Surg 241:715–724

Pelletier G, Ink RA et al (1990) A randomized trial of hepatic arterial chemoembolization in patients with unresectable hepatocellular carcinoma. J Hepatol 11:181–184

Penna C (2002) Colorectal metastasis (liver and lung). Surg Clin N Am 82:1075–1090

Poon R, Lau C et al (2007) High serum vascular endothelial growth factor levels predict poor prognosis after radiofrequency ablation of hepatocellular carcinoma: Importance of tumor biomarker in ablative therapies. Ann Surg Oncol 14:1835–1845

Prasad B, Hendrickson LM et al (1977) Irradiation of hepatic metastases. Int J Radiat Oncol Biol Phys 2:129–132

Reed GB (1966) The human liver after radiation injury. Am J Pathol 48:597–611

Reuter NP, Scoggins WC et al (2009) Radiofrequency ablation vs. resection for hepatic colorectal metastasis: therapeutically equivalent? J Gastrointest Surg 13:486–491

Ries L, Kosary EM et al (2004) SEER Cancer statistics review, 1975–2001. National Cancer Institute, Bethesda

Robertson JM, Walker LT et al (1995) The treatment of colorectal liver metastases with conformal radiation therapy and regional chemotherapy. Int J Radiat Oncol Biol Phys 32:445–450

Robertson JM, Walker M et al (1997) A phase I trial of hepatic arterial bromodeoxyuridine and conformal radiation therapy for patients with primary hepatobiliary cancers or colorectal liver metastases. Int J Radiat Oncol Biol Phys 39:1087–1092

Rule W, Timmerman R et al (2011) Phase I dose-escalation study of stereotactic body radiotherapy in patients with hepatic metastases. Ann Surg Oncol 18:1081–1087

Russell AH, Wasserman CC et al (1993) Accelerated hyperfractionated hepatic irradiation in the management of patients with liver metastases: results of the RTOG dose escalating protocol. Int J Radiat Oncol Biol Phys 27:117–123

Rusthoven K, Kavanagh B et al (2009) Multi-institutional phase I/II trial of stereotactic body radiation therapy for liver metastases. J Clin Oncol 27:1572–1578

Salem R, Lewandowski RJ et al (2011) Radioembolization results in longer time-to-progression and reduced toxicity compared with chemoembolization in patients with hepatocellular carcinoma. Gastroenterology 140:497–507

Schefter TE, Kavanagh BD et al (2005) A phase I trial of stereotactic body radiation therapy (SBRT) for liver metastases. Int J Radiat Oncol Biol Phys 62:1371–1378

Schefter TE, Kavanagh BD (2011) Radiation therapy for liver metastases. Semin Radiat Oncol 21:264–270

Seo Y, Kim M et al (2010) Preliminary result of stereotactic body radiotherapy as a local salvage treatment for inoperable hepatocellular carcinoma. J Surg Oncol 102:209–214

Seong J, Lee I et al (2009) A multicenter retrospective cohort study of practice patterns and clinical outcome on radiotherapy for hepatocellular carcinoma in Korea. Liver Int 29:147–152

Shah S, Coates BR et al (2007) Survival after liver resection for metastatic colorectal carcinoma in a large population. J Am Coll Surg 205:676–683

Shannon AM, Williams KJ (2008) Antiangiogenics and radiotherapy. J Pharm Pharmacol 60:1029–1036

Sherman DM, Order S (1978) Palliation of hepatic metastasis. Cancer 41:2013–2017

Simmonds P, Primrose J et al (2006) Surgical resection of hepatic metastases from colorectal cancer: a systematic review of published studies. Br J Cancer 20:982–999

Son SH, Choi BO et al (2010) Stereotactic body radiotherapy for patients with unresectable primary hepatocellular carcinoma: Dose-volumetric parameters predicting the hepatic complication. Int J Radiat Oncol Biol Phys 78:1073–1080

Spradling P, Rupp L et al (2012) Hepatitis B and C virus infection among 1.2 million persons with access to care: factors associated with testing and infection prevalence. Clin Infect Dis 55:1047–1055

Stenmark M, Liu E et al (2011) SBRT outcomes for primary and metastatic liver lesions. ASCO Gastrointestinal Cancers Symposium, San Francisco

Stillwagon GB, Guse OS et al (1989) 194 hepatocellular cancers treated by radiation and chemotherapy combinations: toxicity and response: a Radiation Therapy Oncology Group Study. Int J Radiat Oncol Biol Phys 17:1223–1229

Taniai N, Yoshida H et al (2006) Outcome of surgical treatment of synchronous liver metastases from colorectal cancer. J Nippon Med Sch 73:82–88

Timmerman R, Kavanagh B et al (2007) Stereotactic body radiation therapy in multiple organ sites. J Clin Oncol 25:947–952

Timmerman R, Galvin PR et al (2010) Stereotactic body radiation therapy for inoperable early stage lung cancer. JAMA 303:1070–1076

Timmerman R, Bizekis C et al (2009) Local surgical, ablative, and radiation treatment of metastases. CA: Cancer J Clinicians 59:145–170

Tomizawa N, Ohwada S et al (2006) Factors affecting prognosis of anatomical liver resection for liver metastases from colorectal cancer. Hepatogastroenterology 53:89–93

Tsai MS, Su YH et al (2007) Clinicopathological features and prognosis in resectable synchronous and metachronous colorectal liver metastasis. Ann Surg Oncol 14:786–794

Tse R, Hawkins M et al (2008) Phase I study of individualized stereotactic body radiotherapy for hepatocellular carcinoma and intrahepatic cholangiocarcinoma. J Clin Oncol 26:657–664

Van Cutsem E, Adam NB et al (2006) Towards a pan-Europen consensus on the treatment of patients with colorectal liver metastases. Eur J Cancer 42:2212–2221

Wang X, Zhang K et al (2008) Proton radiotherapy for liver tumors: dosimetric advantages over photon plans. Med Dosim 33:259–267

Wei AC, Grant GP et al (2006) Survival after hepatic resection for colorectal metastases: a 10-year experience. Ann Surg Oncol 13:668–676

Weichselbaum RR, Hellman S (2011) Oligometastases revisited. Nat Rev Clin Oncol 8:378–382

Wong S, Mangu P et al (2010) American Society of Clinical Oncology 2009 clinical evidence review on radiofrequency ablation of hepatic metastases from colorectal cancer. J Clin Oncol 28:493–508

Woody NM, Videtic GM et al (2012) Predicting chest wall pain from lung stereotactic body radiotherapy for different fractionation schemes. Int J Radiat Oncol Biol Phys 83:427–434

Xu ZY, Liang SX et al (2006) Prediction of radiation-induced liver disease by Lyman normal-tissue complication probability model in three-dimensional conformal radiation therapy for primary liver carcinoma. Int J Radiat Oncol Biol Phys 65:189–195

Zhang BH, Tang YB et al (2004) Randomized controlled trial of screening for hepatocellular carcinoma. J Cancer Res Clin Oncol 130:417–422

Rectal and Anal Cancer

Joanna Y. Chin, Nataliya Kovalchuk, and Lisa A. Kachnic

Contents

J. Y. Chin
Harvard Radiation Oncology Program, Boston, MA, USA

N. Kovalchuk
Department of Radiation Oncology, Boston Medical Center, Boston University School of Medicine, Boston, MA, USA

L. A. Kachnic (✉)
Department of Radiation Oncology, Boston Medical Center, Boston University School of Medicine, Moakley Building, LL, 830 Harrison Avenue, Boston, MA 02118, USA
e-mail: Lisa.kachnic@bmc.org

Abstract

Rectal adenocarcinoma and anal canal squamous cell cancer represent two distinct diseases that arise from the distal gastrointestinal tract and utilize radiation concurrent with chemotherapy as a component of care for localized presentations. While chemoradiation is administered preoperatively for rectal cancer, and as definitive treatment for anal cancer, localized management decisions and determination of prognosis are currently based on the assessment of clinical stage. For these cancers, the role of imaging to guide radiotherapy is critical and further investigation into the identification of biomarkers and other predictors for individualized patient care is warranted.

Abbreviations

CEA	Carcinoembryonic antigen
TME	Total mesorectal excision
APR	Abdominoperineal resection
5-FU	5-fluorouracil
FOLFOX	Folinic acid (leucovorin), Fluorouracil (5-FU), OXaliplatin (Eloxatin)
MMC	Mitomycin-C
pCR	Pathologic complete response
HR	Hazard ratio
EUS	Endoscopic ultrasound
MRI	Magnetic resonance imaging
CT	Computerized tomography
PET	Positron emission tomography
N+	Metastatic regional nodal disease
3D-CRT	Three-dimensional conformal radiation therapy

C. Nieder and L. E. Gaspar (eds.), *Decision Tools for Radiation Oncology*, Medical Radiology. Radiation Oncology,
DOI: 10.1007/174_2013_844, © Springer-Verlag Berlin Heidelberg 2013
Published Online: 12 June 2013

IMRT	Intensity modulated radiation therapy
NCI-CTC v3	National Cancer Institute Common Terminology Criteria for Adverse Events version 3.0
RTOG	Radiation Therapy Oncology Group
HPV	Human papilloma virus
HIV	Human immunodeficiency virus
HARRT	Highly active antiretroviral therapy
PTV	Planning tumor volume

1 Rectal Cancer Introduction

Colorectal cancer is the third most common new cancer diagnosis in the U.S., with an estimated 103,170 of new cases of colon cancer and 40,290 of rectal cancer in 2012 (Siegel et al. 2012). The median age of onset is 62, with a male predominance. Its incidence has decreased from 60.5 per 100,000 in 1976 to 46.4 in 2008, in large part due to screening, and mortality has decreased due to improvements in early detection and treatment. Although colorectal cancer mortality has been progressively declining since 1990 at a rate of about 3 percent per year, it still remains the second most common cause of cancer death in the U.S. (Siegel et al. 2012). While the majority of cases are sporadic, 10 % have an inherited predisposition, including hereditary non-polyposis colorectal cancer and familial adenomatous polyposis (Jasperson et al. 2010). Environmental risk factors for developing colorectal cancer include a diet rich in animal fat and low in fiber, smoking, alcohol, and prior radiation (Ahmed 2003).

Colon and rectal cancers have different patterns of failure after surgery and are therefore also managed differently. Clinically, a lesion from the dentate line to within 12–16 cm from the anal verge by proctoscopy is considered rectal cancer, although the precise anatomic division of the rectum and sigmoid colon is the peritoneal reflection. As the location of the rectum is deep within the pelvis, surgical access to rectal lesions, in contrast to colon cancers, is often limited by the anatomical boundaries of the pelvis. Local recurrence in rectal cancer, therefore, is more of a concern than in colon cancer, and adjuvant radiation-based treatment is often necessary to reduce this risk.

2 General Treatment Paradigm

Preoperative staging has an important role to play in guiding initial treatment decisions in rectal cancer. In addition to digital rectal examination, serum carcinoembryonic antigen (CEA), complete colonoscopy to rule out cancers elsewhere in the bowel, and full-body CT or PET/CT to rule out distant metastatic disease, the current treatment paradigm for localized rectal cancer requires a detailed imaging work-up for accurate clinical staging. Both endoscopic ultrasound (EUS) and pelvic MRI are currently employed and are used to determine the depth of invasion of the primary tumor, the distance of the tumor from the sphincter complex, the potential for achieving negative circumferential margins with total mesorectal excision (TME), any involvement of mesorectal or iliac lymph nodes, and any invasion of adjacent organs such as the prostate or vagina. EUS is extremely accurate for assessing invasion of tumors within the bowel wall, but less accurate for staging tumors beyond the wall, as it is not able to well visualize the mesorectal fascia. EUS is also of low value in obstructed rectums where the scope is not able to pass the tumor. High resolution MRI predicts the circumferential margin (positive or negative) with high accuracy and T2-weighted sequences are recommended. The accuracy of EUS ranges from 80 to 95 %, compared with 75–85 % for MRI and 65–75 % for CT in determining local staging of the primary tumor (Siddiqui et al. 2006). In a meta-analysis of 84 studies, all three imaging modalities were equivalent in staging nodal status (Lahaye et al. 2005).

Figures 1 and 2 summarize preoperative and postoperative decisions regarding the use of radiation. In clinical stage I patients (T1N0, T2N0), definitive local surgery with nodal dissection is appropriate. If pathology reveals pT3/T4 or N1-2 disease, then postoperative chemoradiation followed by adjuvant chemotherapy is recommended. In select clinical stage I patients, such as those with medical co-morbidities or other contraindications to a larger surgery, or tumors with very favorable pathology, local excision using a full thickness resection with negative margins may be utilized, followed by 50.4–54 Gy chemoradiation for pT1 tumors with poor histopathologic features and for all pT2 cancers (Schmoll et al. 2012). If pathology at local excision reveals pT3/4 disease, then 50.4 Gy chemoradiation, followed by consideration of TME, and then additional systemic therapy should be administered. Additionally, select patients with low-lying distal cT2 lesions may be considered for preoperative chemoradiation in attempts to convert an abdominoperineal resection (APR) to a sphincter sparing TME.

For clinical stage II–III rectal cancers (T3-T4N0 or N +) implying locally advanced disease, preoperative treatment is indicated. The German Rectal Cancer Study Group CAO/ARO/AIO-94 phase III trial compared preoperative long-course radiotherapy (50.4 Gy in 28 fractions) followed by TME, with TME followed by postoperative standard chemoradiation (54 Gy over 6 weeks with concurrent 5-FU). Patients in the preoperative radiation arm had a decreased risk of local recurrence at 10 years (7.1 vs. 10 %, $p = 0.048$), improved acute and late morbidity, enhanced

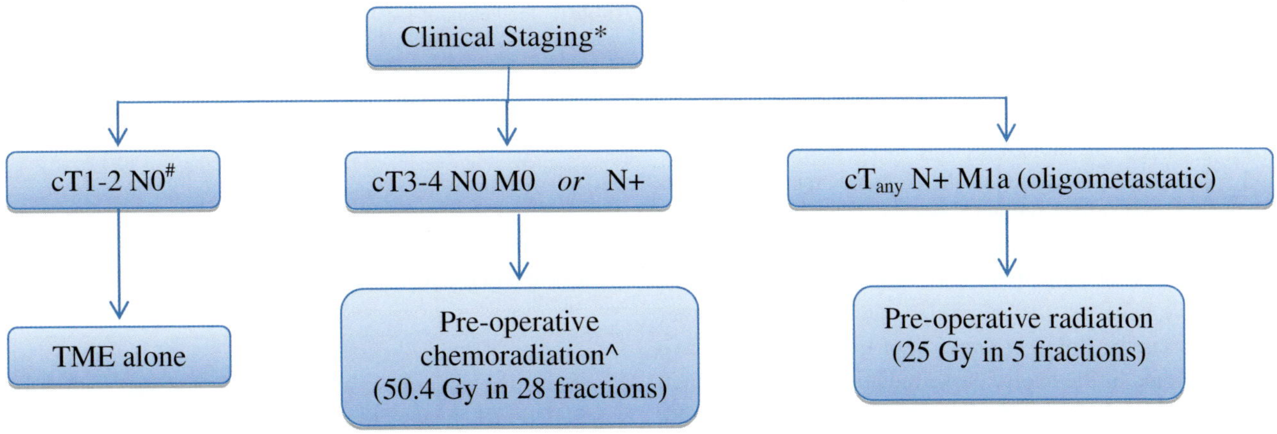

Fig. 1 Preoperative chemoradiation for rectal cancer: decisions based on clinical staging (* Local clinical staging based on exam, EUS and MRI; distant disease staging based on full body PET/CT or CT of chest, abdomen and pelvis. # Select patients with low-lying distal cT2 lesions may be considered for preoperative chemoradiation in attempts to convert an APR to a sphincter sparing TME ^ Chemotherapy concurrent with long-course radiation may be 5-FU or capecitabine). Of note, all clinical stage II and III patients receive additional postoperative chemotherapy

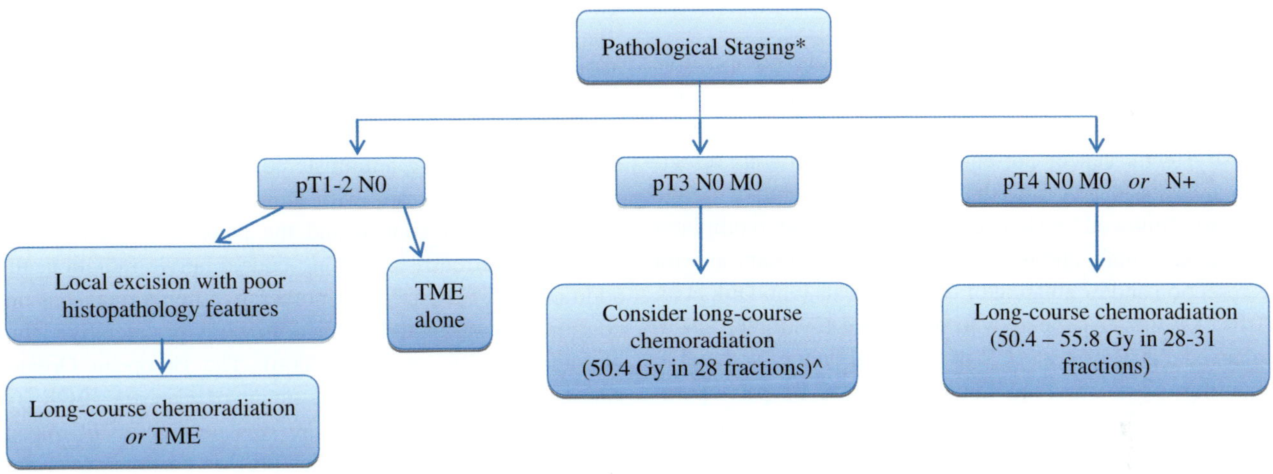

Fig. 2 Postoperative chemoradiation for rectal cancer: decisions based on pathologic staging (* No preoperative chemoradiation was administered ^ If high lesion with negative margins and good histopathology features, may consider omitting chemoradiation). Of note, may consider adjuvant chemoradiation for any margin positive status, and all stage II and III patients receive additional postoperative chemotherapy

tumor downstaging, and an increased rate of sphincter-preserving surgery for those declared upfront to have required an APR, relative to the postoperative chemoradiation arm (Sauer et al. 2004, 2012). There was, however, no difference in overall or disease-free survival between preoperative and postoperative chemoradiation. Of note, both arms received 4 cycles of chemotherapy outback, and the rate of distant failures was the same in both of these groups (29.8 and 29.6 % at 10 years, $p = 0.9$) (Sauer et al. 2012).

In the United States, preoperative treatment for stage II–III cancers is long-course chemoradiation to 50.4 Gy with concurrent 5-FU-based chemotherapy (continuous infusion 5-FU or oral capecitabine), rather than short-course radiation (5 Gy $\times$ 5 fractions) to 25 Gy, which is commonly used in Europe, because of the concern for heightened late effects with one week of hypofractionated radiation. These two preoperative regimens were compared head-to-head in the recently published Tasman Radiation Oncology Group (TROG) 01.04 trial; 326 patients with T3N0-2M0 ultrasound or MRI staged rectal cancer were randomized to receive either standard fractionated long-course chemoradiation followed by TME 4–8 weeks later or short-course radiation followed by TME one week later (Ngan et al. 2012). No statistical difference in rates of local or distant recurrence or overall survival was reported at a relatively short follow-up of 3 years. However, in a subset analysis of patients with distal (<5 cm from the anal verge) tumors, there was an observed difference in local recurrence rate favoring long-course preoperative chemoradiation (12.5 % in the short-course arm compared with 0 % in the long-course arm, $p = 0.21$). Pathologic downstaging was also significantly more common in the long-course preoperative arm (45 vs. 28 %), though the rate of APR was similar (79 and 77 %). An increased risk of local recurrence was associated with older patients, poorer ECOG performance status, positive lymph nodes, and increased CEA level. Notable, 56 % of patients in both arms had T3N0 disease, which may have led to the similar outcomes, and another criticism was the different duration of treatment in the two arms (patients in the short-course radiation arm go through approximately 1 week of preoperative treatment before surgery versus the 2–4 months before surgery in the long-course arm). It is unclear whether this difference in timing affected outcome, and this is anticipated to be one of the analyses performed for the ongoing Stockholm III three arm randomized trial comparing short-course radiation followed by TME one week later, with short-course radiation or long course–chemoradiation followed by TME 4–8 weeks later (Pettersson et al. 2010).

One clinical scenario potentially favoring preoperative short-course radiation is oligometastatic disease. In a phase II study by the Dutch Colorectal Group, 50 patients with primary rectal cancer presenting with synchronous resectable metastasis received short-course preoperative pelvic radiation followed by six cycles of capecitabine, oxaliplatin and bevacizumab, and then resection of the primary as well as resection and/or ablation of the metastasis (van Dijk et al. 2010). Of the 41 patients who proceeded to surgery, 44 % achieved a pCR or near-pCR of the rectal tumor. No notable toxicities were observed during radiation or peri-operatively, and no progression was noted during chemotherapy. Another phase II trial for patients with cT3-4, any N and any M rectal cancer examined preoperative short course radiation followed by 4 cycles of mFOLFOX6 chemotherapy prior to surgery (Myerson et al. 2012). Of the 44 evaluable cases, 33 had ypT0-2 residual disease. These two studies suggest that short-course preoperative radiation may be a reasonable strategy to achieve durable disease-free survival and local palliation in patients with low burden metastatic disease. Some institutions also consider neoadjuvant short-course radiation a valid alternative in patients with cT3N0 rectal cancer whose disease does not need downsizing (not threatened by a close circumferential margin; located in the upper and mid rectum) (Mohiuddin et al. 2008). Adjuvant chemotherapy decisions are then made based on pathological data.

In the U.S., concurrent adjuvant postoperative chemotherapy is administered for patients with clinical stage II or III cancer that received preoperative chemoradiation or for those that underwent upfront TME and had pathologic stage II or III disease receiving chemoradiation postoperatively. The efficacy of postoperative radiation therapy and 5-FU-based chemotherapy for stage II and III rectal cancer was established by a series of prospective, randomized clinical trials from the Gastrointestinal Tumor Study Group (GITSG-7175), the Mayo/North Central Cancer Treatment Group (NCCTG-794751), and the National Surgical Adjuvant Breast and Bowel Project (NSABP-R-01) (Thomas and Lindblad 1988; Krook et al. 1991; Wolmark et al. 1988). These studies demonstrated an increase in both disease-free and overall survival when postoperative chemoradiation and four additional cycles of adjuvant 5-FU were administered.

Table 1 Predictors of local recurrence in rectal cancer

Prognostic factor
Clinical
T stage
Node-positive
Pathologic
Circumferential margins <2 mm
Treatment response to preoperative chemoradiation

While chemotherapy with fluoropyramidines has shown to enhance local control and the pCR rate when administered concurrently with long course pelvic radiation, the addition of 5-FU based chemotherapy after surgery has not conferred a survival benefit following preoperative chemoradiation (Bosset et al. 2006). The European Organization for Research and Treatment of Cancers (EORTC) 22921 study showed that there was no significant impact on overall survival with either pre- or postoperative chemotherapy (HR for death in the preoperative chemoradiation group was 1.02 compared with the preoperative radiation group; and the 5-year overall survival rate was 63.2 % for patients that did not receive adjuvant chemotherapy as compared to 67.2 % for patients receiving 5-FU postoperatively). However, an unplanned subset analysis of patients who underwent complete resection with negative margins and had M0 disease at surgery showed that ypT0-2 patients appeared to experience a survival benefit from adjuvant 5-FU as compared with ypT3-4 patients; patients in whom no downstaging was achieved did not benefit (Collette et al. 2007). Despite these findings, many academic oncologists recommend that 5-FU and more recently FOLFOX be considered as adjuvant chemotherapy in rectal cancer. However, there are no data in preoperatively treated clinical stage II or III rectal cancer to support this consideration.

3 Prognostic Factors

The prognosis of patients with localized rectal cancer is associated with several factors including the depth of tumor penetration through the bowel wall, involvement of pelvic lymph nodes, positive circumferential (radial) margin, and response to preoperative chemoradiation. However, only disease stage and circumferential margin status has been validated in multi-institutional prospective studies (Table 1).

3.1 Disease Stage (Tumor and Nodal)

The American Joint Committee on Cancer (AJCC) staging system is universally recommended and describes the anatomical extension of rectal tumors (American Joint Committee on Cancer 2010), Table 2. Its prognostic value is based on data derived from the outcome of patients after complete surgical resection with or without combined modality therapy. Both tumor penetration of the bowel wall (the T stage) and lymph node involvement (the N stage) are associated with an increased risk of local recurrence, distant relapse and overall survival (Gunderson et al. 2002, 2004). In pooled analyses of 2551 patients from three phase III North American postoperative localized rectal cancer trials, both overall and disease-free survival were dependent on TN stage, and treatment method (Gunderson et al. 2002). Three patient risk groups were defined: intermediate- (T1-2N1, T3N0), moderately high- (T1-2N2, T3N1, T4N0), and high- (T3N2, T4N1, T4N2) risk. Patients with a single high-risk factor (T1-2N1, T3N0) had better overall survival, disease-free survival, and local disease control than patients with both high-risk factors; surgery and chemotherapy (without radiation) for these patients resulted in a 5-year overall survival rate of approximately 85 %.

The Intergroup 0114 adjuvant trial for rectal cancer, comparing the addition of leucovorin and/or levamisole to 5-FU chemotherapy, demonstrated that even in the TME era, adjuvant therapy was beneficial in patients with resectable T3-4 or N1-3 disease, with no distant metastases (Tepper et al. 2002). Within this locally advanced group of patients, those with T4 or T3N+ disease had significantly lower overall survival (55 % at 5 years) and disease-free survival (44 %), compared to patients with T1-2N+ or T3N0 disease who had a 5-year overall survival of 76 % (RR 2.1, $p < 0.0001$) and disease-free survival of 67 % (RR 2.0, $p < 0.0001$). Local recurrence also varied by stage: the higher risk group of T4 or T3N+ disease had double the local failure rate at 5 years than did the T1-2N+ or T3N0 patients (18 vs. 9 %, respectively, $p < 0.0001$). Interestingly, this prospective study also found that males had a worse overall survival than females (RR 1.2, $p = 0.03$), though disease-free survival or local recurrence was not significantly different by gender. There was no interaction between gender and stage, although it was found that females experienced more toxicity than males (81 % females reported grade 3–5 toxicity compared with 69 % of males).

Table 2 AJCC TNM classification of rectal cancer (clinical or pathological)

Stage	Description
Primary tumor (T)[a]	
TX	Primary tumor cannot be assessed
T0	No evidence of primary tumor
Tis	Carcinoma *in situ*, intraepithelial or invasion of the lamina propria
T1	Tumor invades submucosa
T2	Tumor invades muscularis propria
T3	Tumor invades through the muscularis propria into perirectal tissue
T4a	Tumor penetrates to the surface of the visceral peritoneum
T4b	Tumor directly invades or is adherent to other organs or structures
Regional lymph nodes (N)[b]	
NX	Regional lymph nodes cannot be assessed
N0	No regional lymph node metastasis
N1a	Metastasis in 1 node
N1b	Metastasis in 2–3 regional nodes
N1c	Tumor deposits in the subserosa, mesentery, or nonperitonealized perirectal tissues without regional nodal metastasis
N2a	Metastasis in 4–6 regional nodes
N2b	Metastasis in 7 or more regional nodes
Distant metastasis (M)	
MX	Distant metastasis cannot be assessed
M0	No distant metastasis
M1a	Metastasis confined to one organ site (liver, lung, ovary, nonregional lymph node)
M1b	Metastases in more than one organ/site or the peritoneum

[a] The use of "m" denotes multiple primaries; "r" denotes recurrent disease; "y" if tumor is staged after neoadjuvant chemoradiation (and not at initial presentation); "L0" or "L1" denotes with or without lymphatic vessel invasion, respectively; "V0," "V1," or "V2" denotes no, microscopic, or macroscopic venous invasion, respectively
[b] Regional nodes include perirectal, presacral, lateral sacral, inferior mesenteric, internal iliac, sacral promontory, superior rectal, middle rectal, and inferior rectal; at least 10–14 nodes should be studied for accurate pN staging in patients who have not undergone neoadjuvant therapy

3.2 Surgical Margins

Another important prognostic factor is the circumferential or radial surgical margin status. The circumferential margin is a surgically created plane of dissection produced during the removal of the mesorectum and rectum from its surroundings during a TME. Retrospective studies have confirmed a strong association between the presence of microscopic tumor cells within 1 mm of the circumferential margin and increased risks of both local recurrence and disease-free survival, even with meticulous TME surgery (Wibe et al. 2002). Macroscopic or microscopic margin radial positivity was recently shown to be a significant risk factor for local recurrence, resulting in a hazard ratio of 6.46 ($p < 0.001$) in the randomized TROG study previously described (Ngan et al. 2012).

3.3 Tumor Downstaging Following Preoperative Chemoradiation

The degree of tumor regression following preoperative chemoradiation has also been demonstrated to be prognostic for outcome. In the experience of the German Rectal Cancer Study Group, using a histology grading system that analyzes cytologic alterations in response to neoadjuvant treatment, patients whose tumors have no evidence of viable tumor cells in the rectal wall (tumor regression grade 4) had improved disease-free survival (86 % at 5 years) and metastases-free survival, compared with patients whose tumors showed no regressive changes post-treatment (Rödel et al. 2005). Patients with tumors showing intermediate tumor regression yielded an intermediate prognosis (disease-free survival 75 % at 5 years), and poor tumor regression predicted for an unfavorable outcome (disease-free survival 63 % at 5 years). As all stage II and III rectal cancers are recommended to receive adjuvant chemotherapy following resection, tumor downstaging is currently not used to determine chemotherapy-based management decisions.

3.4 Molecular Markers

Preoperative chemoradiation for localized rectal cancer also provides investigators with the opportunity to identify predictive and prognostic markers for treatment response. This may lead to the potential for individualizing treatment regimens. Although there are many biomarkers that have been evaluated in this regard, none have been validated for clinical use. This is an area that warrants continued research. In terms of response to systemic therapy, some molecular markers that are known to confer a poorer prognosis include microsatellite instability, 18q loss of homozygosity, epidermal growth factor overexpression, KRAS mutations, and the BRAF V600E mutation (Tol et al. 2009; Di Nicolantonio et al. 2008; Fallik et al. 2003; Des Guetz et al. 2009; Khambata-Ford et al. 2007).

4 Investigations into Selective Treatment

4.1 Omission of Pelvic Radiation

While several clinical trials have established that trimodality therapy (surgery with chemoradiation) improves local recurrence rates over surgery alone, there is ongoing investigation to identify patients who are at low-risk for pelvic recurrence, in whom preoperative radiation may be omitted. In a retrospective review of patients with pathologic stage T3N0 rectal cancer who underwent resection without pelvic radiation or chemotherapy, patients with favorable histologic features (well- or moderately well-differentiated carcinomas invading <2 mm into perirectal fat, without lymphatic or venous vessel involvement) experienced a local control and recurrence-free survival advantage (95 and 87 %, respectively), relative to patients whose tumors exhibited deep perirectal fat invasion, vessel involvement, or poor differentiation (71 and 55 %, respectively) (Willett et al. 1999).

In Europe, rectal MRI findings (the extramural extent of the tumor, the relation of the tumor to the mesorectal fascia, and the presence of suspicious lymph nodes) have been used to stratify patients into low-, intermediate-, and high-risk groups for preoperative radiation management decisions. Patients with MRI determined low-risk disease are treated with surgery alone, while those with intermediate-risk rectal tumors receive short course radiotherapy, and patients with high-risk tumors are administered long course preoperative chemoradiation (Smith and Brown 2008).

Perhaps pelvic radiation may be omitted in patients who have a good response to induction chemotherapy. A Phase II study at Memorial Sloan Kettering Cancer Center assessed 6 cycles of preoperative FOLFOX with bevacizumab in 30 patients with stage II-T3N0-any rectal cancer (Schrag et al. 2010). At preoperative restaging with sigmoidoscopy and EUS, all patients were deemed to have a complete response and underwent TME without pelvic radiation. An R0 resection (complete resection with negative margins) was performed in all patients, and the pCR rate was 27 %. Follow-up thus far is limited; so information on pelvic control and survival are not yet available. However, based on this encouraging pilot data, the PROSPECT trial, a large U.S. phase II/III randomized trial, is actively accruing patients to determine whether those with locally advanced rectal cancer undergoing low anterior resection with TME may be treated with preoperative chemotherapy and selective, rather than routine, use of pelvic radiotherapy prior to resection. Pelvic radiation will be omitted in those patients having a good response to FOLFOX therapy as determined by imaging studies (N1048, Schrag 2012).

4.2 Wait-and-See Approach for Surgery

Preoperative chemoradiation may lead to pCR in approximately 20 % of patients. As such, the option of nonoperative therapy is being evaluated in patients who have a clinical complete response to neoadjuvant therapy. The feasibility of this approach was initially reported by investigators from Brazil, who observed 99 patients with a clinical complete response to preoperative chemoradiation without radical resection (Habr-Gama et al. 2006). The local recurrence rate was remarkably low (5 %), and all recurrences have been salvaged. This "wait-and-see" policy has also been studied prospectively by a group from the Netherlands in 21 patients who achieved clinical complete response following standard chemoradiation for T4 or T3N1-2 rectal cancer, based on MRI, endoscopy, digital rectal exam, and biopsies (Maas et al. 2011). Patients with node-positive disease at initial staging (16 of the 21 patients) had adjuvant chemotherapy (capecitabine and oxaliplatin). With a median follow-up of 15 months, only one patient in the wait-and-see group developed a local recurrence at 22 months of follow-up that was successfully salvaged. All other 20 of the patients were alive and disease-free, with better bowel function than a control group of patients who had pathologic complete response at surgery. Overall survival and disease-free survival were comparable in the wait-and-see and control groups, suggesting that surgery may be avoided in a very carefully selected group of patients following chemoradiation.

5 Toxicity

5.1 Acute and Late Morbidity from Long-Course Chemoradiation

Pelvic chemoradiation can be associated with both acute and long-term toxicities due to the radiosensitivity of the surrounding normal structures including bowel, bladder, genitalia and bone. The German Rectal Cancer Study demonstrated that both physician-reported acute and late toxicity was improved with a preoperative chemoradiation approach (Sauer et al. 2004). Grade 3 or 4 acute toxic effects occurred in 27 % of the patients in the preoperative treatment group, as compared with 40 % of the patients in the postoperative treatment group ($p = 0.001$); the corresponding rates of long-term toxic effects were 14 and 24 %, respectively ($p = 0.01$). They have not yet determined any predictors for radiation-related morbidity.

The most common toxicity of pelvic chemoradiation is gastrointestinal. Acute symptoms resulting from adverse effects of the gastrointestinal tract include gas, diarrhea, rectal emptying problems, frequent bowel movements and incontinence, with late effects of obstruction due to stenosis or adhesions and more rarely malabsorption, necrosis, perforation, and fistulation (Coia et al. 1995; Sauer et al. 2004). Physician-reported grade 3 and higher diarrhea was demonstrated in 36 % of patients in the preoperative chemoradiation arm of the NSABP R-03 trial, while Bosset and colleagues reported $\geq$ grade 2 diarrhea in 38 % of patients treated with preoperative 5-FU and pelvic radiation (Roh et al. 2009; Bosset et al. 2006). The incidence of small bowel obstruction requiring surgery following adjuvant pelvic radiation for rectal cancer is 4–15 % in historical series (Collette et al. 2007), with a risk of late anastomotic strictures of 4–12 % (Sauer et al. 2004). Investigations have attempted to determine predictors of physician-reported small bowel toxicity. The primary predictor is increasing radiation dose. Dose-volume relationships between the amount of small bowel receiving low- and intermediate-doses of radiation and the rates of severe diarrhea have been demonstrated, but not validated in prospective multi-institutional studies (Tho et al. 2006; Baglan et al. 2002).

Interestingly, it has also been demonstrated that gastrointestinal toxicity rates may be interpreted differently by patients. Seventy-seven consecutive patients receiving preoperative chemoradiation at Harvard radiation oncology departments completed a 7-item Bowel Problems Scale immediately before weekly physician visits (Chen et al. 2010). By week 5 of long-course chemoradiation, approximately 40 % of all patients developed clinically meaningful pain, bowel urgency, or tenesmus that was not present during week 1; 30 % developed diarrhea, abdominal cramping, and passing mucus. Within each physician-assessed grade of diarrhea, patient experience varied widely. The same group also evaluated dose-volume predictors of gastrointestinal toxicity from the patient's perspective in this patient cohort (Chen et al. 2012). The amount of small bowel receiving at least 15 Gy was significantly associated with acute symptoms ($p = 0.01$). These studies highlight the importance of including patient-reported morbidity and associated dose-volume predictors in prospective trials.

Urogenital dysfunction after chemoradiation for rectal cancer is also common, but to a much lesser degree than gastrointestinal toxicity. Acute morbidity may include incontinence, retention, dysuria, frequency and urgency. Late urinary tract symptoms have been reported in 2–4 % of all patients in the German study (Sauer et al. 2004).

Pelvic radiation for rectal cancer may also lead to increased sexual dysfunction, although rates of this toxicity are not well defined. In males, a long-term deterioration of ejaculatory and erectile function is due to late radiation damage to the seminal vesicles and small vessels, respectively. In females, radiation leads to vaginal dryness as well as varying degrees of vaginal fibrosis, with a resultant diminished sexual satisfaction (Marijnen et al. 2005). Dose-volume predictors for sexual dysfunction have not been reported. In females, vaginal dilators following completion of pelvic radiation are often recommended, although their efficacy has not been confirmed in randomized trial data.

Additionally, femoral head and pelvic fractures are a late complication of pelvic radiation that appears to be significantly increased in irradiated patients (Bruheim et al. 2010). In the Norwegian study by Bruheim et al. the incidence of pelvic fracture was five times higher in the irradiated patients (5 vs. 1 %) and suggested to be dose-related (Bruheim et al. 2010). However, female sex appears to be the only independent predictor for fracture likely due to age and hormone-related bone loss (Baxter et al. 2005).

5.2 Role of Conformal Radiotherapy

While there is an advantage of neoadjuvant chemoradiation followed by TME over postoperative adjuvant therapy in terms of tolerability and local control, acute gastrointestinal toxicity remains a limiting factor (Sauer et al. 2004). For example, 36 % of patients in the preoperative arm of the NSABP R-03 trial experienced $\geq$ grade 3 diarrhea, while Bosset et al. reported $\geq$ grade 2 diarrhea in 38 % of patients treated with preoperative 5-fluorouracil and pelvic radiation (Roh et al. 2009; Bosset et al. 2006).

These rates of acute gastrointestinal toxicity are due, in part, to the large amount of normal small bowel that is in the standard pelvic radiation field. Dose-volume relationships between the amount of small bowel receiving low- and intermediate-doses of radiation and the rates of severe diarrhea have been demonstrated (Tho et al. 2006; Baglan et al. 2002). Finding strategies to reduce acute gastrointestinal toxicity may potentially lead to unplanned chemoradiation treatment breaks, which has been shown to confer untoward local control and survival outcomes (Fietkau et al. 2007).

One technique to reduce the volume of irradiated small bowel is the use of prone positioning with a bowel displacement device (belly-board) (Gunderson et al. 1985). More recently, there has been investigation in the use of highly conformal treatment approaches, such as intensity modulated radiation therapy (IMRT). Compared to conventional two- or three-dimensional conformal radiation therapy (3D-CRT) planning methods, IMRT allows discriminatory dose escalation to the target volume while minimizing radiation exposure to adjacent normal tissues. Improvements in treatment-related morbidity have been described in patients treated with IMRT for other pelvic malignancies including anal, gynecologic and prostate (Kachnic et al. 2012a, b, c; Ashman et al. 2005; Mundt et al. 2002).

To this end, we performed a retrospective analysis of 48 consecutive patients treated with preoperative chemoradiation for rectal cancer to a planned dose of 45–50 Gy using 3D-CRT or IMRT while prone on a bowel displacement device (Parekh et al. 2010). There was a significant reduction in grade $\geq$2 gastrointestinal toxicity (NCI-CTC v3) between IMRT (30 %) and 3D-CRT (60.7 %), ($p = 0.036$), and grade $\geq$2 diarrhea: IMRT (10 %) and 3D-CRT (42.8 %), ($p = 0.014$). Radiation duration was significantly less with IMRT, 35 versus 39 days using 3D-CRT, ($p = <0.0001$). While pCR rates were 16.7 % for 3D-CRT and 21.4 % for IMRT, when also including patients with only microscopic residual disease, pCR plus microscopic rates were 57.1 % for IMRT and 27.8 % for 3D-CRT, ($p = 0.093$). These results are consistent with the published observations from the Mayo Clinic, which showed a similar reduction in grade 2+ gastrointestinal toxicity with the use of IMRT (Samuelian et al. 2011).

The Radiation Therapy Oncology Group (RTOG) recently completed the phase II 0822 trial examining the role of preoperative IMRT in combination with capecitabine and oxaliplatin. Preliminary results presented only in abstract form have suggested a small, but insignificant benefit in GI toxicity with IMRT as compared to patients treated with 3D-CRT on the RTOG 0247 trial (Garofalo et al. 2011). Although these data require further analysis, they may be due to the lack of maximal bowel displacement and heterogeneous method of contouring small bowel. Despite these early results, the optimization and further analysis of this IMRT approach in the combined modality management of locally advanced rectal cancer is warranted.

6 Anal Cancer Introduction

Anal squamous cell cancer is a rare malignancy and accounts for only 4 % of all cancers of the lower gastrointestinal tract. The estimated new cases from anal cancer in the United States in 2013 are 7,060 resulting in approximately 880 deaths (American Cancer Society 2013 Facts and Figures). In the last decade, the incidence of anal cancer is increasing due to the association with human papilloma virus (HPV) infection (Johnson et al. 2004). The incidence of anal cancer is also higher in those who are Human Immunodeficiency Virus (HIV) positive due to immunosuppression, and in transplant recipients (Johnson et al.

2004). In contrast to other gastrointestinal tract malignancies, anal cancers are highly sensitive to chemoradiation alone. Preservation of anorectal function occurs in the majority of cases, preserving APR for local–regional recurrences.

The anal canal begins at the narrowing of the rectal ampulla at the anorectal junction where the rectum enters the puborectalis sling at the apex of the anal sphincter complex, and extends distally for approximately 3–4 cm and ends at the anal verge. This is in distinction from an anal margin or skin cancer.

7 General Treatment Paradigm

Whereas surgical management with a permanent colostomy was the first-line approach to treating anal canal cancer prior to the 1980s, organ preservation with chemoradiation is now the mainstay of treatment due to the contributions of Dr. Norman Nigro from Wayne State University (Nigro et al. 1977). Dr. Nigro initially evaluated chemoradiation, 30 Gy concurrent with 5-FU and mitomycin-C (MMC) chemotherapy, as neoadjuvant therapy prior to an APR in an effort to improve pelvic control. When it was shown that pathologic complete responses were induced in 24 of 28 patients, surgery was then reserved for salvage of local–regional persistent or recurrent cancer.

Four randomized clinical trials have since validated chemoradiation with both 5-FU and MMC as the standard treatment of anal canal cancer (Northover et al. 2010; Bartelink et al. 1997; Flam et al. 1996; Ajani et al. 2008). The United Kingdom Coordinating Committee on Cancer Research (UKCCCR) Anal Cancer Trial (ACT I) and the European Organization for Research and Treatment of Cancer (EORTC) phase III studies had similar designs, comparing 5-FU, MMC and radiation to radiation alone, but employed higher radiation doses (45 Gy plus a boost) than the original Nigro trial (Northover et al. 2010; Bartelink et al. 1997). Both studies demonstrated improved local–regional control with the addition of doublet chemotherapy over radiation alone, which translated into higher cancer-specific survival in the ACT I trial and improved colostomy-free survival in the EORTC investigation. There was no statistically significant survival difference in either study between the two arms, likely in part due to the ability of APR to salvage persistent or recurrent local–regional disease.

Further investigative attempts focusing on reducing the acute toxicity, particularly myelosuppression of chemoradiation, by removing or replacing the MMC from the Nigro regimen, have been unsuccessful. Elimination of MMC in the RTOG 87-04 phase III trial, which randomized patients to radiation (45–54 Gy) and 5-FU (delivered as continuous infusion in week 1) with or without MMC (delivered weeks 1 and 5) resulted in an almost doubling of 5-year local recurrence, an increase in colostomy rate (23 vs. 9 % at 4 years, $p = 0.002$), and a decrease in 5 year disease-free survival (from 64 % in the 5-FU/MMC arm to 50 % in the 5-FU alone arm, $p < 0.003$) (Flam et al. 1996). Moreover, the addition of MMC to 5-FU and radiation appeared to be most beneficial to patients with T3-4 or N0 disease, in terms of colostomy rate reduction.

More recently, cisplatin has been studied as a substitute for MMC in the RTOG 98-11 trial. Six hundred and eighty-two patients with stage T2N0 and above non-metastatic anal canal cancer were randomized to receive either radiation with 5-FU/MMC (per the RTOG 87-04 study), or to receive induction 5-FU/cisplatin for 2 cycles followed by radiation with 5-FU/cisplatin. Radiation was in general a two-dimensional delivery approach with 45 Gy to the pelvis followed by a boost to gross disease at the discretion of the physician to up to 59.4 Gy. Although there was no statistically significant difference in 3-year overall or disease-free survival between the two groups, local–regional relapse rates were higher in the cisplatin-treated patients (33 vs. 25 %; $p = 0.07$), while colostomy-free survival was significantly lower (90 vs. 81 %; $p = 0.02$) (Ajani et al. 2008). In the most recent update, the use of cisplatin was now shown to be inferior to MMC in terms of both overall survival and disease-free survival (5-year disease-free survival: 67.8 vs. 57.8 %, $p = 0.006$; 5-year overall survival: 78.3 vs. 70.7 %, $p = 0.026$), (Gunderson et al. 2012). One potential limitation of the RTOG 98–11 trial was the use of induction chemotherapy, which may have accounted for the poorer outcomes as it delayed the initiation of definitive chemoradiation. To this end, neither induction or outback 5-FU and cisplatin chemotherapy, nor higher radiation doses, have been proven effective in enhancing outcomes in anal canal cancer (Peiffert et al. 2012; James et al. 2009).

To guide chemoradiation treatment decisions in anal canal cancer, preoperative staging, which is based on gross tumor volume and nodal involvement, is critical. As such, anal canal cancers are staged by physical examination and imaging studies. Digital rectal examination can determine the sphincter tone, size (which is a main indicator for AJCC T staging), location, and degree of fixation to adjacent structures of the primary tumor, while palpation of the groins can indicate nodal enlargement (AJCC N staging), (American Joint Committee on Cancer 2010), Table 3. Female patients should undergo a gynecological examination to exclude other HPV-associated cancers. Sigmoidoscopy is also warranted as it provides additional information about the primary and its mucosal spread. Exam under anesthesia is sometimes necessary due to pain upon the digital rectal evaluation. Determination of HIV status is also important in guiding clinical treatment decisions and will be discussed in Sect. 3.

Table 3 Predictors of local recurrence in anal canal cancer

Adverse prognostic factor
Clinical
Lymph node involvement
Tumor diameter >5 cm
Male sex
Treatment breaks during chemoradiation
Limited clinical response to chemoradiation

Imaging studies should be performed to further assess the local extent of the disease and to detect regional adenopathy and/or distant metastases. Local–regional staging investigations include CT or MRI of the pelvis. MRI has become the imaging modality of choice for local–regional staging as it provides high-resolution multiplanar information concerning the location, size and extent of the primary tumor, as well as data regarding the involvement of adjacent structures (Koh et al. 2008). PET/CT has an increasing role in staging and radiation treatment planning of anal canal cancers, as up to 98 % are fluorodeoxyglucose (FDG)-avid (Grigsby 2009; Saboo et al. 2012). FDG PET/CT is used to evaluate primary tumor size, lymph node status, and whether distant metastases are present. It may also be useful for radiation therapy planning by defining sites of metabolically active tumor. Several studies have shown that PET/CT (in comparison with CT or MRI imaging) alters staging of anal canal cancer in approximately 20–30 % of cases, which has important implications on treatment field design and radiation dose (Grigsby 2009; Saboo et al. 2012). Due to these advances in imaging, histologic confirmation of enlarged inguinal or pelvic nodes is not necessary if the morphologic and/or metabolic characteristics of the suspicious nodes are consistent with metastatic disease.

Figure 3 summarizes treatment decisions regarding the use of radiation for anal canal cancer. In patients with clinical stage T1 (primary tumor ≤2 cm) N0 disease, local surgery with wide negative margins alone is appropriate if the disease is distal and not involving the sphincter muscle. If this cannot be achieved, chemoradiation with 5-FU and MMC appears to be more effective than radiation therapy alone (Northover et al. 2010), and doses of approximately 45–50.4 Gy to the gross tumor with 30.6–45 Gy to the elective inguinal, internal and external iliac, mesorectal and presacral nodal groups are recommended. One single institution series showed good local–regional control in a small cohort of these patients with lower total radiation doses and more limited elective nodal fields (Hatfield et al. 2008). In patients with clinical stage T2N0 cancer, definitive chemoradiation is warranted with total radiation doses of 50.4–54 Gy to gross disease. With two-dimensional radiation delivery, total radiation doses of 54 Gy or higher have been shown to be associated with improved local control (Fung et al. 1994). For patients with higher stages of non-metastatic disease, a total radiation dose of 54–59.6 Gy is employed. Additionally, as in rectal cancer, patients who present with oligometastatic disease, are managed with curative intent. Modifications of these clinical treatment approaches may be made in frail patients or in patients with HIV who have CD4 counts of less than 200/mcL.

8 Prognostic Factors

The prognosis of patients with localized anal canal cancer is associated with several factors including the size of the primary anal tumor, involvement of local–regional lymph nodes, gender, treatment breaks, response to chemoradiation, as well as HIV status, and p16 and epidermal growth factor expression. However, only disease stage, gender, treatment breaks, and clinical response to chemoradiation have been validated in multi-institutional prospective studies (Table 4).

8.1 Disease Stage (Tumor and Nodal)

The prognostic value of T and N status in patients treated with primary chemoradiation is demonstrated in randomized trials. In the multivariate secondary analysis of the RTOG 98-11 trial, tumor-related prognosticators for poorer survival included large (>5 cm) tumor diameter nodal positivity, and male gender (Ajani et al. 2009, 2010). Tumor diameter >5 cm resulted in poorer 5-year disease-free survival ($p = 0.0003$) and poorer 5-year overall survival ($p = 0.0031$). The presence of clinically involved lymph nodes is also a significant negative prognostic factor for locoregional failure and overall survival. In the ACT I trial previously described, patients with palpable lymph nodes had almost double the risk of local–regional failure and death from anal cancer (HR 1.87 and HR 1.83, respectively), than did patients with non-palpable lymph nodes (Glynne-Jones et al. 2013). In the EORTC phase III study, lymph node involvement was a significant negative prognostic factor for both local control and survival (Bartelink et al. 1997). However, the prognosis of N2/N3 disease was not different from that of N1, nor did the size of involved nodes (e.g. >2 cm) carry a worse prognosis. In the recent update of RTOG 98-11, patients with clinically negative nodes carries an adjusted HR of 1.88 for overall survival, and 1.82 for disease-free survival, compared with patients with clinically positive nodes at diagnosis (Gunderson et al. 2012).

Patients with either of these unfavorable characteristics, that is, tumors over 5 cm in size and/or node positive

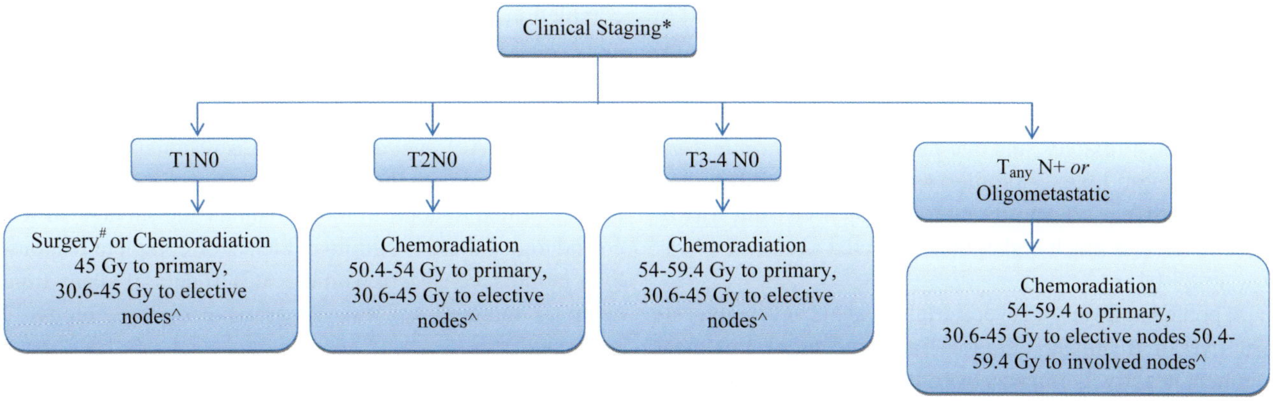

Fig. 3 Definitive chemoradiation for anal canal cancer: decisions based on clinical staging (* Local clinical staging based on exam, CT, MRI and PET/CT; distant disease staging based on full body PET/CT or CT of chest, abdomen and pelvis. # Select patients with distal small lesions may be considered for excision. ^ Elective nodal irradiation doses depend on the method of radiation delivery)

Table 4 AJCC TNM classification of anal cancer

Stage description	
Primary tumor (T)	
TX	Primary tumor cannot be assessed
T0	No evidence of primary tumor
Tis	Carcinoma *in situ*
T1	Tumor ≤2 cm in greatest dimension
T2	Tumor >2 cm but ≤5 cm in greatest dimension
T3	Tumor >5 cm in greatest dimension
T4	Tumor of any size invades adjacent organ(s), e.g., vagina, urethra, bladder
Regional lymph nodes (N)	
NX	Regional lymph nodes cannot be assessed
N0	No regional lymph node metastasis
N1	Metastasis in perirectal lymph node(s)
N2	Metastasis in unilateral internal iliac and/or inguinal lymph node(s)
N3	Metastasis in perirectal and inguinal lymph nodes and/or bilateral internal iliac and/or bilateral internal iliac and/or inguinal lymph nodes
Distant metastasis (M)	
MX	Distant metastasis cannot be assessed
M0	No distant metastasis
M1	Distant metastasis (including seeding of the peritoneum and positive peritoneal cytology)

Source Edge et al. (2009)

disease, were analyzed in a subgroup analysis of RTOG 98-11, and fared worse in terms of disease-free survival (Ajani et al. 2010). These "advanced or bulky disease" patients had a local–regional recurrence rate of 40–64 %, significantly higher than in patients with T2N0 or T3N0 disease (~20 %). The very high rate of local–regional recurrence in patients with bulky disease following concurrent chemoradiation suggests that more aggressive treatment may be necessary, such as radiation dose escalation or adoption of a lower threshold for planned or early surgical resection. As outlined in Fig. 3, the total radiation dose is increased for clinically positive nodes and/or larger primary tumors.

8.2 Gender

Interestingly, female gender is associated with improved survival and local control in the randomized trials described above. The ACT I trial demonstrated a HR of 1.6 for local–regional failure, an HR of 1.8 for death from anal cancer, and 1.56 for overall survival in favor of women, while RTOG 98-11 showed a HR of 1.38 for overall survival in favor of women, $p = 0.031$ (Glynne-Jones et al. 2013; Ajani et al. 2008). Perhaps wild type p16 status confers an improved outcome in anal canal cancers, as with squamous cell cancer of the head and neck, however, such biomarker data is not available at this time.

8.3 Treatment Breaks

Treatment breaks during chemoradiation, or overall prolonged treatment duration, has been shown in several cancers to lead to a detriment in overall survival and local regional control. RTOG 92-08 investigated split course therapy, or a planned treatment break, to reduce radiation-related toxicity associated with dose escalation. In this phase II trial, forty-six patients with anal tumors more than 2 cm in size received 5FU and MMC on day 1 of each course of 5-FU. The radiation dose used was 59.4 Gy in 1.8 Gy fractions over 9 weeks with a two-week mandatory rest (John et al. 1996; Konski et al. 2008). The results were compared to the RTOG 87-04 trial previously described in which patients were treated with 45 Gy in a continuous schedule plus the same chemotherapy regimen (Flam et al. 1996). On 92-08, 40 % of patients suffered Grade 3 toxicity, 23 % Grade 4 toxicity, and one patient died from infection. Although these toxicity profiles were similar to RTOG 87-04, the two-year colostomy rate with 59.4 Gy and a two-week break was much higher than expected (30 % 92-08 vs. 9 % in 87-04).

A pooled analysis of several trials in anal cancer suggests that overall treatment duration, independent of treatment regimen, negatively impacts overall survival possibly due to accelerated repopulation during fractionated radiotherapy (Ben-Josef et al. 2010). In multivariate modeling, there was a trend toward an association between chemoradiation duration of >44 days and colostomy failure (HR = 1.57; 95 % CI, 0.98–2.50; p = 0.06), and a statistically significant association with local failure (HR = 1.96; 95 % CI, 1.34–2.87; p = 0.0006). Prolonged treatment duration is also one major criticism of the RTOG 98-11 study, as patients in the 5-FU/cisplatin arm had a lead-in time to radiation of an additional two months compared with the 5-FU/MMC arm. The median total treatment duration for the 5FU/cisplatin arm was 101 days, compared with a median of 49 days for the 5-FU/MMC arm (even though more patients in the 5FU/MMC arm needed treatment breaks due to treatment-related toxicity). In effect, this induction period with 5-FU/cisplatin clinically delayed the time to definitive treatment with chemoradiation.

8.4 Tumor Response

Determination of clinical response to chemoradiation is generally based on digital rectal examination and exam under anesthesia, as there is no prospective multi-institutional data to support the ability of imaging to accurately predict clinical outcome. Tumor response or regression at 11 weeks, 18 weeks and 26 weeks post chemoradiation on the ACT II study (a multicenter, randomized factorial trial that compared cisplatin versus MMC when combined with 5-FU concurrent chemoradiotherapy, and two cycles of 5-FU and cisplatin maintenance chemotherapy versus no maintenance) was associated with statistically significant improvement in progression-free survival (11 weeks: 3-year progression-free survival: 80 % complete response vs. 72 % no complete response, p = 0.02; 26 weeks 3-year progression-free survival: 83 % complete response vs. 45 % no complete response, p < 0.001) and overall survival (26 weeks: 3-year overall: 93 % complete response vs. 61 % no complete response, p < 0.001) (Glynne-Jones et al. 2012).

At our institution, clinical assessment with digital rectal examination is routinely performed at 4 week intervals after completion of chemoradiation. We also perform a PET/CT at 12 weeks (3 months) after chemoradiation, as metabolic regression at this time has been shown to predict treatment response at our institution and others (Day et al. 2011). If exam or PET/CT suggest that there is residual disease, then an examination with the patient under anesthesia and biopsy are performed to confirm these findings and salvage APR is considered if there is still no evidence of complete response by 6 months, consistent with the ACT II data. If at any time, exam or imaging suggests progressive disease, biopsy is warranted.

8.5 HIV Status

As discussed above, the incidence of invasive anal cancer appears to be rising in the HIV-positive population, even in the highly active antiretroviral therapy (HAART) era. It is believed the increased anal cancer risk is due to the high prevalence of HPV infection in this population. Though there is no prospective randomized clinical trial, several single-institution series suggest that patients with HIV who develop squamous cell carcinoma of the anal canal are at increased risk of significant treatment morbidity (acute grade 3/4 toxicities) and worse local control, as compared to the immunocompetent population, when treated with chemotherapy concurrent with non-conformal radiation (Chiao et al. 2008; Oehler-Janne et al. 2008). With the concern for morbidity, especially in patients with low CD4 counts, oncologists often substitute or omit the standard MMC chemotherapy, which may adversely affect outcomes. More recently, for patients well controlled on HAART, we and other groups have shown that HIV-infected patients treated with concurrent 5-FU, MMC and full dose radiation have similar disease-free and overall survival as in HIV negative patients (Romesser et al. 2012). As such, current clinical practice recommendations are to treat HIV-positive patients with anal canal cancers at standard chemotherapy and radiation doses, with added surveillance of treatment-related toxicities, most notably hematologic. Treatment modifications are then based on the severity of the acute complications. For HIV-positive patients with CD4 counts less than 200/mcL, some oncologists consider using cisplatin instead of MMC.

8.6 Molecular Markers

HPV, particularly HPV genotype 16, is recognized as an important etiologic factor for anal squamous cell carcinoma and is also implicated in the development of cervical and head and neck cancers. Recently, several studies demonstrate that the p16 expression status determined by immunohistochemical staining is a useful surrogate biomarker for HPV integration and predicts the treatment outcome of chemoradiation in patients with HPV-associated oropharyngeal cancers (Ang et al. 2010; Rischin et al. 2010). In anal cancer, only one small retrospective series suggests improved treatment outcome in HPV16-positive patients after chemoradiation (Yhim et al. 2011). Patients whose tumors were p16-positive had significantly better 4-year progression-free survival (63.1 vs. 15.6 %, $p < 0.001$) and overall survival (84.6 vs. 39.8 %, $p = 0.008$) than p16-negative tumors. Currently, RTOG investigators are assessing p16 expression in tissue collected from the 98-11 study.

Anal cancers have been shown to also express epidermal growth factor (EGFR). One single institution series performed immunohistochemical analysis of EGFR and reported expression in 86 % of patients with anal cancer, but no significant correlation was observed between the degree of EGFR staining and disease-free survival (Ajani et al. 2009). Currently, RTOG investigators are assessing EGFR expression in tissue collected from the 98-11 study. The EGFR protein may also serve as a potential treatment target in this disease, similar to the approach in head and neck cancer. Cetuximab, a monoclonal chimeric antibody against EGFR, is effective in combination with radiotherapy in treating squamous cell carcinoma of the head and neck (Bonner et al. 2006). Two phase II studies of cetuximab combined with 5-FU and cisplatin chemoradiation for anal canal cancer are being conducted by the Eastern Cooperative Oncology Group and the AIDS Malignancy Clinical Trials Consortium (AMC-045, Sparano 2006; ECOG-E3205, Garg 2006).

9 Toxicity

9.1 Acute and Late Morbidity from Definitive Chemoradiation

Although many of the acute and late effects from chemoradiation for anal canal cancer are similar to those reported above for rectal cancer, the acute dermatologic and hematologic morbidities are heightened due to the use of MMC. On the RTOG 98-11 trial, conventional radiation therapy techniques were employed to deliver a total dose of 55–59 Gy for T3, T4, node positive disease or T2 tumors with residual disease after 45 Gy without a planned treatment break (Ajani et al. 2008). For patients randomized to the 5-FU/MMC arm, acute toxicity was significant, most notably grade 3-4 gastrointestinal, skin and hematologic morbidity rates of 48, 36, and 61 % respectively. Similarly, preliminary results of the ACT II trial reported a 61 % grade 3–4 non-hematologic toxicity rate in the MMC arm (James et al. 2009). Such morbidity often leads to unscheduled treatment breaks, which may confer untoward local control and survival outcomes (Ben-Josef et al. 2010).

While radiation-dose volume predictors of gastrointestinal toxicity have already been described in the discussion of treatment decisions for rectal cancer, the association between acute hematologic toxicity and the volume of pelvic bone marrow irradiated for anal cancer is under evaluation. Investigators from Stanford have recently demonstrated, in a retrospective analysis of 33 patients receiving IMRT and chemotherapy for anal cancer, that maintaining a pelvic bone marrow mean radiation dose of <22.5 and <25 Gy is associated with a 5 and 10 % risk of a hematologic event (grade 3 or higher hematologic morbidity or any grade $\geq$2 event with a modification in chemotherapy dose), respectively (Bazan et al. 2012). Additionally, Mell and colleagues described, in a cohort of 48 consecutive patients with anal cancer treated with concurrent chemoradiotherapy using IMRT, that the volume of pelvic bone marrow (defined as the region extending from the iliac crests to the ischial tuberosities, including the os coxae, lumbosacral spine, and proximal femora) irradiated was associated with acute grade 3–4 hematologic toxicity (Mell et al. 2008). To date, dose volume predictors of dermatologic morbidity for anal cancer have not been identified, but prior to the use of IMRT, radiation doses as low as 30.6 Gy with concurrent MMC, yielded grade 2 and higher rates of moist desquamation in the majority of patients.

9.2 Role of Conformal Radiotherapy

As in the discussion for rectal cancer, conformal radiation delivery, specifically IMRT, holds the potential to reduce the significant acute and late toxicities associated with 5-FU/MMC chemoradiation for anal canal cancer. Figure 4 demonstrates the normal tissue sparing with IMRT over a 3D-CRT approach for a patient with clinical T2N0 disease.

To date, the only prospective trial of IMRT, RTOG 0529, has recently been reported (Kachnic et al. 2012a, b, c). This phase II study combined concurrent 5-FU/MMC with IMRT to evaluate acute toxicity, and employed real-time pretreatment evaluation of all IMRT plans. The primary endpoint was to determine if the combined rate of acute grade $\geq$2 gastrointestinal and genitourinary toxicity may be decreased by 15 % with the use of IMRT, compared to the data reported with non-conformal delivered radiation on the MMC arm of the RTOG 98-11 trial as the benchmark (Ajani et al. 2008). Planned secondary endpoints assessed all adverse events, the investigator's ability to perform IMRT, and long-term outcomes. All patients received 5-FU and MMC days 1 and 29 of IMRT. IMRT dose was prescribed based on tumor stage. For T2N0 cancers, the plan

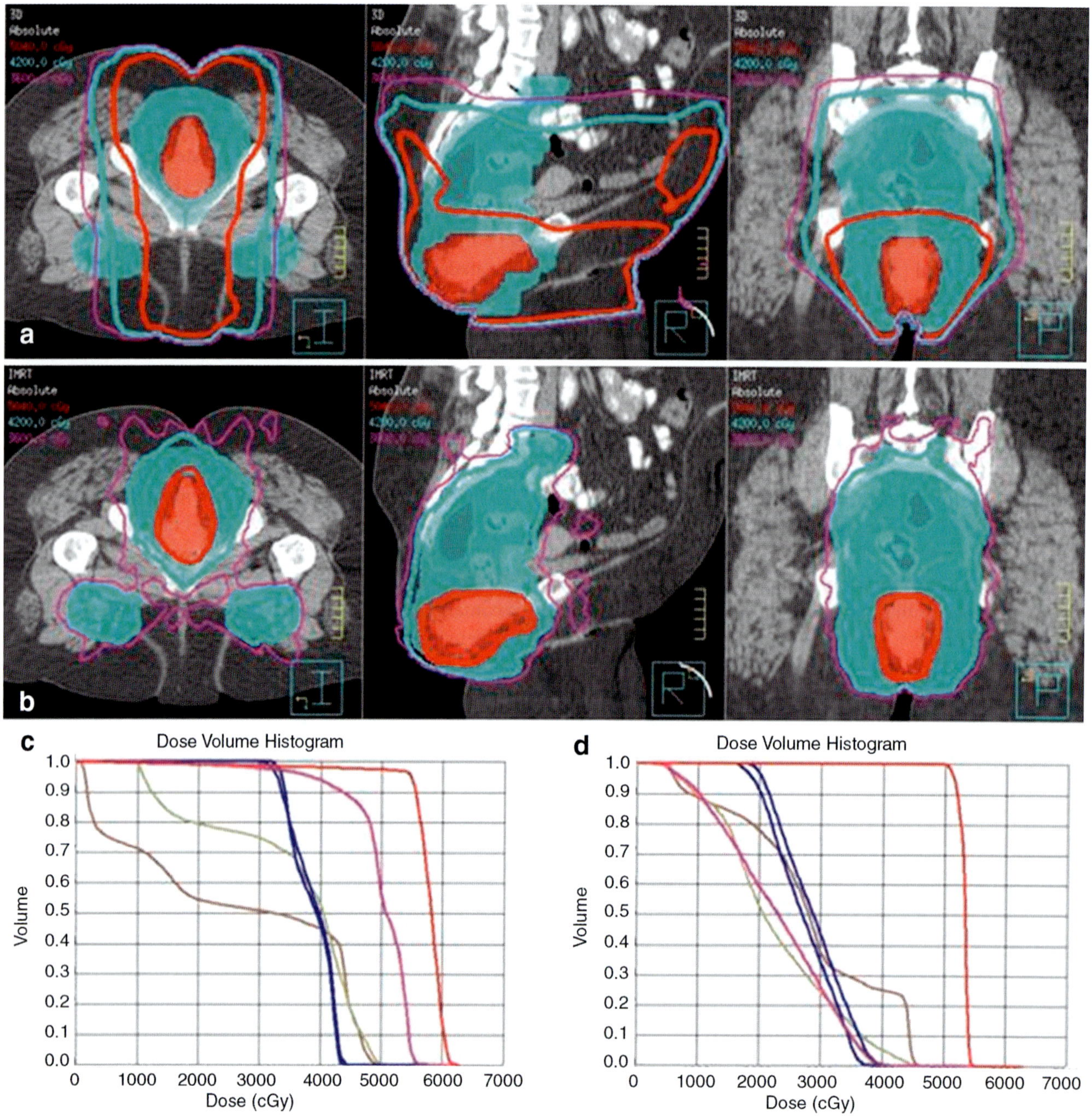

Fig. 4 Comparison of IMRT and 3D-CRT radiation for anal canal cancer. Example of 3D-CRT plan **a** and IMRT plan **b** for a patient with clinical T2N0 anal cancer. From left to right: treatment fields and coronal, sagittal and axial views. Planning target volume (PTV) for anal primary (*red*), with PTV for elective nodes (*light blue*). Isodose lines demonstrate the volumes receiving 50.4 Gy (*red*), 42 Gy (*light blue*), and 36 Gy (*magenta*). Note the under-coverage of the superior iliac nodal region in the 3D-CRT plan, and the sparing of the anterior bowel and femoral heads in the IMRT plan. Dose-volume histograms are shown in **c** and **d** for the 3D-CRT and IMRT plans, respectively. Anal primary PTV (*red*), femoral heads (*blue*), genitals (*magenta*), small bowel (*olive*) and large bowel (*brown*). Compared with 3D, IMRT shows better high-dose sparing of the critical normal structures

was for 42 Gy in 1.5 Gy per fractions to the elective nodal planning tumor volume (PTV) and 50.4 Gy in 1.8 Gy per fraction to the anal tumor PTV. For T3-4N0-3 cancer, the dose was increased to 45 Gy in 1.5 Gy per fractions to the elective nodal PTV, and 54 Gy, 1.8 Gy per fraction, to the anal tumor. Patients with nodal involvement included PTVs that received 50.4 Gy in 1.68 Gy per fraction for nodes $\leq$3 cm, and 54 Gy in 1.8 Gy per fraction for >3 cm in size. Of 63 accrued patients, 52 were analyzable. The stage of cancer was 54 % stage II, 25 % IIIA, and 21 % IIIB. In primary endpoint analysis, 77 % experienced grade 2 and higher gastrointestinal/genitourinary acute similar to that reported on RTOG 98-11 (also 77 %). IMRT however yielded a statistically significant reduction in acute grade 2 and higher hematologic, 73 % (98-11 85 %, $p = 0.032$), and grade 3 and higher gastrointestinal, 21 % (98-11 36 %, $p = 0.0082$) and dermatologic morbidity, 23 % (98-11 49 %, $p < 0.0001$). Treatment interruptions due to toxicity were less frequent with IMRT. The median duration of IMRT on RTOG 0529 was 43 days, compared with 49 days for the RTOG 98-11 MMC arm ($p < 0.0001$).

Critical to the use of IMRT is an understanding of the elective clinical target volumes. On initial pretreatment review, incorrect investigator contouring was identified in approximately 80 % of RTOG 0529's plans, with under-contouring of the mesorectum in >50 %. It was, however, reassuring that major deviations to the radiation planning directives were identified in only 3 cases, demonstrating that IMRT for anal cancer is feasible in a cooperative group setting. It is important to note that target volumes for anal cancer differ from those appropriate for other pelvic malignancies. While the rectum and its associated mesentery are to be avoided for IMRT planning of cervical or prostate cancers, they represent the first echelon of nodal drainage for anal cancer, and therefore must be carefully contoured. As the mesorectal contouring had proven to be challenging for the investigators participating in RTOG 0529, two atlases are now available to assist radiation oncologists in IMRT contouring and planning (Myerson et al. 2009; Ng et al. 2012).

Analysis of efficacy, patterns of failure, and late effects for the RTOG 0529 study will be forthcoming in attempts to validate this approach. If local–regional control appears equivalent or superior to RTOG 98-11 historical rates, as has been reported by large retrospective series (Kachnic et al. 2012a,, b, c), IMRT (with 5-FU and MMC) will become the standard arm for future RTOG studies and may likely become standard practice.

References

Ahmed FE (2003) Colon cancer: prevalence, screening, gene expression and mutation, and risk factors and assessment. J Environ Sci Health C Environ Carcinog Ecotoxicol Rev 21(2):65–131

Ajani JA, Winter KA, Gunderson LL, Pedersen J, Benson AB 3rd, Thomas CR Jr, Mayer RJ, Haddock MG, Rich TA, Willett C (2008) Fluorouracil, mitomycin, and radiotherapy vs fluorouracil, cisplatin, and radiotherapy for carcinoma of the anal canal. A randomized controlled trial. JAMA 299:1914–1921

Ajani JA, Winter KA, Gunderson LL, Pedersen J, Benson AB 3rd, Thomas CR Jr, Mayer RJ, Haddock MG, Rich TA, Willett CG (2009) US intergroup anal carcinoma trial: tumor diameter predicts for colostomy. J Clin Oncol 27(7):1116–1121

Ajani JA, Winter KA, Gunderson LL, Pedersen J, Benson AB 3rd, Thomas CR Jr, Mayer RJ, Haddock MG, Rich TA, Willett CG (2010) Prognostic factors derived from a prospective database dictate clinical biology of anal cancer: the intergroup trial (RTOG 98–11). Cancer 116(17):4007–4013. doi:10.1002/cncr.25188

American Cancer Society (2013) Cancer facts and figures 2013. American Cancer Society, Atlanta

American Joint Committee on Cancer (2010) Colon and rectum. In: Edge SB, Byrd DR, Compton CC, Fritz AG, Greene FL, Trotti AE (eds). AJCC cancer staging manual. 7th edn. Springer, New York

Ang KK, Harris J, Wheeler R, Weber R, Rosenthal DI, Nguyen-Tân PF, Westra WH, Chung CH, Jordan RC, Lu C, Kim H, Axelrod R, Silverman CC, Redmond KP, Gillison ML (2010) Human papilloma virus and survival of patients with oropharyngeal cancer. N Engl J Med 363(1):24–35. doi:10.1056/NEJMoa0912217

Ashman JB, Zelefsky MJ, Hunt MS, Leibel SA, Fuks Z (2005) Whole pelvic radiotherapy for prostate cancer using 3D conformal and intensity-modulated radiotherapy. Int J Radiat Oncol Biol Phys 63(3):765–771

Baglan KL, Frazier RC, Yan D, Huang RR, Martinez AA, Robertson JM (2002) The dose-volume relationship of acute small bowel toxicity from concurrent 5-FU-based chemotherapy and radiation therapy for rectal cancer. Int J Radiat Oncol Biol Phys 52(1): 176–183

Bartelink H, Roelofsen F, Eschwege F, Rougier P, Bosset JF, Gonzalez DG, Peiffert D, van Glabbeke M, Pierart M (1997) Concomitant radiotherapy and chemotherapy is superior to radiotherapy alone in the treatment of locally advanced anal cancer: results of a phase III randomized trial of the European organization for research and treatment of cancer radiotherapy and gastrointestinal cooperative groups. J Clin Oncol 15:2040–2049

Baxter NN, Habermann EB, Tepper JE, Durham SB, Virnig BA (2005) Risk of pelvic fractures in older women following pelvic irradiation. JAMA 294(20):2587–2593

Bazan JG, Luxton G, Mok EC, Koong AC, Chang DT (2012) Normal tissue complication probability modeling of acute hematologic toxicity in patients treated with intensity-modulated radiation therapy for squamous cell carcinoma of the anal canal. Int J Radiat Oncol Biol Phys 84(3):700–706. doi:10.1016/j.ijrobp.2011.12.072

Ben-Josef E, Moughan J, Ajani JA, Flam M, Gunderson L, Pollock J, Myerson R, Anne R, Rosenthal SA, Willett C (2010) Impact of overall treatment time on survival and local control in patients with anal cancer: a pooled data analysis of radiation therapy oncology group trials 87–04 and 98–11. J Clin Oncol 28(34):5061–5066. doi: 10.1200/JCO.2010.29.1351

Bonner JA, Harari PM, Giralt J, Azarnia N, Shin DM, Cohen RB, Jones CU, Sur R, Raben D, Jassem J, Ove R, Kies MS, Baselga J, Youssoufian H, Amellal N, Rowinsky EK, Ang KK (2006) Radiotherapy plus cetuximab for squamous-cell carcinoma of the head and neck. N Engl J Med 354(6):567–578

Bosset JF, Collette L, Calais G, Mineur L, Maingon P, Radosevic-Jelic L, Daban A, Bardet E, Beny A, Ollier JC, EORTC Radiotherapy Group Trial 22921 (2006) Chemotherapy with preoperative radiotherapy in rectal cancer. N Engl J Med 355(11):1114–1123

Bruheim K, Guren MG, Skovlund E, Hjermstad MJ, Dahl O, Frykholm G, Carlsen E, Tveit KM (2010) Late side effects and quality of life after radiotherapy for rectal cancer. Int J Radiat Biol Phys 76(4):1005–1011. doi:10.1016/j.ijrobp.2009.03.010

Chen RC, Mamon HJ, Chen YH, Gelman RS, Suh WW, Talcott JA, Clark JW, Hong TS (2010) Patient-reported acute gastrointestinal symptoms during concurrent chemoradiation treatment for rectal cancer. Cancer 116(8):1879–1886. doi:10.1002/cncr.24963

Chen RC, Mamon HJ, Ancukiewicz M, Killoran JH, Crowley EM, Blaszkowsky LS, Wo JY, Ryan DP, Hong TS (2012) Dose–volume effects on patient-reported acute gastrointestinal symptoms during chemoradiation therapy for rectal cancer. Int J Radiat Oncol Biol Phys 83(4):e513–e517. doi:10.1016/j.ijrobp.2012.01.013

Chiao EY, Giordano TP, Richardson P, El-Serag HB (2008) Human immunodeficiency virus-associated squamous cell cancer of the anus: epidemiology and outcomes in the highly active antiretroviral therapy era. J Clin Oncol 26:474–479

Coia LR, Myerson RJ, Tepper JE (1995) Late effects of radiation therapy on the gastrointestinal tract. Int J Radiat Oncol Biol Phys 31(5):1213–1236

Collette L, Bosset JF, den Dulk M, Nguyen F, Mineur L, Maingon P, Radosevic-Jelic L, Piérart M, Calais G, European Organisation for Research and Treatment of Cancer Radiation Oncology Group (2007) Patients with curative resection of cT3-4 rectal cancer after preoperative radiotherapy or radiochemotherapy: does anybody benefit from adjuvant fluorouracil-based chemotherapy? A trial of the European organisation for research and treatment of cancer radiation oncology group. J Clin Oncol 25(28):4379–4386

Day FL, Link E, Ngan S, Leong T, Moodie K, Lynch C, Michael M, Ed Winton, Hogg A, Hicks RJ, Heriot A (2011) FDG-PET metabolic response predicts outcomes in anal cancer managed with chemoradiotherapy. Br J Cancer 105(4):498–504. doi: 10.1038/bjc.2011.274

Des Guetz G, Schischmanoff O, Nicolas P, Perret GY, Morere JF, Uzzan B (2009) Does microsatellite instability predict the efficacy of adjuvant chemotherapy in colorectal cancer? A systematic review with meta-analysis. Eur J Cancer 45(10):1890–1896

Di Nicolantonio F, Martini M, Molinari F, Sartore-Bianchi A, Arena S, Saletti P, De Dosso S, Mazzucchelli L, Frattini M, Siena S, Bardelli A (2008) Wild-type BRAF is required for response to panitumumab or cetuximab in metastatic colorectal cancer. J Clin Oncol 26(35):5705–5712

Edge SB, Byrd DR, Compton CC et al (2009) American Joint Committee on Cancer, American Cancer Society. AJCC cancer staging manual, 7th edn. Springer, Berlin

Fallik D, Borrini F, Boige V, Viguier J, Jacob S, Miquel C, Sabourin JC, Ducreux M, Praz F (2003) Microsatellite instability is a predictive factor of the tumor response to irinotecan in patients with advanced colorectal cancer. Cancer Res 63(18):5738–5744

Fietkau R, Rödel C, Hohenberger W, Raab R, Hess C, Liersch T, Becker H, Wittekind C, Hutter M, Hager E, Karstens J, Ewald H, Christen N, Jagoditsch M, Martus P, Sauer R, German Rectal Cancer Study Group (2007) Rectal cancer delivery of radiotherapy in adequate time and with adequate dose is influenced by treatment center, treatment schedule, and gender and is prognostic parameter for local control: results of study CAO/ARO/AIO-94. Int J Radiat Oncol Biol Phys 67(4):1008–1019

Flam M, John M, Pajak TF, Petrelli N, Myerson R, Doggett S, Quivey J, Rotman M, Kerman H, Coia L, Murray K (1996) Role of mitomycin in combination with fluorouracil and radiotherapy, and of salvage chemoradiation in the definitive nonsurgical treatment of epidermoid carcinoma of the anal canal: results of a phase III randomized intergroup study. J Clin Oncol 14:2527–2539

Fung CY, Willett CG, Efird JT, Shellito PC, Kaufman DS (1994) Chemoradiotherapy for anal carcinoma: what is the optimal radiation dose? Radiat Oncol Investig 2(3):152–156. doi: 10.1002/roi.2970020307

Garg M (2006) Cetuximab, cisplatin, fluorouracil, and radiation therapy in treating patients with stage I, stage II, or stage III anal cancer. http://clinicaltrials.gov/ct2/show/NCT00316888. Accessed 11 March 2013

Garofalo MC, Moughan J, Hong TS, Bendell J, Berger AC, Lerma F, Lee RJ Anne PR, Sharma NK, Crane CH (2011) RTOG 0822: a phase II evaluation of preoperative chemoradiotherapy (CRT) utilizing IMRT in combination with capecitabine (C) and oxaliplatin (O) for patients with locally advanced rectal cancer. Poster presentation at the American Society for Therapeutic Radiology and Oncology 53rd annual meeting, Miami Beach

Glynne-Jones R, James R, Meadows H, Begum R, Cunningham D, Northover J, Ledermann JA, Beare S, Kadalayil L, Sebag-Montefiore D, ACT II Study Group (2012) Optimum time to assess complete clinical response (CR) following chemoradiation (CRT) using mitomycin (MMC) or cisplatin (CisP), with or without maintenance CisP/5FU in squamous cell carcinoma of the anus: results of ACT II. J Clin Oncol 30 (suppl; abstr 4004)

Glynne-Jones R, Sebag-Montefiore D, Adams R, Gollins S, Harrison M, Meadows HM, Jitlal M; United Kingdom Coordinating Committee on Cancer Research Anal Cancer Trial Working Party (2013) Prognostic factors for recurrence and survival in anal cancer: generating hypotheses from the mature outcomes of the first United Kingdom Coordinating Committee on Cancer Research Anal Cancer Trial (ACT I). Cancer 119(4):748–755. doi: 10.1002/cncr.27825

Grigsby PW (2009) FDG-PET/CT: new horizons in anal cancer. Gastroenterol Clin Biol 33:456–458

Gunderson LL, Russell AH, Llewellyn HJ, Doppke KP, Tepper JE (1985) Treatment planning for colorectal cancer: radiation and surgical techniques and value of small-bowel films. Int J Radiat Oncol Biol Phys 11(7):1379–1393

Gunderson LL, Sargent DJ, Tepper JE, O'Connell MJ, Allmer C, Smalley SR, Martenson JA, Haller DG, Mayer RJ, Rich TA, Ajani JA, Macdonald JS, Goldberg RM (2002) Impact of T and N substage on survival and disease relapse in adjuvant rectal cancer: a pooled analysis. Int J Radiat Oncol Biol Phys 54:386–396

Gunderson LL, Sargent DJ, Tepper JE, Wolmark N, O'Connell MJ, Begovic M, Allmer C, Colangelo L, Smalley SR, Haller DG, Martenson JA, Mayer RJ, Rich TA, Ajani JA, MacDonald JS, Willett CG, Goldberg RM (2004) Impact of T and N stage and treatment on survival and relapse in adjuvant rectal cancer: a pooled analysis. J Clin Oncol 22(10):1785–1796

Gunderson LL, Winter KA, Ajani JA, Pedersen JE, Moughan J, Benson AB, Thomas CR Jr, Mayer RJ, Haddock MG, Rich TA, Willett CG (2012) Long-term update of US GI intergroup RTOG 98-11 phase III trial for anal carcinoma: survival, relapse, and colostomy failure with concurrent chemoradiation involving fluorouracil/mitomycin versus fluorouracil/cisplatin. J Clin Oncol 30(35):4344–4351. doi:10.1200/JCO.2012.43.8085

Habr-Gama A, Perez RO, Proscurshim I, Campos FG, Nadalin W, Kiss D, Gama-Rodrigues J (2006) Patterns of failure and survival for nonoperative treatment of stage c0 distal rectal cancer following neoadjuvant chemoradiation therapy. J Gastrointest Surg 10:1319–1328

Hatfield P, Cooper R, Sebag-Montefiore D (2008) Involved-field, low-dose chemoradiotherapy for early-stage anal carcinoma. Int J Radiat Oncol Biol Phys 70(2):419–424

James R, Wan S, Glynne-Jones R, Sebag-Montefiore D, Kadalayil L, Northover J, Cunningham D, Meadows H, Ledermann J, National Cancer Research Institute (NCRI) ACT II Trial Management Group (2009) A randomized trial of chemoradiation using mitomycin or cisplatin, with or without maintenance cisplatin/5FU in squamous cell carcinoma of the anus (ACT II). J Clin Oncol 27(suppl):18s(abstr LBA4009)

Jasperson KW, Tuohy TM, Neklason DW, Burt RW (2010) Hereditary and familial colon cancer. Gastroenterol 138(6):2044–2058. doi: 10.1053/j.gastro.2010.01.054

John M, Pajak T, Flam M, Hoffman J, Markoe A, Wolkov H, Paris K (1996) Dose escalation in chemoradiation for Anal Cancer: preliminary results of RTOG 92-08 Cancer J Sci Am 2(4): 205–211

Johnson LG, Madeleine MM, Newcomer LM, Schwartz SM, Daling JR (2004) Anal cancer incidence and survival: the surveillance, epidemiology, and end results experience, 1973–2000. Cancer 101(2):281–288

Kachnic LA, Tsai HK, Coen JJ, Blaszkowsky LS, Hartshorn K, Kwak EL, Willins JD, Ryan DP, Hong TS (2012a) Dose-painted intensity-modulated radiation therapy for anal cancer: A multi-institutional report of acute toxicity and response to therapy. Int J Radiat Oncol Biol Phys 82(1):153–158. doi:10.1016/j.ijrobp.2010.09.030

Kachnic LA, Winter K, Myerson R, Goodyear M, Willins J, Esthappan J. Haddock M, Rotman M, Parikh P, Safran H, Willett C (2012b) RTOG 0529: a phase II evaluation of dose-painted IMRT in combination with 5-Fluorouracil and Mitomycin-C for the reduction of acute morbidity in carcinoma of the Anal Canal. Int J Radiat Oncol Biol Phys pii:S0360–3016(12)03601-2. doi: 10.1016/j.ijrobp.2012.09.023

Kachnic LA, Winter K, Myerson RJ, Goodyear MD, Willins J, Esthappan J, Haddock MG, Rotman M, Parikh PJ, Safran H, Willett CG (2012c) RTOG 0529: a phase 2 evaluation of dose-painted intensity modulated radiation therapy in combination with 5-Fluorouracil and Mitomycin-C for the reduction of acute morbidity in carcinoma of the Anal Canal. Int J Radiat Oncol Biol Phys. doi: 10.1016/j.ijrobp.2012.09.023

Khambata-Ford S, Garrett CR, Meropol NJ, Basik M, Harbison CT, Wu S, Wong TW, Huang X, Takimoto CH, Godwin AK, Tan BR, Krishnamurthi SS, Burris HA 3rd, Poplin EA, Hidalgo M, Baselga J, Clark EA, Mauro DJ (2007) Expression of epiregulin and amphiregulin and K-ras mutation status predict disease control in metastatic colorectal cancer patients treated with cetuximab. J Clin Oncol 25(22):3230–3237

Koh DM, Dzik-Jurasz A, O'Neill B, Tait D, Husband JE, Brown G (2008) Pelvic phased-array MR imaging of anal carcinoma before and after chemoradiation. Br J Radiol 81(962):91–98. doi: 10.1259/bjr/96187638

Konski A, Garcia M Jr, John M, Krieg R, Pinover W, Myerson R, Willett C (2008) Evaluation of planned treatment breaks during radiation therapy for anal cancer: update of RTOG 92–08. Int J Radiat Oncol Biol Phys 72:114–118

Krook JE, Moertel CG, Gunderson LL, Wieand HS, Collins RT, Beart RW, Kubista TP, Poon MA, Meyers WC, Mailliard JA, Twito DI, Morton RF, Veeder MH, Witzig TE, Cha S, Vidyarthi SC (1991) Effective surgical adjuvant therapy for high-risk rectal carcinoma. N Engl J Med 324(11):709–715

Lahaye MJ, Engelen SM, Nelemans PJ, Beets GL, van de Velde CJ, van Engelshoven JM, Beets-Tan RG (2005) Imaging for predicting the risk factors-the circumferential resection margin and nodal disease–of local recurrence in rectal cancer: a meta-analysis. Semin Ultrasound CT MR 26(4):259–268

Maas M, Beets-Tan RG, Lambregts DM, Lammering G, Nelemans PJ, Engelen SM, van Dam RM, Jansen RL, Sosef M, Leijtens JW, Hulsewé KW, Buijsen J, Beets GL (2011) Wait-and-see policy for clinical complete responders after chemoradiation for rectal cancer. J Clin Oncol 29(35):4633–4640. doi:10.1200/JCO.2011.37.7176

Marijnen CA, van de Velde CJ, Putter H, van den Brink M, Maas CP, Martijn H, Rutten HJ, Wiggers T, Kranenbarg EK, Leer JW, Stiggelbout AM (2005) Impact of short-term preoperative radiotherapy on health-related quality of life and sexual functioning in primary rectal cancer: report of a multicenter randomized trial. J Clin Oncol 23(9):1847–1858

Mell LK, Schomas DA, Salama JK, Devisetty K, Aydogan B, Miller RC, Jani AB, Kindler HL, Mundt AJ, Roeske JC, Chmura SJ (2008) Association between bone marrow dosimetric parameters and acute hematologic toxicity in anal cancer patients treated with concurrent chemotherapy and intensity-modulated radiotherapy. Int J Radiat Oncol Biol Phys 70(5):1431–1437

Mohiuddin M, Marks J, Marks G (2008) Management of rectal cancer: short- versus long-course preoperative radiation. Int J Radiat Oncol Biol Phys 72(3):636–643. doi:10.1016/j.ijrobp.2008.05.069

Mundt AJ, Lujan AE, Rotmensch J, Waggoner SE, Yamada SD, Fleming G, Roeske JC (2002) Intensity-modulated whole pelvic radiotherapy in women with gynecologic malignancies. Int J Radiat Oncol Biol Phys 52(5):1330–1337

Myerson RJ, Garofalo MC, El Naqa I, Abrams RA, Apte A, Bosch WR, Das P, Gunderson LL, Hong TS, Kim JJ, Willett CG, Kachnic LA (2009) Elective clinical target volumes for conformal therapy in anorectal cancer: a radiation therapy oncology group consensus panel contouring atlas. Int J Radiat Oncol Biol Phys 74(3): 824–830. doi:10.1016/j.ijrobp.2008.08.070

Myerson RJ, Parikh PJ, Tan B, Hunt S, Fleshman JW, Birnbaum EH, Mutch MG, Kodner IJ, Safar B, Naughton M, Picus J, Sorscher S, Lockhart AC, Rigden C, Suresh R, Wang-Gillam A, Hall L (2012) A single-institution phase II trial of five fractions of radiotherapy followed by four courses of FOLFOX chemotherapy as preoperative therapy for rectal adenocarcinoma. J Clin Oncol 30(suppl 4; abstr 553)

Ng M, Leong T, Chander S, Chu J, Kneebone A, Carroll S, Wiltshire K, Ngan S, Kachnic L (2012) Australasian Gastrointestinal Trials Group (AGITG) contouring atlas and planning guidelines for intensity-modulated radiotherapy in anal cancer. Int J Radiat Oncol Biol Phys 83(5):1455–1462. doi:10.1016/j.ijrobp.2011.12.058

Ngan SY, Burmeister B, Fisher RJ, Solomon M, Goldstein D, Joseph D, Ackland SP, Schache D, McClure B, McLachlan SA, McKendrick J, Leong T, Hartopeanu C, Zalcberg J, Mackay J (2012) Randomized trial of short-course radiotherapy versus long-course chemoradiation comparing rates of local recurrence in patients with T3 rectal cancer: Trans-Tasman Radiation Oncology Group trial 01.04. J Clin Oncol 30(31):3827–3833. doi:10.1200/JCO.2012.42.9597

Nigro ND, Vaitkevicius VK, Considine B Jr (1977) Combined therapy for cancer of the anal canal: a follow-up report. Dis Colon Rectum 20:677–678

Northover J, Glynne-Jones R, Sebag-Montefiore D, James R, Meadows H, Wan S, Jitlal M, Ledermann J (2010) Chemo- radiation for the treatment of epidermoid anal cancer: 13-year follow-up of the first randomized UKCCCR Anal Cancer Trial (ACT I). Br J Cancer 102(7):1123–1128. doi:10.1038/sj.bjc.6605605

Oehler-Jänne C, Huguet F, Provencher S, Seifert B, Negretti L, Riener MO, Bonet M, Allal AS, Ciernik IF (2008) HIV-specific differences in outcome of squamous cell carcinoma of the anal canal: a multicentric cohort study of HIV-positive patients receiving highly active antiretroviral therapy. J Clin Oncol 26:2550–2557

Parekh A, Truong MT, Quresh MM, Orlina LA, Hartshorn K, Kachnic LA (2010) Comparison of acute toxicity with three-dimensional versus intensity modulated radiotherapy in patients treated preoperatively for rectal cancer. Poster presentation at the American Society for Therapeutic Radiology and Oncology. 52nd annual meeting, San Diego

Peiffert D, Tournier-Rangeard L, Gérard JP, Lemanski C, François E, Giovannini M, Cvitkovic F, Mirabel X, Bouché O, Luporsi E, Conroy T, Montoto-Grillot C, Mornex F, Lusinchi A, Hannoun-Lévi JM, Seitz JF, Adenis A, Hennequin C, Denis B, Ducreux M (2012) Induction chemotherapy and dose intensification of the radiation boost in locally advanced anal canal carcinoma: final analysis of the randomized UNICANCER ACCORD 03 trial. J Clin Oncol 30(16):1941–1948. doi:10.1200/JCO.2011.35.4837

Pettersson D, Cedermark B, Holm T, Radu C, Påhlman L, Glimelius B, Martling A (2010) Interim analysis of the Stockholm III trial of preoperative radiotherapy regimens for rectal cancer. Br J Surg 97(4):580–587. doi:10.1002/bjs.6914

Rischin D, Young RJ, Fisher R, Fox SB, Le QT, Peters LJ, Solomon B, Choi J, O'Sullivan B, Kenny LM, McArthur GA (2010) Prognostic significance of p16INK4A and human papilloma virus in patients with oropharyngeal cancer treated on TROG 02.02 phase III trial. J Clin Oncol 28:4142–4148

Rödel C, Martus P, Papadoupolos T et al (2005) Prognostic significance of tumor regression after preoperative chemoradiotherapy for rectal cancer. J Clin Oncol 23:8688–8696

Roh MS, Colangelo LH, O'Connell MJ, Yothers G, Deutsch M, Allegra CJ, Kahlenberg MS, Baez-Diaz L, Ursiny CS, Petrelli NJ, Wolmark N (2009) Preoperative multimodality therapy improves disease-free survival in patients with carcinoma of the rectum: NSABP R-03. J Clin Oncol 27(31):5124–5130

Romesser PB, Mancias JD, Qureshi MM, Hartshorn KL, Willins JD, Hong TS, Kachnic LA (2012) Dose-painted intensity-modulated radiation therapy (DP-IMRT) for anal cancer: No differences in treatment toxicity and early outcomes between human immunodeficiency virus (HIV) positive and negative patients. J Clin Oncol 30(suppl 4; abstr 565)

Saboo SS, Zukotynski K, Shinagare AB, Krajewski KM, Ramaiya N (2012) Anal carcinoma: FDG PET/CT in staging, response evaluation, and follow-up. Abdom Imaging. doi:10.1007/s00261-012-9958-3

Samuelian JM, Callister MD, Ashman JB, Young-Fadok TM, Borad MJ, Gunderson LL (2011) Reduced acute bowel toxicity in patients treated with intensity-modulated radiotherapy for rectal cancer. Int J Radiat Oncol Biol Phys 82(5):1981–1987. doi:10.1016/j.ijrobp.2011.01.051

Sauer R, Becker H, Hohenberger W, Rödel C, Wittekind C, Fietkau R, Martus P, Tschmelitsch J, Hager E, Hess CF, Karstens JH, Liersch T, Schmidberger H, Raab R, German Rectal Cancer Study Group (2004) Preoperative versus postoperative chemoradiotherapy for rectal cancer. N Engl J Med 351(17):1731–1740

Sauer R, Liersch T, Merkel S, Fietkau R, Hohenberger W, Hess C, Becker H, Raab HR, Villanueva MT, Witzigmann H, Wittekind C, Beissbarth T, Rödel C (2012) Preoperative versus postoperative chemoradiotherapy for locally advanced rectal cancer: results of the German CAO/ARO/AIO-94 randomized phase III trial after a median follow-up of 11 years. J Clin Oncol 30(16):1926–1933. doi:10.1200/JCO.2011.40.1836

Schmoll HJ, Van Cutsem E, Stein A, Valentini V, Glimelius B, Haustermans K, Nordlinger B, van de Velde CJ, Balmana J, Regula J, Nagtegaal ID, Beets-Tan RG, Arnold D, Ciardiello F, Hoff P, Kerr D, Köhne CH, Labianca R, Price T, Scheithauer W, Sobrero A, Tabernero J, Aderka D, Barroso S, Bodoky G, Douillard JY, El Ghazaly H, Gallardo J, Garin A, Glynne-Jones R, Jordan K, Meshcheryakov A, Papamichail D, Pfeiffer P, Souglakos I, Turhal S, Cervantes A (2012) ESMO consensus guidelines for management of patients with colon and rectal cancer. A personalized approach to clinical decision making. Ann Oncol 23(10):2479–2516

Schrag D (2012) Chemotherapy alone or chemotherapy plus radiation therapy in treating patients with locally advanced rectal cancer undergoing surgery. ClinicalTrials.gov. http://clinicaltrials.gov/show/NCT01515787. Accessed 11 March 2013

Schrag D, Weiser MR, Goodman KA, Gonen M, Cercek A, Reidy DL, Temple LK, Wong WD, Paty P, Saltz L (2010) Neoadjuvant FOLFOX-bev, without radiation, for locally advanced rectal cancer. J Clin Oncol 28(suppl):15s(abstr 3511)

Siddiqui AA, Fayiga Y, Huerta S (2006) The role of endoscopic ultrasound in the evaluation of rectal cancer. Int Semin Surg Oncol 3:36

Siegel R, DeSantis C, Virgo K, Stein K, Mariotto A, Smith T, Cooper D, Gansler T, Lerro C, Fedewa S, Lin C, Leach C, Cannady RS, Cho H, Scoppa S, Hachey M, Kirch R, Jemal A, Ward E (2012) Cancer treatment and survivorship statistics. Cancer J Clin 62(4):220–241. doi:10.3322/caac.21149

Smith N, Brown G (2008) Preoperative staging of rectal cancer. Acta Oncol 47:20–31

Sparano (2006) Cisplatin, fluorouracil, cetuximab, and radiation therapy in treating patients with HIV and Stage I, Stage II, or Stage III anal cancer. ClinicalTrials.gov. http://clinicaltrials.gov/show/NCT00324415. Accessed 11 March 2013

Tepper JE, O'Connell M, Niedzwiecki D, Hollis DR, Benson AB 3rd, Cummings B, Gunderson LL, Macdonald JS, Martenson JA, Mayer RJ (2002) Adjuvant therapy in rectal cancer: analysis of stage, sex, and local control—final report of intergroup 0114. J Clin Oncol 20:1744–1750

Tho LM, Glegg M, Paterson J, Yap C, MacLeod A, McCabe M, McDonald AC (2006) Acute small bowel toxicity and preoperative chemoradiotherapy for rectal cancer: investigating dose-volume relationships and role for inverse planning. Int J Radiat Oncol Biol Phys 66(2):505–513

Thomas PR, Lindblad AS (1988) Adjuvant postoperative radiotherapy and chemotherapy in rectal carcinoma: a review of the Gastrointestinal Tumor Study Group experience. Radiother Oncol 13(4):245–252

Tol J, Koopman M, Cats A, Rodenburg CJ, Creemers GJ, Schrama JG, Erdkamp FL, Vos AH, van Groeningen CJ, Sinnige HA, Richel DJ, Voest EE, Dijkstra JR, Vink-Börger ME, Antonini NF, Mol L, van Krieken JH, Dalesio O, Punt CJ (2009) Chemotherapy, bevacizumab, and cetuximab in metastatic colorectal cancer. N Engl J Med 360(6):563–572

van Dijk TH, Havenga K, Beukema J, Beets GL, Gelderblom H, de Jong KP, Rutten HJ, Van De Velde CJ, WIggers T, Hospers G (2010) Short-course radiation therapy, neoadjuvant bevacizumab, capecitabine and oxaliplatin, and radical resection of primary tumor and metastases in primary stage IV rectal cancer: a phase II multicenter study of the Dutch colorectal cancer group. J Clin Oncol 28(suppl 15):295s(abstr 3638)

Wibe A, Rendedal PR, Svensson E, Norstein J, Eide TJ, Myrvold HE, Søreide O (2002) Prognostic significance of the circumferential resection margin following total mesorectal excision for rectal cancer. Br J Surg 89:327–334

Willett CG, Badizadegan K, Ancukiewicz M, Shellito PC (1999) Prognostics factors in stage T3N0 rectal cancer: do all patients require postoperative pelvic irradiation and chemotherapy? Dis Colon Rectum 42:167–173

Wolmark N, Fisher B, Rockette H, Redmond C, Wickerham DL, Fisher ER, Jones J, Glass A, Lerner H, Lawrence W, Prager D, Wexler M, Evans J, Cruz A, Dimitrov N, Jochimsen P et al (1988) Postoperative adjuvant chemotherapy or radiation therapy for rectal cancer: results from NSABP protocol R-01. J Natl Cancer Inst 80(1):21–29

Yhim HY, Lee NR, Song EK, Kwak JY, Lee ST, Kim JH, Kim JS, Park HS, Chung IJ, Shim HJ, Hwang JE, Kim HR, Nam TK, Park MR, Shim H, Park HS, Kim HS, Yim CY (2011) The prognostic significance of tumor human papilloma virus status for patients with anal squamous cell carcinoma treated with combined chemoradiotherapy. Int J Cancer 129(7):1752–1760. doi:10.1002/ijc.25825

Gynecologic Cancer

Melissa R. Young, Susan A. Higgins, William Yuh, and Nina A. Mayr

Contents

M. R. Young · S. A. Higgins (✉)
Department of Therapeutic Radiology,
Yale University School of Medicine,
New Haven, CT 06520, USA
e-mail: Susan.Higgins@yale.edu

W. Yuh
Department of Diagnostic Radiology,
University of Washington School of Medicine,
Seattle, WA 98195-6043, USA

N. A. Mayr
Department of Radiation Oncology,
University of Washington School of Medicine,
Seattle, WA 98195-6043, USA

Abstract

The management of gynecologic cancers has historically been guided by a clinically-oriented staging system, based largely on physical examination and standard imaging studies including CT of the abdomen and pelvis. This has more recently been supplemented by pre-treatment MRI and functional imaging, as well as imaging biomarkers. This chapter will focus on the most common gynecologic malignancies, discussing the clinical, pathological, and treatment-related factors that influence clinical outcome as well as the influence of biomarkers on prognosis.

1 Introduction

Gynecologic cancers are a diverse group of tumors which are characterized by an orderly pattern of loco-regional spread that is correlated with prognosis. This is reflected in the International Federation of Gynecology and Obstetrics (FIGO) staging system. In addition to the traditional staging system, biologic and molecular markers reflecting angiogenesis, hypoxia and tumor cell proliferation are emerging that correspond to treatment response and prognosis. However, their use in clinical decision-making remains limited. Imaging-based predictors are easier to utilize in clinical management, and show promise in predicting outcome and risk of failure both before and during therapy.

At present, in patients treated primarily with surgery, histopathologic factors can be highly predictive of treatment outcomes, and these variables can dictate the need for

C. Nieder and L. E. Gaspar (eds.), *Decision Tools for Radiation Oncology*, Medical Radiology. Radiation Oncology,
DOI: 10.1007/174_2013_956, © Springer-Verlag Berlin Heidelberg 2014
Published Online: 13 February 2014

Table 1 FIGO and TNM staging of cervical cancer

FIGO	TNM	Description
–	TX	Primary tumor cannot be assessed
–	T0	No evidence of primary tumor
–[a]	Tis	Carcinoma in situ (pre-invasive carcinoma)
I	T1	Cervical carcinoma confined to uterus (extension to corpus should be disregarded)[a]
IA	T1a	Invasive carcinoma diagnosed only by microscopy (*all macroscopically visible lesions are stage IB/T1b tumors*). Stromal invasion with a maximum depth of 5.0 mm measured from the base of the epithelium and a horizontal spread of 7.0 mm or less. Vascular space involvement, venous or lymphatic, does not affect classification
IA_1	$T1a_1$	Measured stromal invasion 3.0 mm or less in depth and 7.0 mm or less in horizontal spread
IA_2	$T1a_2$	Measured stromal invasion more than 3.0 mm and not more than 5.0 mm, with a horizontal spread 7.0 mm or less
IB	T1b	Clinically visible lesion confined to the cervix or microscopic lesion greater than IA_1/IA_2
IB_1	$T1b_1$	Clinically visible lesion 4.0 cm or less in greatest dimension
IB_2	$T1b_2$	Clinically visible lesion more than 4.0 cm in greatest dimension
II	T2	Cervical carcinoma invades beyond uterus but not to pelvic wall or to lower third of vagina
IIA	T2a	Tumor without parametrial invasion
IIA_1	$T2a_1$	Lesion 4.0 cm or less in greatest dimension
IIA_2	$T2a_2$	Lesion more than 4.0 cm in greatest dimension
IIB	T2b	Tumor with parametrial invasion
III	T3	Tumor extends to pelvic wall and/or involves lower third of vagina, and/or causes hydronephrosis or nonfunctioning kidney
IIIA	T3a	Tumor involves lower third of vagina, no extension to pelvic wall
IIIB	T3b	Tumor extends to pelvic wall and/or causes hydronephrosis or nonfunctioning kidney
IV	T4	Bladder and/or rectal invasion or distant spread
IVA	T4a	Tumor invades mucosa of bladder or rectum, and/or extends beyond true pelvis (bullous edema is not sufficient to classify a tumor as IVA)
IVB	T4b	Distant metastasis (including peritoneal spread, involvement of supraclavicular or mediastinal lymph nodes, lung, liver, or bone)
3/4	Nx	Regional lymph nodes cannot be assessed regional lymph node metastasis
3/4	N0	No regional lymph node metastasis
3/4	N1	Regional lymph node metastasis
3/4	M0	No distant metastasis (no pathologic M0; use clinical M to complete stage group)
3/4	M1	Distant metastasis (including peritoneal spread, involvement of supraclavicular or mediastinal lymph nodes, lung, liver, or bone)

[a] FIGO staging no longer includes stage 0 (Tis)
Source Edge et al. (2009)

adjuvant radiation therapy and/or chemotherapy. For example, histopathologic variables such as margin status, lymphovascular invasion, and positive lymph nodes are commonly factored into adjuvant therapy decisions (Sedlis et al. 1999; Peters et al. 2000). In the future, there may be a role for biomarkers in this regard. However, to date, there has not been substantial progress in the use of biomarkers for use in the post-operative setting.

2 Cancer of the Cervix

The prognosis and treatment outcome for patients with cervical cancerare largely determined by local tumor extent, tumor size and regional lymphatic spread, which follows predictable pathways along anatomic routes and lymph node echelons. In general, the extent of loco-regional spread will guide the selection of therapy—tumors confined to the cervix are managed primarily by surgical therapy, while those with extension to the parametrium, distal vagina or adjacent organs are treated by primary radiation and chemotherapy.

2.1 Staging

The loco-regional tumor extent is only partially reflected by the traditional FIGO staging system (Pecorelli 2009). The FIGO staging system (Table 1) relies on findings from clinical examination and invasive investigations, including cystoscopy and proctoscopy, with biopsy. It also allows the use of radiographic information from plain X-ray films. However, information regarding lymph node involvement, a strong determinant of outcome, is not incorporated. In addition, findings from CT, MRI and functional imaging, namely PET-CT, are not utilized. This results in inherent limitations in assessing well validated prognostic factors, including tumor volume, involvement of adjacent structures, and parametrial extension, that are challenging to assess by palpation and visual inspection alone. In addition, the detection of regional lymph node spread and sites of distant metastatic disease, that can be detected with cross-sectional imaging, can be missed (Eifel 1994). Due to these inherent limitations, FIGO staging has been shown to result in under-staging of 20–60 % of cervical cancer patients, when compared with surgical staging (Averette et al. 1975). This explains why significant variations in treatment failure rates and survival are observed within each FIGO stage category (Eifel et al. 1994; Perez et al. 1992a).

Despite the fact that the FIGO staging system suffers from the aforementioned limitations, it remains the current standard of practice, and provides the major entrance criteria utilized in determining the eligibility of patients for cooperative group trials. Thus, most current cooperative group trials enroll patients across almost the entire FIGO stage spectrum, from stage IB2-IVA, and accession them to largely uniform treatment regimens. Of note, although cross-sectional imaging is not "permitted" to influence FIGO stage assignment, the use of CT, MRI and molecular imaging with fluorodeoxyglucose (^{18}F)FDG PET imaging is likely to result in "stage migration" by excluding patients with subtle imaging-based evidence of regional or distant metastatic involvement from cooperative group trials (Fig. 1). This will make any improvements of therapy with newer interventions difficult to compare to historic controls. However, the incorporation of functional imaging into future clinical trials will potentially enhance our ability to accurately stratify patients and tailor therapy to the "true" clinical stage (i.e. locally advanced vs. metastatic disease).

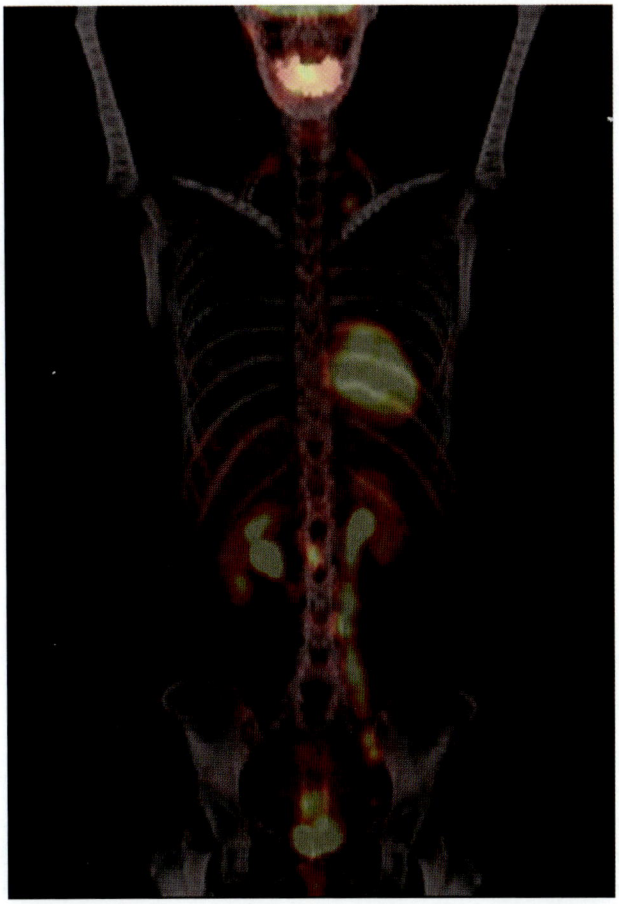

Fig. 1 PET-CT and Staging of Cervical Cancer: A 43 year old woman with invasive squamous cell carcinoma of the cervix underwent PET-CT revealing retroperitoneal and supraclavicular adenopathy, consistent with Stage IV disease

2.2 Clinical Factors

Eligibility for primary surgical therapy is determined by regional tumor extent to adjacent structures and significantly influences prognosis. Patients with stage I disease (tumor limited to the cervix) and selected patients with stage II disease (including patients with upper vaginal involvement), are candidates for radical hysterectomy. The overall survival of surgically treated patients with stage IB tumors ranges from 85 to 90 % (Morley and Seski 1976; Hopkins and Morley 1991; Landoni et al. 1997). However, large tumor size, deep cervical invasion, lymphovascular space invasion, as well as involved lymph nodes and parametrial involvement have been recognized as risk factors for pelvic recurrence after radical hysterectomy. Depending on the number and extent of these factors present, adjuvant therapy can improve outcomes, albeit at the cost of increased risk of toxicity from adjuvant radiation and/or chemotherapy (Sedlis et al. 1999; Peters et al. 2000; Rotman et al. 2006). Thus, if imaging modalities or other factors could identify the presence of these pathologic features during workup leading to upstaging, definitive radiation and chemotherapy could be considered instead of primary surgery, thus potentially reducing the morbidity of treatment.

2.2.1 Stage

In patients with cervical cancer treated with definitive radiation therapy, FIGO stage remains an important prognostic factor. Due to the relative rarity of cervical cancer in western nations, phase III cooperative group trials do not subclassify patients by stage, nor do they group patient cohorts as stages IB–II versus III–IVA for subgroup

Table 2 Tumor diameter versus disease free survival for stage IB cervical cancer

Size (cm)	NP	1	2	3	4	5	6	7	8	>8
Eifel et al. (1994) n = 1,526	94	87				86	72	69	64	47
Lowrey et al. (1992) n = 130	93				77		67			
Perez et al. (1992b) n = 384	90				65		~60			
Homesley et al. (1980) n = 45	95					67				

NP Not palpable

Table 3 Tumor diameter versus disease free survival for stage IIB cervical cancer

Size (cm)	NP	1	2	3	4	5	6	7	8	>8
Mendenhall et al. (1984) n = 83	–				84		66			
Lowrey et al. (1992) n = 130	100				85		61			

NP Not palpable

analyses, because analysis by individual stage categories would require unachievably large patient cohorts. Based on large single-institution series in which contemporary radiation techniques and concurrent chemotherapy were utilized, reported local control rates, disease free survival rates, and overall survival rates for patients with Stage IB–IIA and III–IVA are 87 and 79 %, 74 and 54 %, and 79 and 59 %, respectively (Whitney et al. 1999; Eifel et al. 2004; Rose et al. 2007).

2.2.2 Tumor Volume

In addition to FIGO stage, tumor size has profound prognostic significance (Eifel et al. 1994; Kovalic et al. 1991). In 1988 FIGO added tumor diameter as a stratifying factor for stage I disease, with tumors less than or greater than 4 cm classified as stage IB1 versus IB2 respectively. In the 2009 revision of the staging system, tumor size of greater or less than 4 cm was also incorporated into the stage IIB category (Pecorelli et al. 2009). Tables 2 and 3 shows the profound significance of tumor size, measured as largest or average palpated diameter, for local control and survival. Within the same stage category of IB, tumor size of <4 cm in diameter was associated with a disease-free survival of 87 %, compared to 72 % for 6 cm, 69 % for 7 cm, 64 % for 8 cm and 47 % for >8 cm tumors (Table 2). Similar relationship exists for tumor size and outcomes within the stage IIB category (Table 3) (Eifel et al. 1994; Hansgen and Dunst 1996; Hockel et al. 1996; Homesley et al. 1980; Lowrey et al. 1992; Perez et al. 1992b; Mendenhall et al. 1984).

2.2.3 Lymph Node Status

For any given FIGO stage, lymph node involvement reduces overall survival by approximately 50 % (Stehman et al. 1991). Furthermore, among patients with positive lymph nodes, prognosis declines with increasing extent of lymph node involvement (Macdonald et al. 2009; Hsu et al. 1972; Tsai et al. 1999; Takeda et al. 2002; Morice et al. 1999). In a pooled study by the Gynecologic Oncology Group (GOG), para-aortic involvement was associated with an 11-fold risk of recurrence and sixfold risk of death, and was also associated with extrapelvic failures (Berman et al. 1984). However, even with para-aortic lymph node involvement, survival in the range of 20–50 % has been reported for patients with locally advanced disease (Komaki et al. 1983; Rotman et al. 1994), justifying aggressive therapy for patients with regional lymphatic spread.

Although controversy exists whether surgical excision of suspicious lymph nodes improves outcomes, a large retrospective study of patients treated in the pre-chemo-radiation era showed among patients who underwent lymphadenectomy and postoperative radiation, patients with macroscopically involved lymph nodes had similar regional and distant tumor control as those with microscopic lymph node involvement, and significantly better than those patients with unresectable lymph nodes (Cosin et al. 1998). This supports the use of imaging for identification of involved nodes, thus allowing for a tumor directed combined modality approach. Increasing use of molecular imaging in cervix cancer will facilitate this approach and will also likely lead to stage migration as lymph nodes with more subtle involvement can be identified and treated more aggressively.

2.3 Patient Factors

2.3.1 Hemoglobin

Over the past 50 years, numerous studies have provided indirect evidence that the effects of poor tumor blood supply have an adverse impact on radiation response. Early studies of morphologic parameters of angiogenesis, such as microvessel density, have been shown to correlate with radioresponsiveness and clinical outcome in cervical cancer (Awwad et al. 1986; Cooper et al. 1998). Cervical cancer patients with high inter-capillary distances locally within their tumors measured by colposcopy were found to have increased tumor recurrence rates after radiation therapy (Kolstad 1968).

Similarly cervical cancer patients with low hemoglobin levels have been reported to have higher recurrence rates after radiotherapy (Mendenhall et al. 1984; Bush et al. 1978; Evans and Bergsjo 1965; Diesche et al. 1983; Thomas 2001; Dunst et al. 2003). This supports the concept that poor "systemic" oxygenation is clinically significant for treatment outcome. Haensgen et al. analyzed hemoglobin levels of 70 patients, and reported survival was 27 % for patients with low hemoglobin (<11 g/dL), compared to 62 % in those with higher levels (Haensgen et al. 2001). Dunst et al. mirrored these results, showing overall survival of 64 and 32 %, respectively and local recurrence rates of 15 % versus 67 %, respectively (Dunst et al. 2003). Hemoglobin *during* the course of therapy, when the actual cytotoxic events occur, may also be relevant. Thomas et al. showed in 605 patients that the average weekly hemoglobin nadir <12 g/dL was associated with a higher incidence of local failure and metastases (Thomas 2001). In a recent study, weekly mean hemoglobin levels measured during the course of radiotherapy was more predictive of outcome than pre-therapy or nadir hemoglobin (Mayr et al. 2009). In all, the thresholds value for this effect of hemoglobin level appears to be in the range of 11–12 g/dL.

Although the impact of blood transfusion on outcome in patients treated with definitive radiation therapy remains controversial, the Canadian experience suggests that maintaining hemoglobin levels above 12 g/dL is associated with improved 5-year survival. Pre-treatment hemoglobin, which may not reflect the longitudinal status of hemoglobin levels, did not have any impact on outcome (Grogan et al. 1999). Interestingly, in one retrospective study of 204 patients at a single institution where departmental practice was to transfuse for hemoglobin <11 g/dL, it was noted that only 18.5 % of patients who received transfusion had a sustained response to transfusion, although outcomes for these patients were equivalent to those presenting with normal hemoglobin (Kapp et al. 2002). However, for patients who did not have a sustained response to blood transfusion, outcomes were significantly worse compared to those with response or with normal hemoglobin pre-therapy. While there was a therapeutic benefit to transfusion for those patients with sustained response, the low rate of response of 18.5 % was disappointing, and it was proposed that finding and treating the underlying cause of the anemia may be more beneficial.

2.4 Histologic Factors

2.4.1 Histology

Approximately 90 % of cervical cancers are squamous cell carcinomas. Squamous cell carcinomas arise from epithelial precursors, and can be classified into one of three cell types: large cell keratinizing, large cell nonkeratinizing, and small cell. Tumor grade is based on the degree of differentiation, and is reported as well, moderately, or poorly differentiated. Adenocarcinoma is the second most common, accounting for 10–15 % depending on region and age. More recently, the incidence of adenocarcinomas appears to be increasing, especially in younger patients (Liu et al. 2001; Smith et al. 2000). Adenocarcinomas arise from the mucus-secreting endocervical glands of the cervix or the cylindrical mucosa. The most common subtype of adenocarcinoma of the cervix is endometrioid adenocarcinoma, where cells have characteristic features of the endometrium and grading is based on the degree of gland formation. It is critical to differentiate this from primary endometrioid endometrial adenocarcinoma as recommended therapy would change, thus clinical presentation, such as absence or presence of an endometrial tumor with extension into the cervix, is incorporated to determine the true site of primary disease. The next most common subtype of adenocarcinoma is adenosquamous histology, comprising 21–30 % of adenocarcinomas (Farley et al. 2003; Kleine et al. 1989), and is characterized by epithelial cell cores mixed with glandular structures. Other histologies, such as clear cell, small cell carcinoma, basaloid carcinoma, lymphoma, and sarcomas occur, but are rare and have varying prognostic impact.

The prognosis of adenocarcinoma versus squamous cell histology is debated. While adenocarcinoma is associated with an increased risk of failure, particularly metastatic failure in some retrospective reports (Eifel et al. 1995; Huang et al. 2011, 2012), many show no significant impact on outcome between adenocarcinoma and squamous cell carcinoma (Shingleton et al. 1995; Look et al. 1996; Davidson et al. 1989). Interestingly, adenosquamous carcinoma may be associated with poorer recurrence free and overall survival (Farley et al. 2003; Look et al. 1996;

Lea et al. 2003; Grisaru et al. 2001; Galic et al. 2012). In all, the differences in outcomes among these studies may be in part due to regional variation in Human Papilloma Virus (HPV) genotype distribution, changes in etiology and incidence of histologic type, differences in treatment approach, and overall study sizes, making it difficult to draw any definitive conclusion about subtype implications in the absence of prospective data.

2.4.2 Histopathologic Risk Factors in Postoperative Patients

In surgically treated stage I-IIA patients, lymph node involvement, parametrial invasion and involved margins have long been recognized as *high risk factors* for local recurrence and death (Morrow 1980). In those with involved lymph nodes, number of involved nodes (<3 vs. >3), bilaterality, level (common iliac vs. pelvic) and size (micro- vs. macroscopic) impact outcome (van Bommel et al. 1987; Tanaka et al. 1984). Therefore, adjuvant therapy based on histopathologic risk factors is paramount because salvage therapy for recurrent cervical cancer after hysterectomy has dismal results with a 5–45 % survival (Thomas et al. 1993). Postoperative radiation has been the hallmark in adjuvant therapy.

Tumor size, depth of invasion and capillary-lymphatic space invasion have also been shown to impact prognosis in surgically treated stage I-IIA patients. However, until the completion of the phase III GOG 92 study, the impact of adjuvant therapy on survival was not well established. GOG 92 (Sedlis et al. 1999; Rotman et al. 2006) established a set of *intermediate risk factors* (commonly referred to as "Sedlis criteria") for poor outcome in stage IB patients treated with radical hysterectomy. Patients with two of the three features (capillary lymphatic space invasion, large clinical tumor diameter, or more than one-third cervical stromal invasion) were randomized to pelvic radiotherapy versus no further therapy (Table 4). At 10 years median follow-up, postoperative radiation reduced the risk of recurrence by 46 % (HR 0.54) with the greatest benefit in patients with a combination of *deep 1/3 invasion plus tumor size >4 cm* (HR 0.16) or *capillary lymphatic space invasion plus deep 1/3 invasion with any tumor size* (HR 0.53) (Rotman et al. 2006). There was no significant improvement in overall survival (Table 5). On subgroup analysis, proportionally greater improvement was noted among 44 patients with adenosquamous or adenocarcinoma, where adjuvant radiation therapy reduced the recurrence rate from 44 to 9 % (Rotman et al. 2006). A current GOG study is underway to evaluate whether postoperative radiation with concurrent chemotherapy can further improve upon this outcome.

Improvement of adjuvant therapy with the addition of concurrent chemotherapy to radiation has also been demonstrated for some select patients. The intergroup trial GOG 109 randomized stage IA2-IIA patients treated with radical hysterectomy and pelvic lymphadenectomy and high risk features, defined as positive pelvic lymph nodes and/or positive margins, and/or microscopic involvement of the parametrium, to pelvic radiotherapy versus pelvic radiotherapy with chemotherapy (cisplatin/5-FU for 4 cycles during and after radiation) (Peters et al. 2000). Addition of chemotherapy resulted in significant improvement of overall survival at 81 % versus 71 % (HR 1.96, p = 0.007). The greatest benefit was observed for patients with larger tumors and multiple involved lymph nodes, underscoring the importance of identification of involved lymph nodes in order to offer the optimal adjuvant therapy. Table 6 summarizes the results of five randomized trials that show improved survival with concurrent chemotherapy and radiotherapy (Peters et al. 2000; Whitney et al. 1999; Rose et al. 2007; Keys et al. 1999; Morris et al. 1999).

Table 4 Inclusion criteria for GOG 92: randomization to postoperative pelvic radiotherapy versus no further therapy in stage IB intermediate risk cervical cancer

LVSI	Depth of invasion	Tumor size (cm)
Positive	Deep 1/3	Any
Positive	Middle 1/3	≥2
Positive	Superficial 1/3	≥5
Negative	Deep or middle 1/3	≥4

Adapted from Sedlis et al. (1999). For inclusion into GOG 92, patients fit one of the above set of criteria. *LVSI* lymphovascular space invasion

Table 5 GOG 92 results: postoperative radiotherapy improves recurrence-free, but not overall survival, in intermediate risk stage IB cervix cancer

	RT (n = 137) (%)	Observation (n = 140) (%)	p value
Recurrences (all)	17.5	30.7	0.007
AC, AS	8.8	44.0	0.019[a]
Squamous cell	20.4	27.8	
Survival	80.3	71.4	n.s.

Adapted from Rotman et al. (2006)

[a] Adenocarcinoma and Adenosquamous histology had a statistically significant improvement in recurrence free survival with RT compared to other histologic subtypes treated with RT. *RT* radiotherapy, *AC* Adenocarcinoma, *AS* Adenosquamous carcinoma, *n.s.* not significant

2.4.3 Molecular Tumor Markers

2.4.3.1 HPV

HPV is found in an estimated 93–99.7 % of invasive cervical cancer (Bosch et al. 1995; Walboomers et al. 1999). Further, the prevalence of different genotypes varies in

Table 6 Estimates of the relative risk of death in five clinical trials of radiotherapy and concurrent chemotherapy

Study	FIGO stage	Control group	Comparison group	Relative risk of death	p value
Peters et al. (2000)	IB or IIA	RT	RT plus cisplatin and 5-FU	0.5	0.007
Whitney et al. (1999)	IIB–IVA	RT plus hydroxyurea	RT plus cisplatin and 5-FU	0.72	0.018
Rose et al. (2007)	IIB–IVA	RT plus hydroxyurea	RT plus weekly cisplatin RT plus cisplatin, 5-FU, hydroxyurea	0.61 0.58	<0.025 <0.025
Keys et al. (1999)	IB2	RT	RT plus weekly cisplatin	0.54	0.008
Morris et al. (1999)	IB–IVA	Extended field RT	RT plus cisplatin and 5-FU	0.52	0.004

RT radiotherapy, *5-FU* 5-fluorouracil

cellular histology. HPV16 is identified in the majority of squamous cell carcinomas, and HPV18 is the predominant genotype in adenocarcinomas and adenosquamous carcinomas (Bosch et al. 1995). HPV may be a prognostic indicator for outcomes. Several studies have shown HPV18 and HPV16 is associated with more advanced cervical cancers at presentation and poorer outcomes (Schwartz et al. 2001; Pilch et al. 2001; Burger et al. 1996). Further, HPV18 has been associated with increased radioresistance and increased recurrence rates compared to other HPV genotypes in patients receiving only radiation therapy (Wang et al. 2010). However, HPV18 has subsequently been shown to be predictive of improved disease specific survival when concurrent chemotherapy and radiotherapy was used in place of radiotherapy alone (Wang et al. 2012). The clinical utility of this association is an area of active investigation.

2.4.3.2 Angiogenesis

Angiogenesis-related molecular markers would be expected to be of great importance for radiation and chemotherapy because of the critical dependence of the cytotoxic effect on tumor microcirculation and oxygenation (Tannock 1972). It is postulated that poorly-perfused, hypoxic, endophytic tumors are associated with radio-resistance and resulting poor treatment outcome in cervical cancer. Angiogenic factors have been shown to correlate with tumor recurrence and survival in surgically treated patients (Cheng et al. 2000; Dellas et al. 1997; Dinh et al. 1996; Hawighorst et al. 1997; Lee et al. 2011; Mayr et al. 1999; Kainz et al. 1995; Obermair et al. 1998; Tjalma et al. 2000). Therefore, there has been increasing interest in molecular markers of angiogenesis and cytokines in cervical cancer. Cooper et al. (Cooper et al. 1998) reported that patients with high MVD had significantly poorer local control and survival. Although Gaffney et al. (2003) found increased VEGF and EGFR expression to be associated with poor survival, inconsistent results have been observed in regard to VEGF association with tumor progression, stage (Loncaster et al. 2000), histologic type (Cheng et al. 2000; Loncaster et al. 2000, 2002) and microvessel density (MVD) (Mayr et al. 1999; Hawighorst et al. 1998). High expression of another angiogenic marker, carbonic anhydrase IX (CA IX) correlates with poor survival (Loncaster et al. 2002). More recently the GOG evaluated a panel of angiogenesis markers including MVD, VEGF, CD31 (non-specific endothelial marker), TSP-1 (thrombospondin-1 an anti-angiogenesis factor), and CD105 (tumor-specific endothelial marker) and association with clinical outcome (Randall et al. 2009). Expression of each was determined in tumors from patients included in GOG 109, including stage IA2-IIA patients with positive lymph nodes, parametrial involvement, or positive surgical margins (Peters et al. 2000). Of these, only high expression CD31 was independently predictive of improved disease free and overall survival. Authors posit that this may be representative of CD31 as a surrogate marker for improved tumor flow and oxygenation, thus improving response to adjuvant therapy.

2.4.3.3 Alternate Candidate Molecules

There has been increasing interest in evaluation of molecular mechanisms of radiation response through candidate gene approach and microarray analysis. Studies in cervical cancer cell lines have found that genes related to angiogenesis, apoptosis and tumor cell invasion correlate with radio-resistance (Harima et al. 2004; Kitahara et al. 2002; Tewari et al. 2005; Wong et al. 2003). A pilot study of 12 patients in 2008 used microarray analysis and demonstrated immortalization upregulated protein (IMUP), IGF-2, and ARHD were associated with tumor recurrence in patients treated with radiation and concurrent chemotherapy (Klopp et al. 2008). Proteins that have been shown to correlate with clinical outcome include Ku80, GADD45 (Harima et al. 2003), bax, bcl-2 (Harima et al. 1998), intracellular adhesion molecule-3 (ICAM-3) (Chung et al. 2005), and hypoxia inducible factor (HIF)-1a (Bachtiary et al. 2003; Burri et al. 2003). However, to date, none of these molecular markers has been incorporated into clinical care.

2.5 Imaging Prognostic/Predictive Markers

2.5.1 Morphologic Imaging

Improvements in spatial and temporal resolution of cross-sectional imaging have broadened the capabilities of both anatomical and functional imaging in cervical cancer. Three-dimensional tumor volume can be quantified, and tumor extent and involvement of adjacent structures more accurately assessed than by clinical palpation (Hricak et al. 1988; Hricak 1991; Bhosale et al. 2010; Balleyguier et al. 2011). Higher temporal and spatial resolution also allows for functional imaging, such as dynamic contrast-enhanced (DCE) MRI and diffusion-weighted imaging, in addition to the morphologic/anatomical imaging. Beyond pre-therapy assessment, repeated imaging throughout the course of definitive chemoradiotherapy with an intact cervix provides longitudinal information on functional changes in response to ongoing therapy. Such on-therapy imaging shows promise for deriving imaging biomarkers to predict therapeutic response and disease outcome.

Tumor size in cervical cancer is best assessed with MRI (Bhosale et al. 2010; Balleyguier et al. 2011), which was demonstrated in imaging-histologic correlation studies (Burghardt et al. 1989; Greco et al. 1989). For on-therapy assessments, the velocity of tumor regression, assessed by 3D tumor volumetry (not diameter-based measurement) allows an indirect measure of therapy responsiveness (Mayr et al. 2006), which has been shown to be predictive of treatment outcome in cervical cancer patients treated with radiation/chemotherapy (Hatano et al. 1999; Mayr et al. 1996, 2010; Sethi et al. 2005; Lim et al. 2008). Using 3D volumetric measurements, Mayr et al. found that patients with <20 % of residual tumor volume at 40–50 Gy delivered over 4–5 weeks had excellent local control and disease free survival of 90.5 and 88.4 %, compared to 23.1 and 45.4 % in patients with slower tumor regression (Mayr et al. 1996). Similarly, Hatano et al. (1999) found 100 % local control in patients with rapid tumor volume regression to less than 30 % of the original volume at 30 Gy over 3 weeks. Further, the velocity of tumor shrinkage directly correlates with patients' risk for local failure and death of disease (Mayr et al. 2010). Such early predictive information, available *during* the ongoing therapy course, may open a window of opportunity to adapt and intensify therapy. For post-therapy assessment in the early follow-up period, complete resolution of the tumor 3–6 months after therapy is associated with better outcome (Hricak 1991; Flueckiger et al. 1992).

2.5.2 Functional Imaging

Among the functional imaging modalities, DCE MRI provides an in vivo imaging biomarker that indirectly reflects tumor perfusion and the delivery of oxygen and therapeutic agents to the tumor. Low perfusion, indicative of poor vascularity and oxygenation, before or early during the course of radiation therapy (at approximately 20 Gy, ~2 weeks), significantly predicts unfavorable local tumor control (73 % vs. 100 %, $p = 0.006$) and survival (47 % vs. 79 %, $p = 0.001$, respectively). The 2-week intra-treatment time point may be superior to the pre-therapy time point likely because the 2-week DCE MRI incorporates early therapy-specific information of responsiveness to the ongoing treatment (Yuh et al. 2009).

Diffusion-weighed imaging, which indirectly assesses tumor cellularity (Hamstra et al. 2008; Ross et al. 2003) provides another imaging biomarker in cervix cancer. The apparent diffusion coefficient (ADC) measures the magnitude of diffusion (of water molecules) within tissues. A low ADC value is indicative of increased tissue cellularity, and an increase in the ADC suggests cell death. Such an ADC increase can occur very early, within days of therapy start, prior to any morphologic changes (e.g. tumor volume) (Charles-Edwards and DeSouza 2006; Charles-Edwards et al. 2008; Chenevert et al. 2000). Early clinical experience shows that increase in ADC during ongoing radiation and chemotherapy correlates with improved tumor response (Harry et al. 2008; Naganawa et al. 2005; Liu et al. 2009). These studies suggest that both DCE-MRI and DW-MRI may have value as early imaging biomarkers of radioresponsiveness in cervical cancer.

In addition to being the most accurate assessment of lymph node involvement, FDG-PET/CT has also been used to assess the primary tumor during/after therapy. Persistent metabolic activity of the tumor 3 months after therapy has been correlated with poor outcome (Kidd et al. 2007). However, the optimal imaging timing for FDG-PET is a subject of active investigation.

3 Cancer of the Uterine Corpus

Endometrial cancer is the most common gynecologic malignancy in the United States. In 2013, 49,500 cases of endometrial cancer are expected, accounting for approximately 6 % of female malignancies, with approximately 8,200 deaths anticipated, accounting for 3 % of all female cancer deaths (Siegel et al. 2013). Mean age at diagnosis in the United States is approximately 62 years old, consistent with a disease largely occurring in postmenopausal women. SEER data show approximately 70 % of cases are diagnosed as localized disease, with an 81.5 % 5-year survival for all stages, and 95.3 % for localized disease (Howlader et al. 2013). Risk factors for endometrial cancer include diabetes, obesity, hyperestrogenic state, nulliparity, tamoxifen use, early menarche or late menopause, and anovulatory cycles (Brinton et al. 1992). Certain genetic diseases,

Table 7 FIGO and American Joint Committee on Cancer (AJCC 7th edition) TNM staging for endometrial cancer

FIGO staging (2008)	AJCC 7th edn (2009) TNM staging[a]			Description
Group	T	N	M	
IA	T1a	0	0	Limited to the endometrium or invades less than half of the myometrium
IB	T1b	0	0	Invades half or more of the myometrium
II	T2	0	0	Invades cervical stromal tissue but does not extend beyond the uterus
IIIA	T3a	0	0	Involves serosa and/or adnexa
IIIB	T3b	0	0	Vaginal involvement or parametrial involvement
IIIC1	T1–3	1	0	Metastasis to pelvic lymph nodes
IIIC2	T1–3	2	0	Metastasis to para-aortic lymph nodes
IVA	T4	Any	0	Invades bladder mucosa and/or bowel mucosa
IVB	Any	Any	1	Distant metastasis

Source Edge et al. (2009)
[a] Changes from the AJCC 6th edition and the previous FIGO staging recommendations (1988):
No longer includes uterine sarcoma (now staged with a new staging system)
Positive peritoneal cytology is no longer considered (previously was T3a/IIIA)
Involvement of the endocervical glands is not longer considered (previously was stage IIA)
Stages IA and IB combined (now: IA). IC moved to IB
Stage IIIC subdivided into IIIC1 and IIIC2

such as hereditary nonpolyposis colon cancer (HNPCC) or Lynch syndrome and Cowden disease, are associated with increased risk for endometrial cancer, with lifetime risks ranging from 10 to 60 % depending on disease and specific genetic mutation (Aarnio et al. 1995; Gustafson et al. 2007).

Most endometrial cancers are diagnosed during the workup of abnormal, or postmenopausal, vaginal bleeding. Pathologic diagnosis is essential, as both FIGO stage and FIGO histologic grade are prognostic for outcome and determine treatment. Thus, diagnosis is often made via endometrial biopsy or dilation and curettage for those patients in which endometrial biopsy is not possible or non-diagnostic. Endometrial cancers often arise within the endometrial layer, and spread by invasion into the myometrium. In more advanced disease, tumor can spread to the uterine serosa, adnexa, endocervical canal, peritoneal cavity, bowel, bladder, and other adjacent structures. Lymphatic drainage is to the pelvic lymph nodes (including the internal/external iliacs, common iliacs, obturator, presacral and parametrial), with direct spread to the para-aortic lymph nodes possible. FIGO staging requires surgical staging based on the at-risk areas of spread, therefore total hysterectomy and bilateral salpingo-oopherectomy, with or without lymph node dissection, is performed in most patients. Adjuvant therapy is then based on pathologic information that determines the stage and grade of each endometrial cancer, both of which are prognostic for patient outcome.

3.1 Staging

The gold standard for staging in endometrial cancer remains surgical staging as defined by FIGO (Creasman 2009), Table 7. Prior to the 1988 FIGO staging system, staging was clinical evaluation for tumor size, extent of disease (confined to uterus or pelvic extension), and bowel or bladder involvement. However, this was found to under-stage patients approximately 23 % of the time (Creasman et al. 1987). Therefore, FIGO staging was changed to incorporate surgical evaluation and subsequent pathologic information for staging which improved the prognostic accuracy of staging. Initially, myometrial invasion, cervical invasion (including endocervical glandular involvement), adnexal involvement, serosal involvement, positive peritoneal cytology, and lymph node status were factored into staging. On the last revision of the FIGO surgical staging for endometrial cancer (2009), peritoneal cytology and isolated endocervical glandular involvement have been removed from the criteria. Further, myometrial invasion, previously stratified into three levels of involvement, is now subdivided into only two categories; invasion of less than one-half or invasion of one-half or more of the myometrium. Lymph node positive disease is substratified to pelvic lymph node only, or para-aortic lymph node disease (IIIC1 vs. IIIC2). In summary, under 2009 FIGO staging, stage I disease now includes endometrial/myometrial only disease; stage II disease invades cervical stroma; stage III disease is a heterogenous group with IIIA including uterine serosa or adnexal involvement, IIIB involving the vagina, and IIIC1 versus IIIC2 denoting pelvic lymph node only versus any para-aortic lymph node positive disease; stage IV represents metastatic disease to other sites not included above.

Surgical staging at minimum is to include total hysterectomy and bilateral salpingo-oopherectomy (BSO). The role of extended surgical staging, with sampling and/or dissection of the pelvic and para-aortic lymph nodes, is still debated. Given the significant prognostic importance of lymph node metastasis, many advocate for lymph node histologic evaluation, and some have suggested a possible therapeutic benefit to lymphadenectomy, although not been proven in a prospective manner. While older techniques for extended surgical staging required laparotomy, more modern techniques with laparoscopic assisted methods have yielded equivalent nodal yields with reduced morbidity for many experienced gynecologic oncologists (Eltabbakh 2002; Scribner et al. 2002). Given the fact that many women with endometrial cancer are elderly, obese, and have co-morbidities such as diabetes, hypertension, and coronary artery disease, concerns exist for increased risks of deep venous thrombosis, vascular injury, or pulmonary emboli in the postoperative setting. Further, extended surgical staging followed by adjuvant radiation therapy is reported by some to carry higher enteric morbidity than hysterectomy and radiation alone (Lewandowski et al. 1990). Thus, some point to the experience of PORTEC and ASTEC trials as data to support omission of routine lymphadenectomy in low and intermediate risk patients without clinical/palpable adenopathy. PORTEC-1 included intermediate risk stage I patients, all undergoing total hysterectomy and BSO without lymphadenectomy randomized to adjuvant radiotherapy versus observation with 80–85 % overall survival at 5 years (Creutzberg et al. 2000). In ASTEC, intermediate risk patients underwent total hysterectomy-BSO, pelvic washings, and para-aortic lymph node palpation and were randomized to lymphadenectomy or no further surgery, with no statistically significant difference on overall survival at 3 years (ASTEC study group et al. 2009). Conversely, several studies support the role of maximal surgical debulking and resection of gross nodal disease, with improvement in median survival in some cohorts from 8.8 to 37.5 months (Bristow et al. 2003; Chi et al. 1997; Lambrou et al. 2004).

Of note, the American College of Obstetricians Gynecologists (ACOG) recommends comprehensive surgical staging including total hysterectomy and BSO, pelvic washings, bilateral pelvic and paraaortic lymphadenectomy, and complete resection of all disease, with exceptions considered for young or perimenopausal women with grade 1 endometrioid adenocarcinoma associated with atypical endometrial hyperplasia and those at increased risk of morbidity/mortality secondary to comorbidities (American College of Obstetricians and Gynecologists 2005). Omental sampling is also often performed, especially in papillary serous and clear cell histology due to the risk of upper abdominal spread.

Table 8 GOG 33: Rate of pelvic lymph node metastasis based on extent of myometrial invasion and FIGO grade

	Grade 1 (%)	Grade 2 (%)	Grade 3 (%)
Endometrium only	0	3	0
Inner 1/3 myometrial invasion	3	5	9
Middle 1/3 myometrial invasion	0	9	4
Deep 1/3 myometrial invasion	11	19	34

Adapted from Morrow et al. (1991). Rates of pelvic lymph node metastasis observed in 621 Stage I endometrial cancers treated primarily with surgery

3.2 Clinical Factors

3.2.1 Stage

Surgical stage continues to be one the most important clinical factors predictive of outcomes. The outcomes of 81,900 patients with endometrial cancer from 1988 to 2006 in a SEER database and a cohort of 1,268 patients from the MoMaTEC study were shown to verify the improved prognostic utility of the current 2009 FIGO staging in comparison to the FIGO 1988 staging schema (Lewin et al. 2010; Werner et al. 2012). Five year overall survival rates in early stage disease were 90–96 %, 78–87 %, and 74–80 %, respectively, for stage IA and IB and stage II. In locally advanced disease, 5-year overall survival was 48–56 %, 36–53 %, 57–60 %, and 49–53 % for stage IIIA (serosa/adnexa), IIIB (vaginal), IIIC1 (pelvic lymph node), and IIIC2 (para-aortic lymph node), respectively. Survival in stage IV disease ranged from 16 to 57 %.

3.2.2 Lymph Node Status

Lymph node status is incorporated in the staging classification above. A drop in 5-year overall survival from 74 to 96 % for stage I/II patients to 49–60 % for node positive patients is observed (Lewin et al. 2010; Werner et al. 2012). A variety of features are associated with increased risk for lymph node metastasis. The strong association of tumor grade, depth of myometrial invasion and pelvic lymph node involvement was first demonstrated in the results of GOG study 33 (Tables 8, 9) (Creasman et al. 1987). In this clinical-pathologic study, 621 stage I endometrial cancer patients, accrued from 1977 to 1983, prospectively underwent hysterectomy, selective pelvic and para-aortic lymph node dissection and peritoneal cytology. Increasing FIGO grade and increasing depth of invasion correlated with progressively higher probability of pelvic lymph node

Table 9 GOG 33: rate of para-aortic lymph node metastasis based on extent of myometrial invasion and FIGO grade

	Grade 1 (%)	Grade 2 (%)	Grade 3 (%)
Endometrium only	0	3	0
Inner 1/3 myometrial invasion	1	4	4
Middle 1/3 myometrial invasion	5	0	0
Deep 1/3 myometrial invasion	6	14	23

Adapted from Morrow et al. (1991). Rates of para-aortic lymph node metastasis observed in 621 Stage I endometrial cancers treated primarily with surgery

involvement, ranging from less than 5 % in patients without myometrial invasion, to 34 % in those with both outer third myometrial invasion and FIGO grade 3 histology.

While node positive patients as a whole have poorer survival compared to stage I and II patients, it should be noted that the predictive outcome of node positive disease should be considered in the context of the extent of other extrauterine disease. Mariani et al. examined the outcomes of 51 patients with surgically staged IIIC disease. In this cohort, it was noted that the 5-year recurrence free survival (RFS) for node positive only disease was 68 %, but dropped to 25 % in patients with node positive disease in combination with other extrauterine disease such as adnexal, vaginal, serosal involvement or positive peritoneal cytology (Mariani et al. 2002a). While this study is limited in its correlation to today's practice as few patient received chemotherapy, this poorer outcome in "higher burden" disease suggests these patient may require a more aggressive treatment approach. The overall nodal disease burden, as described by absolute number of positive lymph nodes and ratio of positive nodes to total nodes on lympadenectomy has also been shown to be prognostic in some studies (Chan et al. 2007a). Five-year disease-specific survival for those with 1, 2–5, and >5 positive nodes were 68.1, 55.1, and 46.1 %, respectively ($p < 0.001$). Percentage of positive lymph nodes was also evaluated, with 5-year disease-specific survival of 77.3 to 60.7 to 40.9 % in those with $\leq$0, >10 to $\geq$50 %, and >50 % nodes involved, respectively. Both factors were independently prognostic on multivariate analysis.

3.2.3 Adnexal and Serosal Involvement

FIGO stage IIIA is defined by serosal and/or adnexal disease spread. Adnexal involvement is associated with poorer outcomes, but is highly correlated with other adverse features such as high tumor grade, other metastatic sites, and unfavorable histology. When considering adnexal involvement in the absence of other factors, outcomes are more favorable than for all stage IIIA patients taken as a whole, with 5-year disease-free survival ranging from 71 to 86 % (Connell et al. 1999; Greven et al. 1989). Serosal involvement is associated with high risk of distant failure, owing in part to its association with other risk factors such as other sites of metastatic disease and higher stage presentation (Greven et al. 1989; Ashman et al. 2001). Similar to adnexal involvement, however, isolated serosal involvement portends an improved prognosis over all patients with serosal involvement, with 5-year disease-free survival of 41.5 % versus 20 % (Ashman et al. 2001).

3.3 Patient Factors

3.3.1 Age

Age has long been considered a risk factor for development of endometrial cancer, as well as prognostic of outcomes. In general, endometrial cancer is a disease of postmenopausal women. Younger women who develop endometrial cancer tend to have improved survival, often with risk factors such as estrogen or other hormone related-disorders, including but not limited to, infertility, polycystic ovarian syndrome, ovarian dysfunction, anovulatory cycles, and obesity (Ota et al. 2005). Young patients tend to have low grade endometrioid histology, correlating to more favorable outcomes.

While many studies have shown advanced age to be an independent predictor of worse outcomes (Kosary 1994; Abeler and Kjorstad 1991; Irwin et al. 1998), many small studies have found this to not be a prognostic factor. Some of been concerned that patient comorbidities, potential de-escalation of therapy in the elderly, or narrow cohorts, or propensity for more advanced stage at diagnosis, or more aggressive histology at diagnosis, among a multitude of other confounding factors, may explain the apparent discrepancy. Regardless, age is still part of the risk stratification of patients for selection of adjuvant therapy as is discussed below.

3.3.2 Serum CA-125

CA-125 is a serum tumor marker that can readily be tested, commonly used to monitor ovarian cancer. The role of CA-125 in endometrial cancer has been proposed to be prognostic, with elevated preoperative CA-125 levels associated with increased risk of lymph node metastasis (Chung et al. 2006). Many suggest measurement of preoperative serum CA-125 given several studies suggestive of prognostic utility (Powell et al. 2005); although no change in therapy is offered based on this value. Some have also proposed an age stratified CA-125 cutoff to improve the predictive value of CA-125 levels, with higher cutoffs proposed in younger patients (Chao et al. 2013). The NCCN guidelines designate CA-125 as an optional test in both workup and surveillance, while the American Society of Gynecologists Oncologists does not endorse the routine use of CA-125 during surveillance in the absence of clinical findings concerning for metastatic disease (Salani et al. 2011). Future studies regarding the use of CA-125 are warranted and will likely focus on its potential as a tool for prediction of extrauterine disease in early stage patients or its use during surveillance for early detection of disease recurrence and whether this translates to improved patient outcomes.

3.4 Histologic Factors

While tumor stage is the most important prognostic indicator, many of the other confirmed prognostic features relate to information from the histology of the tumor itself. Tumor cell type, grade of differentiation, and LVSI are significantly important, and assist with stratification of patients within surgical staging groups into risk categories. Thus, the results of each can have significant influence on the adjuvant therapy given, as patients with early stage, low risk histology may not require adjuvant therapy, the same stage patient with high risk histology or tumor grade may have poorer outcomes if adjuvant therapy is not offered.

3.4.1 Histology

Given that surgical staging predominates for endometrial cancer, characteristics found on pathologic evaluation are highly prognostic. Cell type and tumor grade are highly predictive of patient outcomes, and carry significant weight in determining if adjuvant therapy after hysterectomy should be offered. Additional information regarding myometrial invasion, cervical stromal invasion, lymphovascular invasion, and others have also been shown to be prognostic and are used to help stratify risk of recurrence in patients with early stage disease. The following section on histology relates to histologic factors studied largely in endometrioid adenocarcinomas. In general, non-endometrioid histologies such as papillary serous and clear cell adenocarcionoma are highly correlated with many of these adverse pathologic factors, thus are deemed high risk in even early stage disease, and are offered more aggressive adjuvant therapy.

3.4.1.1 Histologic Type

The vast majority of endometrial cancers arise within the endometrial layer of the uterus, with subsequent growth and spread, usually into the myometrium, as it progresses. Adenocarcinoma accounts for the majority of endometrial cancer cases diagnosed. The most common histologic subtype is endometrioid histology, accounting for nearly 75–80 % of endometrial cancer cases. This is a gland forming variant of adenocarcinoma, often with appearance similar to that of the endometrium. Overall prognosis for low grade endometrioid adenocarcinoma is favorable. By some reports, approximately 25 % of adenocarcinomas can have squamous differentiation, where the grade of the glandular component is prognostic (Abeler and Kjorstad 1992). Villoglandular and mucinous adenocarcinomas are infrequently identified, with no significant effect on outcomes with villoglandular (Zaino et al. 1998a), and improved outcomes with mucinous features (Ross et al. 1983). Two less common, yet clinically significant subsets of adenocarcinoma, include papillary serous and clear cell adenocarcinoma, accounting for a majority of the remaining non-endometrioid cases. Papillary serous carcinomas histologically have a complex papillary architecture, resembling serous carcinoma of the ovary. Nuclear atypia is common, and psammoma bodies can be present. Clear cell carcinomas have 3 types of growth patterns, tubulocystic, papillary, or solid patterns, and are less likely to contain psammoma bodies. Any tumor that contains 10 % or more of either papillary serous or clear cell adenocarcinoma features are classified as mixed histology, although prognosis tends to correlate with the most advanced histology in the tumor.

Endometrial cancer is subdivided into type 1 or type 2 tumors; type 1 defined as low grade (FIGO grade 1 and 2) endometrioid tumors (nearly 80 % of adenocarcinoma), and type 2 encompassing FIGO grade 3 endometroid tumors, papillary serous, and clear cell adenocarcinomas. A different etiology of tumorigenesis has been proposed in these two subgroups. Type 1 tumors are generally associated with the classical risk factors for endometrial cancer including nulliparity, obesity, unopposed estrogen, early menarche/late menopause, tamoxifen therapy, among others. It has been proposed that elevated estrogenic state experienced in these situations can stimulate the endometrial layer, leading to hyperplasia, a likely precursor to endometrial cancer in some settings. Type 2 tumors, on the other hand, are not associated with hyperestrogenism or endometrial hyperplasia. Stage by stage, more aggressive histology is associated with poorer clinical outcomes (Boruta et al. 2004). As such, type 2 tumors are often included as a risk factor warranting intensification of adjuvant therapy as discussed below.

Uterine sarcomas (endometrial stromal sarcomas, leiomyosarcomas, and other mesenchymal tumors), and mixed epithelial and mesenchymal tumors (adenosarcomas and malignant mixed mullerian tumors), are much less common types of uterine cancer. As a group, they all confer very poor prognosis at diagnosis. They tend to be associated with higher stage at diagnosis, and dismal disease free and overall survival (Prat 2009; Callister et al. 2004). More aggressive therapy is generally favored in this group of patients given their significantly higher risk for failure and death, however given the relative rarity, poor response to proposed interventions, and paucity of prospective data, there is no clearly defined guideline in management (Rauh-Hain and Del Carmen 2013; Kanthan and Senger 2011).

3.4.1.2 Tumor Grade

Across a multitude of studies, tumor grade has been shown to be strongly associated with prognosis, degree of myometrial invasion, and risk for lymph node metastasis. FIGO grading of endometrioid carcinomas incorporate the degree of gland formation and nuclear grade. The percent solid (nonglandular) growth is scored as increased solid growth is associated with more aggressive behavior. Grade 1 is defined as no more than 5 % solid growth, grade 2 with 6 to 50 percent solid growth, and grade 3 with more than 50 percent solid growth. If glandular grade is different from nuclear grade, nuclear grade predominates. Non-endometrioid tumors are graded by nuclear grade alone. Zaino et al. reported 5-year survival rates of 94 % for grade 1, 84 % for grade 2, and 72 % for grade 3 tumors (Zaino et al. 1998a). Given the significant prognostic feature of tumor grade, it is incorporated into risk stratification of patients within a given stage to help direct adjuvant therapy.

3.4.1.3 Myometrial Invasion

Degree of myometrial invasion has been shown to be an independent predictor for outcome in a multitude of studies (Creasman et al. 1987; Morrow et al. 1991). This has been validated since originally described and continues to be incorporated as part of the current FIGO staging. While risk factor groups have been described based on thirds of invasion, the most recent revision of FIGO staging has established 50 % as the cutoff between stage IA and stage IB endometrial cancer.

3.4.1.4 Cervical Stromal Invasion

Cervical stromal invasion is included in FIGO staging, given its prognostic significance in outcomes with reduced 5-year disease-free survival of 74–80 % for stage II disease compared to 90–96 % for stage IA. Previously, any cervical invasion was classified as stage II disease in the 1988 FIGO schema, with stage IIA defined as isolated endocervical epithelial involvement and stage IIB for deeper stromal invasion. However, several reports failed to demonstrate a difference in survival between the two groups (Orezzoli et al. 2009; Eltabbakh and Moore 1999). Thus, this subclassification was eliminated with the recent 2009 revision of FIGO staging and currently cervical *stromal* invasion only constitutes stage II disease. This has been shown to be independently prognostic for patient outcomes, with a 44 % increase in risk of progression or death and a 33 % increase in risk of death (Tewari et al. 2012).

3.4.1.5 Lymphovascular Space Invasion

Lymphovascular space invasion (LVSI) has been shown to be a predictor of risk of relapse and poorer survival, independent from tumor grade or depth of myometrial involvement (Morrow et al. 1991; Mariani et al. 2002b, c). LVSI has been shown to increase the rate of pelvic lymph node metastasis (Creasman et al. 1987). LVSI continues to be used as one of several histologic criteria for risk stratification for adjuvant therapy selection and clinical trial inclusion.

3.4.1.6 Peritoneal Cytology

In previous 1988 FIGO staging, the presence of malignant cells in peritoneal fluid was designated stage IIIA disease. However, multiple studies failed to show this as an independent prognostic factor (Hirai et al. 1989; Tebeu et al. 2004; Takeshima et al. 2001). The revised 2009 FIGO staging has eliminated positive peritoneal cytology as a factor in staging. However, recently Milgrom et al. showed that in stage III patients, positive peritoneal cytology was predictive of outcome and associated with distant relapse (Milgrom et al. 2013). This is consistent with the observation that positive peritoneal cytology, while not independently prognostic, may enhance the negative impact of other adverse factors (Takeshima et al. 2001). Peritoneal cytology is still obtained at most institutions during hysterectomy, as it may have some effect on adjuvant therapy selection, and is used as inclusion criteria of some ongoing phase III trials.

3.4.2 Implications of Postoperative Histology on Adjuvant Treatment

As previously discussed, multiple histologic and clinical factors have been found to be independently prognostic of clinical outcome. While some of these are directly used for staging, others are used for risk stratification to help predict a benefit from adjuvant therapy and aid in the selection of adjuvant therapy.

3.4.2.1 Risk Group Stratification in Early Stage Endometrial Cancer

Adjuvant therapy in endometrial cancer is dictated in large part by stage and risk factors within each stage. This is specifically true for early stage endometrial cancer where the extent and method of adjuvant radiotherapy has evolved.

Observation is reasonable for patients with stage IA, grade 1, favorable histology disease, otherwise deemed low risk. In patients with stage I disease, and any risk factor, including Grade 2–3 disease, LVSI, lower uterine segment involvement, deep myometrial invasion, or advanced age > 50–70, adjuvant therapy has traditionally been considered. Previously, the GOG 33 data demonstrated advanced grade or deep myometrial invasion were risk factors for lymph node positive disease, which was associated with worse disease free survival. These risk factors had been employed to determine the need for postoperative pelvic radiation, but how to much weight to assign these risk factors has evolved.

The traditional indications for pelvic radiation in early stage disease have been challenged by the results of the Post-Operative Radiation Therapy in Endometrial Cancer (PORTEC) (Creutzberg et al. 2003, 2004) and GOG 99 (Keys et al. 2004) studies, resulting in identification of a new set of risk factors. This paradigm change has also been fueled by advances in surgical approach over the past 2 decades, with a more comprehensive degree of lymph node dissection, even in co-morbid patients. Based on both trials' results, a new high-intermediate risk group was defined by each cooperative group and a more multi-faceted algorithm was developed that incorporated grade, depth of myometrial invasion, LVSI, and age. PORTEC's and GOG 99's results are highly consistent showing an incidence of failure in the 30 % range for the GOG-defined high-intermediate-risk group and for the grade 3 group in PORTEC. The high-intermediate-risk group was defined by GOG as (1) grade 2–3 with deep third myometrial invasion and LVSI; or (2) age > 50 and two of the risk factors in (1); or (3) age > 70 and one of the risk factors in (1). The definition based on the PORTEC data is similar: <50 % myometrial invasion and grade 3 (any age); or >50 % invasion and grade 1–2 and age > 60 years. However, the combination of <50 % myometrial invasion, grade 3 and LVSI is considered a high-risk feature by PORTEC-2 due to the significantly lower 5-year overall survival of 58 % observed in the PORTEC 1 study (Creutzberg et al. et al. 2004). These overall results are supported by a metaanalysis by Kong et al. (2007) of all four randomized trials (Creutzberg et al. 2000, 2004; Keys et al. 2004; Aalders et al. 1980) that shows adjuvant radiotherapy improved disease specific and overall survival for patients with grade 3 tumors and stage IB (>50 % invasion) disease. The failure pattern in the high-intermediate-risk group has been found to consist largely of vaginal recurrences, therefore, while the high risk patients are often recommended pelvic radiotherapy, high-intermediate risk group patients are often offered vaginal cuff brachytherapy and/or pelvic radiotherapy as vaginal recurrences are the most likely site of failure. This group has been studied by PORTEC-2, and vaginal cuff brachytherapy was found to be equivalent in preventing pelvic recurrence to whole pelvic radiation (Nout et al. 2010).

Adjuvant therapy for high risk disease is an area of active research as there is data to suggest intensifying therapy with chemotherapy is warranted, and currently practiced at many institutions. PORTEC-3 is currently enrolling patients with the high risk criteria and randomizing patients postoperatively to pelvic radiation or pelvic radiation with concurrent and post-radiation chemotherapy. Eligible patients include those with <50 % myometrial invasion plus grade 3 and LVSI; >50 % myometrial invasion with grade 3, or advanced endometrial cancer, including stage II–III disease, papillary serous or clear cell histologies. The results are eagerly anticipated.

3.4.2.2 Locally Advanced Endometrial Cancer

Stage III and IVA endometrial cancer is often described as locally advanced endometrial cancer. This group represents a heterogenous group of patients, with varying degrees of tumor burden and tumor histology, with the best adjuvant therapy not clearly defined. GOG 122 established a role for chemotherapy over whole abdominal radiation owing to improved disease free and overall survival of 38–50 %, and 42–55 %, respectively (Randall et al. 2006). More recently, Hogberg et al. compiled the data from two randomized European trials, NSGO-EC-9501/EORTC-55991 and MaNGO ILIADE-III, which randomized patients to adjuvant radiotherapy alone or sequential chemotherapy and radiation therapy. This indicated a significant improvement in 5-year progression-free survival from 69 to 78 %, with a trend for improved overall survival (Hogberg et al. 2010). The extent of radiotherapy, timing with chemotherapy, and patient selection is still an area of active study.

3.4.3 Molecular Markers

Molecular markers are an area of active interest. In most cases, markers are correlated with established prognostic indicators, such as tumor histology and grade. Some of the most studied factors are briefly reviewed. To date, the clinical utility of these markers is limited.

3.4.3.1 DNA Ploidy

DNA content, or more specifically, aneuploidy, has been studied by many groups. The frequency of aneuploidy has been shown to increase with increased tumor grade (Lundgren et al. 2002). Papillary serous carcinoma has been shown to exhibit aneuploidy, as well (Prat et al. 1994). Further, DNA aneuploidy has been shown to be an independent predictor for disease free survival (Zaino et al. 1998b; Nordstrom et al. 1996).

3.4.3.2 Microsatellite Instability

Microsatellite instability (MSI) is strongly associated with endometrial cancer in patient with HNPCC, occurring in nearly 75 % of such patients, and occurs in approximately 25–45 % of sporadic endometrial carcinomas. Microsatellites are short repeats of DNA that are integrated throughout the genome, and MSI is associated with deficits in DNA mismatch repair. In some studies, MSI is associated with improved clinical outcome (Maxwell et al. 2001). However, there is discrepancy in the published literature, with several reports showing no correlation with clinical outcome (Zighelboim et al. 2007; Baldinu et al. 2002), while others have shown MSI to be an independent prognostic indicator for poorer survival (Mackay et al. 2010; Nout et al. 2012; Steinbakk et al. 2011). This disagreement may be related to sample size, cohort selection, different adjuvant therapies, confounding variables, or may indicate identification of the specific downstream genetic alterations is actually more relevant (Steinbakk et al. 2011).

3.4.3.3 Ki-67 Proliferation Index

Cellular proliferation is an area of interest in most cancer cell types. This has also been evaluated by many groups for endometrial cancer. Nuclear Ki-67 antigen is a marker of proliferating cells, and has been shown to be associated with histological grade and depth of myometrial invasion, as well as other risk factors (Kudela et al. 2012). High levels of Ki-67 expression have also been associated with increased risk of recurrence and poorer survival in some studies (Salvesen et al. 1998).

3.4.3.4 Oncogenes

HER2 and EGFR are both members of the ErbB/HER signaling family, a group of tyrosine kinase receptors critical in cellular proliferation and differentiation, and are implicated in tumorigenesis in many tumor models. HER2 expression was associated with higher tumor grade and depth of myometrial invasion but not independently prognostic for survival, whereas EGFR overexpression in endometrioid adenocarcinoma decreased survival from 89 to 69 % ($p < 0.04$), and in serous papillary and clear cell from 86 to 27 % ($p < 0.03$) (Khalifa et al. 1994; Konecny et al. 2009). There is continued interest in this pathway as inhibitors of EGFR and HER2 are actively used in other cancer treatment and exploitation of this pathway with these pharmaceuticals theoretically may improve patient outcomes.

P53 has been reported to be more highly expressed in type 2 tumors (Kudela et al. 2012). Not surprisingly, this has also been correlated with poorer patient outcomes (Mariani et al. 2000; Saffari et al. 2005; Silverman et al. 2000). Currently, clinical utility of this marker is uncertain as no targeted therapies are readily available.

The evaluation of PTEN as a prognostic factor is also controversial. PTEN is a tumor suppressor gene that down regulates the PI3-Kinase pathway, thus slowing down cellular proliferation. PTEN is mutated in approximately 20–80 % of endometrial cancers, but with less frequency in serous carcinoma. Results regarding the effect of PTEN on patient outcomes is mixed (Latta and Chapman 2002).

3.4.3.5 Cell Adhesion Molecules

Cell adhesion molecules have been widely studied in tumor biology, and are responsible in part for coordinating cell–cell interaction, cellular proliferation, and metastasis. E-cadherin is a cell membrane protein that complexes with cytoplasmic B-catenin regulating cellular adhesion and growth. The loss of E-cadherin expression results in release of B-catenin, which is then able to induce a subset of genes responsible for endothelial to mesenchymal transition which is one mechanism by which tumorigenesis and metastasis is thought to occur. Loss of E-cadherin expression is commonly seen in non-endometrioid endometrial carcinoma, but occasionally in endometrioid histology (Holcomb et al. 2002; Mell et al. 2004). Although in the same pathway, B-catenin has not been found to be independently prognostic of clinical outcomes (Nout et al. 2012; Singh et al. 2011).

3.4.3.6 Steroid Receptors

Expression of estrogen receptor (ER) and progesterone receptor (PR) has been extensively examined, given hormonally directed therapy is of particular interest in patients who may not be surgical candidates or have otherwise limited treatment options. Some studies indicate ER and PR expression are associated with less aggressive tumor behavior/grade (Ferrandina et al. 2005; Geisinger et al. 1986; Kadar et al. 1993; Jeon et al. 2006). While progestins are often used in relapsed or advanced disease, a recent metaanalysis indicates there is no data at present to support its use in primary disease (Martin-Hirsch et al. 2011); prospective evaluation of receptor expression and treatment response is warranted.

3.5 Imaging Prognostic Factors

FIGO staging for endometrial cancer by definition requires surgical staging. In the United States, a majority of centers include routine pelvic lymphadenectomy and para-aortic lymph node sampling at the time of hysterectomy. Morbidity is associated with such extended surgery, although has improved with advances in surgical technology. Further, the ASTEC trial, albeit with relatively limited follow-up, to date has not shown a survival benefit to lymphadenectomy in early stage disease (ASTEC study group et al. 2009). Thus, there is great interest in developing new ways to predict risk of lymph node involvement, and to identify those patients with acceptably low risk of involvement in order to identify patients where omission of lymphadenectomy is reasonable. While clinical exam prior to 1988 was shown to understage endometrial cancer in 13–22 % of patients, newer imaging technology is now available, and may be promising in identification of factors such as myometrial invasion, extrauterine involvement, as well as risk of pelvic lymph node disease. These are briefly reviewed here.

3.5.1 Morphologic Imaging

Computed tomography (CT) has been used for preoperative assessment in endometrial cancer, but its role is with limitations. The ability of CT to delineate endometrial cancer in the uterus is relatively insensitive, especially for small endometrial cancers (i.e. stage IA), with overall sensitivity of 53 % (Grossman et al. 2008). Accuracy of CT for myometrial invasion has been reported to be 61 % with sensitivity of 40 % in one study comparing ultrasound, CT, and MRI for depth of myometrial invasion assessment (Kim et al. 1995). Multidetector CT has improved accuracy for depth of myometrial invasion and cervical involvement at 95 and 81 %, respectively (Tsili et al. 2008). The applicability of this modality is limited given this single experience in 16 patients, thus warrants further evaluation. Sensitivity and specificity of CT for lymph node involvement has been reported at 52 and 92 %, respectively (Connor et al. 2000). Chest CT can be considered in high risk patients, such as advanced stage or high grade tumors who are at increased risk for pulmonary metastasis.

The accuracy of ultrasound for myometrial invasion has been described by many groups. The accuracy of transvaginal ultrasound (TVUS) for predicting stage IA versus stage IB endometrial cancer reportedly ranges from 69 to 93 % (Kim et al. 1995; DelMaschio et al. 1993; Prompeler et al. 1994). High-frequency TVUS has been shown to have accuracy of 73 % for assessment of myometrial invasion (Arko and Takac 2000). The reported experience of ultrasonography to predict cervical involvement has also been limited, with only 7 of 10 patients with pathologic cervical involvement reported pretherapy to have involvement based on ultrasound (Akbayir et al. 2011; Szantho et al. 2001). The use of 3D ultrasonography with volume contrast imaging has also been described. Jantarasaengaram et al. reported accuracy of 92 % for predicting myometrial invasion and 90 % for cervical involvement (Jantarasaengaram et al. 2013). Sonohysterography, which involves intracavitary infusion of saline followed by evaluation with TVUS, has been employed in some settings, with accuracies of 84–89 % for assessing deep myometrial invasion (Chang et al. 2010; Valenzano et al. 2001; Dessole et al. 2006). The use of this modality is controversial, however, due to concern of tumor spillage into the peritoneal cavity with saline infusion, which has been documented by some investigators (Dessole et al. 2006; Alcazar et al. 2000).

The use of ultrasound has been compared to MRI in multiple investigations, and consistently has been found to be superior to ultrasound for evaluation of cervical involvement and depth of myometrial invasion (Kim et al. 1995; DelMaschio et al. 1993; Arko and Takac 2000; Antonsen et al. 2013a; Yamashita et al. 1993a). Further, contrast enhanced MRI, compared to unenhanced MRI, results in significantly improved accuracy, ranging from 85 to 92 % accuracy for depth of myometrial invasion versus 55–78 % for non-contrasted imaging (Kinkel et al. 1999; Ito et al. 1994; Saez et al. 2000; Sironi et al. 1992; Yamashita et al. 1993b; Sala et al. 2009). Accuracy rates for determination of cervical involvement range from 86 to 95 % (Manfredi et al. 2004; Takahashi et al. 1995; Nagar et al. 2006). The use of MRI for pelvic and para-aortic lymph node involvement is comparable to CT, with sensitivity and specificity reported at 44–66 % and 73–98 %, respectively. Thus, given MRI's superior assessment of depth of myometrial invasion and cervical involvement, it is generally preferred over CT and ultrasound for preoperative workup.

3.5.2 Functional Imaging

The use of PET/CT in endometrial cancer is an area of active investigation. A recent meta-analysis of 18F-FDG PET or PET/CT for identification of metastatic lymph nodes in endometrial cancer reported the pooled estimates for 243 patients, indicating sensitivity and specificity of 63 % (95 % CI, 48.7–75.7 %) and 94.7 % (95 % CI, 90.4–97.4 %), respectively (Chang et al. 2012). The relatively low sensitivity is uncertain, but may be related to low glucose metabolism in low grade lesions, as well as limited ability to detect subcentimeter metastases. Further, PET imaging is limited in ability to detect intraperitoneal tumor implants and parenchymal implants. Due to these limitations, CT and MRI are preferable for detection of extrauterine disease, although FDG-PET may be appropriate in patients with high grade tumor that is likely to be FDG avid (Lee et al. 2011).

The role for PET/CT for assessment of myometrial invasion and cervical invasion is uncertain. Antonsen et al. recently reported the results of 318 patients with endometrial cancer who preoperatively underwent 2D ultrasonography, MRI, and PET/CT imaging. Sensitivity, specificity, and accuracy for PET/CT for myometrial invasion were 93, 49, and 61 %, and 43, 94, and 83 %, respectively for cervical invasion, which were similar to MRI (Antonsen et al. 2013a).

SUVmax has been evaluated by some groups, with limited data suggesting SUVmax may be able to predict higher stage disease, higher grade tumors, risk of deeper myometrial invasion, and lymph node metastatic risk (Antonsen et al. 2013b; Nakamura et al. 2010). Other studies have indicated SUVmax can also predict for poor disease free survival (Kitajima et al. 2012) and overall survival (Nakamura et al. 2011, 2013).

Finally, 18F-FDG PET or PET/CT has also been used for detection of recurrent disease (Park et al. 2008; Belhocine et al. 2002; Chung et al. 2008; Kitajima et al. 2008).

Saga et al. assessed the use of 18F-FDG PET in 21 patients for detection of recurrence and evaluation of treatment response. Compared to conventional imaging and serum tumor markers, FDG-PET combined with CT or MRI was more accurate and had comparable or better sensitivity and specificity (Saga et al. 2003). Currently, the ACR guidelines indicate that FDG-PET is usually appropriate over MRI pelvis or CT pelvis if recurrence is suspected clinically (Lee et al. 2011).

4 Cancer of the Vulva

Vulvar cancer is a rare disease, accounting for only 5 % of malignancies of the female genital tract (Siegel et al. 2012). It is estimated that in 2013 there will be approximately 4,700 new cases and 900 deaths due to this disease in the United States (Siegel et al. 2012). The mean age at diagnosis for vulvar cancer is 65 years, and clinical risk factors for this disease include immunodeficiency, prior history of cervical cancer, cigarette smoking, vulvar dystrophy, vulvar or cervical intraepithelial neoplasia, and HPV infection (Ansink 1996; Madsen et al. 2008).

Vulvar cancer is a disease of the skin, arising from squamous epithelium, and tumor spread occurs primarily through the lymphatic system. The first station of nodal spread is the inguino-femoral lymph nodes, usually superficial first then deep, which then spreads in a predictable fashion to the pelvic lymph nodes in more advanced cases. Pelvic lymph node involvement without inguinal node involvement is rare (Krupp and Bohm 1978). Locally, vulvar cancer can invade adjacent structures including the vagina, bladder, anus and rectum. Given the propensity of this type of cancer to spread to adjacent structures and metastasize to lymph nodes, standard of care had previously been *en bloc* resection of the primary tumor with inguinofemoral lymph node dissection, resulting in significant risk of morbidity and psychosexual impact. However, the approach to treatment has evolved over the last several decades, with therapy ranging from wide local excision for small, superficial lesions, to definitive or neoadjuvant chemo-radiation which may reduce the extent of surgical resection required, versus pelvic exenteration in advanced disease.

4.1 Staging

Prognostic factors for vulvar cancer include size and local extension of the primary tumor, as well as the degree of lymphatic involvement, as reflected in the most recent (2009) version of the FIGO staging system (Hacker 2009), Table 10. As with other gynecologic malignancies, the FIGO staging system is a clinicopathologic staging system and formal recommendations for the staging evaluation for vulvar cancer have not been established. The extent and size of the primary tumor is established by clinical examination, often by EUA, including colposcopy, excisional biopsy or FNA of clinically positive inguinal nodes, and/or cystoscopy and proctoscopy based on presentation in advanced disease. Clinical palpation alone does not have a high degree of specificity or sensitivity for inguino-femoral adenopathy (Homesley et al. 1993; Franklin 1972; Selman et al. 2005). Thus, imaging modalities such as MRI and PET/CT, as well as CT of the chest, abdomen, and pelvis are also typically employed, particularly to evaluate for lymph node involvement. Several studies have shown that MRI may be useful in evaluating the inguinofemoral lymph nodes (Singh et al. 2006; Sohaib et al. 2002). However, it is important to note that radiologic findings cannot be used as a substitute for pathologic assessment of the nodes.

The gold standard for pathologic assessment of the inguinofemoral lymph nodes is lymphadenectomy. However, this carries a significant risk for morbidity. Recently, studies have evaluated the utility of sentinel lymph node biopsy, rather than lymphadenctomy in select patients as this technique carries less morbidity (Hefler et al. 2008). Comparison of sentinel lymph node biopsy to lymphadenectomy in a phase II GOG study showed that a sentinel lymph node can be found in 92 % of patients, and is 92 % sensitive, with a false negative rate of 2 % in patients with tumor less than 4 cm in size (Levenback et al. 2012). Information from sentinel lymphadenectomy has not yet been incorporated into the staging system. However, data from the recent GROINSS-V study indicates that the disease burden identified in the sentinel node is a sensitive indicator of prognosis (Oonk et al. 2010).

4.2 Clinical Factors

Lymph node involvement and size and extent of primary tumor are the strongest prognostic indicators in vulvar cancer, thus the 2009 FIGO staging system incorporates both factors. In the past, wide local excision or en bloc resection with bilateral inguinofemoral lymph node dissection was the standard surgical approach. However, bilateral lymphadenectomy carries significant risk for morbidity, both in the short and long term due to wound complications, infection, and lymphedema. Therefore, efforts are made to identify a cohort of patients that may not require lymph node dissection, albeit with an abundance of caution. In early vulvar cancer, appropriate management of the lymph nodes is the single most important factor in decreasing mortality as recurrence in the undissected inguino-femoral lymph nodes results in higher mortality

Table 10 AJCC TNM and FIGO staging of vulvar cancer

TNM	FIGO	Description
Primary tumor (T)		
TX		Primary tumor cannot be assessed
T0		No evidence of primary tumor
Tis[a]		Carcinoma in situ
T1[a]	IA	Lesions 2 cm or less in size, confi ned to the vulva or perineum and with stromal invasion 1.0 mm or less[b]
T1[b]	IB	Lesions more than 2 cm in size *or* any size with stromal invasion more than 1.0 mm, confined to the vulva or perineum
T2[c]	II	Tumor of any size with extension to adjacent perineal structures (lower/distal third of urethra, lower/distal third vagina, anal involvement)
T3[d]	IVA	Tumor of any size with extension to any of the following: upper/ proximal two thirds of urethra, upper/proximal two thirds of vagina, bladder mucosa, rectal mucosa, or fixed to pelvic bone
Regional lymph nodes (N)[e]		
NX		Regional lymph nodes cannot be assessed
N0		No regional lymph node metastasis
N1[a]	IIIA	One lymph node metastasis each 5 mm or less
N1[b]	IIIB	One lymph node metastasis 5 mm or greater
N2[a]	IIIB	Three or more lymph node metastases each less than 5 mm
N2[b]	IIIB	Two or more lymph node metastases 5 mm or greater
N2[c]	IIIC	Lymph node metastasis with extracapsular spread
N3	IVA	Fixed or ulcerated regional lymph node metastasis
Distant metastasis (M)		
MX		Distant metastasis cannot be assessed
M0		No distant metastasis
M1	IVB	Distant metastasis (including pelvic lymph node metastasis)

Source Edge et al. (2009)

[a] FIGO no longer includes stage 0 (Tis)

[b] The depth of invasion is defined as the measurement of the tumor from the epithelial–stromal junction of the adjacent most superficial dermal papilla to the deepest point of invasion

[c] FIGO used the classification T2/T3. This is defined as T2 in TNM

[d] FIGO used the classification T4. This is defined as T3 in TNM

[e] An effort should be made to describe the site and laterality of lymph node metastasis

(Cormio et al. 2010). Tumor size and depth of invasion can help predict for risk of lymph node involvement, therefore, combined with clinical exam and imaging, the decision for surgical evaluation of lymph nodes is determined.

4.2.1 Stage

In the 1988 FIGO staging system, prognosis was well distributed among the stage categories with 89 % 5-year survival for stage I, 85 % for stage II, 74 % for stage III and 31 % for stage IV (Homesley et al. 1991). However stage III consisted of a heterogeneous group of patients, with survival ranging from 30 to 100 %. The current revised 2009 FIGO staging system improves upon the prior staging schema by including more detailed information regarding the extent of lymph node involvement by subdividing the category into Stage IIIA and IIIB based on size and number of lymph nodes, or extracapsular spread (Stage IIIC), all of which are reported to closely correlate with prognosis (Homesley et al. 1991; Hacker et al. 1983; Lataifeh et al. 2004; Origoni et al. 1992; Raspagliesi et al. 2006; Fons et al. 2009a; Woelber et al. 2009). Several recent studies have validated the prognostic utility of these expanded stage categories (Tan et al. 2012; Tabbaa et al. 2012).

4.2.2 Tumor Volume

While lymph node involvement is the most important outcome predictor in multivariate analysis, tumor size has been shown to be an independent prognostic factor for local recurrence (Rutledge et al. 1970). However, in several larger contemporary series, tumor size does not independently predict disease free and overall survival on multivariate analysis (Raspagliesi et al. 2006; Tantipalakorn et al. 2009), although associations between T-stage and local recurrence-free and disease-free survival are seen in univariate analysis in a large series of 215 patients with reported local recurrence-free survival and disease-free survival rates of 85 and 88 % in T1 lesions, 74 and 61 % in T2 and 69 % and 37 % for T3/4 tumors (Rouzier et al. 2002). Finally, tumor size correlates closely with the probability of lymph node involvement, thereby likely conferring worse prognosis through its association with this unfavorable risk factor. The incidence of lymph node involvement is 5–8 % for tumors <1 cm and increases to 24 % for 1–2 cm, 31 % for 2–3 cm and 36 % for 3–5 cm tumors (Gonzalez Bosquet et al. 2003; Boyce et al. 1985).

4.3 Patient Factors

4.3.1 Age

While the mean age at diagnosis of vulvar cancer is 65, advanced age is a prognostic factor for increased risk of groin node metastasis and worse survival (Homesley et al. 1993; Sznurkowski et al. 2013; Blecharz et al. 2008; Ramanah et al. 2012). However, this variable has not been significant in some cohorts when adjusted for stage, lymph node status, and surgical therapy (Raspagliesi et al. 2006; Woelber et al. 2009; Burger et al. 1995).

4.3.2 Hemoglobin

As in many cancers, tumor hypoxia is thought to be one factor for poor prognosis. Vulvar cancer patients with anemia have been found to have higher incidence of inguinal lymph node metastasis (Stone et al. 2005; van de Nieuwenhof et al. 2010). On univariate analysis, Hefler et al. showed hemoglobin <12 g/dl resulted in shorter survival, similar to van de Nieuwenhof et al. that showed hemoglobin <11.3 g/dl was an independent predictor of poorer survival (van de Nieuwenhof et al. 2010; Hefler et al. 2000). Interestingly, this did not correlate with expression of hypoxia markers GLUT-1 nor CA-IX. Further evaluation of this variable has not been studied, therefore clinical utility is uncertain, as anemia may simply be a marker of poorer overall health.

4.4 Histologic Factors

4.4.1 Histology

Nearly 85–90 % of vulvar malignancies are squamous cell carcinoma. Melanoma is the second most common while other histologies such as basal cell carcinoma, Bartholin's gland adenocarcinoma, Merkel cell and sarcomas are more rare (Hunter 1975; Finan and Barre 2003; Sugiyama et al. 2007; Stang et al. 2005; Ragnarsson-Olding et al. 1993; Weinstock 1994). Squamous cell carcinoma are often classified into one of two types; classic, warty, Bowenoid type or keratinizing, differentiated, simplex type. Squamous cell carcinoma of the vulva often arise in the setting of premalignant conditions such as vulvar intraepithelial neoplasia (VIN) or other areas of chronic inflammation such as lichen sclerosis Bowen's disease, Paget's disease, and erythroplasia of Queyrat (Carlson et al. 1998; Kutlubay et al. 2013). A large subset of premalignant conditions, particularly usual type VIN, are associated with HPV infection and are more likely to be observed in young women or smokers and warty or basaloid type squamous cell tumors. Conversely, keratinizing type is more often reported in older women in the setting of chronic inflammation such as lichen sclerosis (Hildesheim et al. 1997; de Koning et al. 2008; Del Pino et al. 2013). This dichotomy is thought to be a result of two different tumorigenic mechanisms that can result in vulvar squamous cell carcinoma, HPV dependent or independent mechanisms. Several reports indicate patients with HPV positive tumors have better survival than those with HPV negative tumors (Lindell et al. 2010).

Data supporting prognostic implications of tumor grade or LVSI is varied. In multiple studies, higher tumor grade is associated with increased risk for lymph node metastasis and worse overall survival (Homesley et al. 1993; Sznurkowski et al. 2013; Podratz et al. 1983; Lavie et al. 1999). However, it was not a significant variable for survival according to Burger et al. or Lataifeh et al. (Lataifeh et al. 2004; Burger et al. 1995). LVSI is associated with increased risk of lymph node metastasis (Homesley et al. 1993; Husseinzadeh et al. 1990; Binder et al. 1990) and is significant for overall survival on univariate analysis (Lataifeh et al. 2004; Raspagliesi et al. 2006; Burger et al. 1995; Knopp et al. 2004; Paladini et al. 1994), but only retains significance on multivariate analysis in a select few reports (Raspagliesi et al. 2006; Knopp et al. 2004).

4.4.2 Depth of Invasion

Depth of tumor invasion, defined as the distance from the epithelial/stromal junction to the deepest point of invasion, correlates strongly with lymph node involvement. While the risk of lymph node involvement for tumors with < 1 mm invasion is essentially nil, it increases to 6 % for 1–2 mm depth of invasion, 8 % for 2–3 mm, 22 % for 3–4 mm, 25 % for 4–5 mm and 38 % for > 5 mm depth of invasion. Lymph node dissection is therefore recommended for tumors with a depth of invasion of >1 mm (Berek and Hacker 1989). Similar criteria should be applied for the decision of adjuvant radiation in un-dissected groins. Other investigators observed variable threshold level of 3 mm (Woelber et al. 2009) and 9 mm as predictors of relapse and survival (Nicoletto et al. 2010).

4.4.3 Surgical Margins

A clear association between surgical margins and local failure has been shown. Microscopic margins of <8 mm (in formalin fixed tissue) are associated with a local recurrence rate of 48 %, compared to no recurrences with wider

Table 11 The effect of positive lymph nodes on cancer specific survival

	Negative LN	1–2 + LN	3 + LN
Homesley et al. (1993)	91 %	75 %	36 %, [*5–6 LN:24 %, *7 LN: 0 %]
Hacker et al. (1983)	94 % (0–1 LN)	80 % (2 LN)	12 % (≥ 3 LN)
Origoni et al. (1992)	–	55 % (≤3 LN)	22 % (> 3 LN)
Chan et al. (2007b)	–	92 % (≤2 LN)	30 % (> 2: LN)

LN lymph node

margins (Heaps et al. 1990). This correlation has been substantiated in a more recent study showing a 23 % incidence of local recurrence in patients with margin distance of < 8 mm, compared to no recurrences in those with >8 mm margins (Chan et al. 2007b). Adjuvant radiotherapy significantly reduces local recurrence rates for both close and positive margins and improved survival (Faul et al. 1997; Viswanathan et al. 2013).

4.4.4 Histopathologic Lymph Node Status

Lymph node status is the single most significant prognostic factor in vulvar cancer. Lymph node positivity has a profoundly adverse effect on treatment outcome, with survival declining from >90 % in patients with negative lymph nodes to as low as 30 % or less in those with involved lymph nodes (Homesley et al. 1993; Hacker et al. 1983; Origoni et al. 1992; Rutledge et al. 1970; Podratz et al. 1983; Chan et al. 2007b; Iversen et al. 1980).

Number and pathologic extent of the lymph node involvement are of paramount importance for prognosis (Table 11). Patients with involvement of one lymph node and small primary tumors tend to have a survival above 90 %, whereas survival is reduced below 35 % in those with 2 or more nodes (Homesley et al. 1991). In a large single institution study of 389 patients, nodal status was the most significant independent prognostic factor, followed by LVSI. Within the node-positive group, percentage of nodal replacement and extracapsular spread independently predicted outcome (Raspagliesi et al. 2006).

The prognostic significance of bilaterality of LN involvement has remained controversial, some suggesting that it influences outcome (Burger et al. 1995; Fons et al. 2009b), while others find no correlation when the number of lymph nodes is also considered (Hacker et al. 1983; Raspagliesi et al. 2006). Of note, the most recent revision of the FIGO staging has eliminated laterality of lymph node involvement in favor or number and size, and the presence or absence of extracapsular extension.

Recommendations regarding adjuvant therapy have been informed in part by GOG 37, in which 114 patients who underwent radical vulvectomy and bilateral inguino-femoral lymph node dissection, and with positive lymph nodes were randomized to adjuvant bilateral inguinal and pelvic radiation versus pelvic node dissection (Homesley et al. 1986). Patients with >2 involved inguinal nodes showed a significant benefit from adjuvant radiotherapy over surgery. The study was underpowered to draw clear conclusions on involvement of one or two lymph nodes. However, single-institution studies suggest that gross involvement of a single node also has a substantial recurrence risk, particularly if extranodal extension is present, and warrants consideration of adjuvant therapy (Origoni et al. 1992; Ansink et al. 1991).

4.4.5 Molecular Markers

4.4.5.1 DNA Ploidy

Aneuploidy has been reported to correlate with other poor prognostic factors, and has been reported to predict for worse outcome (Lerma et al. 1999; Mariani et al. 1998), although other studies have shown no significant relationship (Knopp et al. 2004; Dolan et al. 1993).

4.4.5.2 HPV Dependence and Independence

HPV positive tumors, which occurs more commonly in younger patients, may be associated with a better prognosis (Monk et al. 1995; Ansink et al. 1994). Given that vulvar cancer is thought to be driven by HPV-dependent and independent pathways, several groups have looked at associated markers. Basaloid and warty tumors, often considered HPV-dependent tumors, often express p16, and are p53 negative, whereas keratinized tumors, classically HPV-independent tumors, are p16 negative and p53 positive (Santos et al. 2004; Kruse et al. 2008). Investigators have also explored if markers of HPV infection, such as $p16^{INK4a}$, a protein that is increased due to HPV E7 oncogene activity, is prognostic in vulvar cancer. Knopp et al. and Tringler et al. showed high expression was associated with improved survival on univariate, but not multivariate analysis (Knopp et al. 2004; Tringler et al. 2007). The expression of p53 has also been associated with poorer overall survival in several studies (Hoffmann et al. 1999; Scheistroen et al. 1999; Kohlberger et al. 1995). Of note, in Scheistrøen et al., this was only found in stage III vulvar cancer, and not stage I and II disease. Kagie et al. and McConnell et al. did not find p53 overexpression to be a significant prognostic indicator, but did note its presence in adjoining premalignant lesions, such as VIN, perhaps indicating it as a marker for malignant transformation from precursor lesions (Kagie et al. 1997; McConnell et al. 1997).

4.4.5.3 ErbB/HER Signaling Family

HER2 and EGFR expression have also been identified in a variety of small studies as prognostic indicators for clinical outcome. HER2 and EGFR overexpression has been identified in 47 and 67 % of vulvar cancers, respectively (Hantschmann et al. 2005; Johnson et al. 1997). Further, both HER2 and EGFR expression has been associated with increased risk for lymph node metastasis, while EGFR overexpression, in the absence of HPV infection, is associated with decreased survival (Johnson et al. 1997; Gordinier et al. 1997; Woelber et al. 2012; Growdon et al. 2008). Given that small molecule EGFR tyrosine kinase inhibitors and HER2 directed therapies are available, this may represent a cohort of patients that may benefit from targeted therapies in the future.

4.4.5.4 Angiogenic Factors

Increased VEGF expression is associated with increased microvessel density, and has been associated with poorer survival (Jach et al. 2011; Obermair et al. 1996). CA IX, often associated with hypoxia, is up-regulated in various solid tumors, including vulvar cancer. High intratumoral expression has been associated with unfavorable disease-free survival (Kock et al. 2011; Choschzick et al. 2010). Interestingly, higher serum CA IX preoperatively was also associated with unfavorable prognosis (HR 7.2 $p = 0.02$) (Kock et al. 2011). The clinical utility of such measurements is uncertain.

4.4.5.5 Microarray Identified Factors

Several groups have employed microarray techniques to try to identify prognostic markers, or therapeutic targets, in vulvar cancer (Kowalewska et al. 2012; Fons et al. 2007), some of which were significantly associated with worse disease free survival including cyclooxygenase 2 and Caspase 3, (Fons et al. 2007) and SFN, CA12 and JUP which are associated with increased nodal recurrence risk and earlier time to recurrence (Kowalewska et al. 2012). However, given the limited number of cases, and unknown mechanism of these markers, further studies will be needed in order to verify any prognostic or therapeutic potential.

4.5 Treatment Related Factors

Vulvar cancer is primarily surgically treated disease, while radiation therapy plays a major role in adjuvant therapy and in locally advanced unresectable disease. Over time, the surgical approach has become more tailored toward clinical stage at presentation, with wide local excision acceptable for stage IA lesions, and the use of sentinel lymph node biopsy instead of lymphadenectomy in lateralized, clinically negative, early stage patients at the time of primary treatment with vulvectomy result in reduced morbidity without compromise in local control (Levenback et al. 2012; Van der Zee et al. 2008).

The approach to locally advanced disease has also evolved. More recently, the use of neoadjuvant chemotherapy and/or radiation or definitive chemoradiotherapy have been investigated. Patients with locally advanced unresectable vulvar cancer treated on the GOG 101 and 205 studies received neoadjuvant concurrent radiation and chemotherapy prior to resection of residual disease (Moore et al. 2012; Montana et al. 2000). Response to neoadjuvant therapy was a powerful predictor of local control and survival. In GOG 205, among the patients who completed therapy, 64 % achieved a complete clinical response and 50 % of patients achieved a complete pathological response (Moore et al. 2012). Among those with pathological response, local control was 75 % (22/29), and 3 local failures were salvageable with surgical resection; thus 25/29 patients with complete pathologic response are disease free. Conversely, only 43 % (9/21) of patients with incomplete response survived. Among those who did not undergo resection of persistent tumor, none survived.

4.6 Imaging Prognostic Factors

As treatment of vulvar cancer has evolved from radical vulvectomy and bilateral inguino-femoral lymphadenectomy to a more tailored surgical and neoadjuvant chemoradiation approach, the accuracy of pre-treatment staging is increasingly important.

Imaging prognostic factors have not been clearly identified in vulvar cancer. However molecular imaging is emerging as a useful tool to identify lymph node involvement, location and extent. Given the rarity of vulvar cancer, diagnostic imaging utility is extrapolated from experience in cervical and anal cancer. In a small prospective study, PET/CT has been shown to have a sensitivity of 67 % and specificity of 95 % in indentifying lymph node involvement, and was particularly useful in detecting extranodal involvement (Cohn et al. 2002), which all constitute powerful prognostic factors. Thus patients may be triaged to more aggressive therapy based on the imaging findings, however at present, imaging cannot substitute for histologic information obtained with invasive lymph node evaluation.

MRI has also become common for evaluation of vulvar cancer at diagnosis. While early stage vulvar cancers can often be staged on clinical exam, the extent of involvement of adjacent structures may be more difficult in locally advanced disease. MRI has been shown to be 70–85 % accurate with particular utility in defining the extent of invasion of adjacent structures and outlining tumor size, thus aiding in pretreatment surgical or radiotherapeutic planning (Kataoka et al. 2010; Sohaib et al. 2002).

5 Cancer of the Vagina

Primary vaginal cancer, defined as a lesion arising from the vagina, without involvement of the vulva or cervix, is a rare entity comprising only 1–2 % of gynecologic malignancies. The incidence of invasive vaginal cancer in the US has been reported at 0.69 per 100,000 women, with approximately 1,100 invasive cases annually. The median age at diagnosis is 68 years (Wu et al. 2008). Greater than 90 % are of squamous cell etiology. Risk factors for vaginal carcinoma include history of HPV infection, cervical intraepithelial neoplasia, prior hysterectomy, first intercourse before 17 years of age, five or more sexual partners, genital warts, chronic irritant vaginitis, and immunosuppression (Daling et al. 2002; Okagaki et al. 1983; Brinton et al. 1990; Bouma et al. 1994; Sillman et al. 1997).

Vaginal cancer is often found to be multifocal and often arises in the upper vagina. Tumor spread can be by local extension, lymphatic spread or hematogenous dissemination. Current FIGO staging is by clinical exam, chest and skeletal radiography. By definition, vaginal cancer cannot involve the vulva or cervix, therefore, multiple biopsies are performed to rule out involvement as this may change the diagnosis of the primary lesion. The lymphatic drainage of the vagina is very complex, with the upper vagina draining primarily via cervical lymphatics to the interiliac and parametrial nodes. The posterior vagina drains into the presacral, anorectal and inferior gluteal nodes, while the distal vagina drains in a vulvar pattern to the inguinal and femoral nodes, and subsequently to the pelvic nodes. Thus, all regional nodal stations are at risk for spread in vaginal carcinoma within the mid vagina, or tumors spanning several areas of the vagina.

Given the rarity of this disease, phase III trials have not been conducted, with guidelines drawn from retrospective studies and extrapolated from cervical and anal cancer experience given similarities in histology and preference for organ preservation. Similarly, prognostic and predictive factors are more challenging to elucidate in vaginal cancer due to limited data and relatively non-standardized treatment.

5.1 Staging

FIGO staging is the major prognostic indicator of disease outcome (2009). A thorough bimanual and rectovaginal exam is the most important tool for evaluation of local extent of disease, and often is carried out under anesthesia at which time biopsies can also be performed. Clinical exam focuses on differentiating vaginal wall only (stage I), extension to subvaginal tissue (stage II), or extension to the pelvic wall (stage III). In advanced disease, cystoscopy, proctoscopy, and IV pyelogram to rule out hydronephrosis may be indicated to rule out direct extension of tumor which would constitute stage IVA disease. Biopsies of the cervix or any other suspicious lesions should be performed to rule out cervical, urethral, or vulvar primaries, as these must be excluded for the diagnosis of vaginal cancer by FIGO criteria. Chest and skeletal radiography are also allowed. The results of biopsy or fine-needle aspiration of the inguinal/femoral or other nodes may be included in the clinical staging, although FIGO does not specify staging stratification for lymph node positive disease.

5.2 Clinical Prognostic Factors

5.2.1 Stage

Clinical stage is the major prognostic factor for overall survival. Most patients, except those with very limited involvement, are treated with primary radiation therapy. Based on NCDB data, one of the largest retrospective reviews of survival by stage, 5-year overall survival was 73 % for stage I, 58 % for stage II, and 36 % for stage III–IV (Creasman and Menck 1998). Similarly, in a SEER analysis by Shah et al., 5 year disease specific survival was 84 % for stage I tumors, 75 % for stage II tumors, and 57 % for stage III/IV (Shah et al. 2009).

5.2.2 Tumor Volume

Tumor size is an important predictor of outcome. In one of the largest series of patients treated with primary radiation, pelvic control was 85 % in tumors <4 cm versus 75 % in those >4 cm, and disease-specific survival was 82 and 60 % respectively (Frank et al. 2005). In a series of 301 patients by Chyle et al., lesions <5 cm maximum dimension had a 10-year local recurrence rate of 20 % compared to 40 % for >5 cm, which was significant on univariate analysis (Chyle et al. 1996). Perez et al. demonstrated tumor size was only predictive of pelvic control and disease free survival in stage II patients without parametrial involvement (Perez et al. 1999). Length of vaginal involvement has been implicated as an adverse prognostic factor (Kirkbride et al. 1995), which may also be linked to tumor size.

5.2.3 Tumor Location

While location of the tumor is important, particularly in consideration of nodal regions at risk, the utility of location as a prognostic factor is unclear. Several studies have indicated better survival and decreased risk for recurrence for patients with tumors located in the proximal half compared to those of the entire vagina or distal portion (Chyle et al. 1996; Kucera and Vavra 1991; Urbanski et al. 1996; Ali et al. 1996). Lesions of the posterior vagina wall also have worse prognosis than other locations (Chyle et al. 1996; Dixit et al. 1993). Counter to these studies, however, Perez et al. did not show any prognostic value to tumor location in the posterior vaginal wall (Perez et al. 1988).

5.2.4 Lymph Node Status

Surgical series have reported rates of pathologic nodal involvement that range from 6 %-14 % for stage I disease and 26–32 % for stage II disease (Al-Kurdi and Monaghan 1981; Davis et al. 1991). Al-Kurdi and Monaghan noted that 12 % survived when pelvic or inguinal lymph nodes were involved as compared to 47 % survival in node negative patients. However, these are small studies, and given the fact FIGO staging does not include lymph node disease, it is difficult to assess its prognostic utility.

5.3 Histologic Factors

5.3.1 Histology

The majority of invasive vaginal cancers are squamous cell histology at >90 %. Approximately 5 % of primaries are adenocarcinoma, most commonly clear cell adenocarcinoma, and 3–5 % are malignant melanoma. Other less common histologies include sarcomas, lymphoma, leukemia, and neuroendocrine small cell.

Among the histopathologic factors, correlation between histologic tumor grade and outcome has been controversial although two studies have demonstrated increased rates of recurrence with higher tumor grade (Chyle et al. 1996; Vavra et al. 1991). Adenocarcinaomas appear to confer a less favorable prognosis than squamous cell carcinomas, particularly those unrelated to DES exposure (Frank et al. 2007). DES induced clear cell adenocarcinomas in younger women arising from in utero exposure have a generally better prognosis than squamous cell carcinoma, but are unlikely to be seen today, as the use of DES during pregnancy has been banned in 1975.

5.3.2 Molecular Markers

Squamous cell carcinoma of the vagina, much like other gynecologic malignancies, are associated with HPV-dependent and independent pathways. HPV-negative tumors tend to occur in older women, with classical keratinizing, verrucous features. HPV-positive tumors are associated with basaloid, non-keratinizing lesions, tend to occur in younger patients, and present with earlier stage disease (Daling et al. 2002; Larsson et al. 2013). Larsson et al. showed significantly improved 5 year overall survival in HPV-positive tumors compared to HPV-negative tumors at 51.1 and 10.7 %, respectively ($p = 0.0008$). Owing to the rarity of vaginal cancer, evaluation of other molecular markers has been limited.

5.4 Treatment Related Factors

Stage is an important determinant of therapy selection, as stage I patients and selected stage II patients may be amenable to surgical therapy alone, ranging from wide local excision to vaginectomy with reported survival rates of 90 % or greater (Creasman and Menck 1998). Some population based studies have also reported improved survival with surgery over radiotherapy for early stage disease of 90 % versus 38 %, but is likely confounded due to patient selection bias and the use of radiotherapy in patients deemed poor surgical candidates due to comorbid disease (Creasman and Menck 1998). Similar results were observed in a SEER analysis that identified an adjusted hazard ratio of 1.5 for increased mortality risk in stage I patients undergoing radiotherapy in place of definitive surgery (Shah et al. 2009).

Given that organ preservation is desirable if outcomes are equivalent to surgery, the utility of definitive radiotherapy has also been explored. Superficial stage I tumors can be treated with brachytherapy alone. However several investigators have observed higher local recurrence rates in stage I patients with infiltrating lesions or higher grade tumors, thus external beam radiation has been advocated in such patients (Nori et al. 1983; Leung 1993). Definitive radiotherapy for early stage disease has reported cause specific survival of 40–90 % for stage I and 35–78 % for stage II disease (Frank et al. 2005; Perez et al. 1999; Kucera and Vavra 1991; Urbanski et al. 1996; Kirkbride et al. 1995; de Crevoisier et al. 2007; Tran et al. 2007; Prempree and Amornmarn 1985; Pingley et al. 2000). In more advanced disease, the combination of external beam radiotherapy with brachytherapy has been shown to improve pelvic control and survival in stage II vaginal cancer (Pingley et al. 2000).

Locally advanced disease is often approached with external beam radiotherapy with or without chemotherapy, given to the extremely morbid exenteration that would be necessary to remove surgically.

Although the influence of tumor location within the vagina on prognosis has not been substantiated (Chyle et al. 1996; Perez et al. 1999; Kirkbride et al. 1995), tumor location has profound impact of radiation therapy planning, and treatment algorithms have been based on location and depth of invasion to optimize therapy and minimize toxicity. Following external beam therapy, upper vaginal and apical tumors are treated with intracavitary radiation, if their residual thickness is 5 mm but require more invasive interstitial therapy for thicker lesions. Anterior mid-vaginal lesions are treated with interstitial therapy, and posterior mid-vaginal lesions with a highly conformal or IMRT external beam boost due to the poor tolerance of interstitial therapy in the perirectal region. Confined distal vaginal lesions can be treated with interstitial brachytherapy, whereas massive lesions require external beam boost (Frank et al. 2005).

The role of addition of chemotherapy is still evolving. No randomized trials evaluating radiotherapy with or without chemotherapy have been performed, although chemotherapy is used concurrently in some settings given the experience of improved outcomes in locally advanced cervical cancer (Morris et al. 1999; Lanciano et al. 2005; Rose et al. 1999). Feasibility has been demonstrated in several small institutional studies. Concurrent 5-fluorouracil (5-FU) with bolus cisplatin or mitomycin C in patients with early stage disease resulted in 93 % cause specific survival at 5 years (Dalrymple et al. 2004). Five year cause specific survival of 50 % and pelvic control rate of 31 % were reported in 26 locally advanced patients treated with definitive radiotherapy and concurrent 5-FU and mitomycin C or single agent cisplatin (Kirkbride et al. 1995). A small series reporting outcomes for neoadjuvant paclitaxel and cisplatin prior to radical surgery in 11 stage II patients resulted in 27 % complete clinical response and 64 % partial clinical response with chemotherapy, and 18 % rate of disease recurrence at median follow up of 75 months (Benedetti Panici et al. 2008).

5.5 Imaging Prognostic Factors

Delineation of tumor size and degree of infiltration or spread is of critical importance, especially in the setting of definitive radiotherapy. Therefore, information obtained from radiographic workup guides treatment approach and delivery.

Given the inaccuracy of clinical palpation findings, MRI is a very useful tool for delineating extent of disease. MRI can be used in determining tumor thickness and paravaginal infiltration on T2-weighted imaging, identified as hyperintense lesions (Taylor et al. 2007). This is in line with the superior soft tissue resolution described with MRI from cervical cancer literature Bipat et al. 2003; Hricak et al. 2005. Visualization of the vaginal tumor may be improved with the instillation of vaginal gel or a dry vaginal tampon (Young et al. 2012).

Similar to its utility in cervical cancer, PET has shown high sensitivity in identifying inguinal or pelvic lymph node involvement in advanced vaginal cancer and by some reports is more accurate than CT scan (Lamoreaux et al. 2005). In practice, PET can be critical for defining target volumes for accurate external beam and brachytherapy planning. Taken together, MRI and/or PET imaging is often obtained to identify tumor size and predict lymph node involvement and MRI is often recommended in the setting of surveillance to distinguish between tumor recurrence or radiation change. These modalities appear more sensitive than CT alone, therefore 3D CT information is often used primarly for radiotherapy treatment planning.

6 Summary

Gynecologic malignancies are somewhat unique in regard to the methods of staging and treatment compared to more commonly encountered cancers such as lung, breast, or prostate. Clinical and surgical staging have long dominated how gynecologic cancers are evaluated and substratified. With the advent of new imaging modalities and molecular diagnostic abilities, more information is available prior to selection of therapy, and the prognostic utility of these factors is evolving. As more research focuses on validating prognostic utility of imaging, histopathologic characteristics, and molecular footprints, treatment approach will likely continue to evolve.

References

Aalders J, Abeler V, Kolstad P, Onsrud M (1980) Postoperative external irradiation and prognostic parameters in stage I endometrial carcinoma: clinical and histopathologic study of 540 patients. Obstet Gynecol 56(4):419–427

Aarnio M, Mecklin JP, Aaltonen LA, Nystrom-Lahti M, Jarvinen HJ (1995) Life-time risk of different cancers in hereditary non-polyposis colorectal cancer (HNPCC) syndrome. Int J Cancer 64(6):430–433

Abeler VM, Kjorstad KE (1991) Endometrial adenocarcinoma in Norway. A study of a total population. Cancer 67(12):3093–3103. Epub 1991/06/15

Abeler VM, Kjorstad KE (1992) Endometrial adenocarcinoma with squamous cell differentiation. Cancer 69(2):488–495

Akbayir O, Corbacioglu A, Numanoglu C, Guleroglu FY, Ulker V, Akyol A et al (2011) Preoperative assessment of myometrial and cervical invasion in endometrial carcinoma by transvaginal ultrasound. Gynecol Oncol 122(3):600–603 Epub 2011/06/28

Alcazar JL, Errasti T, Zornoza A (2000) Saline infusion sonohysterography in endometrial cancer: assessment of malignant cells dissemination risk. Acta Obstet Gynecol Scand 79(4):321–322

Ali MM, Huang DT, Goplerud DR, Howells R, Lu JD (1996) Radiation alone for carcinoma of the vagina: variation in response related to the location of the primary tumor. Cancer 77(9):1934–1939

Al-Kurdi M, Monaghan JM (1981) Thirty-two years experience in management of primary tumours of the vagina. Br J Obstet Gynaecol 88(11):1145–1150

American College of Obstetricians and Gynecologists. ACOG practice bulletin, clinical management guidelines for obstetrician-gynecologists, number 65, August 2005: management of endometrial cancer. Obstet Gynecol 106(2):413–425

Ansink A (1996) Vulvar squamous cell carcinoma. Semin Dermatol 15(1):51–59

Ansink AC vTH, Aartsen EJ, Heintz AP (1991) Outcome, complications and follow-up in surgically treated squamous cell carcinoma of the vulva 1956-1982. Eur J Obstet Gynecol Reprod Biol 42(2):137–143

Ansink ACKM, De Weger RA, Kleyne JA, Pijpers H, Van Tinteren H, De Kraker EW, Helmerhorst TJ, Heintz AP (1994) Human papillomavirus, lichen sclerosus, and squamous cell carcinoma of the vulva: detection and prognostic significance. Gynecol Oncol 52(2):180–184

Antonsen SL, Jensen LN, Loft A, Berthelsen AK, Costa J, Tabor A et al (2013a) MRI, PET/CT and ultrasound in the preoperative staging of endometrial cancer—a multicenter prospective comparative study. Gynecol Oncol 128(2):300–308 Epub 2012/12/04

Antonsen SL, Loft A, Fisker R, Nielsen AL, Andersen ES, Hogdall E et al (2013b) SUVmax of 18FDG PET/CT as a predictor of high-risk endometrial cancer patients. Gynecol Oncol 129(2):298–303

Arko D, Takac I (2000) High frequency transvaginal ultrasonography in preoperative assessment of myometrial invasion in endometrial cancer. J Ultrasound Med 19(9):639–643 Epub 2000/09/06

Ashman JB, Connell PP, Yamada D, Rotmensch J, Waggoner SE, Mundt AJ (2001) Outcome of endometrial carcinoma patients with involvement of the uterine serosa. Gynecol Oncol 82(2):338–343 Epub 2001/09/05

ASTEC study group, Kitchener H, Swart AM, Qian Q, Amos C, Parmar MK (2009) Efficacy of systematic pelvic lymphadenectomy in endometrial cancer (MRC ASTEC trial): a randomised study. Lancet 373(9658):125–136

Averette HE, Ford JH Jr, Dudan RC, Girtanner RE, Hoskins WJ, Lutz MH (1975) Staging of cervical cancer. Clin Obstet Gynecol 18:215–232

Awwad HK, el Naggar M, Mocktar N, Barsoum M (1986) Intercapillary distance measurement as an indicator of hypoxia in carcinoma of the cervix uteri. Int J Radiat Oncol Biol Phys 12(8):1329–1333 Epub 1986/08/01

Bachtiary B, Schindl M, Pötter R, Dreier B, Knocke TH, Hainfellner JA, Horvat R, Birner P (2003) Overexpression of hypoxia-inducible factor 1alpha indicates diminished response to radiotherapy and unfavorable prognosis in patients receiving radical radiotherapy for cervical cancer. Clin Cancer Res 9(6):2234–2240

Baldinu P, Cossu A, Manca A, Satta MP, Pisano M, Casula M et al (2002) Microsatellite instability and mutation analysis of candidate genes in unselected Sardinian patients with endometrial carcinoma. Cancer 94(12):3157–3168 Epub 2002/07/13

Balleyguier C, Sala E, Da Cunha T, Bergman A, Brkljacic B, Danza F et al (2011) Staging of uterine cervical cancer with MRI: guidelines of the European Society of Urogenital Radiology. Eur Radiol 21(5):1102–1110 Epub 2010/11/11

Belhocine T, De Barsy C, Hustinx R, Willems-Foidart J (2002) Usefulness of (18)F-FDG PET in the post-therapy surveillance of endometrial carcinoma. Eur J Nucl Med Mol Imaging 29(9):1132–1139

Benedetti Panici P, Bellati F, Plotti F, Di Donato V, Antonilli M, Perniola G et al (2008) Neoadjuvant chemotherapy followed by radical surgery in patients affected by vaginal carcinoma. Gynecol Oncol 111(2):307–311. Epub 2008/08/19

Berek JS, Hacker NF (1989) Practical gynecologic oncology, 2nd edn. Williams & Wilkins, Philadelphia

Berman MLKH, Creasman W, DiSaia P, Bundy B, Blessing J (1984) Survival and patterns of recurrence in cervical cancer metastatic to periaortic lymph nodes (a Gynecologic Oncology Group study). Gynecol Oncol 19(1):8–16

Bhosale P, Peungjesada S, Devine C, Balachandran A, Iyer R (2010) Role of magnetic resonance imaging as an adjunct to clinical staging in cervical carcinoma. J Comput Assist Tomogr 34(6):855–864 Epub 2010/11/19

Binder SW, Huang I, Fu YS, Hacker NF, Berek JS (1990) Risk factors for the development of lymph node metastasis in vulvar squamous cell carcinoma. Gynecol Oncol 37(1):9–16

Bipat S, Glas AS, van der Velden J, Zwinderman AH, Bossuyt PM, Stoker J (2003) Computed tomography and magnetic resonance imaging in staging of uterine cervical carcinoma: a systematic review. Gynecol Oncol 91(1):59–66

Blecharz P, Karolewski K, Bieda T, Klimek M, Pudelek J, Kojs E et al (2008) Prognostic factors in patients with carcinoma of the vulva—our own experience and literature review. Eur J Gynaecol Oncol 29(3):260–263

Boruta DM 2nd, Gehrig PA, Groben PA, Bae-Jump V, Boggess JF, Fowler WC Jr et al (2004) Uterine serous and grade 3 endometrioid carcinomas: is there a survival difference? Cancer 101(10):2214–2221

Bosch FX, Manos MM, Munoz N, Sherman M, Jansen AM, Peto J et al (1995) Prevalence of human papillomavirus in cervical cancer: a worldwide perspective. International biological study on cervical cancer (IBSCC) Study Group. J Natl Cancer Inst 87(11):796–802. Epub 1995/06/07

Bouma J, Burger MP, Krans M, Hollema H, Pras E (1994) Squamous cell carcinoma of the vagina: a report of 32 cases. Int J Gynecol Cancer 4(6):389–394

Boyce J, Fruchter R, Kasambilides E, Nicastri AD, Sedlis A, Remy JC (1985) Prognostic factors in carcinoma of the vulva. Gynecol Oncol 20(3):364–377

Brinton LA, Nasca PC, Mallin K, Schairer C, Rosenthal J, Rothenberg R et al (1990) Case-control study of in situ and invasive carcinoma of the vagina. Gynecol Oncol 38(1):49–54

Brinton LA, Berman ML, Mortel R, Twiggs LB, Barrett RJ, Wilbanks GD et al (1992) Reproductive, menstrual, and medical risk factors for endometrial cancer: results from a case-control study. Am J Obstet Gynecol 167(5):1317–1325

Bristow RE, Zahurak ML, Alexander CJ, Zellars RC, Montz FJ (2003) FIGO stage IIIC endometrial carcinoma: resection of macroscopic nodal disease and other determinants of survival. Int J Gynecol Cancer 13(5):664–672

Burger MPHH, Emanuels AG, Krans M, Pras E, Bouma J (1995) The importance of the groin node status for the survival of T1 and T2 vulval carcinoma patients. Gynecol Oncol 57(3):327–334

Burger RA, Monk BJ, Kurosaki T, Anton-Culver H, Vasilev SA, Berman ML et al (1996) Human papillomavirus type 18: association with poor prognosis in early stage cervical cancer. J Natl Cancer Inst 88(19):1361–1368 Epub 1996/10/02

Burghardt E, Hofmann H, Ebner F et al (1989) Magnetic resonance imaging in cervical cancer: a basis for objective classification. Gynecol Oncol 33:61–67

Burri P, Djonov V, Aebersold DM, Lindel K, Studer U, Altermatt HJ, Mazzucchelli L, Greiner RH, Gruber G (2003) Significant correlation of hypoxia-inducible factor-1alpha with treatment outcome in cervical cancer treated with radical radiotherapy. Int J Radiat Oncol Biol Phys 56(2):494–501

Bush RS, Jenkin RDT, Allt WEC (1978) Definitive evidence for hypoxic cells influencing cure in cancer therapy. Br J Cancer 37(Suppl 3):302–306

Callister M, Ramondetta LM, Jhingran A, Burke TW, Eifel PJ (2004) Malignant mixed Mullerian tumors of the uterus: analysis of patterns of failure, prognostic factors, and treatment outcome. Int J Radiat Oncol Biol Phys 58(3):786–796

Carlson JA, Ambros R, Malfetano J, Ross J, Grabowski R, Lamb P et al (1998) Vulvar lichen sclerosus and squamous cell carcinoma: a cohort, case control, and investigational study with historical perspective; implications for chronic inflammation and sclerosis in the development of neoplasia. Hum Pathol 29(9):932–948

Chan JK, Kapp DS, Cheung MK, Osann K, Shin JY, Cohn D et al (2007a) The impact of the absolute number and ratio of positive lymph nodes on survival of endometrioid uterine cancer patients. Br J Cancer 97(5):605–611 Epub 2007/08/02

Chan JKSV, Pham H, Gu M, Rutgers J, Osann K, Cheung MK, Berman ML (2007b) PJ D. Margin distance and other clinicopathologic prognostic factors in vulvar carcinoma: a multivariate analysis. Gynecol Oncol 104(3):636–641

Chang SJ, Lee EJ, Kim WY, Yoo SC, Yoon JH, Chang KH et al (2010) Value of sonohysterography in preoperative assessment of myometrial invasion for patients with endometrial cancer. J Ultrasound Med 29(6):923–929

Chang MC, Chen JH, Liang JA, Yang KT, Cheng KY, Kao CH (2012) 18F-FDG PET or PET/CT for detection of metastatic lymph nodes in patients with endometrial cancer: a systematic review and meta-analysis. Eur J Radiol 81(11):3511–3517

Chao A, Tang YH, Lai CH, Chang CJ, Chang SC, Wu TI et al (2013) Potential of an age-stratified CA125 cut-off value to improve the prognostic classification of patients with endometrial cancer. Gynecol Oncol 129(3):500–504 Epub 2013/03/06

Charles-Edwards EM, DeSouza NM (2006) Diffusion-weighted magnetic resonance imaging and its application to cancer. Cancer Imaging 6:135–143

Charles-Edwards EMMC, Morgan VA, De Silva SS, McWhinney NA, Katesmark M, Attygalle AD, DeSouza NM (2008) Diffusion-weighted imaging in cervical cancer with an endovaginal technique: potential value for improving tumor detection in stage Ia and Ib1 disease. Radiology 249(2):541–550

Chenevert TLSL, Taylor JM, Robertson PL, Greenberg HS, Rehemtulla A, Ross BD (2000) Diffusion magnetic resonance imaging: an early surrogate marker of therapeutic efficacy in brain tumors. J Natl Cancer Inst 92(24):2029–2036

Cheng W, Chen C, Lee C (2000) Vascular endothelial growth factor and prognosis in cervical carcinoma. Obstet Gynecol 96:721–726

Chi DS, Welshinger M, Venkatraman ES, Barakat RR (1997) The role of surgical cytoreduction in Stage IV endometrial carcinoma. Gynecol Oncol 67(1):56–60

Choschzick M, Woelber L, Hess S, zu Eulenburg C, Schwarz J, Simon R et al (2010) Overexpression of carbonic anhydrase IX (CAIX) in vulvar cancer is associated with tumor progression and development of locoregional lymph node metastases. Virchows Arch 456(5):483–490

Chung YMKB, Park CS, Huh SJ, Kim J, Park JK, Cho SM, Kim BS, Kim JS, Yoo YD, Bae DS (2005) Increased expression of ICAM-3 is associated with radiation resistance in cervical cancer. Int J Cancer 117(2):194–201

Chung HH, Kim JW, Park NH, Song YS, Kang SB, Lee HP (2006) Use of preoperative serum CA-125 levels for prediction of lymph node metastasis and prognosis in endometrial cancer. Acta Obstet Gynecol Scand 85(12):1501–1505 Epub 2007/01/30

Chung HH, Kang WJ, Kim JW, Park NH, Song YS, Chung JK et al (2008) The clinical impact of [(18)F]FDG PET/CT for the management of recurrent endometrial cancer: correlation with clinical and histological findings. Eur J Nucl Med Mol Imaging 35(6):1081–1088

Chyle V, Zagars G, Wheeler JA, Wharton JT, Delclos L (1996) Definitive radiotherapy for carcinoma of the vagina: outcome and prognostic factors. Int J Radiat Oncol Biol Phys 35(5):191–905

Cohn DE, Dehdashti F, Gibb RK, Mutch DG, Rader JS, Siegel BA et al (2002) Prospective evaluation of positron emission tomography for the detection of groin node metastases from vulvar cancer. Gynecol Oncol 85(1):179–184

Connell PP, Rotmensch J, Waggoner S, Mundt AJ (1999) The significance of adnexal involvement in endometrial carcinoma. Gynecol Oncol 74(1):74–79 Epub 1999/07/01

Connor JP, Andrews JI, Anderson B, Buller RE (2000) Computed tomography in endometrial carcinoma. Obstet Gynecol 95(5): 692–696

Cooper RA, Wilks DP, Logue JP, Davidson SE, Hunter RD, Roberts SA et al (1998) High angiogenesis is associated with poor survival in carcinoma of the cervix treated with radiotherapy. Clin Can Res 4:2795–2800

Cormio G, Loizzi V, Carriero C, Cazzolla A, Putignano G, Selvaggi L (2010) Groin recurrence in carcinoma of the vulva: management and outcome. Eur J Cancer Care 19(3):302–307 Epub 2009/10/17

Cosin JAFJ, Chen MD, Paley PJ, Carson LF, Twiggs LB (1998) Pretreatment surgical staging of patients with cervical carcinoma: the case for lymph node debulking. Cancer 82(11):2241–2248

Creasman W (2009) Revised FIGO staging for carcinoma of the endometrium. Int J Gynaecol Obstet 105(2):109

Creasman WTPJ, Menck HR (1998) The National Cancer Data Base report on cancer of the vagina. Cancer 83(5):1033–1040

Creasman WTMC, Bundy BN et al (1987) Surgical pathologic spread patterns of endometrial cancer: a Gynecologic Oncology Group study. Cancer 60:2035–2041

Creutzberg CL vPW, Koper PC, Lybeert ML, Jobsen JJ, Wárlám-Rodenhuis CC, De Winter KA, Lutgens LC, van den Bergh AC, van de Steen-Banasik E, Beerman H, van Lent M (2000) Surgery and postoperative radiotherapy versus surgery alone for patients with stage-1 endometrial carcinoma: multicentre randomised trial. PORTEC Study Group. Post Operative Radiation Therapy in Endometrial Carcinoma. Lancet 355:1404–1411

Creutzberg CL vPW, Koper PC, Lybeert ML, Jobsen JJ, Wárlám-Rodenhuis CC, De Winter KA, Lutgens LC, van den Bergh AC, van der Steen-Banasik E, Beerman H, van Lent M, PORTEC Study Group (2003) Survival after relapse in patients with endometrial cancer: results from a randomized trial. Gynecol Oncol 89(2):201–209

Creutzberg CL vPW, Wárlám-Rodenhuis CC, van den Bergh AC, de Winter KA, Koper PC, Lybeert ML, Slot A, Lutgens LC, Stenfert Kroese MC, Beerman H, van Lent M (2004) Postoperative Radiation Therapy in Endometrial Carcinoma Trial,. Outcome of high-risk stage IC, grade 3, compared with stage I endometrial carcinoma patients: the Postoperative Radiation Therapy in Endometrial Carcinoma Trial. J Clin Oncol 22(7):1234–1241

Current FIGO (2009) staging for cancer of the vagina, fallopian tube, ovary, and gestational trophoblastic neoplasia. Int J Gynaecol Obstet 105(1):3–4

Daling JR, Madeleine MM, Schwartz SM, Shera KA, Carter JJ, McKnight B et al (2002) A population-based study of squamous cell vaginal cancer: HPV and cofactors. Gynecol Oncol 84(2):263–270

Dalrymple JL, Russell AH, Lee SW, Scudder SA, Leiserowitz GS, Kinney WK et al (2004) Chemoradiation for primary invasive squamous carcinoma of the vagina. Int J Gynecol Cancer 14(1):110–117 Epub 2004/02/07

Davidson SE, Symonds RP, Lamont D, Watson ER (1989) Does adenocarcinoma of uterine cervix have a worse prognosis than squamous carcinoma when treated by radiotherapy? Gynecol Oncol 33(1):23–26 Epub 1989/04/01

Davis KP, Stanhope CR, Garton GR, Atkinson EJ, O'Brien PC (1991) Invasive vaginal carcinoma: analysis of early-stage disease. Gynecol Oncol 42(2):131–136

de Crevoisier R, Sanfilippo N, Gerbaulet A, Morice P, Pomel C, Castaigne D et al (2007) Exclusive radiotherapy for primary squamous cell carcinoma of the vagina. Radiother Oncol 85(3): 362–370 Epub 2007/10/30

de Koning MN, Quint WG, Pirog EC (2008) Prevalence of mucosal and cutaneous human papillomaviruses in different histologic subtypes of vulvar carcinoma. Mod Pathol 21(3):334–344

Del Pino M, Rodriguez-Carunchio L, Ordi J (2013) Pathways of vulvar intraepithelial neoplasia and squamous cell carcinoma. Histopathology 62(1):161–175

Dellas A, Moch H, Schultheiss E, Feichter G, Almendral AC, Gudat F et al (1997) Angiogenesis in cervical neoplasia: microvessel quantitation in precancerous lesions and invasive carcinomas with cliniciopathological correlations. Gynecol Oncol 67:27–33

DelMaschio A, Vanzulli A, Sironi S, Spagnolo D, Belloni C, Garancini P et al (1993) Estimating the depth of myometrial involvement by endometrial carcinoma: efficacy of transvaginal sonography vs MR imaging. Am J Roentgenol 160(3):533–538 Epub 1993/03/01

Dessole S, Rubattu G, Farina M, Capobianco G, Cherchi PL, Tanda F et al (2006) Risks and usefulness of sonohysterography in patients with endometrial carcinoma. Am J Obstet Gynecol 194(2):362–368

Diesche S, Anderson P, Sealy R (1983) Carcinoma of the cervix—anaemia, radiotherapy and hyperbaric oxygen. Br J Radiol 56:251–255

Dinh TV, Hannigan EV, Smith ER et al (1996) Tumor angiogenesis as a predictor of recurrence in stage Ib squamous cell carcinoma of the cervix. Obstet Gynecol 87(5, Part 1):751–754

Dixit S, Singhal S, Baboo HA (1993) Squamous cell carcinoma of the vagina: a review of 70 cases. Gynecol Oncol 48(1):80–87

Dolan JR, McCall AR, Gooneratne S, Walter S, Lansky DM (1993) DNA ploidy, proliferation index, grade, and stage as prognostic factors for vulvar squamous cell carcinomas. Gynecol Oncol 48(2):232–235

Dunst J, Kuhnt T, Strauss HG, Krause U, Pelz T, Koelbl H et al (2003) Anemia in cervical cancers: impact on survival, patterns of relapse, and association with hypoxia and angiogenesis. Int J Radiat Oncol Biol Phys 56(3):778–787

Edge SB, Byrd DR, Compton CC et al (eds) (2009) American Joint Committee on Cancer, American Cancer Society. AJCC Cancer Staging Manual, 7th ed. Springer, Berlin

Eifel PJ (1994) Problems with the clinical staging of carcinoma of the cervix. Semin Radiat Oncol 4:1–8

Eifel PJ, Morris M, Wharton JT, Oswald MJ (1994) The influence of tumor size and morphology on the outcome of patients with FIGO stage IB squamous cell carcinoma of the uterine cervix. Int J Radiat Oncol Biol Phys 29:9–16

Eifel PJ, Burke TW, Morris M, Smith TL (1995) Adenocarcinoma as an independent risk factor for disease recurrence in patients with stage IB cervical carcinoma. Gynecol Oncol 59(1):38–44 Epub 1995/10/01

Eifel PJ, Winter K, Morris M, Levenback C, Grigsby PW, Cooper J et al (2004) Pelvic irradiation with concurrent chemotherapy versus pelvic and para-aortic irradiation for high-risk cervical cancer: an update of radiation therapy oncology group trial (RTOG) 90-01. J Clin Oncol 22(5):872–880 Epub 2004/03/03

Eltabbakh GH (2002) Analysis of survival after laparoscopy in women with endometrial carcinoma. Cancer 95(9):1894–1901

Eltabbakh GH, Moore AD (1999) Survival of women with surgical stage II endometrial cancer. Gynecol Oncol 74(1):80–85

Evans J, Bergsjo P (1965) The influence of anemia and results of radiotherapy in carcinoma of the cervix. Radiology 48:709–717

Farley JH, Hickey KW, Carlson JW, Rose GS, Kost ER, Harrison TA (2003) Adenosquamous histology predicts a poor outcome for patients with advanced-stage, but not early-stage, cervical carcinoma. Cancer 97(9):2196–2202 Epub 2003/04/25

Faul CM, Mirmow D, Huang Q, Gerszten K, Day R, Jones MW (1997) Adjuvant radiation for vulvar carcinoma: improved local control. Int J Radiat Oncol Biol Phys 38(2):381–389 Epub 1997/05/01

Ferrandina G, Ranelletti FO, Gallotta V, Martinelli E, Zannoni GF, Gessi M et al (2005) Expression of cyclooxygenase-2 (COX-2), receptors for estrogen (ER), and progesterone (PR), p53, ki67, and neu protein in endometrial cancer. Gynecol Oncol 98(3):383–389 Epub 2005/06/28

Finan MA, Barre G (2003) Bartholin's gland carcinoma, malignant melanoma and other rare tumours of the vulva. Best Pract Res Clin Obstet Gynaecol 17(4):609–633

Flueckiger F, Ebner F, Poschauko H, Tamussino K, Einspieler R (1992) G. R. Cervical cancer: serial MR imaging before and after primary radiation therapy—a 2-year follow-up study. Radiology 184:89–93

Fons G, Burger MP, Ten Kate FJ, van der Velden J (2007) Identification of potential prognostic markers for vulvar cancer using immunohistochemical staining of tissue microarrays. Int J Gynecol Pathol 26(2):188–193

Fons G, Hyde SE, Buist MR, Schilthuis MS, Grant P, Burger MP et al (2009a) Prognostic value of bilateral positive nodes in squamous cell cancer of the vulva. Int J Gynecol Cancer 19(7):1276–1280

Fons G, Hyde S, Buist MR, Schilthuis MS, Grant P, Burger MP, van der Velden J (2009b) Prognostic value of bilateral positive nodes in squamous cell cancer of the vulva. Int J Gynecol Cancer 19(7):1276–1280

Frank SJJA, Levenback C, Eifel PJ (2005) Definitive radiation therapy for squamous cell carcinoma of the vagina. Int J Radiat Oncol Biol Phys 62(1):138–147

Frank SJDM, Jhingran A, Bodurka DC, Eifel PJ (2007) Primary adenocarcinoma of the vagina not associated with diethylstilbestrol (DES) exposure. Gynecol Oncol 105(2):470–474

Franklin EW 3rd (1972) Clinical staging of carcinoma of the vulva. Obstet Gynecol 40(3):277–286

Gaffney DK, Haslam D, Tsodikov A, Hammond E, Seaman J, Holden J et al (2003) Epidermal growth factor receptor (EGFR) and vascular andothelial factor receptor (VGEF) negatively affect overall survival in carcinoma of the cervix treated with radiotherapy. Int J Rad Oncol Biol Phys 56:922–928

Galic V, Herzog TJ, Lewin SN, Neugut AI, Burke WM, Lu YS et al (2012) Prognostic significance of adenocarcinoma histology in women with cervical cancer. Gynecol Oncol 125(2):287–291 Epub 2012/01/24

Geisinger KR, Marshall RB, Kute TE, Homesley HD (1986) Correlation of female sex steroid hormone receptors with histologic and ultrastructural differentiation in adenocarcinoma of the endometrium. Cancer 58(7):1506–1517 Epub 1986/10/01

Gonzalez Bosquet J, Kinney W, Russell AH, Gaffey TA, Magrina JF, Podratz KC (2003) Risk of occult inguinofemoral lymph node metastasis from squamous carcinoma of the vulva. Int J Radiat Oncol Biol Phys 57(2):419–424

Gordinier ME, Steinhoff MM, Hogan JW, Peipert JF, Gajewski WH, Falkenberry SS et al (1997) S-Phase fraction, p53, and HER-2/neu status as predictors of nodal metastasis in early vulvar cancer. Gynecol Oncol 67(2):200–202

Greco A, Mason P, Leung AWL, Dische S, McIndoe GA, Anderson MC (1989) Staging of carcinoma of the uterine cervix: MRI-surgical correlation. Clin Radiol 40(4):401–405. Epub July

Greven KM, Curran WJ Jr, Whittington R, Fanning J, Randall ME, Wilder J et al (1989) Analysis of failure patterns in stage III endometrial carcinoma and therapeutic implications. Int J Radiat Oncol Biol Phys 17(1):35–39 Epub 1989/07/01

Grisaru D, Covens A, Chapman B, Shaw P, Colgan T, Murphy J et al (2001) Does histology influence prognosis in patients with early-stage cervical carcinoma? Cancer 92(12):2999–3004 Epub 2001/12/26

Grogan M, Thomas GM, Melamed I, Wong FLW, Pearcey RG, Joseph PK et al (1999) The importance of hemoglobin levels during radiotherapy for carcinoma of the cervix. Cancer 86:1528–1536

Grossman J, Ricci ZJ, Rozenblit A, Freeman K, Mazzariol F, Stein MW (2008) Efficacy of contrast-enhanced CT in assessing the endometrium. Am J Roentgenol 191(3):664–669

Growdon WB, Boisvert SL, Akhavanfard S, Oliva E, Dias-Santagata DC, Kojiro S et al (2008) Decreased survival in EGFR gene amplified vulvar carcinoma. Gynecol Oncol 111(2):289–297

Gustafson S, Zbuk KM, Scacheri C, Eng C (2007) Cowden syndrome. Semin Oncol 34(5):428–434

Hacker NF (2009) Revised FIGO staging for carcinoma of the vulva. Int J Gynaecol Obstet 105(2):105–106

Hacker NF, Berek JS, Lagasse LD, Leuchter RS, Moore JG (1983) Management of regional lymph nodes and their prognostic influence in vulvar cancer. Obstet Gynecol 61(4):408–412

Haensgen G, Krause U, Becker A, Stadler P, Lautenschlaeger C, Wohlrab W, Rath FW, Molls M, Dunst J (2001) Tumor hypoxia, p53, and prognosis in cervical cancers. Int J Radiat Oncol Biol Phys 50(4):865–872

Hamstra DA, Rehemtulla A, Ross BD (2008) Diffusion magnetic resonance imaging: a biomarker for treatment response in oncology. J Clin Oncol 25:4104–4109

Hantschmann P, Jeschke U, Friese K (2005) TGF-alpha, c-erbB-2 expression and neoangiogenesis in vulvar squamous cell carcinoma. Anticancer Res 25(3A):1731–1737

Harima Y, Harima K, Shikata N, Oka A, Ohnishi T, Tanaka Y (1998) Bax and Bcl-2 expressions predict response to radiotherapy in human cervical cancer. J Cancer Res Clin Oncol 124(9):503–510

Harima Y, Sawada S, Miyazaki Y, Kin K, Ishihara H, Imamura M, Sougawa M, Shikata N, Ohnishi T (2003) Expression of Ku80 in cervical cancer correlates with response to radiotherapy and survival. Am J Clin Oncol 26(4):e80–e85

Harima Y, Togashi A, Horikoshi K (2004) Prediction of outcome of advanced cervical cancer to thermoradiotherapy according to expression profiles of 35 genes selected by cDNA microarray analysis. Int J Radiat Oncol Biol Phys 60:237–248

Harry VNSS, Gilbert FJ, Parkin DE (2008) Diffusion-weighted magnetic resonance imaging in the early detection of response to chemoradiation in cervical cancer. Gynecol Oncol 111:213–220

Hatano K, Sekiya Y, Araki H, Sakai M, Togawa T, Narita Y et al (1999) Evaluation of the therapeutic effect of radiotherapy on cervical cancer using magnetic resonance imaging. Int J Radiat Oncol Biol Phys 45:639–644

Hawighorst H, Knapstein PG, Weikel W, Knopp MV, Zuna I, Knof A et al (1997) Angiogenesis of uterine cervical carcinoma: characterization by pharmacokinetic magnetic resonance parameters and histological microvessel density with correlation to lymphatic involvement. Cancer Res 57:4777–4786

Hawighorst H, Weikel W, Knapstein PG et al (1998) Angiogenic activity of cervical carcinoma: assessment by functional magnetic resonance imaging-based parameters and a histomorphological approach in correlation with disease outcome. Clin Cancer Res 4(10):2305–2312

Heaps JM, Fu YS, Montz FJ, Hacker NF, Berek JS (1990) Surgical-pathologic variables predictive of local recurrence in squamous cell carcinoma of the vulva. Gynecol Oncol 38(3):309–314

Hefler L, Mayerhofer K, Leibman B, Obermair A, Reinthaller A, Kainz C et al (2000) Tumor anemia and thrombocytosis in patients with vulvar cancer. Tumour Biol 21(5):309–314

Hefler LA, Grimm C, Six L, Seebacher V, Polterauer S, Joura E et al (2008) Inguinal sentinel lymph node dissection vs. complete inguinal lymph node dissection in patients with vulvar cancer. Anticancer Res 28(1B):515–517. Epub 2008/04/04

Hildesheim A, Han CL, Brinton LA, Kurman RJ, Schiller JT (1997) Human papillomavirus type 16 and risk of preinvasive and invasive vulvar cancer: results from a seroepidemiological case-control study. Obstet Gynecol 90(5):748–754

Hirai Y, Fujimoto I, Yamauchi K, Hasumi K, Masubuchi K, Sano Y (1989) Peritoneal fluid cytology and prognosis in patients with endometrial carcinoma. Obstet Gynecol 73(3 Pt 1):335–338

Hansgen G hK, Dunst J (1996) Oxygen status of cervical cancer prior and during definitive radiotherapy: possible impact of pretreatment with INF-a-2a-Retinol acid on oxygenation (abstr). Int J Radiat Oncol Biol Phys 36(Suppl):324

Hockel M, Schlenger K, Aral B, Mitze M, Schaffer U (1996) P V. Association between tumor hypoxia and malignant progression in advanced cancer of the uterine cervix. Cancer Res 56:4509–4515

Hoffmann G, Casper F, Weikel W, Kummerle T, Pollow B, Schaffrath M et al (1999) Value of p53, urokinase plasminogen activator, PAI-1 and Ki-67 in vulvar carcinoma. Zentralbl Gynakol 121(10): 473–478. Untersuchungen zu p53, UPA, PAI-1 und Ki-67 beim Vulvakarzinom

Hogberg T, Signorelli M, de Oliveira CF, Fossati R, Lissoni AA, Sorbe B et al (2010) Sequential adjuvant chemotherapy and radiotherapy in endometrial cancer—results from two randomised studies. Eur J Cancer 46(13):2422–2431

Holcomb K, Delatorre R, Pedemonte B, McLeod C, Anderson L, Chambers J (2002) E-cadherin expression in endometrioid, papillary serous, and clear cell carcinoma of the endometrium. Obstet Gynecol 100(6):1290–1295 Epub 2002/12/07

Homesley H, Raben M, Blake D (1980) Relationship of lesion size to survival in patients with stage IB squamous cell carcinoma of the cervix uteri treated by radiation therapy. Surg Gynecol Obstet 150:529–531

Homesley HD, Bundy BN, Sedlis A, Adcock L (1986) Radiation therapy versus pelvic node resection for carcinoma of the vulva with positive groin nodes. Obstet Gynecol 68(6):733–740 Epub 1986/12/01

Homesley HDBB, Sedlis A, Yordan E, Berek JS, Jahshan A, Mortel R (1991) Assessment of current International Federation of Gynecology and Obstetrics staging of vulvar carcinoma relative to prognostic factors for survival (a Gynecologic Oncology Group study). Am J Obstet Gynecol 164(4):997–1004

Homesley HD, Bundy BN, Sedlis A, Yordan E, Berek JS, Jahshan A et al (1993) Prognostic factors for groin node metastasis in squamous cell carcinoma of the vulva (a Gynecologic Oncology Group study). Gynecol Oncol 49(3):279–283

Hopkins MP, Morley GW (1991) Radical hysterectomy versus radiation therapy for stage IB squamous cell cancer of the cervix. Cancer 68(2):272–277 Epub 1991/07/15

Howlader N, Noone AM, Krapcho M, Garshell J, Neyman N, Altekruse SF, Kosary CL, Yu M, Ruhl J, Tatalovich Z, Cho H, Mariotto A, Lewis DR, Chen HS, Feuer EJ, Cronin KA (eds) (2013) SEER Cancer Statistics Review, 1975–2010. National Cancer Institute, Bethesda. http://seer.cancer.gov/csr/1975_2010. Accessed 13 April 2013, based on November 2 SEER data submission, posted to the SEER web site

Hricak H (1991) Cancer of the uterus: the value of MRI pre-and post-irradiation. Int J Rad Oncol Biol Phys 21:1089–1094

Hricak H, Lacey CG, Sandles LG, Chang YC, Winkler ML, Stern JL (1988) Invasive cervical carcinoma: comparison of MR imaging and surgical findings. Radiology 166:623–631

Hricak H, Gatsonis C, Chi DS, Amendola MA, Brandt K, Schwartz LH, Koelliker S, Siegelman ES, Brown JJ, McGhee RB Jr, Iyer R, Vitellas KM, Snyder B, Long HJ 3rd, Fiorica JV, Mitchell DG (2005) American College of Radiology Imaging Network 6651, Gynecologic Oncology Group 183,. Role of imaging in pretreatment evaluation of early invasive cervical cancer: results of the intergroup study American College of Radiology Imaging Network 6651-Gynecologic Oncology Group 183. J Clin Oncol 23(36):9329–9337

Hsu CT, Cheng YS, Su SC (1972) Prognosis of uterine cervical cancer with extensive lymph node metastases. Special emphasis on the value of pelvic lymphadenectomy in the surgical treatment of uterine cervical cancer. Am J Obstet Gynecol 114(7):954–962. Epub 1972/12/01

Huang YT, Wang CC, Tsai CS, Lai CH, Chang TC, Chou HH et al (2011) Long-term outcome and prognostic factors for adenocarcinoma/adenosquamous carcinoma of cervix after definitive radiotherapy. Int J Radiat Oncol Biol Phys 80(2):429–436 Epub 2010/06/15

Huang YT, Wang CC, Tsai CS, Lai CH, Chang TC, Chou HH et al (2012) Clinical behaviors and outcomes for adenocarcinoma or adenosquamous carcinoma of cervix treated by radical hysterectomy and adjuvant radiotherapy or chemoradiotherapy. Int J Radiat Oncol Biol Phys 84(2):420–427 Epub 2012/03/01

Hunter DJ (1975) Carcinoma of the vulva: a review of 361 patients. Gynecol Oncol 3(2):117–123

Husseinzadeh N, Wesseler T, Schneider D, Schellhas H, Nahhas W (1990) Prognostic factors and the significance of cytologic grading in invasive squamous cell carcinoma of the vulva: a clinicopathologic study. Gynecol Oncol 36(2):192–199

Irwin C, Levin W, Fyles A, Pintilie M, Manchul L, Kirkbride P (1998) The role of adjuvant radiotherapy in carcinoma of the endometrium-results in 550 patients with pathologic stage I disease. Gynecol Oncol 70(2):247–254 Epub 1998/09/19

Ito K, Matsumoto T, Nakada T, Nakanishi T, Fujita N, Yamashita H (1994) Assessing myometrial invasion by endometrial carcinoma with dynamic MRI. J Comput Assist Tomogr 18(1):77–86

Iversen T, Aalders J, Christensen A, Kolstad P (1980) Squamous cell carcinoma of the vulva: a review of 424 patients, 1956-1974. Gynecol Oncol 9(3):271–279

Jach R, Dyduch G, Radon-Pokracka M, Przybylska P, Mika M, Dulinska-Litewka J et al (2011) Expression of vascular endothelial growth factors VEGF- C and D, VEGFR-3, and comparison of lymphatic vessels density labeled with D2-40 antibodies as a prognostic factors in vulvar intraepithelial neoplasia (VIN) and invasive vulvar cancer. Neuro Endocrinol Lett 32(4):530–539

Jantarasaengaram S, Praditphol N, Tansathit T, Vipupinyo C, Vairojanavong K (2013) Three-dimensional ultrasound using volume contrast imaging (VCI) display for the preoperative assessment of myometrial invasion and cervical involvement in endometrial cancer. Ultrasound Obstet Gynecol. Epub 03 Sept 2013

Jeon YT, Park IA, Kim YB, Kim JW, Park NH, Kang SB et al (2006) Steroid receptor expressions in endometrial cancer: clinical significance and epidemiological implication. Cancer Lett 239(2):198–204 Epub 2005/09/20

Johnson GA, Mannel R, Khalifa M, Walker JL, Wren M, Min KW et al (1997) Epidermal growth factor receptor in vulvar malignancies and its relationship to metastasis and patient survival. Gynecol Oncol 65(3):425–429

Kadar N, Malfetano JH, Homesley HD (1993) Steroid receptor concentrations in endometrial carcinoma: effect on survival in surgically staged patients. Gynecol Oncol 50(3):281–286 Epub 1993/09/01

Kagie MJ, Kenter GG, Tollenaar RA, Hermans J, Trimbos JP, Fleuren GJ (1997) p53 protein overexpression, a frequent observation in squamous cell carcinoma of the vulva and in various synchronous vulvar epithelia, has no value as a prognostic parameter. Int J Gynecol Pathol 16(2):124–130

Kainz C, Speiser P, Wanner C (1995) Prognostic value of tumor microvessel density in cancer of the uterine cervix stage IB to IIB. Anticancer Res 15:1549–1551

Kanthan R, Senger JL (2011) Uterine carcinosarcomas (malignant mixed mullerian tumours): a review with special emphasis on the controversies in management. Obstet Gynecol Int 2011:470795

Kapp KS, Poschauko J, Geyer E, Berghold A, Oechs AC, Petru E et al (2002) Evaluation of the effect of routine packed red blood cell transfusion in anemic cervix cancer patients treated with radical radiotherapy. Int J Radiat Oncol Biol Phys 54(1):58–66 Epub 2002/08/17

Kataoka MY, Sala E, Baldwin P, Reinhold C, Farhadi A, Hudolin T et al (2010) The accuracy of magnetic resonance imaging in staging of vulvar cancer: a retrospective multi-centre study. Gynecol Oncol 117(1):82–87

Keys HM, Bundy BN, Stehman FB, Muderspach LI, Chafe WE, Suggs CL 3rd et al (1999) Cisplatin, radiation, and adjuvant hysterectomy compared with radiation and adjuvant hysterectomy for bulky stage IB cervical carcinoma. N Engl J Med 340(15):1154–1161 Epub 1999/04/15

Keys HM, Roberts JA, Brunetto VL, Zaino RJ, Spirtos NM, Bloss JD et al (2004) A phase III trial of surgery with or without adjunctive external pelvic radiation therapy in intermediate risk endometrial adenocarcinoma: a Gynecologic Oncology Group study. Gynecol Oncol 92(3):744–751 Epub 2004/02/27

Khalifa MA, Mannel RS, Haraway SD, Walker J, Min KW (1994) Expression of EGFR, HER-2/neu, P53, and PCNA in endometrioid, serous papillary, and clear cell endometrial adenocarcinomas. Gynecol Oncol 53(1):84–92 Epub 1994/04/01

Kidd EASB, Dehdashti F, Grigsby PW (2007) The standardized uptake value for F-18 fluorodeoxyglucose is a sensitive predictive biomarker for cervical cancer treatment response and survival. Cancer 110(8):1738–1744

Kim SH, Kim HD, Song YS, Kang SB, Lee HP (1995) Detection of deep myometrial invasion in endometrial carcinoma: comparison of transvaginal ultrasound, CT, and MRI. J Comput Assist Tomogr 19(5):766–772 Epub 1995/09/01

Kinkel K, Kaji Y, Yu KK, Segal MR, Lu Y, Powell CB et al (1999) Radiologic staging in patients with endometrial cancer: a meta-analysis. Radiology 212(3):711–718

Kirkbride P, Fyles A, Rawlings GA, Manchul L, Levin W, Murphy KJ, Simm J (1995) Carcinoma of the vagina—experience at the Princess Margaret Hospital (1974–1989). Gynecol Oncol 56(3):435–443 Epub 1995/03/01

Kitahara O, Katagiri T, Tsunoda T (2002) Classification of sensitivity or resistance of cervical cancers to ionizing radiation according to expression profiles of 62 genes selected by cDNA microarrayanalysis. Neoplasia 4:295–303

Kitajima K, Murakami K, Yamasaki E, Hagiwara S, Fukasawa I, Inaba N et al (2008) Performance of FDG-PET/CT in the diagnosis of recurrent endometrial cancer. Ann Nucl Med 22(2):103–109
Kitajima K, Kita M, Suzuki K, Senda M, Nakamoto Y, Sugimura K (2012) Prognostic significance of SUVmax (maximum standardized uptake value) measured by [(1)(8)F]FDG PET/CT in endometrial cancer. Eur J Nucl Med Mol Imaging 39(5):840–845
Kleine W, Rau K, Schwoeorer D, Pfleiderer A (1989) Prognosis of the adenocarcinoma of the cervix uteri: a comparative study. Gynecol Oncol 35(2):145–149 Epub 1989/11/01
Klopp AH, Jingran A, Ramdas L (2008) Gene expression changes in cervical squamous cell carcinoma after initiation of chemoradiation and correlation with clnical outcome. Int J Radiat Oncol Biol Phys 71:226–236
Knopp S, Bjorge T, Nesland JM, Trope C, Scheistroen M, Holm R (2004) p16INK4a and p21Waf1/Cip1 expression correlates with clinical outcome in vulvar carcinomas. Gynecol Oncol 95(1):37–45
Kock L, Mahner S, Choschzick M, Eulenburg C, Milde-Langosch K, Schwarz J et al (2011) Serum carbonic anhydrase IX and its prognostic relevance in vulvar cancer. Int J Gynecol Cancer 21(1):141–148
Kohlberger P, Kainz C, Breitenecker G, Gitsch G, Sliutz G, Kolbl H et al (1995) Prognostic value of immunohistochemically detected p53 expression in vulvar carcinoma. Cancer 76(10):1786–1789
Kolstad P (1968) Intercapillary distance, oxygen tension and local recurrence in cervix cancer. Scand J Clin Lab Invest 106(Suppl): 145–157
Komaki R, Mattingly R, Hoffman RG, Barber SW, Satre R, Greenberg M (1983) Irradiation of para-aortic lymph node metastases from carcinoma of the cervix or endometrium. Preliminary results. Radiology 147(1):245–248
Konecny GE, Santos L, Winterhoff B, Hatmal M, Keeney GL, Mariani A et al (2009) HER2 gene amplification and EGFR expression in a large cohort of surgically staged patients with nonendometrioid (type II) endometrial cancer. Br J Cancer 100(1):89–95 Epub 2008/12/18
Kong A, Simera I, Collingwood M, Williams C, Kitchener H, Cochrane Gynaecological Cancer Group (2007) Adjuvant radiotherapy for stage I endometrial cancer: systematic review and meta-analysis. Ann Oncol 18(10):1595–1604
Kosary CL (1994) FIGO stage, histology, histologic grade, age and race as prognostic factors in determining survival for cancers of the female gynecological system: an analysis of 1973-87 SEER cases of cancers of the endometrium, cervix, ovary, vulva, and vagina. Semin Surg Oncol 10(1):31–46 Epub 1994/01/01
Kovalic JJ, Perez CA, Grigsby PW et al (1991) The effect of volume of disease in patients with carcinoma of the uterine cervix. Int J Radiat Oncol Biol Phys 21:905–910
Kowalewska M, Radziszewski J, Goryca K, Bujko M, Oczko-Wojciechowska M, Jarzab M et al (2012) Estimation of groin recurrence risk in patients with squamous cell vulvar carcinoma by the assessment of marker gene expression in the lymph nodes. BMC Cancer 12:223
Krupp PJ, Bohm JW (1978) Lymph gland metastases in invasive squamous cell cancer of the vulva. Am J Obstet Gynecol 130(8):943–952
Kruse AJ, Bottenberg MJ, Tosserams J, Slangen B, van Marion AM, van Trappen PO (2008) The absence of high-risk HPV combined with specific p53 and p16INK4a expression patterns points to the HPV-independent pathway as the causative agent for vulvar squamous cell carcinoma and its precursor simplex VIN in a young patient. Int J Gynecol Pathol 27(4):591–595
Kucera H, Vavra N (1991) Radiation management of primary carcinoma of the vagina: clinical and histopathological variables associated with survival. Gynecol Oncol 40(1):12–16
Kudela M, Pilka R, Lubusky M, Hejtmanek P, Dzubak P, Brychtova S (2012) Prognostic importance of selected molecular immunohistochemical markers and DNA ploidy in endometrial cancer. Eur J Gynaecol Oncol 33(2):159–163 Epub 2012/05/23
Kutlubay Z, Engin B, Zara T, Tuzun Y (2013) Anogenital malignancies and premalignancies: facts and controversies. Clin Dermatol 31(4):362–373
Lambrou NC, Gomez-Marin O, Mirhashemi R, Beach H, Salom E, Almeida-Parra Z et al (2004) Optimal surgical cytoreduction in patients with Stage III and Stage IV endometrial carcinoma: a study of morbidity and survival. Gynecol Oncol 93(3):653–658
Lamoreaux WTGP, Dehdashti F, Zoberi I, Powell MA, Gibb RK, Rader JS, Mutch DG, Siegel BA (2005) FDG-PET evaluation of vaginal carcinoma. Int J Radiat Oncol Biol Phys 62(3):733–737
Lanciano R, Calkins A, Bundy BN, Parham G, Lucci JA 3rd, Moore DH et al (2005) Randomized comparison of weekly cisplatin or protracted venous infusion of fluorouracil in combination with pelvic radiation in advanced cervix cancer: a gynecologic oncology group study. J Clin Oncol 23(33):8289–8295
Landoni F, Maneo A, Colombo A, Placa F, Milani R, Perego P et al (1997) Randomised study of radical surgery versus radiotherapy for stage Ib-IIa cervical cancer. Lancet 350(9077):535–540 Epub 1997/08/23
Larsson GL, Helenius G, Andersson S, Sorbe B, Karlsson MG (2013) Prognostic impact of human papilloma virus (HPV) genotyping and HPV-16 subtyping in vaginal carcinoma. Gynecol Oncol 129(2):406–411
Lataifeh I, Nascimento MC, Nicklin JL, Perrin LC, Crandon AJ, Obermair A (2004) Patterns of recurrence and disease-free survival in advanced squamous cell carcinoma of the vulva. Gynecol Oncol 95(3):701–705
Latta E, Chapman WB (2002) PTEN mutations and evolving concepts in endometrial neoplasia. Curr Opin Obstet Gynecol 14(1):59–65 Epub 2002/01/22
Lavie O, Comerci G, Daras V, Bolger BS, Lopes A, Monaghan JM (1999) Thrombocytosis in women with vulvar carcinoma. Gynecol Oncol 72(1):82–86
Lea JS, Coleman RL, Garner EO, Duska LR, Miller DS, Schorge JO (2003) Adenosquamous histology predicts poor outcome in low-risk stage IB1 cervical adenocarcinoma. Gynecol Oncol 91(3):558–562 Epub 2003/12/17
Lee JH DT, Andreotti RF, Cardenes HR, Dejesus Allison SO, Gaffney DK, Glanc P, Horowitz NS, Jhingran A, Lee SI, Puthawala AA, Royal HD, Scoutt LM, Small W Jr, Varia MA, Zelop CM (2011) Expert panel on women's imaging and radiation oncology-gynecology. ACR appropriateness Criteria® pretreatment evaluation and follow-up of endometrial cancer of the uterus. Ultrasound Q 27(2):139–145
Lerma E, Matias-Guiu X, Lee SJ, Prat J (1999) Squamous cell carcinoma of the vulva: study of ploidy, HPV, p53, and pRb. Int J Gynecol Pathol 18(3):191–197
Leung SSM (1993) Radical radiation therapy for carcinoma of the vagina—impact of treatment modalities on outcome: Peter MacCallum Cancer Institute experience 1970-1990. Int J Radiat Oncol Biol Phys 25(3):413–418
Levenback CF, Ali S, Coleman RL, Gold MA, Fowler JM, Judson PL et al (2012) Lymphatic mapping and sentinel lymph node biopsy in women with squamous cell carcinoma of the vulva: A Gynecologic Oncology Group Study. J Clin Oncol 30:3786–3791 Epub 04 July 2012
Lewandowski G, Torrisi J, Potkul RK, Holloway RW, Popescu G, Whitfield G et al (1990) Hysterectomy with extended surgical staging and radiotherapy versus hysterectomy alone and radiotherapy in stage I endometrial cancer: a comparison of complication rates. Gynecol Oncol 36(3):401–404

Lewin SN, Herzog TJ, Barrena Medel NI, Deutsch I, Burke WM, Sun X et al (2010) Comparative performance of the 2009 international Federation of gynecology and obstetrics' staging system for uterine corpus cancer. Obstet Gynecol 116(5):1141–1149. Epub 2010/10/23

Lim K, Chan P, Dinniwell R, Fyles A, Haider M, Cho YB, Jaffray D, Manchul L, Levin W, Hill RP, Milosevic M (2008) Cervical cancer regression measured using weekly magnetic resonance imaging during fractionated radiotherapy: radiobiologic modeling and correlation with tumor hypoxia. Int J Radiat Oncol Biol Phys 70(1):126–133

Lindell G, Nasman A, Jonsson C, Ehrsson RJ, Jacobsson H, Danielsson KG et al (2010) Presence of human papillomavirus (HPV) in vulvar squamous cell carcinoma (VSCC) and sentinel node. Gynecol Oncol 117(2):312–316

Liu S, Semenciw R, Mao Y (2001) Cervical cancer: the increasing incidence of adenocarcinoma and adenosquamous carcinoma in younger women. CMAJ 164(8):1151–1152 Epub 2001/05/08

Liu Y, Bai R, Sun H, Liu H, Zhao X, Li Y (2009) Diffusion-weighted imaging in predicting and monitoring the response of uterine cervical cancer to combined chemoradiation. Clin Radiol 64:1067–1074

Loncaster JA, Cooper RA, Logue JP, Davidson SE, Hunter RD, West CM (2000) Vascular endothelial growth factor (VEGF) expression is a prognostic factor for radiotherapy outcome in advanced carcinoma of the cervix. Br J Cancer 83:620–625

Loncaster JA, Carrington BM, Sykes JR, Jones AP, Todd SM, Cooper R et al (2002) Prediction of radiotherapy outcome using dynamic contrast enhanced MRI of carcinoma of the cervix. Int J Rad Oncol Biol Phys 54:759–767

Look KY, Brunetto VL, Clarke-Pearson DL, Averette HE, Major FJ, Alvarez RD et al (1996) An analysis of cell type in patients with surgically staged stage IB carcinoma of the cervix: a Gynecologic Oncology Group study. Gynecol Oncol 63(3):304–311 Epub 1996/12/01

Lowrey GC, Mendenhall MW, Million RR (1992) Stage IB or IIA-B carcinoma of the intact uterine cervix treated with irradiation: a multivariate analysis. Int J Radiat Oncol Biol Phys 24:205–210

Lundgren C, Auer G, Frankendal B, Moberger B, Nilsson B, Nordstrom B (2002) Nuclear DNA content, proliferative activity, and p53 expression related to clinical and histopathologic features in endometrial carcinoma. Int J Gynecol Cancer 12(1):110–118

Macdonald OK, Chen J, Dodson M, Lee CM, Gaffney DK (2009) Prognostic significance of histology and positive lymph node involvement following radical hysterectomy in carcinoma of the cervix. Am J Clin Oncol 32(4):411–416 Epub 2009/05/20

Mackay HJ, Gallinger S, Tsao MS, McLachlin CM, Tu D, Keiser K et al (2010) Prognostic value of microsatellite instability (MSI) and PTEN expression in women with endometrial cancer: results from studies of the NCIC Clinical Trials Group (NCIC CTG). Eur J Cancer 46(8):1365–1373 Epub 2010/03/23

Madsen BS, Jensen HL, van den Brule AJ, Wohlfahrt J, Frisch M (2008) Risk factors for invasive squamous cell carcinoma of the vulva and vagina—population-based case-control study in Denmark. Int J Cancer 122(12):2827–2834

Manfredi R, Mirk P, Maresca G, Margariti PA, Testa A, Zannoni GF et al (2004) Local-regional staging of endometrial carcinoma: role of MR imaging in surgical planning. Radiology 231(2):372–378

Mariani L, Conti L, Atlante G, Sciarretta F, Pozzi M, Vercillo M, Francavilla V, De Franceschi L, Rossi S, Sindico R, Atlante M, Gandolfo GM (1998) Vulvar squamous carcinoma: prognostic role of DNA content. Gynecol Oncol 71(2):159–164

Mariani A, Sebo TJ, Katzmann JA, Keeney GL, Roche PC, Lesnick TG et al (2000) Pretreatment assessment of prognostic indicators in endometrial cancer. Am J Obstet Gynecol 182(6):1535–1544 Epub 2000/06/28

Mariani A, Webb MJ, Keeney GL, Haddock MG, Aletti G, Podratz KC (2002a) Stage IIIC endometrioid corpus cancer includes distinct subgroups. Gynecol Oncol 87(1):112–117 Epub 2002/12/07

Mariani A, Webb MJ, Keeney GL, Aletti G, Podratz KC (2002b) Predictors of lymphatic failure in endometrial cancer. Gynecol Oncol 84(3):437–442

Mariani A, Webb MJ, Keeney GL, Aletti G, Podratz KC (2002c) Assessment of prognostic factors in stage IIIA endometrial cancer. Gynecol Oncol 86(1):38–44

Martin-Hirsch PP, Bryant A, Keep SL, Kitchener HC, Lilford R (2011) Adjuvant progestagens for endometrial cancer. Cochrane Database Syst Rev 6:CD001040. Epub 2011/06/17

Maxwell GL, Risinger JI, Alvarez AA, Barrett JC, Berchuck A (2001) Favorable survival associated with microsatellite instability in endometrioid endometrial cancers. Obstet Gynecol 97(3):417–422 Epub 2001/03/10

Mayr A, Wang JZ, D Z, Montebello JF, Grecula JC, Lo SS et al (2009) Synergistic effects of hemoglobin and tumor perfusion on tumor control and survival in cervical cancer. Int J Radiat Oncol Biol Phys 74(5):1513–1521

Mayr NA, Magnotta VA, Ehrhardt JC, Wheeler JA, Sorosky JI, Wen BC et al (1996) Usefulness of tumor volumetry by magnetic resonance imaging in assessing response to radiation therapy in carcinoma of the uterine cervix. Int J Radiat Oncol Biol Phys 35(5):915–924

Mayr NA, Hawighorst H, Yuh WTC, Essig M, Magnotta VA, Knopp MV (1999) MR microcirculation in cervical cancer: correlations with histomorphological tumor markers and clinical outcome. J Magn Reson Imaging 10:267–276

Mayr NA, Yuh WTC, Taoka T, Wang JZ, Wu DH, Montebello JF et al (2006) Serial therapy-induced changes in tumor shape in cervical cancer and their impact on assessing tumor volume and treatment response. Am J Roentgenol 187:65–72

Mayr NA, Wang JZ, Lo SS, Zhang D, Grecula JC, Lu L et al (2010) Translating response during therapy into ultimate treatment outcome: a personalized 4-dimensional MRI tumor volumetric regression approach in cervical cancer. Int J Radiat Oncol Biol Phys 76:719–727 (23 July 2009, Epub ahead of print)

McConnell DT, Miller ID, Parkin DE, Murray GI (1997) p53 protein expression in a population-based series of primary vulval squamous cell carcinoma and immediate adjacent field change. Gynecol Oncol 67(3):248–254

Mell LK, Meyer JJ, Tretiakova M, Khramtsov A, Gong C, Yamada SD et al (2004) Prognostic significance of E-cadherin protein expression in pathological stage I-III endometrial cancer. Clin Cancer Res 10(16):5546–5553 Epub 2004/08/26

Mendenhall WM, Thar TL, Bova FJ, Marcus RB Jr, Morgan LS, Million RR (1984) Prognostic and treatment factors affecting pelvic control of stage IB and IIA-B carcinoma of the intact uterine cervix treated with radiation therapy alone. Cancer 53:2649–2654

Milgrom SA, Kollmeier MA, Abu-Rustum NR, Makker V, Gardner GJ, Barakat RR et al (2013) Positive peritoneal cytology is highly predictive of prognosis and relapse patterns in stage III (FIGO 2009) endometrial cancer. Gynecol Oncol 130(1):49–53

Monk BJBR, Lin F, Parham G, Vasilev SA, Wilczynski SP (1995) Prognostic significance of human papillomavirus DNA in vulvar carcinoma. Obstet Gynecol 85:709–715

Montana GS, Thomas GM, Moore DH, Saxer A, Mangan CE, Lentz SS et al (2000) Preoperative chemo-radiation for carcinoma of the vulva with N2/N3 nodes: a gynecologic oncology group study. Int J Radiat Oncol Biol Phys 48(4):1007–1013

Moore DH, Ali S, Koh WJ, Michael H, Barnes MN, McCourt CK et al (2012) A phase II trial of radiation therapy and weekly cisplatin chemotherapy for the treatment of locally-advanced squamous cell carcinoma of the vulva: a gynecologic oncology group study. Gynecol Oncol 124(3):529–533

Morice P, Castaigne D, Pautier P, Rey A, Haie-Meder C, Leblanc M et al (1999) Interest of pelvic and paraaortic lymphadenectomy in patients with stage IB and II cervical carcinoma. Gynecol Oncol 73(1):106–110 Epub 1999/03/30

Morley GW, Seski JC (1976) Radical pelvic surgery versus radiation therapy for stage I carcinoma of the cervix (exclusive of microinvasion). Am J Obstet Gynecol 126(7):785–798 Epub 1976/12/01

Morris M, Eifel PJ, Lu J, Grigsby PW, Levenback C, Stevens RE et al (1999) Pelvic radiation with concurrent chemotherapy compared with pelvic and para-aortic radiation for high-risk cervical cancer. N Engl J Med 340:1137–1143

Morrow (1980) Is pelvic radiation beneficial in the postoperative management of stage Ib squamous cell carcinoma of the cervix with pelvic node metastasis treated by radical hysterectomy and pelvic lymphadenectomy? A report from the Presidential Panel at the 1979 Annual Meeting of the Society of Gynecologic Oncologists (1980) Gynecol Oncol 10(1):105–110

Morrow CP, Bundy BN, Kurman RJ, Creasman WT, Heller P, Homesley HD et al (1991) Relationship between surgical-pathological risk factors and outcome in clinical stage I and II carcinoma of the endometrium: a Gynecologic Oncology Group study. Gynecol Oncol 40(1):55–65

Naganawa S, Sato C, Kumada H, Ishigaki T, Miura S, Takizawa O (2005). Apparent diffusion coefficient in cervical cancer of the uterus: comparison with the normal uterine cervix. Eur Radiol 15:71–78

Nagar H, Dobbs S, McClelland HR, Price J, McCluggage WG, Grey A (2006) The diagnostic accuracy of magnetic resonance imaging in detecting cervical involvement in endometrial cancer. Gynecol Oncol 103(2):431–434

Nakamura K, Kodama J, Okumura Y, Hongo A, Kanazawa S, Hiramatsu Y (2010) The SUVmax of 18F-FDG PET correlates with histological grade in endometrial cancer. Int J Gynecol Cancer 20(1):110–115

Nakamura K, Hongo A, Kodama J, Hiramatsu Y (2011) The measurement of SUVmax of the primary tumor is predictive of prognosis for patients with endometrial cancer. Gynecol Oncol 123(1):82–87

Nakamura K, Joja I, Fukushima C, Haruma T, Hayashi C, Kusumoto T et al (2013) The preoperative SUVmax is superior to ADCmin of the primary tumour as a predictor of disease recurrence and survival in patients with endometrial cancer. Eur J Nucl Med Mol Imaging 40(1):52–60

Nicoletto MO, Parenti A, Del Bianco P, Lombardi G, Pedrini L, Pizzi S, Carli P, Della Palma M, Pastorelli D, Corti L, Becagli L (2010) Vulvar cancer: prognostic factors. Anticancer Res 30(6):2311–2317

Nordstrom B, Strang P, Lindgren A, Bergstrom R, Tribukait B (1996) Carcinoma of the endometrium: do the nuclear grade and DNA ploidy provide more prognostic information than do the FIGO and WHO classifications? Int J Gynecol Pathol 15(3):191–201

Nori D, Hilaris B, Stanimir G, Lewis JL Jr (1983) Radiation therapy of primary vaginal carcinoma. Int J Radiat Oncol Biol Phys 9(10):1471–1475

Nout RA, Smit VT, Putter H, Jurgenliemk-Schulz IM, Jobsen JJ, Lutgens LC et al (2010) Vaginal brachytherapy versus pelvic external beam radiotherapy for patients with endometrial cancer of high-intermediate risk (PORTEC-2): an open-label, non-inferiority, randomised trial. Lancet 375(9717):816–823 Epub 2010/03/09

Nout RA, Bosse T, Creutzberg CL, Jurgenliemk-Schulz IM, Jobsen JJ, Lutgens LC et al (2012) Improved risk assessment of endometrial cancer by combined analysis of MSI, PI3 K-AKT, Wnt/beta-catenin and P53 pathway activation. Gynecol Oncol 126(3):466–473

Obermair A, Kohlberger P, Bancher-Todesca D, Tempfer C, Sliutz G, Leodolter S et al (1996) Influence of microvessel density and vascular permeability factor/vascular endothelial growth factor expression on prognosis in vulvar cancer. Gynecol Oncol 63(2):204–209

Obermair A, Wanner C, Bilgi S, Speiser P, Kaider A, Rheinthaller A et al (1998) Tumor angiogenesis in stage IB cervical cancer: correlaion of microvessel density with survival. Am J Obstet Gynecol 178:314–319

Okagaki T, Twiggs LB, Zachow KR, Clark BA, Ostrow RS, Faras AJ (1983) Identification of human papillomavirus DNA in cervical and vaginal intraepithelial neoplasia with molecularly cloned virus-specific DNA probes. Int J Gynecol Pathol 2(2):153–159

Oonk MH, van Hemel BM, Hollema H, de Hullu JA, Ansink AC, Vergote I et al (2010) Size of sentinel-node metastasis and chances of non-sentinel-node involvement and survival in early stage vulvar cancer: results from GROINSS-V, a multicentre observational study. Lancet Oncol 11(7):646–652

Orezzoli JP, Sioletic S, Olawaiye A, Oliva E, del Carmen MG (2009) Stage II endometrioid adenocarcinoma of the endometrium: clinical implications of cervical stromal invasion. Gynecol Oncol 113(3):316–323

Origoni M, Sideri M, Garsia S, Carinelli SG, Ferrari AG (1992) Prognostic value of pathological patterns of lymph node positivity in squamous cell carcinoma of the vulva stage III and IVA FIGO. Gynecol Oncol 45(3):313–316

Ota T, Yoshida M, Kimura M, Kinoshita K (2005) Clinicopathologic study of uterine endometrial carcinoma in young women aged 40 years and younger. Int J Gynecol Cancer 15(4):657–662 Epub 2005/07/15

Paladini D, Cross P, Lopes A, Monaghan JM (1994) Prognostic significance of lymph node variables in squamous cell carcinoma of the vulva. Cancer 74(9):2491–2496

Park JY, Kim EN, Kim DY, Kim JH, Kim YM, Kim YT et al (2008) Clinical impact of positron emission tomography or positron emission tomography/computed tomography in the posttherapy surveillance of endometrial carcinoma: evaluation of 88 patients. Int J Gynecol Cancer 18(6):1332–1338

Pecorelli S (2009) Revised FIGO staging for carcinoma of the vulva, cervix, and endometrium. Int J Gynaecol Obstet 105(2): 103–104

Pecorelli S, Zigliani L, Odicino F (2009) Revised FIGO staging for carcinoma of the cervix. Int J Gynaecol Obstet 105(2):107–108

Perez CA, Camel HM, Galakatos AE, Grigsby PW, Kuske RR, Buchsbaum G et al (1988) Definitive irradiation in carcinoma of the vagina: long-term evaluation of results. Int J Radiat Oncol Biol Phys 15(6):1283–1290

Perez CA, Grigsby P, Nene S et al (1992a) Effect of tumor size on the prognosis of carcinoma of the uterine cervix treated with irradiation alone. Cancer 69:2796–2806

Perez C, Grigsby P, Nene S et al (1992b) Effect of tumor size on the prognosis of carcinoma of the uterine cervix treated with irradiation alone. Cancer 69:2796–2806

Perez CAGP, Garipagaoglu M, Mutch DG, Lockett MA (1999) Factors affecting long-term outcome of irradiation in carcinoma of the vagina. Int J Radiat Oncol Biol Phys 44(1):37–45

Pilch H, Gunzel S, Schaffer U, Tanner B, Brockerhoff P, Maeurer M et al (2001) The presence of HPV DNA in cervical cancer: correlation with clinico-pathologic parameters and prognostic significance: 10 years experience at the Department of Obstetrics and Gynecology of the Mainz University. Int J Gynecol Cancer 11(1):39–48 Epub 2001/04/04

Pingley S, Shrivastava SK, Sarin R, Agarwal JP, Laskar S, Deshpande DD et al (2000) Primary carcinoma of the vagina: Tata Memorial Hospital experience. Int J Radiat Oncol Biol Phys 46(1):101–108 Epub 2000/02/03

Podratz KCSR, Taylor WF, Williams TJ (1983) Carcinoma of the vulva: analysis of treatment and survival. Obstet Gynecol 61(1):63–74

Powell JL, Hill KA, Shiro BC, Diehl SJ, Gajewski WH (2005) Preoperative serum CA-125 levels in treating endometrial cancer. J Reprod Med 50(8):585–590 Epub 2005/10/14

Prat J (2009) FIGO staging for uterine sarcomas. Int J Gynaecol Obstet 104(3):177–178

Prat J, Oliva E, Lerma E, Vaquero M, Matias-Guiu X (1994) Uterine papillary serous adenocarcinoma. A 10-case study of p53 and c-erbB-2 expression and DNA content. Cancer 74(6):1778–1783

Prempree T, Amornmarn R (1985) Radiation treatment of primary carcinoma of the vagina. Patterns of failures after definitive therapy. Acta Radiologica Oncol 24(1):51–56. Epub 1985/01/01

Prompeler HJ, Madjar H, du Bois A, Lattermann U, Wilhelm C, Kommoss F et al (1994) Transvaginal sonography of myometrial invasion depth in endometrial cancer. Acta Obstet Gynecol Scand 73(4):343–346 Epub 1994/04/01

Peters WA r, Liu PY, Barrett RJ 2nd et al (2000) Concurrent chemotherapy and pelvic radiation therapy compared with pelvic radiation therapy alone as adjuvant therapy after radical surgery in high-risk early-stage cancer of the cervix. J Clin Oncol18:1606–1613

Ragnarsson-Olding B, Johansson H, Rutqvist LE, Ringborg U (1993) Malignant melanoma of the vulva and vagina. Trends in incidence, age distribution, and long-term survival among 245 consecutive cases in Sweden 1960-1984. Cancer 71(5):1893–1897

Ramanah R, Lesieur B, Ballester M, Darai E, Rouzier R (2012) Trends in of late-stage squamous cell vulvar carcinomas: analysis of the surveillance, epidemiology, and end results (SEER) database. Int J Gynecol Cancer 22(5):854–859

Randall ME, Filiaci VL, Muss H, Spirtos NM, Mannel RS, Fowler J et al (2006) Randomized phase III trial of whole-abdominal irradiation versus doxorubicin and cisplatin chemotherapy in advanced endometrial carcinoma: a Gynecologic Oncology Group Study. J Clin Oncol 24(1):36–44

Randall LM, Monk BJ, Darcy KM, Tian C, Burger RA, Liao SY et al (2009) Markers of angiogenesis in high-risk, early-stage cervical cancer: a Gynecologic Oncology Group study. Gynecol Oncol 112(3):583–589 Epub 2008/12/27

Raspagliesi F, Hanozet F, Ditto A, Solima E, Zanaboni F, Vecchione F, Kusamura S (2006) Clinical and pathological prognostic factors in squamous cell carcinoma of the vulva. Gynecol Oncol 102(2):333–337

Rauh-Hain JA, Del Carmen MG (2013) Endometrial stromal sarcoma: a systematic review. Obstet Gynecol 122(3):676–683

Rose PG, Bundy BN, Watkins EB, Thigpen JT, Deppe G, Maiman MA et al (1999) Concurrent Cisplatin-based radiotherapy and chemotherapy for locally advanced cervical cancer. N Engl J Med 340:1144–1153

Rose PGAS, Watkins E, Thigpen JT, Deppe G, Clarke-Pearson DL, Insalaco S (2007) Long-term follow-up of a randomized trial comparing concurrent single agent cisplatin, cisplatin-based combination chemotherapy, or hydroxyurea during pelvic irradiation for locally advanced cervical cancer: a Gynecologic Oncology Group Study. J Clin Oncol 25:2804–2810

Ross JC, Eifel PJ, Cox RS, Kempson RL, Hendrickson MR (1983) Primary mucinous adenocarcinoma of the endometrium. A clinicopathologic and histochemical study. Am J Surg Pathol 7(8):715–729

Ross BDMB, Lawrence TS, Mukherji SK, Gebarski SS, Quint DJ, Johnson TD, Junck L, Robertson PL, Muraszko KM, Dong Q, Meyer CR, Bland PH, McConville P, Geng H, Rehemtulla A, Chenevert TL (2003) Evaluation of cancer therapy using diffusion magnetic resonance imaging. Mol Cancer Ther 2(6):581–587

Rotman M, Aziz H, Eifel PJ (1994) Irradiation of pelvic and para-aortic nodes in carcinoma of the cervix. Semin Radiat Oncol 4(1):23–29

Rotman M, Sedlis A, Piedmonte MR, Bundy B, Lentz SS, Muderspach LI, Zaino RJ (2006) A phase III randomized trial of postoperative pelvic irradiation in Stage IB cervical carcinoma with poor prognostic features: follow-up of a gynecologic oncology group study. Int J Radiat Oncol Biol Phys 65(1):169–176

Rouzier R, Haddad B, Plantier F, Dubois P, Pelisse M, Paniel BJ (2002) Local relapse in patients treated for squamous cell vulvar carcinoma: incidence and prognostic value. Obstet Gynecol 100(6): 1159–1167

Rutledge F, Smith J, Franklin EW (1970) Carcinoma of the vulva. Am J Obstet Gynecol 106(8):1117–1130

Saez F, Urresola A, Larena JA, Martin JI, Pijuan JI, Schneider J et al (2000) Endometrial carcinoma: assessment of myometrial invasion with plain and gadolinium-enhanced MR imaging. J Magn Reson Imaging 12(3):460–466

Saffari B, Bernstein L, Hong DC, Sullivan-Halley J, Runnebaum IB, Grill HJ et al (2005) Association of p53 mutations and a codon 72 single nucleotide polymorphism with lower overall survival and responsiveness to adjuvant radiotherapy in endometrioid endometrial carcinomas. Int J Gynecol Cancer 15(5):952–963 Epub 2005/09/22

Saga T, Higashi T, Ishimori T, Mamede M, Nakamoto Y, Mukai T et al (2003) Clinical value of FDG-PET in the follow up of post-operative patients with endometrial cancer. Ann Nucl Med 17(3):197–203

Sala E, Crawford R, Senior E, Shaw A, Simcock B, Vrotsou K et al (2009) Added value of dynamic contrast-enhanced magnetic resonance imaging in predicting advanced stage disease in patients with endometrial carcinoma. Int J Gynecol Cancer 19(1):141–146

Salani R, Backes FJ, Fung MF, Holschneider CH, Parker LP, Bristow RE et al (2011) Posttreatment surveillance and diagnosis of recurrence in women with gynecologic malignancies: Society of Gynecologic Oncologists recommendations. Am J Obstet Gynecol 204(6):466–478 Epub 2011/07/15

Salvesen HB, Iversen OE, Akslen LA (1998) Identification of high-risk patients by assessment of nuclear Ki-67 expression in a prospective study of endometrial carcinomas. Clin Cancer Res 4(11):2779–2785 Epub 1998/11/26

Santos M, Montagut C, Mellado B, Garcia A, Ramon y Cajal S, Cardesa A et al (2004) Immunohistochemical staining for p16 and p53 in premalignant and malignant epithelial lesions of the vulva. Int J Gynecol Pathol 23(3):206–214

Scheistroen M, Trope C, Pettersen EO, Nesland JM (1999) p53 protein expression in squamous cell carcinoma of the vulva. Cancer 85(5):1133–1138

Schwartz SM, Daling JR, Shera KA, Madeleine MM, McKnight B, Galloway DA et al (2001) Human papillomavirus and prognosis of invasive cervical cancer: a population-based study. J Clin Oncol 19(7):1906–1915 Epub 2001/04/03

Scribner DR Jr, Walker JL, Johnson GA, McMeekin DS, Gold MA, Mannel RS (2002) Laparoscopic pelvic and paraaortic lymph node dissection in the obese. Gynecol Oncol 84(3):426–430

Sedlis A, Bundy B, Rotman MZ, Lentz SS, Muderspach LI, Zaino RJ (1999) A randomized trial of pelvic radiation therapy versus no further therapy in selected patients with stage IB carcinoma of the cervix after radical hysterectomy and pelvic lymphadenectomy: A Gynecologic Oncology Group Study. Gynecol Oncol 73(2):177–183

Selman TJ, Luesley DM, Acheson N, Khan KS, Mann CH (2005) A systematic review of the accuracy of diagnostic tests for inguinal lymph node status in vulvar cancer. Gynecol Oncol 99(1):206–214

Sethi TK, Bhalla NK, Jena AN, Rawat S, Oberoi R (2005) Magnetic resonance imaging in carcinoma cervix—does it have a prognostic relevance. J Cancer Res Ther 1(2):103–107

Shah CA, Goff BA, Lowe K, Peters WA 3rd, Li CI (2009) Factors affecting risk of mortality in women with vaginal cancer. Obstet Gynecol 113(5):1038–1045

Shingleton HM, Bell MC, Fremgen A, Chmiel JS, Russell AH, Jones WB et al (1995) Is there really a difference in survival of women with squamous cell carcinoma, adenocarcinoma, and adenosquamous cell carcinoma of the cervix? Cancer 76(10 Suppl):1948–1955 Epub 1995/11/15

Siegel R, Naishadham D, Jemal A (2012) Cancer statistics, 2012. CA Cancer J Clin 62(1):10–29 Epub 2012/01/13

Siegel R, Naishadham D, Jemal A (2013) Cancer statistics, 2013. CA Cancer J Clin 63(1):11–30

Sillman FH, Fruchter RG, Chen YS, Camilien L, Sedlis A, McTigue E (1997) Vaginal intraepithelial neoplasia: risk factors for persistence, recurrence, and invasion and its management. Am J Obstet Gynecol 176(1 Pt 1):93–99

Silverman MB, Roche PC, Kho RM, Keeney GL, Li H, Podratz KC (2000) Molecular and cytokinetic pretreatment risk assessment in endometrial carcinoma. Gynecol Oncol 77(1):1–7 Epub 2000/03/31

Singh K, Orakwue CO, Honest H, Balogun M, Lopez C, Luesley DM (2006) Accuracy of magnetic resonance imaging of inguinofemoral lymph nodes in vulval cancer. Int J Gynecol Cancer 16(3):1179–1183 Epub 2006/06/29

Singh M, Darcy KM, Brady WE, Clubwala R, Weber Z, Rittenbach JV et al (2011) Cadherins, catenins and cell cycle regulators: impact on survival in a Gynecologic Oncology Group phase II endometrial cancer trial. Gynecol Oncol 123(2):320–328 Epub 2011/08/05

Sironi S, Colombo E, Villa G, Taccagni G, Belloni C, Garancini P et al (1992) Myometrial invasion by endometrial carcinoma: assessment with plain and gadolinium-enhanced MR imaging. Radiology 185(1):207–212

Smith HO, Tiffany MF, Qualls CR, Key CR (2000) The rising incidence of adenocarcinoma relative to squamous cell carcinoma of the uterine cervix in the United States—a 24-year population-based study. Gynecol Oncol 78(2):97–105 Epub 2000/08/06

Sohaib SA, Richards PS, Ind T, Jeyarajah AR, Shepherd JH, Jacobs IJ et al (2002) MR imaging of carcinoma of the vulva. Am J Roentgenol 178(2):373–377

Stang A, Streller B, Eisinger B, Jockel KH (2005) Population-based incidence rates of malignant melanoma of the vulva in Germany. Gynecol Oncol 96(1):216–221

Stehman FBBB, DiSaia PJ, Keys HM, Larson JE, Fowler WC (1991) Carcinoma of the cervix treated with radiation therapy. I. A multivariate analysis of prognostic variables in the Gynecologic Oncology Group. Cancer 67(11):2776–2785

Steinbakk A, Malpica A, Slewa A, Skaland I, Gudlaugsson E, Janssen EA et al (2011) Biomarkers and microsatellite instability analysis of curettings can predict the behavior of FIGO stage I endometrial endometrioid adenocarcinoma. Mod Pathol 24(9):1262–1271 Epub 2011/05/10

Stone JE, Parker R, Gilks CB, Stanbridge EJ, Liao SY, Aquino-Parsons C (2005) Intratumoral oxygenation of invasive squamous cell carcimoma of the vulva is not correlated with regional lymph node metastasis. Eur J Gynaecol Oncol 26(1):31–35

Sugiyama VE, Chan JK, Shin JY, Berek JS, Osann K, Kapp DS (2007) Vulvar melanoma: a multivariable analysis of 644 patients. Obstet Gynecol 110(2 Pt 1):296–301

Szantho A, Szabo I, Csapo ZS, Balega J, Demeter A, Papp Z (2001) Assessment of myometrial and cervical invasion of endometrial cancer by transvaginal sonography. Eur J Gynaecol Oncol 22(3):209–212 Epub 2001/08/15

Sznurkowski JJ, Milczek T, Emerich J (2013) Prognostic factors and a value of 2009 FIGO staging system in vulvar cancer. Arch Gynecol Obstet 287(6):1211–1218

Tabbaa ZM, Gonzalez J, Sznurkowski JJ, Weaver AL, Mariani A, Cliby WA (2012) Impact of the new FIGO 2009 staging classification for vulvar cancer on prognosis and stage distribution. Gynecol Oncol 127(1):147–152

Takahashi K, Yoshioka M, Kosuge H, Iizuka Y, Musha T, Yamauchi I et al (1995) The accuracy of computed tomography and magnetic resonance imaging in evaluating the extent of endometrial carcinoma. Nihon Sanka Fujinka Gakkai Zasshi. 47(7):647–654

Takeda N, Sakuragi N, Takeda M, Okamoto K, Kuwabara M, Negishi H et al (2002) Multivariate analysis of histopathologic prognostic factors for invasive cervical cancer treated with radical hysterectomy and systematic retroperitoneal lymphadenectomy. Acta Obstet Gynecol Scand 81(12):1144–1151 Epub 2003/01/10

Takeshima N, Nishida H, Tabata T, Hirai Y, Hasumi K (2001) Positive peritoneal cytology in endometrial cancer: enhancement of other prognostic indicators. Gynecol Oncol 82(3):470–473

Tan J, Chetty N, Kondalsamy-Chennakesavan S, Crandon A, Garrett A, Land R et al (2012) Validation of the FIGO 2009 staging system for carcinoma of the vulva. Int J Gynecol Cancer 22(3):498–502

Tanaka Y, Sawada S, Murata T (1984) Relationship between lymph node metastases and prognosis in patients irradiated postoperatively for carcinoma of the uterine cervix. Acta Radiologica Oncology 23(6):455–459

Tannock IF (1972) Oxygen diffusion and the distribution of cellular radiosensitivity in tumors. Br J Radiol 45:515–524

Tantipalakorn C, Robertson G, Marsden DE, Gebski V, Hacker NF (2009) Outcome and patterns of recurrence for FIGO stages I and II squamous cell vulvar cancer. Obstet Gynecol 113(4):895–907

Taylor MBDN, Davidson SE, Carrington BM (2007) Magnetic resonance imaging of primary vaginal carcinoma. Clin Radiol 62(6):549–555

Tebeu PM, Popowski Y, Verkooijen HM, Bouchardy C, Ludicke F, Usel M et al (2004) Positive peritoneal cytology in early-stage endometrial cancer does not influence prognosis. Br J Cancer 91(4):720–724

Tewari D, Monk BJ, Al-Ghazi MS (2005) Gene expression profiling of in vitro radiation resistance in cervical carcinoma: a feasibility study. Gynecol Oncol 99:84–91

Tewari KS, Filiaci VL, Spirtos NM, Mannel RS, Thigpen JT, Cibull ML et al (2012) Association of number of positive nodes and cervical stroma invasion with outcome of advanced endometrial cancer treated with chemotherapy or whole abdominal irradiation: a Gynecologic Oncology Group study. Gynecol Oncol 125(1):87–93

Thomas G (2001) The effect of hemoglobin level on radiotherapy outcomes: the Canadian experience. Semin Oncol 28(S8):60–65

Thomas GM, Dembo AJ, Myhr T, Black B, Pringle JF, Rawlings G (1993) Long-term results of concurrent radiation and chemotherapy for carcinoma of the cervix recurrent after surgery. Int J Gynecol Cancer 3(4):193–198

Tjalma W, Weyler J, Weyn B (2000) The association between vascular endothelial growth factor and, microvessel density and clinicopathologic features in invasive cervical cancer. Eur J Obstet Gynecol 92:251–257

Tran PT, Su Z, Lee P, Lavori P, Husain A, Teng N et al (2007) Prognostic factors for outcomes and complications for primary squamous cell carcinoma of the vagina treated with radiation. Gynecol Oncol 105(3):641–649 Epub 2007/03/17

Tringler B, Grimm C, Dudek G, Zeillinger R, Tempfer C, Speiser P et al (2007) p16INK4a expression in invasive vulvar squamous cell carcinoma. Appl Immunohistochem Mol Morphol 15(3):279–283

Tsai CS, Lai CH, Wang CC, Chang JT, Chang TC, Tseng CJ et al (1999) The prognostic factors for patients with early cervical cancer treated by radical hysterectomy and postoperative radiotherapy. Gynecol Oncol 75(3):328–333 Epub 1999/12/22

Tsili AC, Tsampoulas C, Dalkalitsis N, Stefanou D, Paraskevaidis E, Efremidis SC (2008) Local staging of endometrial carcinoma: role of multidetector CT. Eur Radiol 18(5):1043–1048

Urbanski K, Kojs Z, Reinfuss M, Fabisiak W (1996) Primary invasive vaginal carcinoma treated with radiotherapy: analysis of prognostic factors. Gynecol Oncol 60(1):16–21

Valenzano M, Podesta M, Giannesi A, Corticelli A, Nicoletti L, Costantini S (2001) The role of transvaginal ultrasound and sonohysterography in the diagnosis and staging of endometrial adenocarcinoma. Radiol Med 101(5):365–370. Ecografia transvaginale e isterosonografia nella diagnosi e nella stadiazione dell'adenocarcinoma dell'endometrio

van de Nieuwenhof HP, de Hullu JA, Kaanders JH, Bulten J, Massuger LF, van Kempen LC (2010) Hemoglobin level predicts outcome for vulvar cancer patients independent of GLUT-1 and CA-IX expression in tumor tissue. Virchows Arch 457(6):693–703

Van der Zee AG, Oonk MH, De Hullu JA, Ansink AC, Vergote I, Verheijen RH et al (2008) Sentinel node dissection is safe in the treatment of early-stage vulvar cancer. J Clin Oncol 26(6):884–889 Epub 2008/02/19

Vavra N, Seifert M, Kucera H, Weghaupt K (1991) Radiotherapy of primary vaginal carcinoma and effects of histological and clinical factors on the prognosis. Strahlenther Onkol 167(1):1–6

Viswanathan AN, Pinto AP, Schultz D, Berkowitz R, Crum CP (2013) Relationship of margin status and radiation dose to recurrence in post-operative vulvar carcinoma. Gynecol Oncol 130(3):545–549 Epub 2013/06/12

van Bommel PF vLA, Kock HC, Leers WH, Neijt JP (1987). A review of prognostic factors in early-stage carcinoma of the cervix (FIGO I B and II A) and implications for treatment strategy. Eur J Obstet Gynecol Reprod Biol 26(1):69–84

Walboomers JM, Jacobs MV, Manos MM, Bosch FX, Kummer JA, Shah KV et al (1999) Human papillomavirus is a necessary cause of invasive cervical cancer worldwide. J Pathol 189(1):12–19 Epub 1999/08/19

Wang CC, Lai CH, Huang HJ, Chao A, Chang CJ, Chang TC et al (2010) Clinical effect of human papillomavirus genotypes in patients with cervical cancer undergoing primary radiotherapy. Int J Radiat Oncol Biol Phys 78(4):1111–1120 Epub 2010/03/17

Wang CC, Lai CH, Huang YT, Chao A, Chou HH, Hong JH (2012) HPV genotypes predict survival benefits from concurrent chemotherapy and radiation therapy in advanced squamous cell carcinoma of the cervix. Int J Radiat Oncol Biol Phys 84(4):e499–e506 Epub 2012/08/15

Weinstock MA (1994) Malignant melanoma of the vulva and vagina in the United States: patterns of incidence and population-based estimates of survival. Am J Obstet Gynecol 171(5):1225–1230

Werner HM, Trovik J, Marcickiewicz J, Tingulstad S, Staff AC, Amant F et al (2012) Revision of FIGO surgical staging in 2009 for endometrial cancer validates to improve risk stratification. Gynecol Oncol 125(1):103–108

Whitney CWSW, Bundy BN, Malfetano JH, Hannigan EV, Fowler WC Jr, Clarke-Pearson DL, Liao SY (1999) Randomized comparison of fluorouracil plus cisplatin versus hydroxyurea as an adjunct to radiation therapy in stage IIB-IVA carcinoma of the cervix with negative para-aortic lymph nodes: a Gynecologic Oncology Group and Southwest Oncology Group study. J Clin Oncol 17:1339–1348

Woelber L, Mahner S, Voelker K, Eulenburg CZ, Gieseking F, Choschzick M, Jaenicke, F Schwarz J (2009) Clinicopathological prognostic factors and patterns of recurrence in vulvar cancer. Anticancer Res 29(2):545–552

Woelber L, Hess S, Bohlken H, Tennstedt P, Eulenburg C, Simon R et al (2012) EGFR gene copy number increase in vulvar carcinomas is linked with poor clinical outcome. J Clin Pathol 65(2):133–139

Wong YF, Selvanayagam ZE, Wei N (2003) Expression genomis of cervical cancer: molecular classification and predicton of radiotherapy response by DNA microarray. Clin Cancer Res 9:5486–5492

Wu X, Matanoski G, Chen VW, Saraiya M, Coughlin SS, King JB et al (2008) Descriptive epidemiology of vaginal cancer incidence and survival by race, ethnicity, and age in the United States. Cancer 113(10 Suppl):2873–2882

Yamashita Y, Mizutani H, Torashima M, Takahashi M, Miyazaki K, Okamura H et al (1993a) Assessment of myometrial invasion by endometrial carcinoma: transvaginal sonography vs contrast-enhanced MR imaging. Am J Roentgenol 161(3):595–599

Yamashita Y, Harada M, Sawada T, Takahashi M, Miyazaki K, Okamura H (1993b) Normal uterus and FIGO stage I endometrial carcinoma: dynamic gadolinium-enhanced MR imaging. Radiology 186(2):495–501

Young P, Daniel B, Sommer G, Kim B, Herfkens R (2012) Intravaginal gel for staging of female pelvic cancers—preliminary report of safety, distention, and gel-mucosal contrast during magnetic resonance examination. J Comput Assist Tomogr 36(2):253–256

Yuh WTC, Mayr NA, Jarjoura D, Wu DH, Grecula JC, Lo SS et al (2009) Predicting control of primary tumor and survival by DCE MRI during early therapy in cervical cancer. Invest Radiol 44:343–350

Zaino RJ, Kurman RJ, Brunetto VL, Morrow CP, Bentley RC, Cappellari JO et al (1998a) Villoglandular adenocarcinoma of the endometrium: a clinicopathologic study of 61 cases: a gynecologic oncology group study. Am J Surg Pathol 22(11):1379–1385

Zaino RJ, Davis AT, Ohlsson-Wilhelm BM, Brunetto VL (1998b) DNA content is an independent prognostic indicator in endometrial adenocarcinoma. A Gynecologic Oncology Group study. Int J Gynecol Pathol 17(4):312–319

Zighelboim I, Goodfellow PJ, Gao F, Gibb RK, Powell MA, Rader JS et al (2007) Microsatellite instability and epigenetic inactivation of MLH1 and outcome of patients with endometrial carcinomas of the endometrioid type. J Clin Oncol 25(15):2042–2048 Epub 2007/05/22

Bladder Cancer

Ping Jiang and Juergen Dunst

Contents

Abstract

Bladder cancer is the 9th most common cancer diagnosis worldwide. There are more than 330,000 new cases each year and more than 130,000 deaths per year. Although radical cystectomy has been considered as standard for localised muscle-invasive bladder cancer, there is rapidly growing evidence from numerous phase-II-studies that concurrent radiochemotherapy yields survival rates identical to surgical series but with the chance of bladder preservation in 70% to 80% of long-term survivors. Patients treated in organ-sparing protocols should initially undergo a complete transurethral resection of the bladder tumour (TUR-BT), followed by chemoradiotherapy. Major prognostic factor of the overall remission are the completeness of the TUR-BT prior to radiotherapy and the use of chemotherapy. The overall survival of patients lies in the range of about 50% after 5 years which is nearly identical to cystectomy series. Major prognostic factors for overall survival such as age or T-category etc. are reported. The acute toxicity of radiotherapy is moderate. Late toxicity of organ-preserving treatment protocols is low and compares favourably to series with radical cystectomy. A small number of prognostic factors are well established for patients undergoing radiotherapy or radiochemotherapy for bladder cancer (especially age, T-category and completeness of TUR). Currently, there are few nomograms and prognostic models available; all of them include different clinical prognostic factors. New molecular factors have so far not been sufficiently investigated. Nomograms for toxicity (which is low) are not available.

P. Jiang (✉) · J. Dunst
Department of Radiation Oncology,
University Clinic Schleswig-Holstein,
Feldstr. 21, 24105 Kiel, Germany
e-mail: ping.jiang@uksh.de

C. Nieder and L. E. Gaspar (eds.), *Decision Tools for Radiation Oncology*, Medical Radiology. Radiation Oncology,
DOI: 10.1007/174_2013_859,

Published Online: 21 June 2013

1 Major Clinical Facts About Bladder Cancer

1.1 Epidemiology

Bladder cancer is the 9th most common cancer diagnosis worldwide. There are more than 330,000 new cases each year and more than 130,000 deaths per year with an estimated male: female ratio of 3.8:1 (Ploeg et al. 2009). The mean age at diagnosis is about 65 years.

1.2 Histological Subtypes

More than 90 % of all bladder cancers are urothelial carcinoma (also called transitional cell neoplasms), while squamous cell carcinoma (SCC) constitutes 5 % of cases. Adenocarcinoma (most often in dome of bladder; urachal remnant) and small cell cancers make up less than 1 %. An overview over general treatment concepts is given in Table 1. The following paragraphs concentrate on urothelial cancers.

Table 1 Histological subtypes and general treatment recommendations in bladder cancers

Histological type	Remarks	Treatment strategy
Urothelial cancer, transitional cancer	Most frequent subtype (> 90–95 %)	*Superficial tumors*
		TUR ± intravesical therapy is standard
		Radiochemotherapy indicated, if otherwise cystectomy would be performed
		Cystectomy for recurrent and progressive tumors after bladder-sparing initial treatment
		Immediate cystectomy as option in high-risk tumors (T1 G3)
		Muscle-invasive tumors (T2-4)
		Organ-preservation with TUR and radiochemotherapy, salvage-cystectomy only in case of relapse
		Radical cystectomy, (neo)adjuvant chemotherapy for high-risk patients
Squamous cell cancer	Rare (about 5 %), mostly advanced, prognosis slightly inferior to urothelial cancer	Few data. Treatment as muscle-invasive urothelial cancer is recommended
Adenocarcinoma	Rare (<1 %)	Surgery (partial or complete cystectomy) is standard. No data on efficacy of radiotherapy
Undifferentiated small cell cancer	Very rare (≪1 %)	Treatment as extrapulmonary small cell cancer

1.3 TNM Classification

The Tumor, Node, Metastasis (TNM) Classification of Malignant Tumors is the method most widely used to classify the extent of cancer spread (Table 2). Concerning histological grading, the use of the 2004 WHO classification is recommended but still needs to be validated by more clinical trials. Most clinical trials published so far on bladder tumors have been performed using the 1973 WHO Classification.

2 General Treatment Concepts for Urothelial Cancers in Radiation Oncology

2.1 Treatment Concepts in Superficial, Non-muscle Invasive Bladder Cancer (Ta, Tis, T1)

Over 80 % of newly diagnosed cases are classified as Ta, Tis or T1. TUR (transurethral resection) is the cornerstone of initial treatment. In case of risk factors, additional intravesical cytostatic therapy, either with cytotoxic drugs (e.g. mitomycin C) or with Bacillus Calmette-Guérin (BCG) is recommended. The efficacy of intravesical therapy with regard to reduction of local recurrence rate and delaying progression is evident, but a significant impact on long-term outcome and survival remains controversial. Cystectomy is considered as standard therapy in case of poor-prognostic superficial cancers with failure after TUR and intravesical therapy (especially in recurrent T1 G3 cancers).

There are few data on the use of radiotherapy. Some older series from the Netherlands have demonstrated good results with TUR and adjuvant interstitial brachytherapy of the tumor area. Data on external beam radiotherapy are very limited. In a prospective series from Erlangen University, Germany, external beam radiotherapy plus concurrent chemotherapy was used for poor prognostic T1 tumors which otherwise would have been considered candidates for

Table 2 2009 TNM classification of urinary bladder cancer (updated 2012)

T: Primary tumor
TX Primary tumor cannot be assessed
T0 No evidence of primary tumor
Ta Non-invasive papillary carcinoma
Tis Carcinoma in situ: 'flat tumor'
T1 Tumor invades subepithelial connective tissue
T2 Tumor invades muscle
T2a Tumor invades superficial muscle (inner half)
T2b Tumor invades deep muscle (outer half)
T3 Tumor invades perivesical tissue
T3a Microscopically
T3b Macroscopically (extravesical mass)
T4 Tumor invades any of the following: prostate, uterus, vagina, pelvic wall, abdominal wall
T4a Tumor invades prostate, uterus or vagina
T4b Tumor invades pelvic wall or abdominal wall
N: Lymph nodes
NX Regional lymph nodes cannot be assessed
N0 No regional lymph node metastasis
N1 Metastasis in a single lymph node in the true pelvis (hypogastric, obturator, external iliac or presacral)
N2 Metastasis in multiple lymph nodes in the true pelvis (hypogastric, obturator, external iliac, or presacral)
N3 Metastasis in common iliac lymph node(s)
M: Distant metastasis
M0 No distant metastasis
M1 Distant metastasis

cystectomy. The results with regard to overall survival compare favourably to the results of series with cystectomy. The bladder-preservation rate was about 65 % suggesting that an organ-preserving approach is justified even in non-muscle invasive tumors which otherwise would be treated with cystectomy (Weiss et al. 2006).

2.2 Treatment Concepts and Therapy Results in Localised Muscle-Invasive Bladder Cancer (T2-4 N0/1 M0)

Although radical cystectomy has been considered as standard for localised muscle-invasive bladder cancer, there is rapidly growing evidence from numerous phase-II studies that concurrent radiochemotherapy yields survival rates identical to surgical series but with the chance of bladder preservation in 70–80 % of long-term survivors. The most impressive advantage with regard to survival has recently been shown in the British BC 2001-study which demonstrated the superiority of concurrent chemoradiation over radiotherapy alone (James et al. 2012). The absolute difference in survival was 13 % after 5 years which is higher than the increase in survival with adjuvant or neoadjuvant chemotherapy prior or after radical cystectomy. Thus, radiochemotherapy is the standard of care for organ preservation and is, with regard to survival, to be considered as equieffective to cystectomy according to the best available evidence at the moment.

2.3 Indications for Definitive Curative Radiotherapy

Radiotherapy is an attractive curative option for nearly all patients with muscle invasive bladder cancer with the additional advantage of bladder preservation in the majority of patients. Standard treatment for patients with curative approach is radiotherapy plus concurrent chemotherapy. The best chemotherapy regimen is not yet clear. The most widely used drug has been cisplatin (Roedel et al. 2002). However, a combination of 5-FU and mitomycin C has also demonstrated significant efficacy in the BC 2001-trial and is surely an evidence-based alternative to cisplatin (James et al. 2012). A further drug for radiosensitization is paclitaxel which has been shown to be safe and efficacious in patients with contraindications to cisplatin (Mueller AC et al. 1977). There are no obvious contraindications against an organ-preserving approach with combined radiochemotherapy except patients with previous pelvic radiation treatment or other situations that limit the administration of a curative radiation dose.

All patients should initially undergo a complete transurethral resection of the bladder tumor (TUR-BT). The TUR should be complete, if possible; a macroscopically complete TUR-BT is a major prognostic factor. TUR-BT is followed by chemoradiotherapy. About 6 weeks after chemoradiotherapy, a control cystoscopy is recommended. A pathologically complete remission (pCR) can be achieved in about 70 % of all patients and a pCR is a prognostic factor for survival, long-term tumor control in the bladder and bladder preservation (Jenkins et al. 1988; Shipley et al. 1997; Mameghan et al. 1995; Roedel et al. 2002). Patients with residual invasive tumor on control cystoscopy should undergo salvage cystectomy, if there are no contraindications to major surgery.

Start of radiotherapy is recommended 4–6 weeks after TUR-BT because some time is normally required until local symptoms after TUR (dysuria, urgency) have been solved.

2.4 Adjuvant Radiotherapy

The role of adjuvant radiotherapy is not well defined with very limited data. Preoperative radiotherapy has been used in historical studies but is not considered as standard in contemporary guidelines. Preoperative chemoradiation followed by cystectomy is, from a theoretical point of view, an attractive concept, but should only be used in clinical trials.

2.5 Palliative Radiotherapy

Palliative radiotherapy is useful for the relief of symptoms such as bleeding and reduces the pain for patients with T4 bladder tumors, pelvic nodal disease, bone and other distant metastases. Short courses of palliative pelvic radiotherapy may be beneficial for elderly patients who have significant comorbidities precluding radical treatment.

3 Efficacy and Toxicity of Radiotherapy

3.1 Remission Rate and Local Control

In several large prospective series, efficacy of therapy has been determined by cystoscopic evaluation of remission rates. The overall remission rates that have been reported are in the range of 60–70 %. Major prognostic factor that have consistently been reported are the completeness of the TUR-BT prior to radiotherapy and the use of chemotherapy. The completeness of TUR has in some series been classified as visibly complete or incomplete. In one large prospective series, visibly complete TUR was further subdivided in pathologically complete (R0) or incomplete (R1). This subdivision enabled the definition of a very favourable group (T2-3 R0) with a very high rate of clinical remission (90 %) and overall survival (Dunst et al. 2001). Moreover, within the group of patients with histologically proven complete TUR (R0-resection), there was no difference between cT2- and cT3-tumors. Thus, the impact of established prognostic factors depends on the parameters which are included in a multivariate model.

3.2 Overall Survival

The overall survival of patients treated in organ-sparing protocols lies in the range of about 50 % after 5 years which is nearly identical to cystectomy series. One might assume that at least a subset of radiotherapy patients is referred to radiotherapy because of contraindication to major surgery. Being unfit for surgery, however, is a major prognostic factor for survival and identical survival figures after radiotherapy as compared to cystectomy despite a possibly negative selection further support the efficacy of radiotherapy.

Major prognostic factors for overall survival are: age, T-category, completeness of TUR, and remission after radiochemotherapy.

3.3 Bladder Preservation

Bladder preservation can be achieved in about 70–80 % of patients undergoing an organ-preserving approach. These figures have very consistently been reported in the literature. The percentage of bladder-preservation in long-term survivors is in the same range resulting in a bladder-intact survival after 5 years of about 40 % (Roedel et al. 2002; Efstathiou et al. 2012).

Major prognostic factors for bladder-preservation are: completeness of TUR, remission after radiochemotherapy and T-category.

3.4 Acute Toxicity

The acute toxicity of radiotherapy is moderate. Most patients experience mild to moderate symptoms, mainly GU-symptoms such as frequency, urgency, increased nocturia and reduced voiding intervals. Severe acute rectal and bowel symptoms (grade 3 to 4) have been reported each in about 5 % of patients. In patients receiving simultaneous chemotherapy, additional chemotherapy-related symptoms occur frequently. Severe symptoms (grade 3 to 4) have been reported in terms of haematological toxicity (leucopenia, thrombocytopenia, each about 20–30 %), nausea and vomiting (about 5 %) and elevation of serum creatinine (about 5 %). An impact of patient-related parameters or tumor characteristics to the frequency or severity of acute reactions has not been reported. The only risk factor is the administration of chemotherapy.

3.5 Late Toxicity

Late toxicity of organ-preserving treatment protocols is low and compares favourably to series with radical cystectomy. The two largest series in the literature (Rödel et al. 2002; Efstathiou et al. 2009) cover more than 700 patients with follow-up times of more than 5 years and have reported consistent data. Moderate late GU-toxicity (mainly increased voiding frequency and intermittent dysuria) were observed in about 20–25 % of all patients. Grade 3 and 4 late toxicity comprises of GU-toxicity (about 15–20 %) and GI-toxicity (about 5–10 %). Grade 4 complications requiring surgery were observed in less than 5 % of patients. Loss of bladder due to complications (cystectomy due to radiation-related side effects like contracted bladder) was noted in 2.5 % of patients with preserved bladder and local tumor control. In both analyses, no prognostic factors for late toxicity have been reported.

4 Nomograms

4.1 Prognostic Factors and Nomograms in Patients Undergoing Cystectomy

For patients who have undergone radical cystectomy, the most important prognostic factors are pT-category, R0-resection or margin status, pathologically proven lymph node involvement or lymph node density, and (in some other series) elevated CRP and age (Ali-El-Dein et al. 2013; Fairey et al. 2012; Fossa et al. 1996; Xylinas et al. 2012; Yafi et al. 2011). Other factors such as grading or specific histological features seem to be less important. Recently, the impact of molecular features has been stressed. On the basis of these data, a variety of nomograms have been proposed (Table 3). The disadvantage of these factors is that most of them (and especially the most relevant ones) can only be derived from pathohistological examination; this, however, is not possible in patients undergoing a non-surgical approach.

It has been suggested that a more radical and extensive lymph node dissection can improve prognosis (Skinner 1982; Leissner et al. 2004). Although this hypothesis has not definitively been confirmed in randomized trials, it is likely that variations in the type of treatment may impact on prognosis and may thereby change the impact of prognostic factors. Therefore, a unique problem of nomograms results from the fact that they reflect the outcome under certain therapeutic conditions.

Precystectomy nomograms have been used to estimate the risk of locally advanced disease, especially perivesical involvement (T3-4) or lymph node involvement which might be important for treatment decision (e.g. the indication for neoadjuvant chemotherapy prior to cystectomy). However, even nomograms that had been validated did not lead to reproducible results when applied to different patient cohorts (May et al. 2011).

Shariat and coworkers (2008) have recently reviewed the literature and found 11 published prediction tools of which 8 had undergone validation. The authors conclude, however, that the current nomograms still need to be refined. On the other hand, nomograms are surely more precise in predicting the prognosis of an individual patient as compared to single prognostic factors, TNM-categories or UICC-stage.

In the last years, molecular prognostic factors have been identified (Schepeler et al. 2012; Mitra et al. 2013). Very recently, some new models and nomograms including other factors and gene expression profils have been published (Ishioka et al. 2012; Riester et al. 2012; Todenhöfer et al. 2012). However, each of these series is based on a limited number of about 250 to less than 600 patients and include patients who have been treated over a broad time range at a single institution.

Table 3 Studies with nomograms and prognostic models in patients undergoing cystectomy for urothelial bladder cancer

Author	Data base	Prognostic factors in multivariate model and/or use of nomogram
Fossa et al. (1996)	Single-institution analysis of 534 patients treated with preop. XRT and cystectomy or definitive radiotherapy	T category, trial participation, treatment, creatinine, haemoglobin, age and time since initial diagnosis
Bochner et al. (2006)	International cohort study, 4462 cystectomy patients, treatment period 1969–2004	Indication for adjuvant chemotherapy can better be predicted by nomogram than by stage, resulting in less chemotherapy without impairment of survival
Yafi et al. (2011)	2287 patients from 8 academic centers in Canada, treatment period 1993 through 2008	Independent factor for OS and DFS: pT-category, R0-resection, receipt of adjuvant chemotherapy, performance of pelvic lymphadenectomy, non-smoker for OS and DFS
Gakis et al. (2011)	246 patients, single institution, treatment period 1999 through 2009	Independent factor for CSS: Elevated CRP, tumor stage, lymph-node density, margin status
Xylinas et al. (2012)	2145 patients with pT1-3 bladder cancer treated with radical cystectomy. Nomogram was developed from data of 1067 US-patients and validated in 1078 European patients	pT-stage, gender, lymphovascular invasion, and positive margin were independent factors for both disease recurrence and cancer-specific mortality

OS = overall survival, *DFS* = disease-free survival, *CSS* = cause-specific survival

4.2 Nomograms in Patients Undergoing Organ-Preservation with Definitive Radio(chemo)therapy

Organ-preserving therapy of muscle-invasive bladder cancer is a highly effective treatment option for the vast majority of patients. In patients suitable for radical cystectomy, this approach is very likely as effective as surgery with regard to overall survival but offers the chance of bladder preservation in three quarters of the patients. In patients who are unsuitable for major surgery (e.g. due to age or comorbidity), it is the only curative approach. However, most of the data on outcome derive from two large mono-institutional prospective series (MGH in the US, Erlangen University in Europe, covering together several hundreds of patients), a variety of smaller phase-II studies (each with less than 100 patients) and one large randomized study from Great Britain with nearly 500 patients. However, the series differ slightly and although a variety of prognostic factors have consistently been reported, their impact varies between series making it difficult to derive precise information.

One of the first multivariate models for patients undergoing definitive radiotherapy for bladder cancer has been reported by Hannisdal and coworkers (1993). They found five variables independently associated with poor prognosis: T4 tumors, blood sedimentation rate ESR >30 mm/h, albumin <35 g/l, serum LDH >400 U/l and age >75 years. The authors concluded that a small number of routine laboratory tests could help to identify poor prognostic patients.

Recently, Coen and coworkers have published a nomogram based on outcome of 325 patients treated at MGH in the period from 1986 to 2009 (Coen et al. 2013). This is the only nomogram so far in the literature for patients undergoing radiotherapy. Prognostic factors included in the development of the nomogram included T-category, completeness of TUR, presence of hydronephrosis, age, sex and tumor grade. Different nomograms for predicting treatment response (CR-rate), disease-specific survival (DSS), and survival with intact bladder (BIS) were developed. The aforementioned prognostic factors contributed in different ways (Table 4); for each outcome item (CR, DSS, BIS), 3 or 4 out of the six parameters were included in the nomogram. Completeness of TUR was the only parameter that was included in all three nomograms supporting the overwhelming impact of this factor. Moreover, the nomograms predicted outcome only over a certain range; for example, a patient with poor prognostic factors (0 points in the nomogram) had a 5-year disease-specific survival of 39 % whereas a patient with the maximum sum of points (and best predictable outcome) had a 5-year DSS of 81 %.

Both prognostic models are not directly comparable because they analysed different outcome parameters based on not exactly the same factors. However, both models highlight the impact of age and hydronephrosis. The impact of hydronephrosis can be explained as an indirect marker for large tumor volume or paravesical extension with uretheral obstruction. The early model of Hannisdal was set up at a time when modern imaging techniques (CT, MRI) were not routinely used and even in the MGH series, it is not clear what imaging modalities had been used in the patients over the period from 1986 through 2009. Thus, the impact of hydronephrosis might result from the fact that it reflects

Table 4 Variables included in nomograms to predict different outcome parameters in patients undergoing transurethral resection and concurrent radiochemotherapy for muscle invasive bladder cancer at Massachusetts General Hospital in the period from 1986 to 2009

Variable	Prediction of CR	Prediction of 5-year DSS	Prediction of 5-year bladder intact survival
Hydronephrosis no/yes	100/0	–	100/0
Age < 65y/≥ 65y	45/0	–	45/0
TUR complete/ incomplete	100/0	100/0	70/0
Gender female/male	35/0	–	–
T-category cT2/cT3-4	–	100/0	60/0
Grade 2/3	–	65/0	–
Maximum points	280	265	275
Probability with 0 points (%)	30	41	11
Probability with maximum points (%)	88	79	56

Modified from Coen et al. (2013). The numbers in the rows are points depending on the expression of a variable. Figures are estimated from the plots in the original publication. The points for all variables are summed up with the sum lying between 0 points and the maximum points. The prediction of a CR would be calculated with the nomogram as follows: for example, a female patient (35 points) with age <65 years (45 points) and a complete TUR (100 points) and no hydronephrosis (100 points) would achieve the maximum number of points (280 points) and therefore the maximum likelihood of a CR (88 %)

the best available information on tumor volume for the whole series. This leads to the problem that nomograms are nearly always based on a certain number of selected variables which are available in the included patients (Table 5).

Moreover, female sex is associated with a slight advantage in the model of Coen et al. (2013). This is in contrast to a variety of other investigations which found no better prognosis or even a slightly lower survival in female patients (Roedel et al. 2002).

Molecular markers have been investigated in patients undergoing cystectomy and have been found to improve the accuracy of nomograms. In patients undergoing definitive radiotherapy, few information on molecular markers is available. Roedel and coworkers found that a high apoptotic index (>median = 1.6 %) and a high Ki-67 expression (>median = 8.8 %) were significantly related to initial complete response (CR) and local control with preserved bladder after 5 years (Roedel et al. 2000). Recently, MRE11-expression was also identified as a prognostic and predictive factor in patients undergoing definitive radiotherapy (Choudbury et al. 2010). These findings have been

Table 5 Comparison of established variables in nomograms and independent prognostic factors for different outcome parameters (survival, remission, bladder-preservation)

	Nomogram of Coen and coworkers	Prognostic model of Hannisdal and coworkers	Additional independent prognostic factors in other investigations
Overall survival	n.d.	T4-tumors; age >75 years; elevated BSR[a]; albumin <35 g/l; serum LDH > 400 U/l	Completeness of TUR; T-category; histologic grade; gender
Cause-specific survival, disease-specific survival	Completeness of TUR; T-category; histologic grade;	n.d.	Age; gender
Complete remission	Completeness of TUR; hydronephrosis; age; gender	n.d.	T-category; Apoptotic index Ki-67-expresssion
Bladder preservation, bladder-intact-survival	Hydronephrosis; completeness of TUR; T-category; age	n.d.	Completeness of TUR ; remission after XRT; T-category

[a] *BSR* blood sedimentation rate, *n.d.* not determined

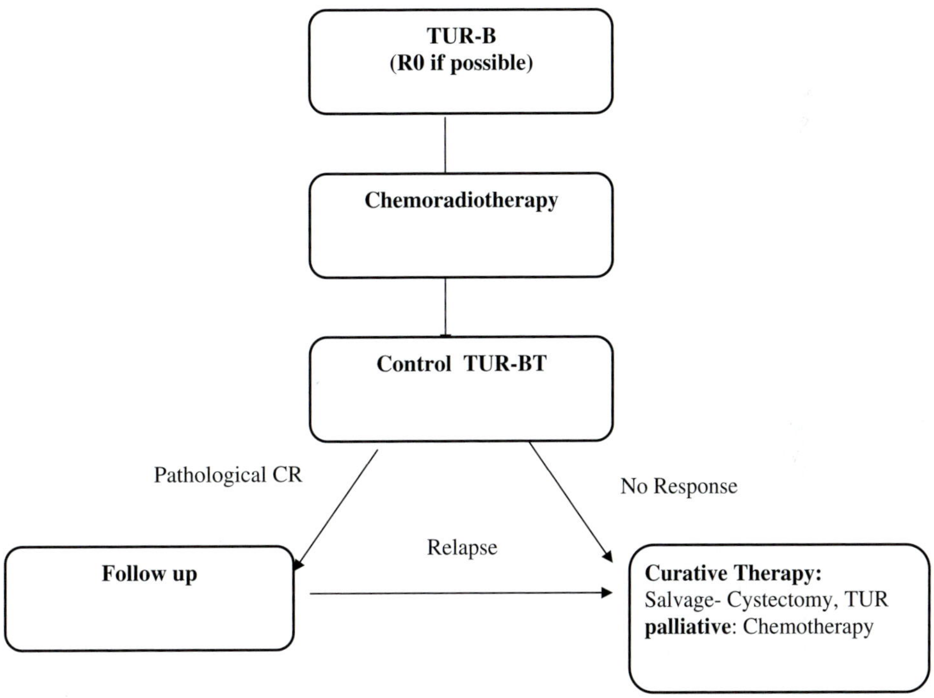

Fig. 1 General treatment concept for an organ-preserving treatment approach

confirmed in another study by Laurberg and coworkers who have demonstrated that a combination of MR11- and TIP60-expression might be able to distinguish two different subgroups of patients of which one had a significant better prognosis after cystectomy as compared to radiotherapy and the other after radiotherapy suggesting that molecular markers might also be able to guide treatment decisions (Laurberg et al. 2012). However, these data have been retrospectively collected and need to be validated in a prospective trial.

Nomograms on toxicity have so far not been published.

5 Summary and Recommendations

Organ-preserving therapy of muscle-invasive bladder cancer is a highly effective treatment option for the vast majority of patients. For patient suitable for radical cystectomy, this approach is very likely as effective as surgery with regard to overall survival but offers the chance of bladder preservation in three quarters of the patients. In patients who are unsuitable for major surgery (e.g. due to age or comorbidity), it is the only curative approach (Fig. 1). However, most of the data on outcome derive from two large mono-institutional prospective series (MGH in the US, Erlangen University in Europe, covering together several hundreds of patients), a variety of smaller phase-II studies (each with less than 100 patients) and one large randomized study from Great Britain with nearly 500 patients. The series differ only slightly in terms of treatment concept and outcome and a variety of prognostic factors have consistently been reported. Nevertheless, their impact varies between series making it difficult to derive precise information. Moreover, established prognostic factors (e.g. hydronephrosis or completeness of TUR) are probably only surrogate parameters for tumor volume and invasiveness and their impact results from the fact that they were the best available information on tumor volume for the majority of patients. Their impact might be smaller or negligible in patients undergoing contemporary imaging techniques such as CT, MRI or PET. Moreover, there are very few reports on the impact of molecular or genomic expression profiles but the very limited data so far suggests that these information might be very helpful to predict prognosis and to guide therapy decisions.

Nomograms are, in general, considered to offer the best information with regard to survival and counseling and decision making (Kattan et al. 2003). This is probably also true for certain clinical situations in bladder cancer (e.g. decision on adjuvant chemotherapy after cystectomy). For patients undergoing radiotherapy, the situation is less clear, mainly due to limited data from prospective bladder-preservation protocols.

In summary, a small number of prognostic factors is well established for patients undergoing radiotherapy or radiochemotherapy for bladder cancer (especially age, T-category and completeness of TUR). Their usefulness for clinical decision making, however, is limited. All patients should be treated with the standard organ-preservation protocol and it can currently not be recommended to change the standard treatment on the basis of any clinical, histological or molecular markers. However, the data on new prognostic factors are increasing and better prediction of outcome might become possible in the future.

References

Ali-El-Dein B, Sooriakumaran P, Trinh QD, Barakat TS, Nabeeh A, Ibrahiem EH (2013) Construction of predictive models for recurrence and progression in >1000 patients with non-muscle-invasive bladder cancer (NMIBC) from a single centre. BJU Int. doi:10.1111/bju.12026

Bochner BH, Kattan MW, Vora KC (2006) Postoperative nomogram predicting risk of recurrence after radical cystectomy for bladder cancer. J Clin Oncol 24:3967–3972

Choudhury A, Nelson LD, Teo MT (2010) MRE11 expression is predictive of cause-specific survival following radical radiotherapy for muscle-invasive bladder cancer. Cancer Res 70:7017–7026

Coen JJ, Paly JJ, Niemierko A, Kaufman DS, Heney NM, Spiegel DY, Efstathiou JA, Zietman A, Shipley WU (2013) Normograms predicting response and outcome after bladder-preserving trimodality therapy in muscle-.invasive bladder cancer. Int J Radiat Oncol Biol Phys 86:311–316

Dunst J, Rödel C, Zietman A, Schrott KM, Sauer R, Shipley WU (2001) Bladder preservation in muscle-invasive bladder cancer by conservative surgery and radiochemotherapy. Semin Surg Oncol 20:24–32

Efstathiou JA, Bae K, Shipley WU, Kaufman DS, Hagan MP, Heney NM, Sandler HM (2009) Late pelvic toxicity after bladder-sparing therapy in patients with invasive bladder cancer: RTOG 89-03, 95-06, 97-06, 99-06. J Clin Oncol. 27(25):4055-4061

Efstathiou JA, Spiegel DY, Shipley WU, Heney NM, Kaufman DS, Niemierko A, Coen JJ, Skowronski RY, Paly JJ, McGovern FJ, Zietman AL (2012) Long-term outcomes of selective bladder preservation by combined-modality therapy for invasive bladder cancer: the MGH experience. Eur Urol 61:705–711

Fairey AS, Kassouf W, Aprikian AG, Chin JL, Izawa JI, Fradet Y, Lacombe L, Rendon RA, Bell D, Cagiannos I, Drachenberg DE, Lattouf JB, Estey EP (2012) Age $\geq$ 80 years is independently associated with survival outcomes after radical cystectomy: results from the canadian bladder cancer network Database. Urol Oncol 30:825–832

Fossa SD, Aass N, Ous S, Waehre H, Ilner K, Hannisdal E (1996). Survival after curative treatment of muscle-invasive bladder cancer. Acta Oncol 35 Suppl 8:59-65

Gakis G, Todenhöfer T, Renninger M, Schilling D, Sievert KD, Schwentner C, Stenzl A (2011) Development of a new outcome prediction model in carcinoma invading the bladder based on preoperative serum C-reactive protein and standard pathological risk factors: the TNR-C score. BJU Int 108:1800–1805

Hannisdal E, Fosså SD, Høst H (1993) Blood tests and prognosis in bladder carcinomas treated with definitive radiotherapy. Radiother Oncol 27:117–122

Ishioka J, Saito K, Sakura M, Yokoyama M, Matsuoka Y, Numao N, Koga F, Masuda H, Fujii Y, Kawakami S, Kihara K (2012) Development of a nomogram incorporating serum C-reactive protein level to predict overall survival of patients with advanced urothelial carcinoma and its evaluation by decision curve analysis. Br J Cancer 107:1031–1036

James ND, Hussain SA, Hall E, Jenkins P, Tremlett J, Rawlings C, Crundwell M, Sizer B, Sreenivasan T, Hendron C, Lewis R, Waters R, Huddart RA (2012) Radiotherapy with or without chemotherapy in muscle-invasive bladder cancer. N Engl J Med 366:1477–1488

Jenkins BJ, Caulfield MJ, Fowler CG, Badenoch DF, Tiptaft RC, Paris AM, Hope-Stone HF, Oliver RT, Blandy JP (1988) Reappraisal of the role of radical radiotherapy and salvage cystectomy in the treatment of invasive (T2/T3) bladder cancer. Br J Urol 62:343–346

Kattan MW (2003) Nomograms are superior to staging and risk grouping systems for identifying high-risk patients: preoperative application in prostate cancer. Curr Opin Urol 13:111–116

Laurberg JR, Brems-Eskildsen AS, Nordentoft I, Fristrup N, Schepeler T, Ulhøi BP, Agerbaek M, Hartmann A, Bertz S, Wittlinger M, Fietkau R, Rödel C, Borre M, Jensen JB, Orntoft T, Dyrskjøt L (2012) Expression of TIP60 (tat-interactive protein) and MRE11 (meiotic recombination 11 homolog) predict treatment-specific outcome of localised invasive bladder cancer. BJU Int 110:E1228–E1236

Leissner J, Ghoneim MA, Abol-Enein H et al (2004) Extended radical lymphadenectomy in patients with urothelial bladder cancer: results of a prospective multicenter study. J Urol 171:139–144

Mameghan H, Fisher R, Mameghan J, Brook S (1995) Analysis of failure following definitive radiotherapy for invasive transitional cell carcinoma of the bladder. Int J Radiat Oncol Biol Phys 31:247–254

May M, Burger M, Brookman-May S, Otto W, Peter J, Rud O, Fritsche HM, Bolenz C, Trojan L, Herrmann E, Michel MS, Wülfing C, Moritz R, Tiemann A, Müller SC, Ellinger J, Buchner A, Stief CG, Tilki D, Wieland WF, Gilfrich C, Höfner T, Hohenfellner M, Haferkamp A, Roigas J, Bretschneider-Ehrenberg P, Müller O, Zacharias M, Gunia S, Bastian PJ (2011) Validation of pre-cystectomy nomograms for the prediction of locally advanced urothelial bladder cancer in a multicentre study: are we able to adequately predict locally advanced tumor stages before surgery? Urologe A 50:706–713

Mitra AP, Castelao JE, Hawes D, Tsao-Wei DD, Jiang X, Shi SR, Datar RH, Skinner EC, Stein JP, Groshen S, Yu MC, Ross RK, Skinner DG, Cortessis VK, Cote RJ (2013) Combination of molecular alterations and smoking intensity predicts bladder cancer outcome: a report from the Los Angeles Cancer Surveillance Program. Cancer 119:756–765

Mueller AC, Diestelhorst A, Kuhnt T, Kühn R, Fornara P, Scholz HJ, Dunst J, Zietman AL (1997) Organ-sparing treatment of advanced bladder cancer: paclitaxel as a radiosensitizer. Strahlenther Onkol 183:177–183

Ploeg M, Aben KK, Kiemeney LA (2009) The present and future burden of urinary bladder cancer in the world. World J Urol 27:289–293

Riester M, Taylor JM, Feifer A, Koppie T, Rosenberg JE, Downey RJ, Bochner BH, Michor F (2012) Combination of a novel gene expression signature with a clinical nomogram improves the prediction of survival in high-risk bladder cancer. Clin Cancer Res 18:1323–1333

Roedel C, Grabenbauer GG, Kuhn R, Papadopoulos T, Dunst J, Meyer M, Schrott KM, Sauer R (2002) Combined-modality treatment and selective organ preservation in invasive bladder cancer: long-term results. J Clin Oncol 20:3061–3071

Roedel C, Grabenbauer GG, Roedel F, Birkenhake S, Kuehn R, Martus P, Zoercher T, Fuersich D, Papadopoulos T, Dunst J, Schrott KM, Sauer R (2000) Apoptosis, p53, bcl-2, and Ki-67 in invasive bladder carcinoma: possible predictors for response to radiochemotherapy and successful bladder preservation. Int J Radiat Oncol Biol Phys 46:1213–1221

Schepeler T, Lamy P, Laurberg JR, Fristrup N, Reinert T, Bartkova J, Tropia L, Bartek J, Halazonetis TD, Pan CC, Borre M, Dyrskjøt L, Orntoft TF (2012). A high resolution genomic portrait of bladder cancer: correlation between genomic aberrations and the DNA damage response. Oncogene. doi:10.1038/onc.2012.381

Shariat SF, Margulis V, Lotan Y, Montorsi F, Karakiewicz PI (2008) Nomograms for bladder cancer. Eur Urol 54:41–53

Shipley WU, Zietman AL, Kaufman DS, Althausen AF, Heney NM (1997) Invasive bladder cancer: treatment strategies using transurethral surgery, chemotherapy and radiation therapy with selection for bladder conservation. Int J Radiat Oncol Biol Phys 39:937–943

Skinner DG (1982) Management of invasive bladder cancer: a meticulous pelvic node dissection can make a difference. J Urol 128:34

Todenhoefer T, Renninger M, Schwentner C, Stenzl A, Gakis G (2012) A new prognostic model for cancer-specific survival after radical cystectomy including pretreatment thrombocytosis and standard pathological risk factors. BJU Int 110:E533–E540

Weiss C, Wolze C, Engehausen DG, Ott OJ, Krause FS, Schrott KM, Dunst J, Sauer R, Roedel C (2006) Radiochemotherapy after transurethral resection for high-risk T1 bladder cancer: an alternative to intravesical therapy or early cystectomy? J Clin Oncol 24(15):2318–2324

Xylinas E, Cha EK, Sun M, Rink M, Trinh QD, Novara G, Green DA, Pycha A, Fradet Y, Daneshmand S, Svatek RS, Fritsche HM, Kassouf W, Scherr DS, Faison T, Crivelli JJ, Tagawa ST, Zerbib M, Karakiewicz PI, Shariat SF (2012) Risk stratification of pT1-3N0 patients after radical cystectomy for adjuvant chemotherapy counselling. Br J Cancer 107:1826–1832

Yafi FA, Aprikian AG, Chin JL, Fradet Y, Izawa J, Estey E, Fairey A, Rendon R, Cagiannos I, Lacombe L, Lattouf JB, Bell D, Drachenberg D, Kassouf W (2011) Contemporary outcomes of 2287 patients with bladder cancer who were treated with radical cystectomy: a Canadian multicentre experience. BJU Int 108: 539–545

Prostate Cancer

Cordula Petersen and Rudolf Schwarz

Contents

Abstract

The knowledge in the field of prostate cancer is rapidly changing. The majority of diagnoses relate to the use of screening prostate-specific antigen (PSA), which remains controversial. A combination of PSA level at diagnosis, clinical stage, and Gleason score is used to stratify patients into prognostic groups, with risk-adapted treatment assignment. The evaluation of treatment options for low-, intermediate- and high-risk prostate cancer has remained difficult primarily because of the lack of randomized trials. Most patients present with curative disease stage. Validated first-line treatment options include radical prostatectomy and radiation therapy, via either interstitial seed implants or external-beam radiation (EBRT). Radiation therapy for localized prostate cancer leads to equivalent oncologic outcomes as compared with radical prostatectomy. Interstitial seed implants and EBRT appear clinically equivalent. Modality-specific toxicity profile and logistics should be incorporated into the decision-making process of the individual patient. Results from randomized studies have established the value of dose-escalated radiotherapy alone in the unimodality setting versus standard-dose irradiation in combination with neoadjuvant and concurrent hormonal treatment. The timing and optimal duration of endocrine therapy in the era of dose escalation remain investigational. Adjuvant radiation therapy improves clinical outcome for pT3 prostate cancer or positive surgical margins.

Abbreviations

ADT	Androgen deprivation therapy
CTV	Clinical target volume
DVH	Dose volume histogram
EBRT	External beam radiotherapy
FFCF	Freedom from clinical failure

C. Petersen (✉) · R. Schwarz
Department of Radiotherapy and Radiooncology,
University Medical Center Hamburg-Eppendorf,
Martinistr. 52, D-20246 Hamburg, Germany
e-mail: cor.petersen@uke.de

C. Nieder and L. E. Gaspar (eds.), *Decision Tools for Radiation Oncology*, Medical Radiology. Radiation Oncology,
DOI: 10.1007/174_2013_855, © Springer-Verlag Berlin Heidelberg 2013
Published Online: 19 June 2013

GTV	Gross tumor volume
IMRT	Intensity modulated radiotherapy
IPSS	International prostatic symptom score
OS	Overall survival
OAR	Organ at risk
PCa	Prostate cancer
PFS	Progression free survival
PLND	Pelvic Lymph Node Dissection
PSA	Prostate specific antigen
PTV	Planning target volume
RT	Radiotherapy

1 Introduction

Cancer of the prostate (PCa) is currently the second most common cause of cancer death in men. The majority of diagnoses relate to the use of screening prostate-specific antigen (PSA), which remains controversial. PCa affects elderly men more often and therefore is a bigger health concern in developed countries. In developed countries, PCa accounts for 15 % of male cancers compared with 4 % of male cancers in developing countries. Within Europe large regional differences exist in the incidence rates of PCa (Brady et al. 2011; Heidenreich et al. 2011, 2012; Mottet et al. 2011).

Risk factors for prostate cancer are multiple. More established factors include increased life expectancy, routine adoption of PSA, ethnicity and family history. Potential but less established factors are obesity, dietary habits, exercise and prostatic inflammation.

Diagnosis and clinical staging depends on findings from history and physical examination, imaging and lab tests. Pathological staging depends on findings during surgical resection and pathological examination, in addition to those required in clinical staging. The 7th edition Union Internationale contre le Cancer (UICC) 2009 Tumour Node Metastasis (TNM) classification is used for staging (Table 1).

Beyond Gleason score, pretreatment serum PSA, and stage at diagnosis, additional pathologic factors including percent positive biopsy cores, PSA density and velocity, length of core involvement by tumor, and presence of perineural invasion also portend prognostic significance.

Since the clinical behavior of prostate cancer might range from indolent to highly aggressive, prognostic assessment is important for predicting outcome and treatment selection. A number of prognostic schemes have been developed. The clinical grouping system developed by the National Comprehensive Cancer Network (NCCN) is summarized, in addition with suggested general risk-adapted treatment recommendations in Table 2. Localized prostate cancer can be treated with surgery, radiation therapy, or the combination of both. In addition, hormonal therapy plays a role in the treatment of locally advanced disease. For selected patients with very low- or low-risk disease, active surveillance may be a valid option. It should be noted that no randomized trial exists comparing modern radiation with prostatectomy techniques, and that oncologic outcomes for localized prostate cancer appear similar, when appropriate radiation doses are employed (Kupelian et al. 2004). In a recent large scale comprehensive review of the literature by Grimm et al. (2012) comparing risk stratified patients by treatment option and with long-term follow-up, the statistical analysis suggested that, in terms of biochemical-free progression, brachytherapy provides superior outcome in patients with low-risk disease. For intermediate-

Table 1 Tumor node metastasis (TNM) classification of cancer of the prostate

T—primary tumor		
TX	Primary tumor cannot be assessed	
T0	No evidence of primary tumor	
T1	Clinically unapparent tumor not palpable or visible by imaging	
	T1a	Tumor incidental histological finding in 5 % or less of tissues resected
	T1b	Tumor incidental histological finding in more than 5 % of tissue resected
	T1c	Tumor identified by needle biopsy (e.g. because of elevated PSA level)
T2	Tumor confined within the prostate	
	T2a	Tumor involves one half of one lobe or less
	T2b	Tumor involves more than half of one lobe, but not both lobes
	T2c	Tumor involves both lobes
T3	Tumor extends through the prostate capsule	
	T3a	Extracapsular extension (unilateral or bilateral)
	T3b	Tumor invades seminal vesicle(s)
T4	Tumor is fixed or invades adjacent structures other than seminal vesicles. External sphincter, rectum, levator ani and/or pelvic wall	
N—regional lymph nodes		
NX	Regional lymph nodes cannot be assessed	
N0	No regional lymph node metastasis	
N1	Regional lymph node metastasis	
M—distant metastasis		
M0	No distant metastasis	
M1	Distant metastasis	
	M1a	Non-regional lymph node(s)
	M1b	Bone(s)
	M1c	Other site(s)

Table 2 NCCN risk groups (2010)

Risk group	Parameter	Suggested treatment strategy
Very low	T1a, Gleason ≤ 6, PSA < 10, <3 positive biopsy cores and <50 % cancer per core	Active surveillance using PSA and DRE, if expected survival <20 years
Low	T1–T2a, Gleason ≤ 6 and PSA < 10	Active surveillance using PSA and DRE if expected survival <10 years, using PSA, DRE, and repeat biopsy if expected survival ≥10 years, or definitive therapy using IG-IMRT, brachytherapy, or radical prostatectomy (RP)
Intermediate	T2b–T2c, Gleason 7, or PSA 10–20	IG-IMRT with or without short-term ADT with or without brachytherapy boost or RP
High	T3a, Gleason 8–10, or PSA > 20	IG-IMRT and long-term ADT or radical prostatectomy plus PLND with or without adjuvant RT
Locally advanced: very high	T3b–T4	IG-IMRT plus long-term ADT or radical prostatectomy plus PLND with or without adjuvant RT or ADT
Locally advanced: LN	N1	ADT or IG-IMRT and long-term ADT
Distant metastases	M1	ADT

risk disease, the combination of EBRT and brachytherapy appears equivalent to brachytherapy alone. For high-risk patients combination therapies involving EBRT and brachytherapy plus or minus androgen deprivation therapy appear superior to more localized treatments such as seed implant alone, surgery alone or EBRT.

2 Treatment of Non-Metastatic Prostate Cancer

External-beam radiation therapy (EBRT) is one of the most important definitive treatment modalities for localized prostate cancer of all stages. Following initial single-institution reports of improved efficacy and therapeutic ratio by Hanks et al. (1998), dose-escalation strategies have become an important focus of prostate cancer research endeavors. Clinical evidence for dose escalation in EBRT is presented in Table 3 for randomized clinical trials.

Several randomized and non-randomized studies have shown that dose escalation with a dose-range of 76–80 Gy has a significant impact on 5-year survival without biochemical relapse. Two randomized trials focused on clinical stages T1-3 N0 M0 and opened the clinical decision for dose escalation. The MD Anderson study (Kuban et al. 2008) compared 78 with 70 Gy conventional radiotherapy. It included 305 patients stage T1b to T3 with a median follow-up of 8.7 years. The results showed a significant increase in freedom from biochemical and/or clinical failure ($p = 0.004$), which was largest for patients with initial PSA > 10 ng/ml ($p = 0.001$) (Table 3).

The PROG 95-09 study (Zietman et al. 2010) evaluated 393 T1b-T2b patients, of whom 75 % had a Gleason score < 6 and a PSA < 15 ng/ml. Patients were randomized to receive an initial boost to the prostate alone, using conformal protons of either 19.8 or 28.8 Gy, and then 50.4 Gy to a larger volume. With a median follow-up of 5.5 years, there was a significant increase in 5-year freedom from biochemical failure ($p < 0.001$) in favour of low-risk patients given a higher dose (79.2 Gy) versus those given a conventional dose (70.2 Gy). There was a strong trend in the same direction for the intermediated-risk patients ($n = 144$, $p = 0.06$). 11 versus 6 % of patients subsequently required ADT for recurrence after conventional versus high-dose RT ($p = 0.047$). There remains no difference in OS (78.4 vs. 83.4 %, $p = 0.41$) and toxicity rates (1–3 % of grade 3–4) between the two arms.

A Dutch randomized phase III trial (Peeters et al. 2006) comparing 68 with 78 Gy showed a significant increase in 5-year freedom from clinical or biochemical failure (FFF or FFCF) for patients in an intermediate risk-group. 669 patients with T1b–T4 diseases were enrolled. With a follow-up of 51 months, 5-year FFF was significantly better after 78 Gy (64 vs. 54 %). No difference in late genitourinary or gastrointestinal toxicity was observed. As a result of these randomized studies, a minimum dose >74 Gy is recommended for EBRT.

Androgen-deprivation therapy (ADT), consisting of a combination of luteinizing-hormone-releasing hormone (LHRH) suppression and an anti-androgen, has been evaluated as an adjunct to standard-dose EBRT as an alternative strategy to improve outcomes in patients with intermediate- and high-risk prostate cancer. The supportive trials, although heterogeneous in their patient selection criteria and radiation treatment volumes, generally demonstrate statistically and clinically significant improvements in overall survival. Evidence in support of androgen suppression is most mature in patients with high-risk disease.

Table 3 Main randomized studies on localized PCa supporting dose escalation

Reference	Number of patients	Dose escalation	Endpoint	Comment
Kuban et al. 2008	301	78 versus 70 Gy	↑ 8-year biochem. DFS: 78 versus 59 %	Largest benefit among patients with pretreatment PSA > 10 ng/ml
Peeters et al. 2006	669	78 versus 68 Gy	5-year FFF sign better after 78 Gy: 64 versus 54 %	No sign differences in FFCF or OS
Zietman et al. 2010	393	70.2 or 79.2 GyE proton RT	10-year ASTRO BF 32.4 versus 16.7 % for high-dose RT	Difference was largely due to low- and intermediate disease

Table 4 Main trials combining RT plus hormonal treatment (intermediate-risk prostate cancer)

Reference	Number of patients	Treatment schedule	Endpoint	Comment
D'Amico et al. 2008	206	70.35 Gy in 36 fractions ±6 months of ADT	All-cause mortality was sign greater in RT alone arm	Sign difference was primarily in patients with no or minimal comorbid illness
Denham et al. 2008	802	RT to 66 Gy alone or RT plus 3 or 6 months of ADT before and during RT	Sign improvement in PCa-specific mortality with 6 but not 3 months of ADT	

Beginning in the 1980s research organizations in the USA and Europe launched a series of trials for which mature follow-up data are now available, and which have systematically evaluated the efficacy, timing and duration of androgen suppression therapy. For overview of studies see Table 4.

Two randomized trials demonstrated clinical evidence on combined EBRT with hormonal therapy for intermediate-risk prostate cancer. D'Amico et al. reported on a phase III clinical trial comparing RT with or without 6 months of ADT. 80 % of 206 randomized patients had intermediate-risk prostate cancer (D'Amico et al. 2004, 2008). Conformal radiation comprised 70.35 Gy in 36 fractions prescribed to the prostate and seminal vesicles with a cone-down boost to the prostate. Initial results at a median follow-up of 4.5 years revealed statistical improvements in prostate cancer-specific survival, survival free of salvage androgen deprivation, and OS rate. Updated results after a median follow-up of 7.6 years showed that all-cause mortality was significantly greater in the RT alone arm (HR 1.8, $p = 0.01$). Subgroup analysis suggested that the significant difference was primarily in patients with no or minimal comorbid illness.

The TROG 96.01 randomized clinical trial (Trans-Tasman Radiation Oncology Group, Australia) studied the optimal duration of short-course hormonal therapy (Denham et al. 2008). This three-arm study compared prostate-only radiation to 66 Gy, versus radiation and 3 or 6 months of androgen deprivation before and during radiation for intermediate-risk patients. Results revealed a significant improvement in prostate-cancer-specific mortality with 6 (HR 0.56) but not 3 (HR 0.95) months of short-term androgen deprivation.

Fortunately, the incidence of locally advanced PCa (T3-4N0M0) has declined as a result of individual or mass screening. Pelvic lymph node irradiation is optional (see Sect. 3), but the results of radiotherapy alone are unsatisfactory. Because of the hormonal dependence of PCa, ADT has been combined with external irradiation in locally advanced PCa (T3-4N0M0) with the aim of reducing the risk of distant metastasis and decreasing the risk of non-sterilisation and/or local recurrence as a source of secondary metastases. Numerous randomized trials have confirmed the value of long-term administration.

The RTOG study 86-10 (Pilepich et al. 2001) included 471 patients with bulky (>5 × 5 cm) tumours T2-4 N0-X M0. Androgen deprivation therapy was administered at 2 months before irradiation and during irradiation, or in the case of relapse in the control arm. 32 % of patients were diagnosed as T2, 70 % as T3-4, and 91 % as N0. The hormone treatment consisted of oral eulexine, 250 mg three times daily, and goserelin acetate (Zoladex) 3.6 mg every 4 weeks by subcutaneous injection. RT target volumes and doses were similar to RTOG 85-31 (Pilepich et al. 1997; Lawton et al. 2001), also including the regional lymphatics to an initial 44–46 Gy, followed by a prostate boost to 65–70 Gy. The 10-year overall survival estimates were 43 % for ADT plus irradiation versus 34 % for hormonal treatment, although the difference was not significant ($p = 0.12$). There was a significant improvement in the 10-year disease-specific mortaliy (23 vs. 36 %; $p = 0.01$), DFS (11 vs. 3 %; $p < 0.0001$) and in biochemical failure

(65 vs. 80 %; $p < 0.0001$). No significant impact on the risk of fatal cardiac events was seen with the addition of ADT.

The RTOG 85-31 trial (Pilepich et al. 1997; Pilepich et al. 2005; Lawton et al. 2001) randomized 977 patients to adjuvant goserelin (Arm I) versus observation (Arm II) with hormones initiated at relapse. Eligible patients had advanced tumor characteristics (T3-4 N0-1 M0) or pathologic penetration (pT3) through the capsule to the resection margin or seminal vesicle involvement after RP. Androgen deprivation therapy was begun in the last week of irradiation and continued up to relapse or was started at recurrence. A total of 15 % of patients in the first group and 29 % in the second group had undergone RP, 14 and 26 % were pN1. Goserelin was administered every 4 weeks. RT portals included treatment of the regional lymphatics to an initial 44–46 Gy (except in node-negative postoperative cases) followed by a prostate boost to 65–70 Gy. With a median follow-up of 7.6 years for all patients, at 10 years, the absolute survival rate was significantly greater for the adjuvant arm than for the control arm: 49 versus 39 % ($p = 0.002$). The 10-year local failure rate for the adjuvant arm was 23 versus 38 % for the control arm ($p < 0.0001$). The corresponding 10-year rates for the incidence of distant metastases and disease-specific mortality was 24 versus 39 % ($p < 0.001$) and 16 versus 22 % ($p = 0.0052$), respectively, both in favour of the adjuvant arm (Lawton et al. 2001, 2008; Pilepich et al. 2005).

The EORTC 22863 was an open-labeled randomized phase 3 trial (Bolla et al. 2002, 2010). Eligible patients were younger than 80 years and had newly diagnosed histologically proven T1–2 prostatic adenocarcinoma with WHO histological grade 3, or T3-4N0M0 and any histological grade. The trial compared EBRT and adjuvant long-term (concurrent and adjuvant) androgen suppression with radiotherapy alone. EBRT initially targeted the prostate and pelvic nodes to 50 Gy, with a subsequent prostate-only boost to an additional 20 Gy. Hormonal therapy consisted of monthly goserelin administration for 3 years, beginning on the first day of EBRT and 1 month of cyproterone acetate. With a median follow-up of 66 months, combination therapy compared with radiotherapy alone yielded significantly better survival (78 % vs. 62 %, $p = 0.001$) (Bolla et al. 2002). At a median follow-up of 9.1 years, the 10-year overall survival remained significantly higher at 58.1 versus 39.8 % ($p < 0.0001$), as did clinical progression-free survival at 47.7 versus 22.7 % ($p < 0.0001$). The 10-year cumulative incidence of PCa mortality was 11 versus 31 % ($p < 0.0001$). No significant difference in cardiovascular mortality was noted between treatment groups both in patients who had cardiovascular problems at study entry and in those who did not. The 10-year cumulative incidence of cardiovascular mortality was 11.1 versus 8.2 % ($p = 0.75$) (Bolla et al. 2010).

In conclusion the trials devoted to locally advanced PCa have shown a significant gain in overall survival of the combination of EBRT and long-term ADT and raised the question of whether the gain was due to ADT alone rather than to the combined approach. However, many trials were launched to assess the value of a long-term ADT plus or minus irradiation.

Mottet et al. (2012) report on the results of a phase 3 multicentric randomized trial devoted to 264 N0-X patients classified as cT3–4 ($n = 254$) or pT2 with positive biopsies of the capsule ($n = 10$), randomly allocated between long-term (3-year) ADT alone or combined with three-dimensional conformal radiotherapy (3D-CRT). ADT was administered with an LHRH-agonist (leuprorelin) given subcutaneously with a 3-monthly depot and an oral anti-androgen (flutamide) for 1 month to inhibit flare-up. In the ADT alone arm, 33 patients received salvage RT for local progression. RT was focused on the pelvis with a four-field box technique (46 ± 2 Gy) followed by a boost on the prostate and periprostatic tissue (22 ± 2 Gy). The patients were <80 year old with a World Health Organization (WHO) performance score (PS) < 2. There was no pathologic central review. 49 % had Gleason score 4–6, and 22.5 % of the patients had a baseline PSA > 20 ng/ml. With a median follow-up of 67 months, there was a significant difference in favor of the combined approach with regard to local–regional control ($p < 0.0001$), metastatic progression ($p = 0.018$), and progression-free survival ($p < 0.001$), but there was no improvement in overall survival or disease-specific survival because of an insufficient target sample size and/or not mature enough results. With the same concept, a life-long ADT, and a greater target sample size, the trials reported by Warde et al. (2011) and Widmark et al. (2009) shared these results but with added value for survival.

Warde et al. (2011) reported on a cohort of 1205 N0-X patients (T3–4) ($n = 1057$), T2 with PSA > 40 ng/ml ($n = 119$), or T2 with PSA > 20 ng and Gleason > 8 ($n = 25$) randomized between life-long ADT (bilateral orchidectomy or LHRH agonist) with or without RT (65–70 Gy to prostate ± 45 Gy to pelvic lymph nodes). With 6-year median follow-up, the combined approach significantly reduced the risk of death ($p = 0.033$) and of disease-specific death ($p = 0.001$). The SPCG-7/SFUO 3 trial (Widmark et al. 2009) accrued a cohort of 875 N0-X M0 patients (T3, any WHO grade ($n = 862$); T1b–T2 G2–3 ($n = 168$); unknown ($n = 5$). Patients were randomly assigned to endocrine treatment alone (3 months of total androgen blockade followed by continuous endocrine treatment using flutamide) or to the same endocrine treatment combined with 3D-CRT (70 Gy to the prostate). With 7.6 years median follow-up, the combined approach halved the 10-year PCa-specific mortality ($p < 0.0001$) and

Table 5 Results of brachytherapy ($^{125}I/^{103}Pd$-Isotopes)

Reference	Patients (*n*)	Risk group	EBRT	Endpoints (years)	Biochemical control (%)	Comment
Buckstein et al. 2013	131	Low and intermediate	Yes	11.5	All: 90	Patients younger than 60 years
Kao et al. 2008	643	Low	No	5	All: 97	Neoadjuvant hormonal treatment
Taira et al. 2010	463	Low and intermediate	No	12	All: 97	
Zelefsky et al. 2007	2693	All	No	8	Low: 82 Intermediate: 70 High: 48	Meta-analysis

decreased overall mortality ($p < 0.004$). These results mimic somehow what was observed for locally advanced breast cancer, with the greatest effect being achieved with the combination of RT and endocrine treatment given concomitantly.

3 Prophylactic Irradiation of Pelvic Lymph Nodes in High-Risk Localized PCa

The optimal strategy for target definition, especially whole-pelvis lymph nodes versus prostate-only radiation therapy, has not been determined. Invasion of the pelvic lymph nodes is a poor prognostic factor. However, randomized trials showed inconclusive results according to what extend patients benefited from prophylactic whole-pelvis irradiation. The RTOG 94-13 four-arm randomized trial (Roach et al. 2003) attempted to discern the relative merits of pelvic nodal irradiation versus prostate-only EBRT in patients with an estimated risk of lymph node involvement of 15 %, and timing (adjuvant versus neoadjuvant and concurrent) of hormonal therapy. The total duration of hormonal treatment was 4 months. An OS difference was seen among all study groups, yet there were no significant differences in PFS or OS between neoadjuvant versus adjuvant hormones, or pelvis versus prostate-only radiation. When neoadjuvant hormone therapy was used in conjunction with EBRT, pelvic nodal irradiation yielded an improved PFS versus prostate-only RT. Neoadjuvant hormones plus pelvic nodal RT improved OS versus adjuvant hormones plus pelvic nodal RT. Late severe GU toxicities were similar in the 4 arms, though severe GI toxicities were more frequent in the neoadjuvant hormone and whole-pelvis arm.

The GETUG-01 randomized phase III trial (Pommier et al. 2007) also studied the role of pelvic and prostate versus prostate-only RT. The trial stratified patients according to risk of lymph node involvement. Initial results with limited follow-up of 42 months demonstrated no significant difference in 5-year PFS between the study groups, either in the high- or low-risk strata.

4 Transperineal Brachytherapy

Transperineal brachytherapy is a safe and effective technique. Modern series continue to demonstrate excellent outcomes for radioactive implantation, either as monotherapy for low-risk cases or selected high-risk patients, or as boost treatment in conjunction with external beam therapy. According to the American Brachytherapy Society there is consensus on the following eligibility criteria: Stage cT1b–T2a N0 M0, a Gleason score ≤ 6 assessed on a sufficient number of random biopsies, an initial PSA level of <10 ng/ml, <50 % of biopsy cores involved with cancer, a prostate volume of <50 cm^3, an International Prostatic Symptom Score ≤ 12 (IPPS) (Nag et al. 1999).

There are no randomized trials comparing brachytherapy with other curative treatment modalities, and outcomes are based on non-randomized case series. Results of permanent implants have been reported from different institutions, with different follow-up. Biochemical control was reported to range from 48 (high risk) to 97 % (low risk) (see Table 5). A significant correlation has been shown between the implant dose and recurrence rates. As demonstrated in a recent multi-institutional study of 2693 men with T1–2 prostate cancer, D90 > 130 Gy emerged as a highly significant predictor of 8-year PSA relapse-free survival (93 vs. 76 %, $p < 0.001$).

5 Immediate and Delayed Post-Operative External Irradiation After Radical Prostatectomy

While prostatectomy provides good control rates for patients with organ-confined disease, failure rates for patients with cancer extensions beyond the capsule are substantial, particularly in cases of high Gleason grade and positive margins. Extracapsular invasion (pT3) is associated with a risk of local recurrence, which can be as high as 30 %. In multifactorial analyses, the predictors of biochemical relapse are: PSA level ($p = 0.005$), Gleason score of the surgical specimen ($p = 0.002$) and positive surgical margins ($p < 0.001$).

Three prospective randomized trials have assessed the role of immediate post-operative radiotherapy (adjuvant radiotherapy). The randomized phase III EORTC trial 22911 (Bolla et al. 2012) recruited patients age 75 or younger with untreated cT0–3 PCa. Eligible patients were randomly assigned centrally (1:1) to postoperative irradiation (60 Gy) to the surgical bed or to a wait-and-see policy until biochemical progression (increase in PSA > 0.2 μg/L confirmed twice at least 2 weeks apart). 1,005 patients were randomly assigned and were followed up for a median of 10.6 years. Postoperative irradiation significantly improved biochemical progression-free survival compared with the wait-and-see group (198 [39.4 %] of 502 patients in postoperative irradiation group vs. 311 [61.8 %] of 503 patients in the wait-and-see group had biochemical or clinical progression or died; HR 0.49 [95 %, CI 0.41–0.59]; $p < 0.0001$). Late adverse effects (any type of any grade) were more frequent in the postoperative irradiation group then in the wait-and-see-group (10-year cumulative incidence 70.8 % [66.6–75.0] vs. 59.7 % [55.3–64.1]; $p = 0.001$). It was concluded that results at median follow-up of 10.6 years show that conventional postoperative RT significantly improved survival and local control compared with a wait-and-see policy, supporting results at 5 year follow up; however, improvements in clinical progression-free survival were not maintained. Exploratory analyses suggested that postoperative RT might improve clinical progression-free survival in patients younger than 70 years and in those with positive surgical margins, but could have a detrimental effect in patients aged 70 years or older.

The most suitable candidates for immediate radiation therapy might therefore be those with multifocal positive surgical margins and a Gleason score >7. The conclusion of the ARO trial 96-02 ($n = 385$) appear to support those of the EORTC study (Wiegel et al. 2009). In this phase III trial patients with pT3N0 disease and (in contrast to the other two studies) an undetectable PSA level after RP were randomized to adjuvant RT (60 Gy) versus observation. After a median follow-up of 54 months, the irradiated group demonstrated a significant improvement in biochemical progression-free survival of 72 versus 54 %, respectively ($p = 0.0015$). This finding demonstrates that adjuvant radiotherapy works even in the setting of undetectable PSA after RP and additional risk factors.

Between 1988 and 1997, SWOG 8794 randomized 425 men with non-organ-confined cancer or positive surgical margins (pT2+N0M0 or pT3N0M0) to immediate adjuvant RT using 60–64 Gy by conventional technique versus observation (Thompson et al. 2009). Because the study did not require men to have an undetectable PSA prior to study entry, 33 % of men in both arms had PSA > 0.2 ng/ml at the time of randomization. The use of salvage RT was not mandated by protocol in the observation arm, and a total of 70 men (33 %) ultimately received postoperative RT (most for a rising PSA). The median PSA at the time of salvage RT in these men was 1.0 ng/ml, which would be considered "late" salvage therapy by current standards. Over a median follow-up of almost 13 years, adjuvant RT was associated with a significant improvement in metastasis-free survival (HR: 0.7, $p = 0.016$) and overall survival (HR: 0.7, $p = 0.023$). Metastases-free survival considers the development of distant metastasis and death from any cause as events. The rate of observed distant metastasis was low (17 % in the observation arm and 9 % in the RT arm), and the majority of events in the analysis of metastasis-free survival and OS were deaths without evidence of metastatic PCa (68 % in the observation arm and 78 % in the RT arm). Adjuvant RT was also associated with reductions in the need of salvage RT. In exploratory analyses, all subgroups (Gleason 2–6 vs. 7–10, pT3a or postoperative surgical margins vs. seminal vesicle invasion, undetectable vs. detectable PSA) appeared to benefit from adjuvant RT with respect to metastasis-free survival. Rectal and urinary toxicity and urethral stricture rates were higher with adjuvant RT, but the overall rates were low.

In conclusion, the decision whether to proceed with adjuvant RT for high-risk PCA (pT3-4 pN0-1) after RP or to postpone RT as an early salvage procedure in case of biochemical relapse remains difficult. In daily practice, the urologist should explain to the patient before RP that adjuvant irradiation could be applied if the patient has negative prognostic risk factors. Ultimately, the decision to treat needs a multidisciplinary approach to determine the optimal timing of radiotherapy when used and to provide justification when not used.

6 The Role of Hypofractionation

In ideal circumstances, the fractionation schedule of radiotherapy should match the fractionation sensitivity of the tumor relative to nearby normal tissues. The alpha–beta (α/β) ratio for most cancers is believed to be about 10 Gy, but for prostate cancer values as low as 1.5 Gy have been suggested, which is smaller than the roughly 3 Gy reported for the late reactions of most normal tissues (including rectum). These findings have potentially important therapeutic implications. Hypofractionated radiotherapy with fewer high-fraction-size treatments would be beneficial for prostate cancer because it would deliver a larger biological-equivalent dose to the tumor than would conventional treatment in 1.8–2.0 Gy fractions, while maintaining a similar or lower incidence of late normal tissue reactions.

Furthermore, improved resource utilization and patient convenience because of short treatment duration would be important gains. Maintenance of few treatment-related side-effects is of paramount importance.

Dearnaley et al. (2012) undertook a multistage, multicenter randomized controlled trial (Conventional or Hypofractionated High-dose Intensity Modulated Radiotherapy in Prostate Cancer: CHHiP). Men with localized prostate cancer were randomized between 2002 and 2006 at 11 UK centres. Patients were randomly assigned in a 1:1:1 ratio to receive conventional or hypofractionated high-dose intensity modulated radiotherapy, and all were given 3–6 months of neoadjuvant androgen suppression. Computer-generated random permuted blocks were used, with risk of seminal vesicle involvement and radiotherapy-treatment centre as stratification factors. The conventional schedule was 37 fractions of 2 Gy to a total dose of 74 Gy. The two hypofractionated schedules involved 3 Gy treatments given either in 20 fractions to a total dose of 60 Gy, or 19 fractions to a total of 57 Gy. The primary endpoint was proportion of patients with grade 2 or worse toxicity at 2 years on the RTOG scale. The primary analysis included all patients who received at least one fraction of radiotherapy and completed a 2-year assessment. 153 men recruited to stages 1 and 2 were randomly assigned to receive conventional treatment of 74 Gy, 153 to receive 60 Gy, and 151 to receive 57 Gy. With 50.5 months median follow-up 4.3 % (95 %, CI 1.6–9.2) of 138 men in the 74 Gy group had bowel toxicity of grade 2 or worse on the RTOG scale at 2 years, as did 3.6 % (1.2–8.3) of 136 men in the 60 Gy group, and 1.4 % (0.2–5.0) of 143 men in the 57 Gy group. For bladder toxicities 2.2 % (0.5–6.2) of 138 men, 2.2 % (0.5–6.3) of 137, and 0.0 % (0.0–2.6) of 143 had scores of grade 2 or worse on the RTOG scale at 2 years. From these results it was concluded that hypofractionated high-dose radiotherapy seems equally well tolerated as conventionally fractionated treatment at 2 years.

In a recent publication by Botrel et al. (2013) a systematic review and meta-analysis of all randomized controlled trials comparing the efficacy and side effect profile of hypofractionated versus conventional EBRT for PCa was conducted. The final analysis included nine trials comprising 2,702 patients. Freedom from biochemical failure was reported in only three studies and was similar in patients who received hypofractionated or conventional radiotherapy. The incidence of acute adverse gastrointestinal events was higher in the hypofractionated group. Acute genitourinary toxicity was similar among the groups. The incidence of all late adverse events was the same in both groups. Hypofractionated radiotherapy in localized prostate cancer was not superior to conventional radiotherapy and showed higher acute gastrointestinal toxicity in this meta-analysis. Because the number of published studies is still small, future assessments should be conducted to clarify better the true role of hypofractionated radiotherapy in patients with prostate cancer.

7 Radiation Therapy Techniques and Target Delineation

IMRT represents the current standard of care for prostate EBRT. According to patient set up and planning, patients should be instructed to present with an empty rectum and comfortably full bladder. Patients are positioned either supine or prone (with or without a rectal balloon depending on institutional practice) on a custom immobilization device. A volumetric CT scan employing a slice thickness < 3 mm is obtained through the volume of interest and imported into a computer for organ segmentation and treatment planning. MRI fusion is employed to delineate the prostate apex. MRI fusion enhances definition of the prostate-rectum interface, the prostatic apex, and neurovascular bundles. The use of a T2-weighted volumetric sequence is suggested. Given susceptibilities for organ deformation, intra- and interfraction organ motion, IMRT is typically combined with daily image guidance. A variety of methods, including ultrasound, fiducial implantation and KV imaging, KV cone-beam CT, MVCT, and intrafraction tracking using transponders are in clinical use. Pelvic radiation using IG-IMRT and incorporating intraprostatic fiducial markers can reduce the volumes of rectum and bladder receiving high doses, thus reducing toxicities. The recently published RTOG consensus documents represent a valuable guideline for postoperative target delineation (Lawton et al. 2009; Michalski et al. 2010). Definitions of gross target volume (GTV), clinical target volume (CTV), and planning target volume (PTV) in IMRT in prostate-only radiation include prostate on imaging studies as GTV, with 0.5–1 cm margins in 3D to achieve PTV. The CTV of seminal vesicles and pelvic lymph node regions (if select to treat) include distal common, internal, and external iliac regions, presacral, and obturator regions. The probability of involvement can be determined by stage, pretreatment PSA, PSA doubling time and/or velocity, high-percent biopsy core involvement, the presence of perineural invasion, and the Roach formulas and/or Partin tables (Roach et al. 1994; Partin et al. 1997; Eifler et al. 2013). These and different nomograms are available on the internet, for example via CaP Calculator. Using a nationally representative mail survey of 1,422 prostate cancer specialists in the United States, Kim et al. queried about self-reported clinical implementation of quality of life instruments, prostate cancer nomograms and life expectancy prediction tools in late 2011. A total of 313 radiation oncologists and 328 urologists completed the survey for a 45 % response rate. Although 55 % of respondents reported using prostate cancer nomograms, only 27 and 23 % reported using quality of life and life expectancy prediction instruments, respectively (Kim et al. 2012). Probably, these variations result from different factors, including time constraints and unresolved issues around the validity of different tools and their applicability in different patient populations, as discussed in the introductory chapters of this textbook. Organs at risk (OARs) in EBRT of prostate cancer, in both adjuvant and definitive settings, include rectum and bladder. Suggested DVH constraints for dose-escalated IMRT are specified in the RTOG active protocols. Efforts towards development of toxicity-prediction nomograms are ongoing (Fiorino et al. 2012; Roeloffzen et al. 2012; Valdagni et al. 2012).

References

Bolla M, Collette L, Blank L, Warde P, Dubois JB, Mirimanoff R-O et al (2002) Long-term results with immediate androgen suppression and external irradiation in patients with locally advanced prostate cancer (an EORTC study): a phase III randomised trial. Lancet 360:103–106

Bolla M, van Poppel H, Collette L, van Cangh P, Vekemans K, Da Pozzo L et al (2012) Postoperative radiotherapy after radical prostatectomy for high-risk prostate cancer: long term results of a randomised controlled trial (EORTC trial 22911). Lancet 380:2018–2027

Bolla M, Van Tienhoven G, Warde P, Dubois JB, Mirimanoff R-O, Storme G et al (2010) External irradiation with or without long-term androgen suppression for prostate cancer with high metastatic risk: 10-year results of an EORTC randomised study. Lancet Oncol 11:1066–1073

Botrel TEA, Clark O, Pompeo ECL, Bretas FFH, Sadi MV, Ferreira U et al (2013) Hypofractionated external-beam radiation (HEBRT) versus conventional external-beam radiation (CEBRT) in patients with localized prostate cancer: a systematic review and meta-analysis. Core Evid 8:1–13

Brady L, Heilmann H-P, Molls M, Nieder C (2011) Foreword. In: Lu JJ, Brady LW (eds) Decision making in radiation oncology (Bd. 2). Springer, Heidelberg

Buckstein M, Carpenter TJ, Stone N, Stock RG (2013) Long-term outcomes and toxicity in patients treated with brachytherapy for prostate adenocarcinoma younger than 60 years of age at treatment with minimum 10 years of follow-up. Urology 81:364–369

D'Amico AV, Chen M-H, Renshaw AA, Loffredo M, Kantoff PW (2008) Androgen suppression and radiation vs. radiation alone for prostate cancer: a randomized trial. JAMA 299:289–295

D'Amico AV, Manola J, Loffredo M, Renshaw AA, DellaCroce A, Kantoff PW (2004) 6-month androgen suppression plus radiation therapy vs. radiation therapy alone for patients with clinically localized prostate cancer: a randomized controlled trial. JAMA 292:821–827

Dearnaley DP, Syndikus I, Sumo G, Bidmead M, Bloomfield D, Clark C et al (2012) Conventional versus hypofractionated high-dose intensity-modulated radiotherapy for prostate cancer: preliminary safety results from the CHHiP randomized controlled trial. Lancet Oncol 13:43–54

Denham JW, Steigler A, Wilcox C, Lamb DS, Joseph D, Atkinson C et al (2008) Time to biochemical failure and prostate-specific antigen doubling time as surrogates for prostate cancer-specific mortality: evidence from the TROG 96.01 randomised controlled trial. Lancet Oncol 9:1058–1068

Eifler JB, Feng Z, Lin BM, Partin MT, Humphreys EB, Han M et al (2013) An updated prostate cancer staging nomogram (Partin tables) based on cases from 2006 to 2011. BJU Int 111:22–29

Fiorino C, Rancati T, Fellin G, Vavassori V, Cagna E, Casanova-Borca V et al (2012) Late fecal incontinence after high-dose radiotherapy for prostate cancer: better prediction using longitudinal definitions. Int J Radiat Oncol Biol Phys 83:38–45

Grimm P, Billiet I, Boswick C, Dicker A, Frank S, Immerzeel J, Keyes M, Kupelian P, Lee W, Machtens S, Mayade J, Moran B, Merrick G, Millar J, Roach M, Stock R, Shinohara K, Scholz M, Weber E, Zietman A, Zelefsky M, Wong J, Wentworth S, Vera R, Langley S (2012) Comparative analysis of prostate-specific antigen free survival outcomes for patients with los, intermediate and high risk prostate cancer treatment by radical therapy. Results from the prostate cancer results study group. BJUI 109:22–29

Hanks GE, Hanlon AL, Schultheiss TE, Pinover WH, Movsas B, Epstein BE et al (1998) Dose escalation with 3D conformal treatment: five year outcomes, treatment optimization, and future directions. Int J Radiat Oncol Biol Phys 41:501–510

Heidenreich A, Bastian P, Bellmunt J, Bolla M, Joniau S, Van der Kwast T, Mason M, Matveev V, Mottet N, Wiegel T, Zattoni F (2012) Guidelines on prostate cancer. http://www.uroweb.org

Heidenreich A, Bellmunt J, Bolla M, Joniau S, Mason M, Matveev V, Mottet N, Schmid H, Van der Kwast T, Wiegel T, Zattoni F (2011) EAU guidelines on prostate cancer. Part 1: screening, diagnosis, and treatment of clinically localised disease. Eur Urol 59:61–71

Kao J, Stone NN, Lavaf A, Dumane V, Cesaretti JA, Stock RG (2008) ^{125}I Monotherapy using D90 implant doses of 180 Gy or greater. Int J Radiat Oncol Biol Phys 70:96–101

Kim SP, Karnes RJ, Nguyen PL, Ziegenfuss JY, Han LC, Thompson RH et al (2012) Clinical implementation of quality of life instruments and prediction tools for localized prostate cancer: results from a national survey of radiation oncologists and urologists. J Urol pii: S0022-5347(12)05806-5. doi: 10.1016/j.juro.2012.11.174

Kuban DA, Tucker SL, Dong L, Starkschall G, Huang EH, Cheung MR et al (2008) Long-term results of the M. D. Anderson randomized dose-escalation trial for prostate cancer. Int J Radiat Oncol Biol Phys 70:67–74

Kupelian PA, Potters L, Khuntia D, Ciezki JP, Reddy CA, Reuther AM et al (2004) Radical prostatectomy, external beam radiotherapy <72 Gy, external beam radiotherapy > or =72 Gy, permanent seed implantation, or combined seeds/external beam radiotherapy for stage T1–T2 prostate cancer. Int J Radiat Oncol Biol Phys 58:25–33

Lawton CA, Bae K, Pilepich M, Hanks G, Shipley W (2008) Long-term treatment sequelae after external beam irradiation with or without hormonal manipulation for adenocarcinoma of the prostate: analysis of radiation therapy oncology group studies 85–31, 86–10, and 92–02. Int J Radiat Oncol Biol Phys 70:437–441

Lawton CA, Michalski J, El-Naqa I (2009) RTOG GU radiation oncology specialists reach consensus on pelvic lymph node volumes for high-risk prostate cancer. Int J Radiat Oncol Biol Phys 74:383–387

Lawton CA, Winter K, Murra K, Machtay M, Mesic J, Hanks G, Coughlin C, Pilepich MV (2001) Updated results of the phase III radiation therapy oncology group (RTOG) trial 85–31 evaluating the potential benefit of androgen suppression following standard radiation therapy for unfavorable prognosis carcinoma of the prostate. Int J Radiat Oncol Biol Phys 49:937–946

Michalski JM, Lawton C, El-Naqa I (2010) Development of RTOG consensus guidelines for the definition of the clinical target volume for postoperative conformal radiation therapy for prostate cancer. Int J Radiat Oncol Biol Phys 76:361–368

Mottet N, Bellmunt J, Bolla M, Joniau S, Mason M, Matveev V, Schmid H, Van der Kwast T, Wiegel T, Zattoni F, Heidenreich A (2011) EAU guidelines on prostate cancer. Part II: treatment of advanced, relapsing, and castration-resistant prostate cancer. Eur Urol 59:572–583

Mottet N, Peneau M, Mazeron J, Molinie V, Richaud P (2012) Addition of radiotherapy to long term androgen deprivation in locally advanced prostate cancer: an open randomized phase 3 trial. Eur Urol 62:213–219

Nag S, Beyer D, Friedland J, Grimm P, Nath R (1999) American Brachytherapy Society (ABS) recommendations for transperineal permanent brachytherapy of prostate cancer. Int J Radiat Oncol Biol Phys 44:789–799

NCCN (2010) NCCN clinical practice guidelines in oncology: prostate cancer v. 1.2010. Available at www.nccn.org/professionals/physicians_gls/pdf/prostate.pdf

Partin AW, Kattan MW, Subong ENP, Walsh PC, Wojno KJ, Oesterling JE (1997) Combination of prostate-specific antigen, clinical stage, and Gleason score to predict pathological stage of localized prostate cancer. JAMA 277:1445–1451

Peeters ST, Heemsbergen WD, Koper PC, van Putten WL, Slot A, Dielwart MF et al (2006) Dose-response in radiotherapy for localized prostate cancer: results of the Dutch multicenter randomized phase III trial comparing 68 Gy of radiotherapy with 78 Gy. J Clin Oncol 24:1990–1996

Pilepich MV, Caplan R, Byhardt RW, Lawton CA, Gallagher MJ, Mesic JB et al (1997) Phase III trial of androgen suppression using goserelin in unfavorable-prognosis carcinoma of the prostate treated with definitive radiotherapy: report of Radiation Therapy Oncology Group Protocol 85–31. J Clin Oncol 15:1013–1021

Pilepich MV, Winter K, John MJ, Mesic JB, Sause W, Rubin P et al (2001) Phase III radiation therapy oncology group (RTOG) trial 86–10 of androgen deprivation adjuvant to definitive radiotherapy in locally advanced carcinoma of the prostate. Int J Radiat Oncol Biol Phys 50:1243–1252

Pilepich MV, Winter K, Lawton CA, Krisch RE, Wolkov HB, Movsas B et al (2005) Androgen suppression adjuvant to definitive radiotherapy in prostate carcinoma—long-term results of phase III RTOG 85–31. Int J Radiat Oncol Biol Phys 61:1285–1290

Pommier P, Chabaud S, Lagrange JL, Richaud P, Lesaunier F, Le Prise E et al (2007) Is there a role for pelvic irradiation in localized prostate adenocarcinoma? Preliminary results of GETUG-01. J Clin Oncol 25:5366–5373

Roach M III, DeSilvio M, Lawton C, Uhl V, Machtay M, Seider MJ et al (2003) Phase III trial comparing whole-pelvic versus prostate-only radiotherapy and neoadjuvant versus adjuvant combined androgen suppression: Radiation Therapy Oncology Group 9413. J Clin Oncol 21:1904–1911

Roach M, Marquez C, You HS et al (1994) Predicting the risk of lymph node involvement using the pre-treatment prostate specific antigen and Gleason score in men with clinically localized prostate cancer. Int J Radiat Oncol Biol Phys 28:33–37

Roeloffzen EM, Crook J, Monninkhof EM, McLean M, van Vulpen M, Saibishkumar EP (2012) External validation of the pretreatment nomogram to predict acute urinary retention after (125)I prostate brachytherapy. Brachytherapy 11:256–264

Taira AV, Merrick GS, Galbreath RW, Wallner KE, Butler W (2010) Natural history of clinically staged low- and intermediate risk prostate cancer treated with monotherapeutic permanent interstitial brachytherapy. Int J Radiat Oncol Biol Phys 76:349–354

Thompson IM, Tangen CM, Paradelo J, Lucia MS, Miller G, Troyer D et al (2009) Adjuvant radiotherapy for pathological T3N0M0 prostate cancer significantly reduces risk of metastases and improves survival: long-term followup of a randomized clinical trial. J Urol 181:956–962

Valdagni R, Kattan MW, Rancati T, Yu C, Vavassori V, Fellin G et al (2012) Is it time to tailor the prediction of radio-induced toxicity in prostate cancer patients? Building the first set of nomograms for late rectal syndrome. Int J Radiat Oncol Biol Phys 82:1957–1966

Warde P, Mason M, Ding K (2011) Combined androgen deprivation therapy and radiation therapy for locally advanced prostate cancer: a randomized phase 3 trial. Lancet 378:2104–2111

Widmark A, Klepp O, Solberg A (2009) Endocrine treatment, with or without radiotherapy, in locally advanced prostate cancer (SPCG-7/SFUO-3): an open randomized phase III trial. Lancet 373: 301–308

Wiegel T, Bottke D, Steiner U, Siegmann A, Golz R, Störkel S et al (2009) Phase III postoperative adjuvant radiotherapy after radical prostatectomy compared with radical prostatectomy alone in pT3 prostate cancer with postoperative undetectable prostate-specific antigen: ARO 96–02/AUO AP 09/95. J Clin Oncol 27:2924–2930

Zelefsky MJ, Kuban D, Levy LB, Potters L, Beyer DC, Blasko JC et al (2007) Multi-institutional analysis of long-term outcome for stages T1–T2 prostate cancer treated with permanent seed implantation. Int J Radiat Oncol Biol Phys 67:327–333

Zietman AL, Bae K, Slater JD, Shipley WU, Efstathiou JA, Coen JJ et al (2010) Randomized trial comparing conventional-dose with high-dose conformal radiation therapy in early-stage adenocarcinoma of the prostate: long-term results from proton radiation oncology group/American college of radiology 95–09. J Clin Oncol 28:1106–1111

Sarcoma

William P. Levin and Thomas F. DeLaney

Contents

W. P. Levin (✉)
Department of Radiation Oncology, Abramson Cancer Center, Hospital of the University of Pennsylvania, PCAM, TRC 2 West, 3400 Civic Center Blvd, Philadelphia, PA, USA
e-mail: Levin@uphs.upenn.edu

T. F. DeLaney
Connective Tissue Oncology Center, Francis H. Burr Proton Therapy Center, Radiation Oncology, Massachusetts General Hospital, 55 Fruit Street, Boston, MA 02114, USA

Abstract

Soft tissue sarcomas are malignant tumors that arise in the mesoderm. There are over 50 subtypes of these tumors that vary greatly in biological behavior. While small, low-grade lesions may be adequately treated by resection alone; larger, higher-grade lesions require adjuvant therapy to maximize local control. We will examine the prognostic factors that predict for disease recurrence and the role of radiation therapy in this setting. We will also examine the toxicities associated with radiation, and how this information is utilized to help or guide decision making for the treatment of soft tissue sarcomas.

Abbreviations

STS	Soft tissue sarcoma
SO	Second opinion
AJCC	American Joint Committee on Cancer
MSKCC	Memorial Sloan-Kettering Cancer Center
DFS	Disease-free survival
OS	Overall survival
MDACC	University of Texas M. D. Anderson Cancer Center
MGH	Massachusetts General Hospital
PMH	The Princess Margaret Hospital
RLNM	Regional lymph node metastases
MPNST	Malignant peripheral-nerve tumor
CI	Concordance index
LS	Liposarcoma
GPS	General postoperative sarcoma nomogram from MSKCC
DSS	Disease-specific survival
pathCR	Greater than or equal to 95 % necrosis

C. Nieder and L. E. Gaspar (eds.), *Decision Tools for Radiation Oncology*, Medical Radiology. Radiation Oncology,
DOI: 10.1007/174_2013_857,
Published Online: 30 June 2013

1 Introduction

The ability to formulate broad treatment algorithms for patients with soft tissue sarcomas (STS) is complicated by the great diversity in biology and clinical behavior across the numerous subtypes that compose this group of mesenchymal tumors. Because of the relatively low incidence (1 % of all adult malignancies), investigators are often forced to group STS's of different histologies and locations in an attempt to draw statistically meaningful conclusions from the data. As we investigate prognostic factors for STS, it will become apparent that lumping instead of splitting is a flawed methodology. Periodic, seismic reclassification of sarcoma subtypes also adds to the confusion. Despite these potential stumbling blocks, we will explore the literature and make some evidence-based comments regarding important prognostic factors, types and sequencing of local therapies, associated toxicities, and predictions of outcome with and without the use of these treatment modalities. Finally, we will touch upon the future directions of STS, in regards to diagnosis, prediction of prognosis, and therapy.

In 2012, more than 220,000 new cases of breast cancer, and 240,000 new prostate cancers were reported in the United States. In comparison, only 11,000 new soft tissue sarcoma cases were identified (SEER Database, NCI., 2013). Not only are STS's rare but the group is incredibly diverse. The World Health Organization (WHO) classification of STS's includes more than 50 different histologic subtypes. These factors taken together can make accurate diagnosis very difficult, even for very experienced pathologists.

Five hundred consecutive cases submitted for expert consultation at an academic pathology department (Emory University) specializing in the diagnosis of STS's were analyzed for concordance between initial diagnosis and diagnosis rendered by expert review (Arbiser et al. 2001). Of 266 cases (53.2 %) accompanied by a diagnosis, essential agreement with the second opinion was noted in 68 %, with a minor discrepancy in 7 %, and major discrepancy in 25 %. A similar study was done in France, where 1463 cases were evaluated for concordance between initial diagnosis and the diagnosis assigned after expert second opinion (SO). Full concordance between primary diagnosis and SO was observed in 824 (56 %) cases, partial concordance (identical diagnosis of connective tumor but different grade or histological subtype) in 518 (35 %) cases and complete discordance (benign vs. malignant, different histological type or invalidation of the diagnosis of sarcoma) in 121 (8 %) cases. The major discrepancies were related to histological grade ($n = 274$, 43 %) and histological type ($n = 144$, 24 %). The authors concluded that more than 40 % of first histological diagnoses were modified at second reading, possibly resulting in different treatment decisions.

2 Staging

The most widely used staging system for soft tissue sarcomas is the TNM system developed by the International Union Against Cancer (UICC) and the American Joint Committee on Cancer (AJCC). The system uses tumor size (T), depth (superficial or deep), lymph node involvement (N), presence or absence of distant metastases (M), and histologic grade (G) in determining the stage grouping for soft tissue sarcomas (Edge et al. 2010). In the most recent 2010 7th edition of the AJCC Manual (Table 1)[1], the staging for GIST has been separated from the staging of other sarcomas for the first time. Another change in the 7th edition is that depth of tumor invasion (either superficial or deep to the investing fascia) is no longer used to differentiate between stages for tumors of the same size. This change is controversial, given that there are data suggesting a better prognosis with superficial lesions (Salas et al. 2009) (Table 2).

Another problematic issue with the current staging system is that it is judged to offer little prognostic value for retroperitoneal sarcomas (Nathan et al. 2009). A review of outcome based on patients in the SEER database who had undergone resection for retroperitoneal sarcoma (RPS) suggested that histological subtype, histological grade, and tumor invasion of adjacent structures were associated with survival on multivariable analysis while tumor size had no prognostic value. Consequently, the AJCC T classification system demonstrated poor discriminatory ability. The authors concluded that the AJCC staging system for RPS is in need of revision.

3 Prognostic Factors

3.1 Histologic Grade

Histologic grade and tumor size are the primary determinants of clinical stage. In turn, overall TNM stage grouping has been shown to be predictive of outcome. Based on data from Memorial Sloan-Kettering Cancer Center (MSKCC), pathologic group stage was correlated with decreased disease-free survival (DFS) and overall survival (OS) for increasing stage in patients with extremity and trunk soft tissue sarcoma. Five-year DFS for Stages I, II, and III were

[1] This corresponds to Table 33.5 and 33.6 (page 950 and 951) "Decision making in radiation oncology" (Lu and Brady)

Table 1 AJCC TNM classification of soft tissue sarcoma and stage grouping

Stage	Description
Primary tumor (T)	
TX	Primary tumor cannot be assessed
T0	No evidence of primary tumor
T1a	Superficial tumor ≤5 cm in greatest dimension
T1b	Deep[a] tumor ≤5 cm in greatest dimension
T2a	Superficial[a] tumor >5 cm in greatest dimension
T2b	Deep[a] tumor >5 cm in greatest dimension
Regional lymph nodes (N)	
NX	Regional lymph nodes cannot be assessed
N0	No regional lymph node metastasis
N1	Regional lymph node metastasis
Distant metastasis (M)	
MX	Distant metastasis cannot be assessed
M0	No distant metastasis
M1	Distant metastasis
Grade (G)	
GX	Primary tumor cannot be assessed
G1	Well differentiated
G2	Moderately differentiated
G3	Poorly or undifferentiated

[a] Superficial tumor is located exclusively above the superficial fascia without invasion of the fascia; deep tumor is located either exclusively beneath the superficial fascia, superficial to the fascia with invasion of or through the fascia, or both superficial yet beneath the fascia
Source Edge et al. (2009)

Table 2 Stage grouping of STS

Group	Stage (group)			
	T	N	M	G
IA	1a plus 1b	0	0	1
IB	2a plus 2b	0	0	1
IIA	1a plus 1b	0	0	2 or 3
IIB	2a plus 2b	0	0	2
III	2a plus 2b	0	0	3
	Any T	1	0	Any G
IV	Any T	Any N	1	Any G

Source Edge et al. (2009)

86, 72, and 52 %. Corresponding values for OS were 90, 81, and 56 % (Edge et al. 2010).

Another change to the 2010 7th edition of the AJCC Staging Manual is the move from a four-tier to a three-tier histologic grading system based on the degree of differentiation, mitotic activity, and necrosis. Investigators at the University of Texas M. D. Anderson Cancer Center (MDACC) reviewed the cases of 1,225 patients with localized sarcoma treated with conservative surgery and radiation (Zagars et al. 2003a, b). Tumor grade was stratified according to a three-tier system. High tumor grade was found to be a negative prognostic factor for local recurrence, metastatic recurrence, and disease specific survival. Patients with high grade tumors of greater than 5 cm fared worse than those with smaller tumors of similar grade (5-year metastatic control was 53 vs. 79 %, respectively).

3.2 Tumor Size

Investigators at Massachusetts General Hospital (MGH) retrospectively analyzed the cases of 220 patients with soft tissue sarcoma managed by radiation and surgery (Suit et al. 1988). They were also able to correlate size and grade with prognosis. For patients with grade 2 or 3 sarcomas, there was an increase in the frequency of distant metastases with size of the primary lesion; 6 % at less than or equal to 2.5 cm, 60 % at 15–20 cm, and 80 % at greater than 20 cm.

3.3 Anatomic Location

Anatomic site is also an important determinate of outcome. Patients with retroperitoneal, head and neck, and visceral sarcomas have an inferior overall prognosis compared with patients with extremity tumors. These were the findings by researchers at The Princess Margaret Hospital (PMH) where the cases of 389 patients with STS where reviewed (Levay et al. 1993). Extremity lesions fared more favorably compared to head and neck and torso lesions ($p = 0.02$) with respect to survival. Extremity and torso lesions had significantly better local control ($p < 0.0001$) than in the head and neck region where local failure was a common cause of death.

Investigators at MDACC also found site of disease to be a determinate of outcome (Pisters et al. 1996). Overall local control rates for STS of the extremity and superficial trunk, combined were 85 and 81 % at 5 years and 15 years, respectively, and were significantly superior to those for STS of the head and neck and the deep trunk (68 and 64 %, respectively). Interestingly, these findings could not be fully explained by margin status alone.

3.4 Lymph Node Status

Regional lymph node metastases (RLNM) are infrequently seen in patients with STS's; on the order of 5 % (Mazeron and Suit 1987). There are, however, certain histologic subtypes with a greater propensity for nodal spread, remembered as the SCARE histologies (synovial, clear cell, angiosarcoma, rhabdosarcoma, epithelioid). The prognostic significance of RLNM has been debated (Fong et al. 1993).

Investigators at the Royal Marsden Hospital, U.K., studied the significance of RLNM's in sarcoma patients entered in their prospective database (Behranwala et al. 2004). A total of 73 (3.4 %) of 2,127 patients had RLNM. The 1-year survival for patients with isolated RLNM was 77 %, compared with 36 % for patients who presented with RLNM and distant metastasis ($p = 0.005$). The 1-year survival for metachronous and synchronous RLNM was 94 and 68 % respectively ($p = 0.05$).

The MSKCC group published a similar analysis from their prospective database (Fong et al. 1993). From the 1,772 sarcoma patients evaluated, 46 (2.6 %) were identified with lymph node metastasis. Median follow-up of all patients from diagnosis of lymph node metastasis was 12.9 months. Median survival for non-survivors was 12.7 months. Thirty-one patients underwent radical, therapeutic lymphadenectomy with curative intent, whereas 15 patients had less than curative procedures, in most cases biopsy only. Patients not treated with radical lymphadenectomy had a median survival of 4.3 months, whereas radical lymphadenectomy was associated with a 16.3 month median survival and the only long-term survivors (46 % 5-year survival by Kaplan–Meier). The authors conclude that radical lymphadenectomy is appropriate treatment for isolated metastasis to regional lymph nodes and may provide long-term survival.

3.5 Age

It has long been postulated that older patients with STS have inferior outcomes because they present with larger, higher grade tumors, and tend to receive definitive surgery, chemotherapy, and RT less often (Farshadpour et al. 2005). However, at least some data suggest that older patients have higher rates of local recurrence and distant metastases not entirely accounted for by worse tumor characteristics at presentation or less aggressive treatment (Biau et al. 2011). In future sections, we will see that increasing age is a negative prognosticator for outcome.

3.6 Histologic Subtype

In a review of their prospective database, the MSKCC group found that patients with histologic subtypes fibrosarcoma and malignant peripheral-nerve tumor (MPNST) were at higher risk for local recurrence. Worse tumor-related survival was seen in patients with leiomyosarcoma (LMS) and MPNST (Pisters et al. 1996). Other investigators have found the subtype angiosarcoma to be associated with inferior survival, as well (Canter et al. 2010).

3.7 Depth of Invasion

In the most recent 2010 7th edition of the AJCC Staging Manual, superficial and deep tumors of equal size are now included in the same stage, eliminating the risk stratification for tumor depth seen in previous editions. This change is controversial, given the fact that numerous studies have revealed depth of invasion to be a risk factor for outcome (Pisters et al. 1996).

3.8 Margin Status

Given that surgical resection of the primary tumor is the mainstay of treatment for STS's, the significance of margin status is an area of active clinical investigation. This topic is worthy of an in-depth discussion, which will take place in the next section on local control.

3.9 Nomogram for Sarcoma-Specific Death

In 2002, investigators at MSKCC published a post-operative nomogram they developed to predict the probability of 12-year sarcoma-specific death (Kattan 2002). Variables for the nomogram were identified from the cases of over 2,000 patients prospectively followed in their adult STS database. All patients were treated with surgical resection. Some patients received chemotherapy or radiation therapy. The variables considered for the basis of the nomogram were age at diagnosis, tumor size (≤5, 5–10, or >10 cm), histologic grade (high or low), histologic subtype (fibrosarcoma, leiomyosarcoma, liposarcoma, malignant fibrous histiocytoma, malignant peripheral nerve tumor, synovial, or other), depth (superficial or deep), and site (upper extremity, lower extremity, visceral, thoracic or trunk, retro intraabdominal, or head or neck).

Three nomogram development approaches were compared. With the first approach, Kaplan–Meier curves were plotted for all possible strata combinations. The second method utilized recursive partitioning. Because of limitations identified with these approaches, a third approach, Cox regression was explored. The advantage of this technique, according to the authors, is that all patients in the data set are potentially considered for each prediction.

The median follow-up overall, and for those patients still alive was 3.2 and 4 years, respectively (maximum follow up of 18 years). The 5- and 10-year disease-specific death probabilities were 25 and 35 %, respectively. The time interval of 12-year disease-specific death was chosen based on the maturity of the data (number of patients at risk). This appeared to be the most distant time point with many patients at risk ($n = 176$). The three modeling approaches were compared for their ability to reliably predict disease-specific death at 12 years. The bootstrap-corrected concordance indices (CI) were as follows: Kaplan–Meier, 0.69; recursive partitioning, 0.74; and Cox regression, 0.77.

Because the Cox regression model seemed to predict disease-specific death most accurately, it was the basis for the prognostic nomogram. Each variable in the Cox model was associated with sarcoma-specific survival ($p \leq 0.01$). The nomogram predicts the probability that the patient will die of sarcoma within 12 years of his initial surgery, assuming he or she does not die of another cause first (Fig. 1).

Not only can the nomogram assist in decision-making regarding the use of adjuvant therapy and enrollment on clinical trial, it can also be employed when formulating a follow-up schedule. Those patients with lower risk disease may require less stringent surveillance. Reducing the number of follow ups and procedures may reduce stress levels for patients and health care costs for society. In their discussion, the authors note the inherent difficulty in studying one predictive variable at a time. In fact, moving a patient on one axis of the nomogram may also move him on another axis as well. Changing one variable, while holding the other constant may not be realistic and requires caution by the interpreter. The authors emphasize that the nomogram is not perfectly accurate, with an 8 % margin of error, on average. They indicate that better accuracy might be achieved with longer follow up, the addition of more patients, and the inclusion of novel predictive factors.

Investigators at UCLA applied the MSKCC nomogram to their own patient cohort in an attempt to validate predictive accuracy (Eilber et al. 2004). A population of 929 patients treated for primary STS at UCLA was used for the validation study. With median follow-up intervals of 48 months for all patients and 60 months for surviving patients, the 5- and 10-year disease-specific survival rates were 77 and 71 %, respectively. Application of the nomogram to the UCLA data set yielded a concordance index of 0.76.

It should be noted that the MSKCC nomogram was constructed using a binary tumor grading system (high grade, vs. low grade). Pathologic specimens at UCLA, however, are graded according to a three tier system. So in the current study, investigators entered patients with intermediate-grade disease into the nomogram twice—once as patients with low-grade disease, and then as patients with high-grade disease. For each patient, the two resulting predictions were averaged to obtain an 'intermediate' value. The implications of this methodology are unclear.

3.10 Retroperitoneal Sarcoma

Approximately 10–15 % of all STS's arise in the peritoneum (Mendenhall et al. 2005). Because the retroperitoneum can often accommodate large tumors without symptoms, tumors tend to be large. In addition to tumor size, invasion into nearby structures makes complete resection difficult. Approximately 10–20 % of patients are found to have distant metastases on initial presentation (Stoeckle et al. 2001). Approximately two-thirds of tumors are either liposarcomas (LS) or leiomyosarcomas, with the remaining tumors distributed among a large variety of histologic subtypes (Lewis et al. 1998). Retroperitoneal liposarcomas are further classified into well-differentiated, dedifferentiated, and myxoid/round cell subtypes (Singer et al. 2003).

MSKCC published the largest series for retroperitoneal sarcoma (Lewis et al. 1998). Five hundred patients with retroperitoneal STS were treated and followed prospectively. Patient, tumor, and treatment variables were correlated with survival endpoints. The median age of patients was 58 years. Two hundred fourteen patients (43 %) were women and 286 (57 %) were men. The median follow-up was 22 months overall (40 months for survivors). Median survival was 72 months for those with primary disease, 28 months for those with local recurrence, and 10 months for those with metastasis. Most tumors ($n = 319$, 64 %) were high grade, and most ($n = 301$, 60 %) were >10 cm. The most common histologic subtype was liposarcoma ($n = 206$, 41 %), followed by leiomyosarcoma ($n = 133$, 27 %).

The analysis of local recurrence-free survival was confined to the 231 patients who presented to MSKCC with primary disease and then underwent resection. Local recurrence-free survival was 81 % at 2 years and 59 % at 5 years. Factors predictive for local recurrence included high histologic grade ($p = 0.01$) and liposarcoma histologic subtype ($p = 0.01$). Median survival after local recurrence was 28 months. Of the 61 patients in whom a first local recurrence developed, 35 (57 %) underwent complete resection. In the remaining 26 patients, there was residual gross disease after resection or their disease was unresectable. Complete resection was a significant variable predicting survival after local recurrence. The resection rate decreased after each subsequent local recurrence. After the second local recurrence the resection rate was 22 %, and after the third local recurrence it was 10 %.

Metastasis-free survival was 88 % at 2 years and 79 % at 5 years. Sites of metastasis included lung in 14 patients, liver in 10 patients, and lung and liver in four patients. Factors predictive for metastasis include high histologic grade ($p = 0.01$) and positive gross and microscopic margins of resection ($p = 0.01$). Median survival after metastasis was 13 months. On both univariate and multivariate analysis, unresectable disease ($p = 0.001$), incomplete resection ($p = 0.001$), and high histologic grade ($p = 0.001$) were predictive of disease-specific death.

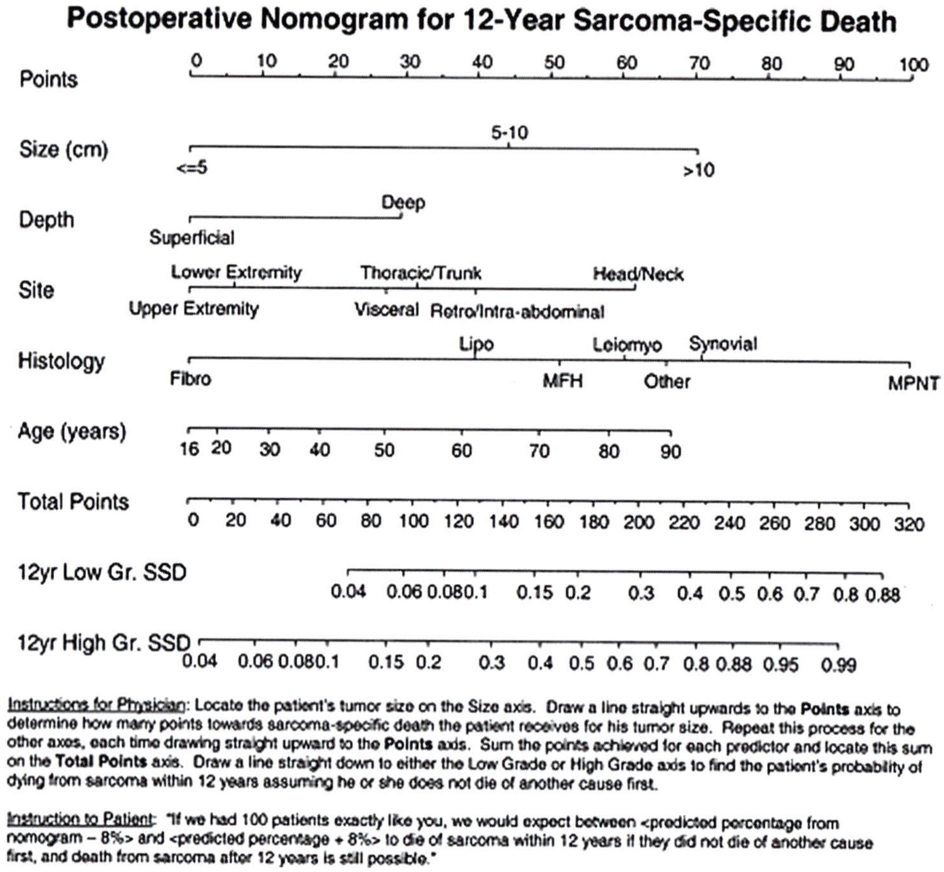

Fig. 1 Postoperative nomogram for 12-year sarcoma-specific death based on 2,163 patients treated at Memorial Sloan-Kettering Cancer Center. Abbreviations: Fibro indicates fibrosarcoma; Lipo, liposarcoma; Leiomyo, leiomyosarcoma; MFH, malignant fibrous histiocytoma; MPNT, malignant peripheral-nerve tumor; GR, grade; SSD, sarcoma-specific death. Kattan (2002)

For the group of patients where complete resection was achieved with gross negative margins ($n = 185$), median survival was 103 months. In contrast, the median survival in patients ($n = 46$) undergoing incomplete resection was 18 months. There was no significant difference in survival between patients whose disease was unresectable and those who underwent incomplete resection ($p = 0.4$). Patients with high-grade tumors had a median survival of 33 months, versus 149 months for those with low-grade tumors. The survival of patients with tumors >10 cm was consistently lower than those with smaller ones.

The MSKCC group carried out an additional analysis of 177 patients with primary retroperitoneal liposarcomas undergoing resection with curative intent (Singer et al. 2003). Breakdown of the histologic subtypes for the patients evaluated was as follows: 99 (56 %) with well-differentiated, 65 (37 %) with dedifferentiated, nine (5 %) with myxoid, and four (2 %) with round cell morphology. Multivariate analysis showed that dedifferentiated liposarcoma subtype was associated with a sixfold increased risk of death compared with well-differentiated histology ($p < 0.0001$). Retroperitoneal dedifferentiated liposarcoma was associated with an 83 % local recurrence rate and 30 % distant recurrence rate at 3 years. Incomplete resection ($p < 0.0001$), contiguous organ resection (excluding nephrectomy; $p = 0.05$), and age ($p = 0.03$) were also important independent prognostic factors for survival in retroperitoneal liposarcoma.

The MSKCC group also published a subtype-specific nomogram for patients with primary liposarcoma of the retroperitoneum extremity, or trunk (Dalal et al. 2006). Like the general postoperative sarcoma (GPS) nomogram discussed above, this one was developed using a Cox regression model. The independent predictors of disease-specific survival (DSS) were age, presentation status, histologic variant, primary site, tumor burden, and gross margin status. When DSS was stratified by primary site, patients with retroperitoneal tumors had a significantly inferior 12-year DSS, compared to tumors in other locations (upper extremity, 87 %; lower extremity, 82 %; truncal, 77 %). For those with LS of the retroperitoneum, the lowest DSS was seen in patients requiring resection of one or more contiguous organs (DSS of 32 %). While patients with retroperitoneal tumors not requiring contiguous organ resection had a 12-year DSS of 53 % ($p = 0.0008$). DSS was not significantly different between patients with microscopically negative and microscopically positive margins, suggesting that even patients in whom the sampled margins were histologically negative likely had tumor cells at the margins of resection if all margins could be histologically assessed with accuracy (12-year DSS of 74 and 68 %, respectively). Patients with grossly positive margins, however, fared worse (12-year DSS of 25 %; $p < 0.0001$). On multivariate analysis, independent predictors of DSS for the entire cohort (all tumor locations) were age ($p = 0.008$), presentation status (biopsy, no prior treatment, prior excision) ($p = 0.004$), primary site ($p = 0.0008$), histologic variant ($p < 0.0001$), tumor burden ($p = 0.0001$), and gross margin status ($p < 0.0001$).

Recall, that when the dataset was applied to the previously established GPS nomogram, the bootstrapping concordance index was 0.776. With the liposarcoma-specific nomogram (Fig. 2), the CI was 0.827. The authors attributed this improved predictive ability to several factors. First, in the LS nomogram, tumor burden was modeled as a continuous variable, as opposed to the three discrete categorical variables (less than 5, 5–10 cm, greater than 10 cm) used in the GPS nomogram. Second, in the LS model, tumor grade was determined by histologic subtype. Well-differentiated and myxoid LS subtypes were classified as low-grade; dedifferentiated, round cell, and pleomorphic LS subtypes were considered to be high grade. Revealed in the analysis, and displayed in the nomogram, is that myxoid LS has a worse prognosis than well-differentiated LS even though both are considered low grade. For high grade LS, the magnitude of worsening prognosis increases as subtype changes from dedifferentiated to round cell to pleomorphic. A third factor thought to be responsible for the improved predictive accuracy in the LS model, is that retroperitoneal LS's were separated according to if contiguous organs were resected. As previously mentioned, patients undergoing these more extensive surgeries tended to fare worse. The inclusion of presentation status was also discussed. Patients with primary liposarcoma who presented with a previous resection/excisional biopsy had a significantly improved DSS. The authors suggested that this reflected a selection bias in that patients who underwent marginal resection due to technical reasons prior to referral to MSKCC were easier to remove completely; thus, reexcision may have been associated with a more favorable prognosis than those patients treated with core/incisional biopsy or referred without prior biopsy. Thus, inclusion of this variable potentially improved the concordance index of the model.

4 Local Control

4.1 Introduction

When the MDACC group analyzed their prospective database for influences on local control, seven factors were identified (Zagars et al. 2003a, b). In order of decreasing significance (favorable feature first), the factors were: final resection margin (negative vs. uncertain/positive), tumor location (extremity/superficial trunk vs. head and neck/deep trunk), presentation (primary vs. locally recurrent), patient age ($\leq$64 years vs. >64 years), histopathology (all others vs. MFH/neurogenic/epithelioid), tumor size ($\leq$10 cm vs. >10 cm), and tumor grade (low and intermediate vs. high).

When investigators at the University of Michigan reviewed their experience in treating STS of the extremity, local control was one of the areas examined (Sabolch et al. 2012). Twenty-five patients (13 %) experienced local recurrence of their disease. The 5-year actuarial estimate for local failure-free survival was 83.7 %. On multivariate analysis, it was found that patients with intermediate/high-grade tumors were 5.6 times more likely to fail locally than patients with low-grade tumors ($p = 0.023$). Patients with multifocally positive surgical margins were nearly 4.3 times more likely to fail locally than patients with negative, close, or focally positive surgical margins ($p = 0.026$).

4.2 Surgical Margins

In an attempt to better understand the significance of resection margin status, the MSKCC group reviewed the cases of over 2,000 patients treated with surgical resection for localized STS (Stojadinovic et al. 2002). After primary resection, 1,624 (78 %) patients had negative and 460 (22 %) had positive resection margins. The risk of local recurrence (LR) with a negative margin was 15 %; the risk with a microscopically positive margin was 28 % ($p < 0.001$). Even with a positive margin, however, 72 % of patients did not have local recurrence.

Additionally, having a positive margin increased the risk of distant recurrence (27 % vs. 23 %, $p < 0.001$) and disease-related death (29 % vs. 18 %, $p < 0.001$). Resection margin did not predict local control for retroperitoneal sarcomas or fibrosarcomas. Because nearly three quarters of the patients with positive margins did not experience a LR, the authors urged clinical judgment when considering adjuvant therapy.

4.3 Local Recurrence and Survival

While the MSKCC group found local recurrence to be correlated with decreased survival, others investigators were not able to draw similar conclusions. Rosenberg et al. (1982) prospectively randomized patients with extremity soft tissue sarcomas and compared amputation with limb-sparing surgery and radiation. There was a 20 % rate of local recurrence in the limb salvage group and none in the amputation group. There was, however, no difference in overall survival, although the small number of patients in

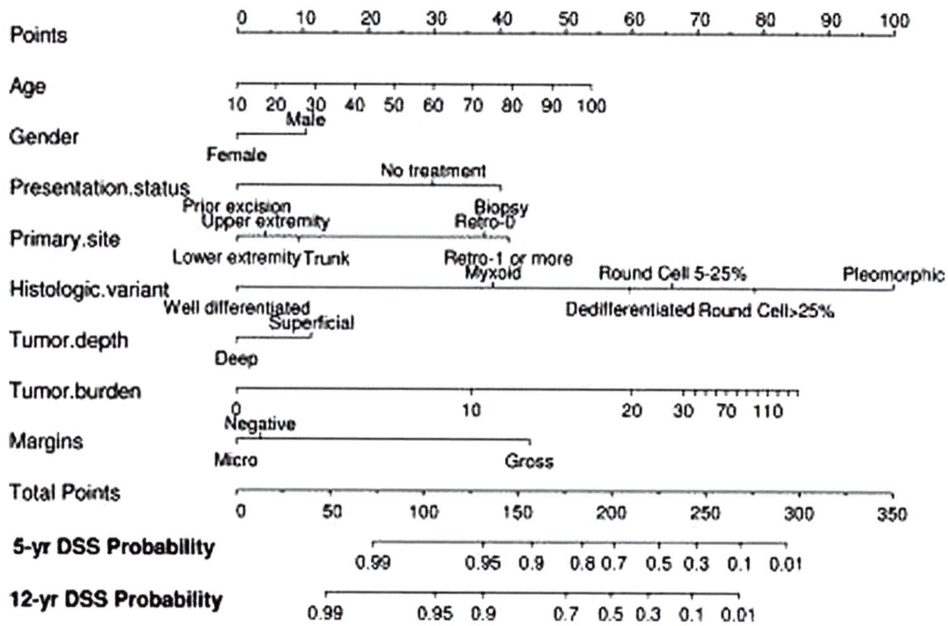

Fig. 2 Nomogram for predicting 5- and 12-year liposarcoma-specific survival probabilities. Dalal et al. (2006)

the study likely reduced the power of the study to detect a difference.

Investigators at the Mayo Clinic explored the impact of microscopic margins on local recurrence, metastasis, and overall survival in 248 of their patients with intermediate- to high-grade STS of the extremity (Novais et al. 2010). The 5-year cumulative incidence of local recurrence was 4.1 %. Patients who presented with positive margins or a margin of 2 mm or less had a worse survival than patients who had margins of greater than 2 mm, or wide margins (5-year survival, 47 % vs. 70 and 72 %).

4.4 Local Recurrence Nomogram

In 2012, investigators at MSKCC published a nomogram based on clinicopathologic factors to quantify the risk of local recurrence after limb-sparing surgery without adjuvant radiation (Cahlon et al. 2012). The nomogram was based on data from 684 patients identified in the prospective database who did not receive adjuvant radiation therapy or chemotherapy. Age, sex, grade, depth, size, site, margin status and histology were analyzed for prognostic significance with respect to local recurrence rates. Variables which were significant in univariate analysis at the 0.05 level were entered into a multivariate competing risk regression model. On the basis of the multivariate analysis, a nomogram for predicting the 3- and 5-year risk of local recurrence was developed (Fig. 3). A concordance index was then calculated to evaluate the discriminatory power of the prognostic model.

With a median follow up of 58 months, a total of 92 patients developed a LR. The 3-, 5-, and 10-year actuarial risk of LR was 11, 13, and 19 %, respectively. On univariate analysis, age >50, size >5 cm, positive/close margin, high grade, and histology other than well-differentiated liposarcoma or atypical lipomatous tumor were all associated with increased risk of LR. Sex, depth and site did not affect the rate of LR. In multivariate analysis, age ($p = 0.02$), size ($p = 0.05$), margin status ($p < 0.01$), histology ($p = 0.01$), and grade ($p < 0.01$) all remained independent prognostic factors for LR. The 5-year rate of LR for AJCC stage 1, 2, and 3 was 8, 15, and 21 %, respectively ($p < 0.001$). The authors claim that the predictive power of the nomogram was actually better than the 2002 AJCC Staging Manual in determining the rate of LR. The CI for the nomogram was 0.74 compared to 0.61 for the AJCC staging system. One cautionary note is that patients who were included in this study are likely to be a lower risk group of patients than an unselected population of soft tissue sarcoma patients, as none of the patients in their study population received either adjuvant radiation or chemotherapy.

5 Adjuvant Therapy

5.1 Introduction

A hallmark study in the era of limb preservation for definitive treatment of STS was performed by Rosenberg and colleagues at the NCI (Rosenberg et al. 1982). In this seminal study, 43 adult patients with high-grade soft tissue sarcomas of the extremities were prospectively randomized to receive either amputation at or above the joint proximal to the tumor, or to receive a limb-sparing resection plus adjuvant radiation therapy. There were four local

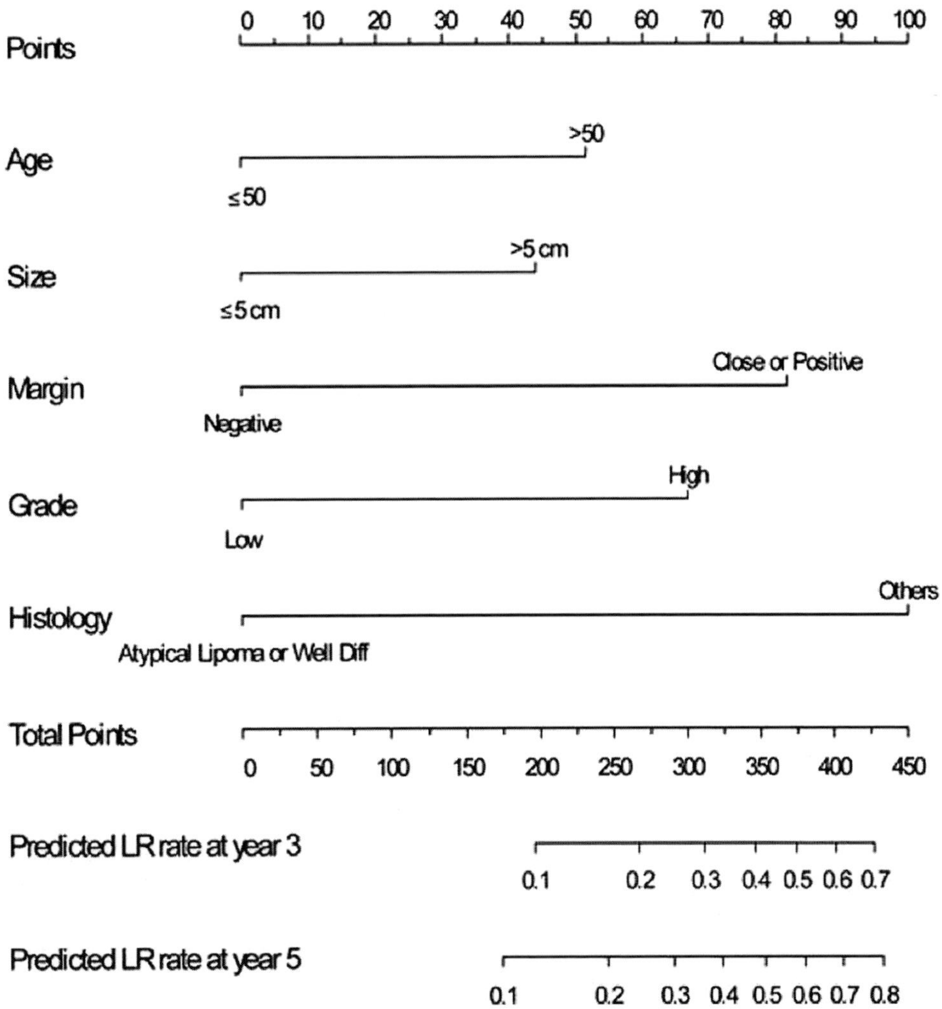

Fig. 3 Nomogram to predict the rate of local recurrence at 3 and 5 years. Cahlon et al. (2012)

recurrences in the limb-sparing group and none in the amputation group ($p = 0.06$). No differences were observed in regards to disease-free survival rates (71 and 78 % at 5 years; $p = 0.75$) or overall survival rates (83 and 88 % at 5 years; $p = 0.99$) between the limb-sparing group and the amputation treatment group.

Multivariate analysis indicated that the only correlate of local recurrence was the final margin of resection. Patients with positive margins of resection had a higher likelihood of local recurrence compared with those with negative margins ($p < 0.0001$) even when postoperative radiotherapy was used. With the results of this study known, definitive therapy for extremity STS shifted away from amputation and towards resection and adjuvant radiation therapy.

5.2 Radiation Therapy and Positive Margins

We previously discussed the significance of surgical margin status in regards to local control and survival. While the goal of any surgical resection is to achieve negative margins, this is not always achieved. Such a scenario is especially concerning when the tumor is of a high grade. Investigators at MSKCC explored the role of adjuvant radiation therapy for patients with high grade soft tissue sarcomas and positive margins (Alektiar et al. 2000).

A total of 110 adult patients with primary high-grade soft tissue sarcoma of the extremity that underwent limb-sparing surgery at MSKCC were found to have histologically positive microscopic surgical margins. Ninety-one (83 %) patients received adjuvant radiation (RT), while 19 (17 %) patients did not. The time frame for the RT group was 1982–1997, and for the no RT group it was 1984–1995. The radiation treatment consisted of brachytherapy alone in 34 (38 %) patients, external beam radiotherapy in 33 (36 %), and a combination of both in 24 (26 %) patients. In patients treated with brachytherapy alone, the median total dose was 45 Gy (range, 30–46 Gy) with a median dose rate of 10 Gy/day (range, 6–14 Gy/day). In the patients treated with external beam radiotherapy alone the median tumor dose was 64 Gy (range, 28–70.2 Gy). The median follow-up time for all 110 patients was 41 months (range, 3–186), but 84 months for those patients that were still alive.

Twenty-six out of 110 patients (24 %) developed local recurrence: 17/91 (19 %) in the RT group and 9/19 (47 %) in the no RT group. Of the 26 patients who developed local recurrence, 11/26 (42 %) were isolated local recurrences and 15/26 (58 %) were associated with synchronous or metachronous distant metastasis. The 5-year actuarial local control for the whole group was 71 %. The 5-year actuarial local control in patients who received adjuvant RT was 74 % compared to 56 % in those who did not receive adjuvant RT ($p = 0.01$). When local control was analyzed according to the type of adjuvant RT received, differences were not significant.

Tumor site and location were also found to be significant predictors of local control. The 5-year local control rate for patients with lower extremity site was 78 % compared to 52 % for upper extremity ($p = 0.03$). A proximal location of the tumor also yielded a superior 5-year local control than distal location (78 % vs. 62 %, $p = 0.03$). Local control was also analyzed according to whether sarcoma cells were present at the inked margins of resection or within less than 1 mm. The 5-year local control rate was 71 % in patients who presented with sarcoma cells at the inked margin compared to 72 % in those with a close margin ($p = 0.6$). On multivariate analysis, only proximal location ($p = 0.003$) and the use of adjuvant radiation ($p = 0.01$) maintained their significance as predictors of improved local control.

The MGH group also published results on patients treated with adjuvant radiation for positive margins (Delaney et al. 2007). A retrospective chart review was performed on 154 patients with STS at various anatomic sites with positive margins. At 5 years, actuarial LC, DFS, and OS rates were: 76, 46.7, and 65.2 %, respectively. LC was highest with extremity lesions ($p < 0.01$), radiation dose >64 Gy ($p < 0.05$), microscopically (vs. grossly visible) positive margin ($p = 0.03$), and superficial lesions ($p = 0.05$). Patients receiving >64 Gy had higher 5-year LC, DFS, and OS rates of 85, 52.1, and 67.8 % versus 66.1, 41.8, and 62.9 % if ≤64 Gy. OS was worse in patients with intermediate and high grade tumors with local failure ($p < 0.001$). Other known prognostic factors, including grade, stage, size, and age (>50), also influenced OS. By multivariate analysis, the best predictors of LC were site (extremity vs. other) and dose (>64 vs. ≤64 Gy); the best predictors for OS were size, gross versus microscopic positive margin, and local failure.

5.3 Toxicity

5.3.1 Timing of Radiotherapy

Another landmark study in the evolution of limb-preservation therapy in the treatment of soft tissue sarcoma comes from Canada. In 2002, O'Sullivan et al. published their results of a prospective study, randomizing patients with extremity STS to receive either preoperative or postoperative radiotherapy (O'Sullivan et al. 2002). A total of 190 patients underwent randomization. Preoperative patients received 50 Gy in 25 fractions, while those in the post-op group were assigned to receive 66 Gy in 33 fractions. Fourteen patients in the pre-op group also received a postoperative dose of 16–20 Gy for positive margins. The primary endpoint was rate of wound complications within 120 days of surgery. Complications were defined as secondary wound surgery, hospital admission for wound care, or the need for deep packing or prolonged wound dressings within 120 days of tumor resection. Secondary endpoints were assessed in all eligible patients, and included local control, metastatic failure, progression-free survival, and overall survival.

The study was terminated when a highly significant result was obtained at the time of a planned interim analysis. With a median follow-up of 3.3 years, acute wound complications were significantly more common with preoperative treatment (35 vs. 17 %). Other factors associated with acute wound complications were the volume of resected tissue and lower limb location of the tumor. Because the post-operative RT fields were larger, and the dose delivered was higher, the investigators indicated that more follow-up would be needed to assess whether these variables would lead to more late treatment effects in these patients. With a median follow-up of 6.9 years, LR rate, regional or distant failure rate, and progression-free survival, was not significantly different between the two treatment arms (O'Sullivan et al. 2004). There was, however, a significant difference between the two groups in terms of late toxicity (Davis et al. 2005). The postoperative RT patients had greater 5-year actuarial rates of grade 2 to grade 4 late toxicity (86 %) when compared with the preoperative patients (68 %) ($p = 0.0002$). Subcutaneous toxicity rated as grade 3 (severe induration and loss of subcutaneous tissue or field contracture greater than 10 % linear measurement) or grade 4 (necrosis) was significantly more common in the postoperative group, 36 % vs. 23 % ($p = 0.02$).

To summarize, a higher rate of generally reversible acute wound healing complications occurred in patients receiving preoperative treatment, which was offset by a higher rate of generally irreversible late complications, including grades 3 and 4 fibrosis, in patients receiving postoperative RT. The authors concluded that for most patients, preoperative RT is favored given that acute wound complications can usually be managed and go on to heal, whereas the late treatment effects are usually permanent. Because no significant difference in the rate of wound healing complications was seen for upper extremity tumors, where wound healing complications were uncommon in either group, patients who are expected to require adjuvant radiotherapy for upper extremity lesions should generally receive preoperative radiation, with postoperative radiation reserved for patients with small, superficial lesions in whom there was an initial expectation that resection alone might be adequate treatment but for whom the final resection margins were close or positive.

5.3.2 Radiation and Bone Fracture

One of the most serious long-term complications associated with radiation and limb salvage surgery is bone fracture. Rates of fracture are generally around 10 %, up to 20 % for patients with known risk factors (Holt et al. 2005). Studies have indicated that both pre- and postoperative radiation can lead to lengthy delays in fracture union beyond 12 months or may prevent osseous union from occurring altogether. Most patients require multiple surgeries to rectify these fractures, consequently increasing their risk of a deep infection. If nonunion persists, total endoprosthetic replacement or amputation may be required (Lin et al. 1998).

Investigators at Princess Margaret Hospital examined the relationship between tumor location, bone dose, and irradiated bone length on the development of radiation-induced fractures in the lower extremity (Dickie et al. 2009). A total of 21 patients with fractures were identified and matched based on tumor size and location, age, beam arrangement, and mean total cumulative RT dose to a sample of 53 non-fracture patients and compared for fracture risk factors. Mean dose to bone, RT field size (FS), maximum dose to bone, and volume of bone irradiated to ≥40 Gy (V40) were compared.

For fracture patients, mean dose to bone was 45 Gy (mean dose at fracture site 59 Gy), mean FS was 37 cm, maximum dose was 64 Gy, and V40 was 76 %, compared with 37 Gy, 32 cm, 59 Gy, and 64 % for non-fracture patients. Differences in mean, maximum dose, and V40 were statistically significant ($p = 0.01$, $p = 0.02$, $p = 0.01$). Leg fractures were more common above the knee joint. The authors concluded that the risk of radiation-induced fracture appears to be reduced if V40 < 64 %. Furthermore, fracture incidence is lower when the mean dose to bone is <37 Gy or maximum dose anywhere along the length of bone is <59 Gy.

Other investigators have linked periosteal stripping to increased fracture risk. The Southern California Kaiser Permanente group analyzed data from their patients who suffered pathologic fractures after undergoing surgery and radiation for treatment of STS (Helmstedter et al. 2001). The fractures occurred at a mean of 40.5 months after treatment. Risk factors associated with the development of fracture included tumor location within the anterior compartment of the thigh, extensive surgical periosteal stripping, and a marginal or intralesional margin of resection. The authors concluded that prophylactic intramedullary fixation of the femur should be considered for patients undergoing resection of large tumors in the anterior compartment of the thigh requiring extensive periosteal stripping and adjuvant radiation therapy.

5.3.3 Intensity Modulated Photon Radiation Therapy

Growing experience suggests that IMRT plans produce dose distributions for patients that are superior to 3-D conformal plans, both in terms of dose conformity around the tumor and dose reduction to the specified critical normal structures, albeit at the cost of irradiating a larger volume of normal tissue with a low-to-moderate dose. In one treatment planning study, IMRT was compared to 3D conformal radiation for treatment of a large extraskeletal chondrosarcoma of the leg (Chan et al. 2001). The IMRT plan produced a superior dose distribution to the patient as compared to the 3D conformal plan both in terms of dose conformity and homogeneity in the target volumes, and reduction of the maximum dose to the bone. Hong and colleagues performed treatment-planning comparisons of IMRT and 3-D conformal RT for 10 patients with STS of the thigh (Hong et al. 2004). They were able to document a reduction in femur dose without compromise in tumor coverage. In addition, IMRT reduced dose inhomogeneity (i.e., hot spots) in the surrounding soft tissues and skin.

5.3.4 Proton Beam Radiation Therapy

As mentioned in the last section, IMRT is able to deliver a highly conformal dose to tumor volumes only by exposing more normal tissue to low-to-moderate doses of radiation. This may be a concern for younger patients who may be at higher risk for a radiation-induced malignancy over the course of their lifetime. The integral dose with IMRT and 3D conformal radiotherapy are similar but the dose distribution is different, with a larger volume of tissue receiving low-moderate dose radiation with IMRT, and the machines requiring higher monitor units increasing the total body exposure, due to leakage radiation with IMRT, both factors expected to increase the risk of secondary, radiation associated cancers. Protons (or other charged particles) may offer up to a 60 % reduction in integral radiation dose to normal tissue, versus photon therapy. Although protons have been extensively used for sarcomas of the skull base and spine/paraspinal tissues, there may be opportunities to use protons with significant sparing of normal tissues in some patients with extremity STS.

Large, medial proximal thigh lesions can be effectively treated with sparing of the femur, hip joint, genitalia, and anorectal tissue (Fig. 4). Lesions around the shoulder can be

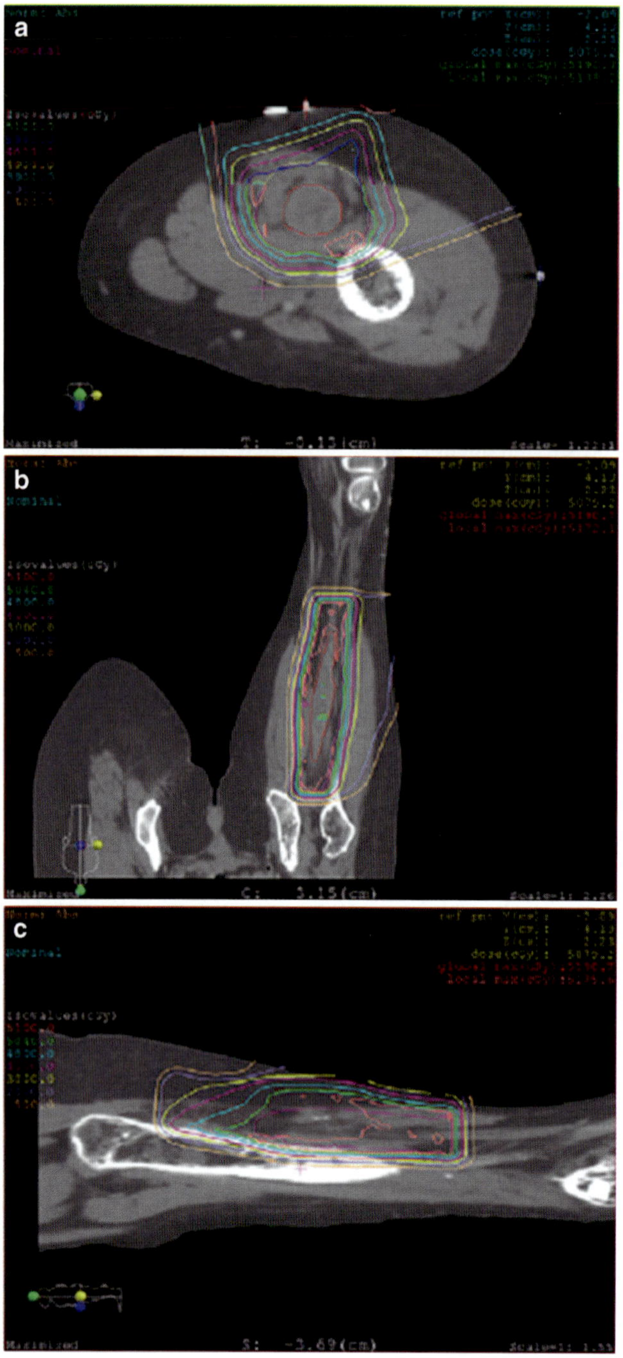

Fig. 4 Proton radiation dose distribution—**a** axial, **b** coronal, **c** sagittal—for a patient with a radiation-associated malignant peripheral nerve sheath tumor arising in the setting of prior RT 18 years earlier for Ewing sarcoma of the femur, metastatic at diagnosis. As it was expected to be difficult to achieve wide margins, preoperative radiation was recommended. Preoperative protons were used to reduce the radiation dose to the normal tissues in the thigh. (Courtesy of Judy Adams, CMD, Massachusetts General Hospital, Boston, MA.)

treated without irradiating the lung apex or shoulder joint. With the recent completion of proton beam facilities at major sarcoma centers in the United States (Massachusetts General Hospital, MD Anderson Cancer Center, University of Florida, and University of Pennsylvania) and Europe (Paul Scherrer Institute in Switzerland and Institute Curie in France as well as other centers in France, Italy, Sweden, and Germany), it is anticipated that a larger proportion of STS patients will be treated with protons, particularly younger patients with large tumors.

5.4 Patients not Requiring Adjuvant Radiation

Because of potential acute and late morbidity from RT, it is important to select patients who may be effectively treated with surgery alone. Several published series have evaluated wide-excision limb-sparing surgery alone. In one study (Rydholm et al. 1991), 70 patients with subcutaneous and intramuscular STS of the extremity were treated by local surgery alone. With a median follow-up of 5 years (range, 3.5–10 years), only four had an LR, despite 84 % having had high-grade tumors. The investigators concluded that postoperative RT may not be necessary in this subgroup.

A similar study at the MD Anderson Cancer Center evaluated LC for T1 tumors after excision alone with negative margins (Pisters et al. 2007). Wide local excision was performed with the intent of including a 1-cm–2-cm margin of normal tissue around the mass. Negative surgical margins were achieved in 84 % of the 88 enrolled patients; the remaining 16 % with microscopically positive margins received postoperative RT. In those with excision alone, the 5-year LR rate was 7.9 %, and the 5-year sarcoma-specific death rate was 3.2 %. This approach may be appropriate for carefully selected patients with small (<5 cm) superficial tumors or small deep tumors that can be resected with all margins greater than or equal to 1 cm (or less if the surgeon is able to resect an intervening fascial barrier.

5.5 Response to Therapy

Previously discussed, was the rationale for using pre-operative radiation therapy in regards to minimizing the long-term morbidity of treatment. Another possible benefit to a neoadjuvant approach is the ability to assess pathologically the response to therapy. This was the basis of an investigation by researchers at UC Davis Cancer Center (Shah et al. 2012). A total of 30 adult patients with localized intermediate- or high-grade primary STS, treated with neoadjuvant external beam RT followed by resection with curative intent were identified for study. Neoadjuvant RT was administered in 2-Gy/day fractions over 25 sessions for a total dose of 50 Gy. Resection was performed 4–6 weeks after completion of RT. There were 22 (73 %) STS of the extremities, seven (23 %) of the retroperitoneum, and one

(3 %) of the trunk. The median tumor size was 8.5 (range 3–35) cm. The majority of tumors were high-grade (87 %) and located deep to the enveloping fascia (97 %). Malignant fibrous histiocytoma/pleomorphic sarcoma (37 %), leiomyosarcoma (20 %), and myxoid/round cell liposarcoma (20 %) comprised the most common histological subtypes.

The median pathological percentage of tumor necrosis for all tumors following neoadjuvant RT was 35 % (range 5–100 %). Eight tumors (27 %) demonstrated greater than 80 % tumor necrosis, and three tumors (10 %) demonstrated pathCR ($\geq$95 % necrosis). The three tumors demonstrating pathCR included an 11-cm high-grade undifferentiated pleomorphic sarcoma of the upper extremity, a 9-cm myxoid/round cell liposarcoma of the lower extremity, and a 7-cm extraskeletal myxoid chondrosarcoma of the upper extremity. With a median follow-up of 40 months, the 5-year LRFS, DRFS, and OS for the entire cohort were 100, 61, and 69 %, respectively. There were no local recurrences, and nine (30 %) patients had distant recurrences. Among the nine patients with distant recurrences, six (67 %) had STS of the extremities, two patients (22 %) had a retroperitoneal STS, and one patient (11 %) had a trunk sarcoma. Five out of the eight patients (62.5 %) with distant recurrence died of their disease.

For the group of three patients (10 %) who exhibited pathological tumor necrosis (pathCR), there were no local recurrences, distant recurrences, or sarcoma deaths. Conversely, all distant recurrences and deaths occurred among patients with less than pathCR. Patients with a pathCR experienced a 3-year DRFS of 100 % compared to 63 % for patients without pathCR ($p = 0.28$). Although this was not a statistically significant difference, patients without pathCR had a 37 % reduction in 3-year DRFS.

In their discussion, the authors point to the fact that the 10 % path CR rate is much lower than that found by other investigators (29–58 %). The discrepancy, they suggest may be due to the fact that chemotherapy was used in some of these studies. Other investigators have achieved high levels of pathologic necrosis using non-conventional fractionation schedules (Willett et al. 1987). Even when a pathCR is achieved, the clinical significance remains unclear. For example, 100 % pathCR after chemoradiation for gastric or rectal cancer does not translate into reduced risk of distant or regional metastasis (Mansour and Schwarz 2009).

6 Relapse of Disease

Previously, we examined the prognostic factors for STS at initial treatment. Few studies have explored variables effecting patient survival for relapsed disease. Such a study was undertaken at MDACC (Zagars et al. 2003a, b). A total of 402 patients with relapsed disease were identified from the prospective STS database. The initial pre-relapse treatment in these patients was a combination of conservative surgery and RT. At the time of the analysis, 328 patients had died and 74 were still alive. The duration of follow-up after relapse among the surviving patients ranged from 3.0 to 308 months (mean 8.7 years, median 6.8 years). The major end point of this study was disease-specific survival from the time of first relapse.

The time to development of the first relapse ranged from 1 day to 11.5 years (mean 21 months, median 12). The time to relapse varied according to the site of relapse, being shortest for nodal relapse (median time 8.1 months), longest for local recurrence (median 18.7 months), and intermediate for distant metastasis (median 13.1 months). All initial relapses were evident by 15 years. The most common site of distance relapse was the lung (84 %), followed by the bone, then liver. Because 94 % (309 of 328) of deaths were due to sarcoma, the overall survival closely paralleled the disease-specific survival. The single most significant determinant of disease-specific survival by univariate and multivariate analyses was the site of first relapse. For a first relapse at the primary site alone—isolated local recurrence—the 5-, 10-, and 15-year disease-specific survival rate was 48, 46, and 39 %, respectively. For a first relapse in the regional nodes with or without local recurrence, but without distant metastasis, the 5- and 10-year disease-specific survival rate was 27 and 20 %, respectively. For a first relapse as distant metastasis with or without other relapse sites, the 5-, 10-, and 15-year disease-specific survival rate was 15, 9, and 8 %, respectively.

The data were analyzed for significant determinants of disease-specific and overall survival for patients with a first relapse as an isolated local recurrence. In multivariate analysis, four individual factors significantly affected disease-specific survival; in order of decreasing significance these were tumor site (extremity and superficial trunk vs. head and neck and deep trunk; $p < 0.001$); tumor grade (low and intermediate vs. high; $p = 0.007$); time to recurrence (>12 vs. $\leq$12 months; $p = 0.027$); and initial tumor size ($\leq$5 vs. >5 cm; $p = 0.044$). There was no evidence that patient age or gender, tumor histologic type, or original resection margin status independently affected the outcome for patients presenting with isolated local recurrence as the first manifestation of relapse.

The authors concluded that patients with localized STS who sustain disease relapse after aggressive initial treatment fare poorly, based in part on the dismal 22 month median disease-specific and overall survival time for the entire group. Having said this, they go on to highlight the fact that the patients who developed isolated local recurrence as the first manifestation of relapse fared much better than those presenting with an initial metastasis, whether nodal or distant. While this study shows that few patients with recurrent STS's of the head and neck or deep trunk are salvaged, aggressive attempts for local control should be considered for all individuals with relapsed disease.

7 Future Directions

French researchers developed a prognostic gene expression signature based on 67 genes profiled in 183 sarcomas (Chibon et al. 2010). With this genetic signature, it was possible to accurately predict metastatic outcome in the initial cohort, as well as in an external validation group. Furthermore, this gene signature was superior to the Fédération Francaise des Centres de Lutte Contre le Cancer grading system in determining metastatic outcome for sarcoma patients.

As with other malignancies, our decision-making in the treatment of soft tissue sarcomas will likely shift dramatically in the near future as the fields of genetics and molecular biology add to our understanding of tumorigenesis and allow for more accurate classification of subtypes. This, in turn, will improve our prognostic abilities and make clearer which patients require aggressive adjuvant therapy or enrollment on an experimental trial.

References

Alektiar KM, Velasco J, Zelefsky MJ et al (2000) Adjuvant radiotherapy for margin-positive high-grade soft tissue sarcoma of the extremity. Int J Radiat Oncol Biol Phys 48:1051–1058

Arbiser ZK, Folpe AL, Weiss SW (2001) Consultative (expert) second opinions in soft tissue pathology. Analysis of problem-prone diagnostic situations. Am J Clin Pathol 116:473–476. doi:10.1309/425H-NW4W-XC9A-005H

Behranwala KA, A'Hern R, Omar A-M, Thomas JM (2004) Prognosis of lymph node metastasis in soft tissue sarcoma. Ann Surg Oncol 11:714–719. doi:10.1245/ASO.2004.04.027

Biau DJ, Ferguson PC, Turcotte RE et al (2011) Adverse effect of older age on the recurrence of soft tissue sarcoma of the extremities and trunk. J Clin Oncol Official J Am Soc Clin Oncol 29:4029–4035. doi:10.1200/JCO.2010.34.0711

Cahlon O, Brennan MF, Jia X et al (2012) A postoperative nomogram for local recurrence risk in extremity soft tissue sarcomas after limb-sparing surgery without adjuvant radiation. Ann Surg 255:343–347

Canter RJ, Beal S, Borys D et al (2010) Interaction of histologic subtype and histologic grade in predicting survival for soft-tissue sarcomas. J Am Coll Surg 210:191–198.e2. doi:10.1016/j.jamcollsurg.2009.10.007

Chan MF, Chui CS, Schupak K et al (2001) The treatment of large extraskeletal chondrosarcoma of the leg: comparison of IMRT and conformal radiotherapy techniques. J Appl Clin Med Phys/Am Coll Med Phys 2:3–8. doi:10.1120/1.1322676

Chibon F, Lagarde P, Salas S et al (2010) Validated prediction of clinical outcome in sarcomas and multiple types of cancer on the basis of a gene expression signature related to genome complexity. Nat Med 16:781–787. doi:10.1038/nm.2174

Dalal KM, Kattan MW, Antonescu CR et al (2006) Subtype specific prognostic nomogram for patients with primary liposarcoma of the retroperitoneum, extremity, or trunk. Ann Surg 244:381–391. doi:10.1097/01.sla.0000234795.98607.00

Davis AM, O'Sullivan B, Turcotte R et al (2005) Late radiation morbidity following randomization to preoperative versus postoperative radiotherapy in extremity soft tissue sarcoma. Radiother Oncol J Eur Soc Ther Radiol Oncol 75:48–53

Delaney TF, Kepka L, Goldberg SI et al (2007) Radiation therapy for control of soft-tissue sarcomas resected with positive margins. Int J Radiat Oncol Biol Phys 67:1460–1469. doi:10.1016/j.ijrobp.2006.11.035

Dickie CI, Parent AL, Griffin AM et al (2009) Bone fractures following external beam radiotherapy and limb-preservation surgery for lower extremity soft tissue sarcoma: relationship to irradiated bone length, volume, tumor location and dose. Int J Radiat Oncol Biol Phys 75:1119–1124. doi:10.1016/j.ijrobp.2008.12.006

Edge SB, Byrd DR, Compton CC et al (2010) American Joint Committee on cancer staging manual 7th edn. Springer, New York, pp 291–300

Edge SB, Byrd DR, Compton CC et al (2009) American Joint Committee on Cancer (AJCC) cancer staging manual, 7th edn. Springer, Berlin

Eilber FC, Brennan MF, Eilber FR et al (2004) Validation of the postoperative nomogram for 12-year sarcoma-specific mortality. Cancer 101:2270–2275. doi:10.1002/cncr.20570

Farshadpour F, Schaapveld M, Suurmeijer AJH et al (2005) Soft tissue sarcoma: why not treated? Crit Rev Oncol/Hematol 54:77–83. doi:10.1016/j.critrevonc.2004.10.006

Fong Y, Coit DG, Woodruff JM, Brennan MF (1993) Lymph node metastasis from soft tissue sarcoma in adults. Analysis of data from a prospective database of 1772 sarcoma patients. Ann Surg 217:72–77

Hall E, Wuu C (2003) Radiation-induced second cancers: the impact of 3D-CRT and IMRT. Int J Radiat Oncol Biol Phys 56(1):83–88

Helmstedter CS, Goebel M, Zlotecki R, Scarborough MT (2001) Pathologic fractures after surgery and radiation for soft tissue tumors. Clin Orthop Relat Res 389:165–172

Holt GE, Griffin AM, Pintilie M et al (2005) Fractures following radiotherapy and limb-salvage surgery for lower extremity soft-tissue sarcomas. A comparison of high-dose and low-dose radiotherapy. J Bone Joint Surg Am 87:315–319. doi:10.2106/JBJS.C.01714

Hong L, Alektiar KM, Hunt M et al (2004) Intensity-modulated radiotherapy for soft tissue sarcoma of the thigh. Int J Radiat Oncol Biol Phys 59:752–759. doi:10.1016/j.ijrobp.2003.11.037

Kattan MW (2002) Postoperative nomogram for 12-year sarcoma-specific death. J Clin Oncol 20:791–796. doi:10.1200/JCO.20.3.791

Levay J, O'sullivan B, Catton C et al (1993) Outcome and prognostic factors in soft tissue sarcoma in the adult. Int J Radiat Oncol Biol Phys 27:1091–1099. doi: 10.1016/0360-3016(93)90529-5

Lewis JJ, Leung D, Woodruff JM, Brennan MF (1998) Retroperitoneal soft-tissue sarcoma: analysis of 500 patients treated and followed at a single institution. Ann Surg 228:355–365

Lin PP, Boland PJ, Healey JH (1998) Treatment of femoral fractures after irradiation. Clin Orthop Relat Res 352:168–178

Mansour JC, Schwarz RE (2009) Pathologic response to preoperative therapy: does it mean what we think it means? Ann Surg Oncol 16:1465–1479. doi:10.1245/s10434-009-0374-z

Mazeron J-J, Suit HD (1987) Lymph nodes as sites of metastases from sarcomas of soft tissue. Cancer 60:1800–1808. doi:10.1002/1097-0142(19871015)60:8<1800:AID-CNCR2820600822>3.0.CO;2-N

Mendenhall WM, Zlotecki RA, Hochwald SN et al (2005) Retroperitoneal soft tissue sarcoma. Cancer 104:669–675. doi:10.1002/cncr.21264

Nathan H, Raut CP, Thornton K et al (2009) Predictors of survival after resection of retroperitoneal sarcoma: a population-based analysis and critical appraisal of the AJCC staging system. Ann Surg 250:970–976. doi:10.1097/SLA.0b013e3181b25183

Novais EN, Demiralp B, Alderete J et al (2010) Do surgical margin and local recurrence influence survival in soft tissue sarcomas? Clin Orthop Relat Res 468:3003–3011. doi:10.1007/s11999-010-1471-9

O'Sullivan B, Davis AM, Turcotte R et al (2002) Preoperative versus postoperative radiotherapy in soft-tissue sarcoma of the limbs: a randomised trial. Lancet 359:2235–2241. doi:10.1016/S0140-6736(02)09292-9

O'Sullivan B, Davis AM, Turcotte R et al (2004) Five-year results of a randomized phase III trial of pre-operative vs. post-operative radiotherapy in extremity soft tissue sarcoma. Proc Am Soc Clin Oncol 23:815

Pisters PW, Leung DH, Woodruff J et al (1996) Analysis of prognostic factors in 1,041 patients with localized soft tissue sarcomas of the extremities. J Clin Oncol Official J Am Soc Clin Oncol 14:1679–1689

Pisters PWT, Pollock RE, Lewis VO et al (2007) Long-term results of prospective trial of surgery alone with selective use of radiation for patients with T1 extremity and trunk soft tissue sarcomas. Ann Surg 246:675–681; discussion 681–2. doi: 10.1097/SLA.0b013e318155a9ae

Rosenberg SA, Tepper J, Glatstein E et al (1982) The treatment of soft-tissue sarcomas of the extremities: prospective randomized evaluations of (1) limb-sparing surgery plus radiation therapy compared with amputation and (2) the role of adjuvant chemotherapy. Ann Surg 196:305–315

Rydholm A, Gustafson P, Rööser B et al (1991) Limb-sparing surgery without radiotherapy based on anatomic location of soft tissue sarcoma. J Clin Oncol Official J Am Soc Clin Oncol 9:1757–1765

Sabolch A, Feng M, Griffith K et al (2012) Risk factors for local recurrence and metastasis in soft tissue sarcomas of the extremity. Am J Clin Oncol 35:151–157. doi:10.1097/COC.0b013e318209cd72

Salas S, Stoeckle E, Collin F et al (2009) Superficial soft tissue sarcomas (S-STS): a study of 367 patients from the French sarcoma group (FSG) database. Eur J Cancer 45:2091–2102 (Oxford, England: 1990). doi: 10.1016/j.ejca.2009.03.006

SEER Database, NCI. In: Surveillance, epidemiology and end results (SEER) program, National Cancer Institute. http://seer.cancer.gov/csr/1975_2009_pops09/results_single/sect_01_table.01.pdf

Shah D, Borys D, Martinez SR et al (2012) Complete pathologic response to neoadjuvant radiotherapy is predictive of oncological outcome in patients with soft tissue sarcoma. Anticancer Res 32:3911–3915

Singer S, Antonescu CR, Riedel E, Brennan MF (2003) Histologic subtype and margin of resection predict pattern of recurrence and survival for retroperitoneal liposarcoma. Ann Surg 238:358–370; discussion 370–1. doi: 10.1097/01.sla.0000086542.11899.38

Stoeckle E, Coindre JM, Bonvalot S et al (2001) Prognostic factors in retroperitoneal sarcoma: a multivariate analysis of a series of 165 patients of the French cancer center federation sarcoma group. Cancer 92:359–368

Stojadinovic A, Leung DHY, Hoos A et al (2002) Analysis of the prognostic significance of microscopic margins in 2,084 localized primary adult soft tissue sarcomas. Ann Surg 235:424–434

Suit HD, Mankin HJ, Wood WC et al (1988) Treatment of the patient with stage M0 soft tissue sarcoma. J Clin Oncol Official J Am Soc Clin Oncol 6:854–862

Willett CG, Schiller AL, Suit HD et al (1987) The histologic response of soft tissue sarcoma to radiation therapy. Cancer 60:1500–1504

Zagars GK, Ballo MT, Pisters PWT et al (2003a) Prognostic factors for patients with localized soft-tissue sarcoma treated with conservation surgery and radiation therapy: an analysis of 1225 patients. Cancer 97:2530–2543. doi:10.1002/cncr.11365

Zagars GK, Ballo MT, Pisters PWT et al (2003b) Prognostic factors for disease-specific survival after first relapse of soft-tissue sarcoma: analysis of 402 patients with disease relapse after initial conservative surgery and radiotherapy. Int J Radiat Oncol Biol Phys 57:739–747

Lymphoma

Chris R. Kelsey and Lynn D. Wilson

Contents

C. R. Kelsey
Duke Cancer Institute, Duke University Medical Center, Morris Building, Room 05125A, 201 Trent Drive, Durham, NC 27710, USA

L. D. Wilson (✉)
Department of Therapeutic Radiology, Yale University School of Medicine, LL 507, 35 Park Street, New Haven, CT 06510, USA
e-mail: lynn.wilson@yale.edu

Abstract

Hodgkin and non-Hodgkin lymphoma represent a diverse spectrum of distinct diseases that arise from the lymphoid system. Lymphomas are characterized by significant biological diversity, heterogeneous presentations, distinct treatment approaches, and ever-changing classification schemes. Prognostic scoring systems have been developed for the most common subtypes using standard clinical and pathological factors. These scoring systems are commonly utilized in clinical practice to guide treatment and assess prognosis. More refined methods of understanding the underlying biology, such as gene expression profiling, are currently being explored. Response to treatment by radiological imaging, particularly positron emission tomography, is instrumental in clinical practice and also has significant prognostic significance.

Abbreviations

HL	Hodgkin lymphoma
NHL	Non-Hodgkin lymphoma
NLPHL	Nodular lymphocyte predominant Hodgkin lymphoma
GHSG	German Hodgkin Study Group
ABVD	Doxorubicine, bleomycin, vinblastine, dacarbazine
BEACOPP	Bleomycin, etoposide, doxorubicin, cyclophosphamide, vincristine, procarbazine, prednisone
DLBCL	Diffuse large B-cell lymphoma
IPI	International prognostic index
FL	Follicular lymphoma
FLIPI	Follicular lymphoma international prognostic index
PET	Positron emission tomography
ALCL	Anaplastic large cell lymphoma
MALT	Mucosa associated lymphoid tissue

C. Nieder and L. E. Gaspar (eds.), *Decision Tools for Radiation Oncology*, Medical Radiology. Radiation Oncology,
DOI: 10.1007/174_2013_830, © Springer-Verlag Berlin Heidelberg 2013
Published Online: 31 March 2013

PCNSL	Primary central nervous system lymphoma
MF	Mycosis fungoides
WBRT	Whole brain radiation therapy
LDH	Lactate dehydrogenase

1 Introduction

Hodgkin lymphoma (HL) and non-Hodgkin lymphoma (NHL) represent a diverse spectrum of distinct diseases that arise from the lymphoid system. Within the HL category there are two distinct entities: nodular lymphocyte predominant HL (NLPHL) and classical HL. The latter consists of four subtypes including nodular sclerosis, mixed cellularity, lymphocyte-rich, and lymphocyte-depleted. Though the immunophenotype is identical between these four subtypes, each has a distinct clinical presentation, pathological findings, and frequency of Epstein-Barr virus infection. NLPHL has a distinct immunophenotype and clinical presentation and is often treated differently. Among NHLs there are numerous subtypes, some of which are still considered provisional entities by the World Health Organization. The most common include diffuse large B-cell lymphoma (DLBCL) and follicular lymphoma (FL), though several other subtypes will also be discussed.

The biological diversity of lymphoma, heterogeneous presentations, distinct treatment approaches, and ever-changing classification schemes can be daunting to an oncologist who does not specialize in their management. This chapter will focus on the more common lymphoma histologies, discussing clinical, pathological, radiological, and treatment-related factors that influence clinical outcomes. Furthermore, since toxicity, particularly long-term toxicity, is a major issue in discussions of lymphoma management, this will be discussed at length as well.

2 Hodgkin Lymphoma

2.1 Clinical Factors

Patients with classical HL are presently distributed into three cohorts- early-stage favorable, early-stage unfavorable, and advanced disease (stages III-IV). The segregation of early-stage disease into favorable and unfavorable cohorts is based on multiple clinical factors which are slightly different among international cooperative groups (Table 1). These factors had particular prognostic importance when radiation therapy was used as a single modality. On the other hand, in the context of a combined modality approach their significance is less. Outcome differences between those with favorable and unfavorable presentations are fading but the intensity of treatment is greater for unfavorable disease. For example, 5-year progression-free survival in patients with early-stage *favorable* disease in the German Hodgkin Study Group (GHSG) HD10 trial was 91.6 % at 5 years with ABVD X 2 (doxorubicin, bleomycin, vinblastine, dacarbazine) + 20 Gy of radiation therapy (Engert et al. 2010). By comparison, 5-year progression-free survival in patients with early-stage, *unfavorable* disease in GHSG HD11 was 87.2 % with ABVD X 4 + 30 Gy radiation therapy (Eich et al. 2010) and 95.4 % with BEACOPP escalated X 2 (bleomycin, etoposide, doxorubicin, cyclophosphamide, vincristine, procarbazine, prednisone)/ABVD X 2 + 30 Gy radiation therapy in GHSG HD14 (von Tresckow et al. 2012). Thus, with more aggressive therapy, the risk of disease recurrence is quite similar.

For patients with advanced HL, the International Prognostic Factors Project on Advanced Hodgkin's Disease evaluated 5141 patients treated with combination chemotherapy, with or without radiation therapy, and identified seven factors that had independent prognostic significance for the outcome freedom from progression These included serum albumin, hemoglobin, male sex, stage, age, and white-cell count (Table 2). The relative risk of each of these factors was relatively similar and ranged from 1.26 (stage IV disease) to 1.49 (hypoalbuminemia). When patients were grouped into 6 prognostic categories based on number of adverse factors (0, 1, 2, 3, 4, and ≥5), 5-year freedom from progression was 84, 77, 67, 60, 51, and 42 % with a similar declining trend in overall survival (Fig. 1). Thus, while clinical factors were able to partition patients into risk groups, the relative differences between risk groups were modest.

Similar to early-stage HL, outcomes in advanced HL have improved with more effective combination chemotherapy regimens. Recent randomized trials have demonstrated excellent outcomes that are approaching those of patients with early-stage disease. For example, 5-year freedom from treatment failure was 88 % with 8 cycles of dose-escalated BEACOPP in the GHSG HD9 study (Engert et al. 2009), 85 % with 4 cycles of dose-escalated BEACOPP and 4 cycles of baseline dose BEACOPP in GHSG HD12 (Borchmann et al. 2011), and 89 % with 6 cycles of dose-escalated BEACOPP in GHSG HD15 (Engert et al. 2012). Radiation therapy was used in all three studies using different criteria.

2.2 Pathological Factors

NLPHL is a rare subtype of HL, accounting for ~5 % of cases. The rarity of this disease has precluded prospective studies, particularly randomized comparisons of differing treatment approaches. The optimal management, particularly for early-stage disease, is controversial and studies in the literature are conflicting (Chen et al. 2010; Nogova et al.

Table 1 Unfavorable Factors in Recent Early-Stage Hodgkin Lymphoma Trials

Factor	GHSG (Eich et al. 2010; Engert et al. 2010)	EORTC (Ferme et al. 2007)	NCI-C (Meyer et al. 2012)
Number of nodal sites	≥3	≥4	≥4
LMA	Present	Present	Present[a]
ESR & B-symptoms	≥50, no "B" symptoms ≥30, "B" symptoms	≥50, no "B" symptoms ≥30, "B" symptoms	ESR ≥ 50
Extranodal involvement	Present	Present	
Age (years)		>50	≥40
Histology		MC/LD	MC/LD
Sex		Male	

GHSG German Hodgkin Study Group; *EORTC* European Organization for Research and Treatment of Cancer; *NCI-C* National Cancer Institute, Canada
LMA large mediastinal adenopathy; *ESR* erythrocyte sedimentation rate
MC mixed cellularity; *LD* lymphocyte depletion
[a] patients with bulky disease were considered "high risk" and not eligible for study

Table 2 International Prognostic Factor Project on Advanced Hodgkin's Disease

Adverse prognostic factor	Relative risk
Serum albumin, <4 g/dL	1.49
White-cell count, ≥15,000/mm^3	1.41
Age, ≥45 years	1.39
Lymphocyte count, <600/mm^3 or <8 % of white-cell count	1.38
Male sex	1.35
Hemoglobin, <10.5 g/dL	1.35
Stage IV disease	1.26

2005; Savage et al. 2011). For localized disease, most patients are treated currently with involved-field radiation therapy alone.

The larger studies that have been performed demonstrate that the risk of relapse after treatment for NLPHL is very similar to classical HL, though patients with classical HL tend to relapse earlier (Nogova et al. 2008; Diehl et al. 1999). However, patients with relapsed NLPHL tend to survive relapse better with a corresponding advantage in long-term overall survival. Indeed, toxicities of treatment are the primary cause of death in patients with NLPHL leading many oncologists to avoid treatment regimens with significant risk. As NLPHL is a CD20 positive lymphoma, ritixumab is often administered. Further studies are necessary to better understand the biology of this rare disease and identify the optimal treatment approach.

2.3 Positron Emission Tomography

Imaging modalities, positron emission tomography (PET) in particular, play a central role in the management of patients with lymphoma. In addition to assessing the extent of disease at diagnosis and for disease surveillance after definitive therapy, PET response also has prognostic impact for both HL and NHLs.

Both interim and post-treatment imaging response with PET have been shown to be a powerful prognostic factors in HL, in all stages of disease and multiple clinical scenarios. Two studies highlight the importance of disease status after chemotherapy but before consolidation radiation therapy. In a Stanford study of 81 patients (73 % with early-stage disease) receiving Stanford V chemotherapy (doxorubicin, vinblastine, mechlorethamine, vincristine, bleomycin, etoposide, prednisone) and consolidation radiation therapy, the presence of PET positive disease after chemotherapy strongly predicted for relapse. Of the six patients who were still PET positive following chemotherapy, four relapses occurred, all within the radiation field (median dose- 33 Gy). Freedom from progression was 96 % in PET negative patients and 33 % in PET positive patients ($p < 0.0003$).

Investigators from the Dana Farber Cancer Institute observed similar findings after ABVD. Among 73 patients with HL (88 % with early-stage disease), 13 were PET positive after chemotherapy. There were four relapses among these 13 patients, three of which were in the radiation field (median dose- 36 Gy). Two-year failure-free survival was 69 and 95 % for PET positive and PET negative cohorts, respectively ($p < 0.01$). While a positive post-chemotherapy PET scan is associated with inferior outcomes, many patients remain disease-free after consolidation radiation therapy. As local failure at the PET positive site is the dominant pattern of failure, higher doses of radiation therapy may be required to sterilize persistent local disease.

Most patients with advanced HL receive chemotherapy alone and post-chemotherapy PET imaging is highly predictive of outcome. In a prospective study by Weihrauch et al. (2001), patients with HL received chemotherapy alone

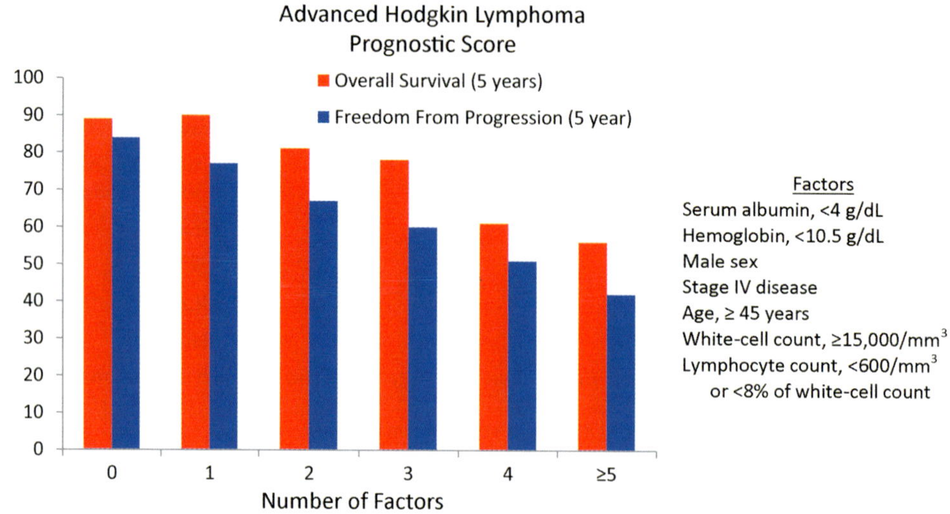

Fig. 1 Prognostic scoring system for advanced Hodgkin lymphoma by the International Prognostic Factors Project on Advanced Hodgkin's Disease. The primary endpoint was 5-year freedom from progression (NEJM 1998; 339:1506)

and were then observed. Of ten patients who were PET positive after chemotherapy, six relapses occurred, all confined to the originally involved site. Compared with the cohort of patients who were PET negative after chemotherapy, the disease-free survival at 1 year was significantly less (40 versus 95 %, $p = 0.004$).

Patients with advanced HL who remain PET positive after chemotherapy appear to be at significantly less risk of relapse when consolidation radiation therapy is administered. In GHSG HD15, patients underwent post-treatment computed tomography (CT) imaging after BEACOPP chemotherapy (Engert et al. 2012). If a residual mass measuring ≥2.5 cm was present then PET imaging was performed. Patients who achieved a complete response by CT imaging and those with residual masses that were PET negative did not receive consolidation radiation therapy. Patients with residual masses that were PET positive did receive RT (30 Gy). Progression-free survival at 4 years was 93 % for PET negative (who did not receive RT) and 86 % for PET positive (who did receive radiation therapy), respectively ($p = 0.02$). This compares favorably with the study by Weihrauch et al. (2001) where no additional treatment was pursued. Patterns of failure were not reported in GHSG HD15. As mentioned previously, higher doses of radiation therapy may be required in the setting of PET positive disease to achieve durable local control.

A positive interim PET also has prognostic significance, though whether the chemotherapy course should be altered if an early complete response is not achieved is unknown. If an interim PET could consistently and accurately identify those patients who would ultimately have refractory or relapsed disease, then this would be a helpful test. However, many patients with a positive interim PET who continue on their current regimen ultimately achieve a complete response and remain disease-free.

The most dramatic study showing the potential prognostic significance of interim PET is from Denmark. Among 77 patients mostly treated with ABVD for all stages of HL, 2-year progression-free survival was 96 % for those who were PET negative after 2 cycles of chemotherapy compared with 0 % for those who were PET positive (Hutchings et al. 2006). A study from Italy showed similar findings, with a 2-year progression-free survival of 95 and 13 % for PET negative and PET positive patients, respectively after ABVD +/− consolidation radiation therapy (Gallamini et al. 2007).

Most studies have not been this dramatic. For example, an Italian study of 304 patients demonstrated 9-year progression-free survival of 95 and 31 % in the presence of a positive and negative interim PET scan, respectively (Zinzani et al. 2012). A study from the Massachusetts General Hospital demonstrated no difference in 4-year progression-free survival for interim PET positive versus PET negative patients (87 versus 91 %, $p = 0.57$), but post-treatment PET was significant (54 versus 94 %, $p < 0.001$). This study only included early-stage patients without bulky disease who largely received combined modality therapy (Barnes et al. 2011). Thus, while interim PET imaging likely has prognostic implications, whether one should alter therapy based on the interim PET response is unclear.

A major issue is PET interpretation. Currently, PET scans are interpreted as positive or negative based on visual analysis alone (Juweid et al. 2007). This leads to some inter-observer and intra-observer variability. An objective method to interpret PET imaging has yet to be validated.

2.4 Treatment-Specific Factors

Chemotherapy is the standard initial treatment for patients with HL in all stages. In early-stage disease, multiple randomized trials have shown that consolidation radiation therapy decreases the risk of relapse (Aviles and Delgado

1998; Laskar et al. 2004; Meyer et al. 2012; Nachman et al. 2002; Noordijk et al. 2005; Pavlovsky et al. 1988; Picardi et al. 2007; Straus et al. 2004) and may improve survival (Franklin et al. 2005). In general, the absolute improvement in progression-free survival is $\sim$10 %. Admittedly, most patients are cured with chemotherapy alone. Identifying the subgroup of patients with residual microscopic disease after chemotherapy that would most benefit from consolidation RT has been challenging.

Currently, most studies attempting to define the subset of patients who are most likely to benefit from consolidation radiation therapy utilize either post-treatment or interim PET imaging. In a study by Picardi et al. (2007), 160 patients with HL (all with disease $\geq$5 cm) received 6 cycles of VEBEP (vinblastine, etoposide, bleomycin, epirubicin, predisone). Those with a good ($\geq$75 % size reduction) but incomplete response by CT imaging but who were negative by PET were randomized to consolidation radiation therapy (32 Gy) or observation. Despite being PET negative, consolidation radiation therapy decreased the risk of relapse. Event-free survival at 5 years was 96 versus 86 %, respectively ($p = 0.03$). Patients who achieved both a negative PET *and* CT ($n = 70$) were not randomized and only received chemotherapy. Of 60 patients with follow-up data, there were seven relapses. Thus, a negative post-treatment PET, even with a negative CT, may lack sufficient sensitivity to indicate a true disease-free state. Interim PET, done after 2–3 cycles, is also being examined, but interim analyses from an EORTC/GELA study (H10) have not been encouraging (Engert 2012). Numerous prospective phase II and phase III studies are currently ongoing by cooperative groups in both the United States and abroad examining the ability of PET to identify patients who would most benefit from consolidation radiation therapy.

Based on the available data, the most effective treatment for early-stage classical HL is combined modality therapy, with the chemotherapy regimen, number of cycles, and dose of radiation therapy dependent on the initial presentation. The standard for advanced HL is chemotherapy. The role of radiation therapy is controversial with conflicting results from randomized studies (Fabian et al. 1994; Aleman et al. 2003).

3 Diffuse Large B-cell Lymphoma

3.1 Clinical Factors

Using data from 2,031 patients with aggressive NHL, two prognostic models were developed as part of the International Non-Hodgkin's Lymphoma Prognostic Factors Project (The International Non-Hodgkin's Lymphoma Prognostic Factors Project 1993). The first model was termed the International Prognostic Index (IPI) and included all patients. Five factors were found to be independently associated with survival including age, performance status, stage, number of extranodal sites, and LDH (Table 3). The relative risks of these factors were relatively low, ranging from 1.47 for stage to 1.96 for age. Five-year survival was 73, 51, 43, and 26 % when 0–1, 2, 3, and 4–5 risk factors were present (Fig. 2).

Table 3 International Non-Hodgkin's Lymphoma Prognostic Factors Project

Adverse prognostic factor	Relative risk
All patients (n = 1385)	
Age, >60 years	1.96
Serum LDH, >1X normal	1.85
Performance status, ECOG 2-4	1.80
Extranodal involvement, >1 site	1.48
Stage, III-IV	1.47
Patients ≤60 years old (n = 885)	
Stage, III-IV	2.17
Serum LDH, >1X normal	1.95
Performance status, ECOG 2-4	1.81

LDH lactate dehydrogenase
ECOG Eastern Cooperative Oncology Group

As age was the most significant risk factor, and 60 is a common age limit for patients receiving more intensive regimens, an Age Adjusted IPI was also developed. When patients were divided by age, three factors remained independently significant- performance status, stage, and lactate dehydrogenase (LDH) (Fig. 3).

The IPI was designed in the pre-rituximab era. In the last 10–15 years, multiple randomized studies have shown that rituximab significantly improves survival when combined with standard combination chemotherapy (Feugier et al. 2005; Pfreundschuh et al. 2006; Habermann et al. 2006). Using data from three prospective trials, the German High-Grade Non-Hodgkin's Lymphoma Study Group found the IPI to retain prognostic significance in the rituximab era (Ziepert et al. 2010).

3.2 Pathological Factors

Classification of lymphomas continues to be based largely on histology and immunohistochemistry. With DLBCL, the heterogeneity of disease presentations and differences in response to therapy indicate that underlying biology plays a dominant role. Similar to breast cancer, the principal genetic changes responsible for this biological diversity are slowly being unraveled and have confirmed that DLBCL is a heterogeneous disease.

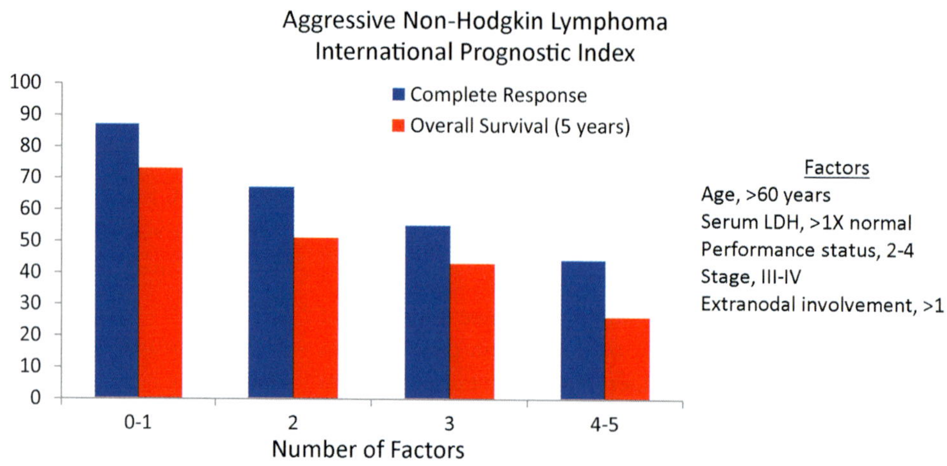

Fig. 2 The International Prognostic Index (IPI) for aggressive non-Hodgkin lymphoma by the International Non-Hodgkin's Lymphoma Prognostic Factors Project. The primary endpoint was 5-year overall survival (NEJM 1993; 329:987)

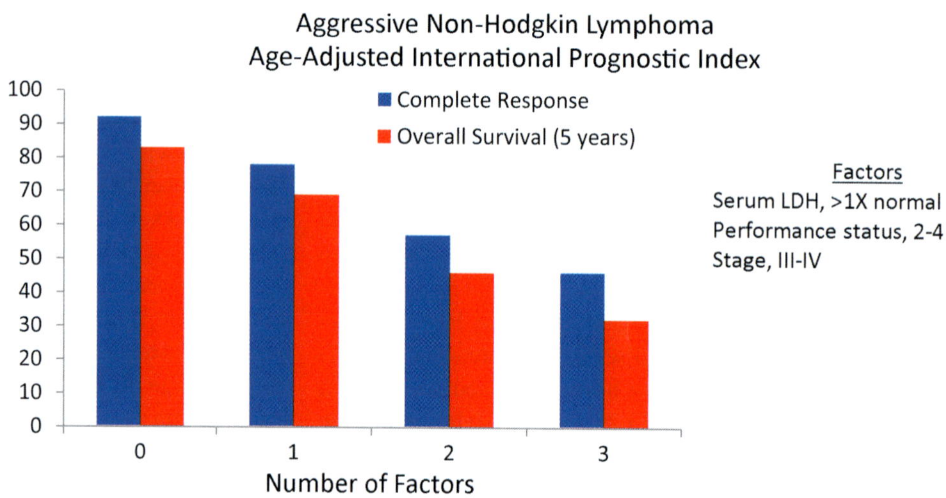

Fig. 3 The age-adjusted ($\leq$60 years old) International Prognostic Index (IPI) for aggressive non-Hodgkin lymphoma by the International Non-Hodgkin's Lymphoma Prognostic Factors Project. The primary endpoint was 5-year overall survival (NEJM 1993; 329:987)

It was first reported by Alizadeh et al. (2000) that distinct subtypes of DLBCL could be identified using gene expression profiling, and that these subtypes were derived from different cells of origin. Germinal center B-cell (GCB) subtype appears to derive from cells actively involved in somatic hypermutation. Lymphomas within this category have a higher prevalence of mutations in pathways involved in apoptosis, often harbor the t(14;18) translocation, and are the more common subtype in cases arising from FL.

On the other hand, the activated B-cell (ABC) subtype derives from cells without ongoing somatic hypermutation. These lymphomas more commonly have constitutively activated nuclear factor κB (*NF-κB*) leading to overexpression of genes under the control of this transcription factor and often involve extranodal sites (e.g., testis, breast). These two subtypes of DLBCL have distinct survival differences (Alizadeh et al. 2000; Lenz et al. 2008; Rosenwald et al. 2002), with the GCB subtype having a better prognosis. Even with the incorporation of rituximab the ABC subtype is associated with an inferior prognosis. Subsequent investigations have proposed additional molecular signatures that appear to influence tumor behavior (Rosenwald et al. 2002; Lenz et al. 2008).

Gene expression profiling is not widely available as a clinical tool. Multiple immunohistochemical algorithms have been designed to predict whether a patient has a GCB or ABC subtype (Hans et al. 2004; Choi et al. 2009; Muris et al. 2006; Natkunam et al. 2008; Nyman et al. 2009; Meyer et al. 2011). No single algorithm is perfect in regards to predicting gene expression profiling results, though each divides patients into groups with different survival outcomes. While personalized therapy may ultimately be based on the molecular subtype of DLBCL, this has not currently been adequately examined.

MYC gene rearrangements are found in approximately 10 % of cases of DLBCL and portends an inferior prognosis (Barrans et al. 2010; Savage et al. 2009). When associated with a concurrent translocation t(14;18) involving *BCL2*, this is referred to as a double-hit DLBCL. The inferior prognosis is felt to be due to the concurrent expression of BCL2 and cMYC (Niitsu et al. 2009; Friedberg 2012). This phenomenon occurs in both GCB and ABC subtypes and retains independent prognostic importance even when the molecular subtype is taken into account (Klapper et al. 2008). Double-hit DLBCL occurs more frequently in the elderly.

3.3 Positron Emission Tomography

Similar to HL, PET has become an important imaging modality in the work-up and response assessment of DLBCL. In terms of the latter, both interim and post-chemotherapy PET assessment provide important prognostic information.

Post-chemotherapy PET response is a powerful prognostic factor, particularly when patients receive chemotherapy without consolidation radiation therapy. In numerous studies, residual PET positive disease after the completion of chemotherapy alone in aggressive NHLs (mostly DLBCL) is associated with a high risk of disease progression (Spaepen et al. 2001; Mikhaeel et al. 2000; Haioun et al. 2005; Juweid et al. 2005). For example, patients with advanced DLBCL with PET positive disease after chemotherapy had a 100 % risk of progression in the series by Mikhaeel et al. (2000) (n = 9) and Spaepen et al. (2001) (n = 26). Thus, observation without further assessment or adjuvant treatment is inappropriate when the PET remains positive after chemotherapy.

The risk of recurrence appears to be much smaller when consolidation radiation therapy is utilized in the setting of a persistently positive PET scan after chemotherapy. In studies from the Dana Farber Cancer Institute (Halasz et al. 2012) and Duke Cancer Institute (Dorth et al. 2011), mostly with early-stage disease, the risk of progression was 10 and 35 % respectively. While this progression risk appears to be higher compared with a negative PET, many patients remained disease free after radiation therapy. As gross residual disease is apparently present, the recommended dose is ~40 Gy.

Similar to HL, the role of interim PET in DLBCL is controversial. As outlined below, the positive predictive value of interim PET is ~50 %. Thus, many patients who have a positive interim PET will achieve a durable complete response after completion of therapy. Further, it is unclear that altering therapy simply because the PET remains positive after 2–3 cycles of chemotherapy improves outcomes. Finally, before embarking on a more aggressive therapy, particularly high-dose chemotherapy and autologous stem cell transplant, a biopsy to confirm persistent disease is generally recommended. This is often neglected in clinical practice. Despite these and other lingering questions, it is clear that interim PET response is prognostic and could potentially play a role in personalizing therapy.

Multiple studies have demonstrated that achievement of a negative PET early in the course of therapy is associated with improved progression-free survival, and often overall survival, compared with a positive interim PET (Zinzani et al. 2011; Cashen et al. 2011; Haioun et al. 2005; Yang et al. 2011; Safar et al. 2012). For example, in a study by Safar et al. (2012), 3-year progression-free and overall survival was 84 and 88 %, respectively, in patients achieving a negative PET after 2 cycles of chemotherapy plus rituximab. This compared with 47 and 62 %, respectively, in patients who were still PET positive. Interim PET response appears to have prognostic significance in both the low and high-risk IPI groups (Haioun et al. 2005; Yang et al. 2011). However, when compared with interim response assessment, post-chemotherapy PET response appears to be better, particularly in terms of the positive predictive value (Pregno et al. 2012; Cashen et al. 2011).

3.4 Treatment-Specific Factors

The addition of rituximab to combination chemotherapy has made the biggest impact on the overall prognosis of patients with DLBCL in the last several decades. On average, rituximab improves overall survival by ~10 % at 5 years (Feugier et al. 2005; Pfreundschuh et al. 2006). Rituximab improves clinical outcomes throughout the spectrum of disease presentations (early stage and advanced stage, younger age and older age, etc.).

Combination chemotherapy is currently considered the backbone of treatment for all stages of DLBCL, most commonly rituximab combined with cyclophosphamide, doxorubicin, vincristine, and prednisone (R-CHOP). Yet, relapses after R-CHOP are common and most frequently involve sites of original involvement. Consolidation radiation therapy has been shown in many (Horning et al. 2004; Miller et al. 1998; Martinelli et al. 2009), but not all (Bonnet et al. 2007), randomized trials to decrease the risk of disease recurrence after CHOP in early-stage disease. Though no randomized trials have been completed in the rituximab era, RT also appears to be beneficial after R-CHOP (Phan et al. 2010). The role of radiation therapy in advanced DLBCL is controversial. Though infrequently employed, both prospective (Aviles et al. 1994, 2004) and retrospective (Ferreri et al. 2000; Schlembach et al. 2000; Dorth et al. 2012) studies have shown that consolidation radiation therapy decreases the overall risk of disease recurrence.

While adjuvant radiation therapy decreases the risk of relapse in patients with DLBCL, many are nonetheless successfully cured with chemotherapy alone and are unnecessarily exposed to the side effects, risks, and costs of treatment. This is not a unique phenomenon. In fact, it is a standard approach for all of oncology, in fact most of medicine, to treat a large number of patients to benefit a

Table 4 Follicular Lymphoma International Prognostic Index (FLIPI)

Adverse prognostic factor	Relative risk
Age, ≥60 years	2.38
Stage, III-IV	2.00
Hemoglobin (<12 g/dL)	1.55
Serum LDH, >1X normal	1.50
Number of nodal sites, >4	1.39

LDH lactate dehydrogenase

few. The challenge in DLBCL, which has thus far been elusive, is to identify those patients who cleared their systemic disease after chemotherapy yet still have residual microscopic local disease. A test to identify these patients has yet to be identified. Thus far, PET imaging after treatment has not been able to successfully identify a population of patients who do not benefit from radiation therapy (Dorth et al. 2012; Phan et al. 2010).

4 Follicular Lymphoma

4.1 Clinical Factors

Similar to the International Non-Hodgkin's Lymphoma Prognostic Factors project for aggressive NHLs, a prognostic scoring system has also been developed for FL (Solal-Celigny et al. 2004). Using patient characteristics from 4,167 patients with FL diagnosed in the pre-rituximab era (1985–1992), five adverse prognostic factors for survival were identified on multivariate analysis. These included age, stage, hemoglobin level, number of nodal areas, and serum LDH. The hazard ratios ranged from 2.38 (age) to 1.39 (number of nodal sites) (Table 4). Three risk groups were identified: low risk (0-1 adverse factor), intermediate risk (2 factors), and poor risk (≥3 adverse factors). Ten-year overall survival was 71, 51, and 36 %, respectively (Fig. 4). This scoring system is known as the Follicular Lymphoma International Prognostic Index or FLIPI.

The FLIPI prognostic scoring system has limitations. It included patients treated before rituximab was available, though the original FLIPI appears to retain prognostic value even when ritixumab is utilized (Nooka et al. 2012). Further, the data were collected retrospectively and limited by missing data and limited available clinical characteristics. Therefore, a prospective study was launched in 2003 in which data from 1,093 patients from 69 institutions were collected (Federico et al. 2009). Using these data the FLIPI2 was created. As opposed to the original FLIPI, the primary endpoint was progression-free survival. The variables used in the model were β2-microglobulin (≤1X normal vs. >1X normal), tumor size (>6 cm versus ≤6 cm), bone marrow involvement, hemoglobin level (<12 g/dL versus ≥12 g/dL) and age (≥60 vs. <60 years). The 3-year progression-free survival was 91, 69, and 51 % for low (0 factors), intermediate (1–2 factors) and high (3–5 factors), respectively (Fig. 5).

4.2 Pathological Factors

Follicular lymphoma is subdivided by the World Health Organization into three histological grades based on the number of centroblasts (large cells) in neoplastic follicles. Grades 1 and 2 are typically considered low grade and contain 0–5 and 6–15 centroblasts per high power field, respectively. Grade 3 FL is subdivided into 3A, where neoplastic follicles have more than 15 centroblasts per high power field but centrocytes (small cells) are still present, while 3B consists of solid sheets of centroblasts. If any diffuse areas are present this is considered DLBCL. Grade 3B FL is rare and most studies only have a small number of such patients, often preventing meaningful comparisons.

The prognostic significance of this grading system, and whether treatment should be modified based on grade, is controversial, with conflicting results in the literature. While some studies have demonstrated better outcomes with grade 1–2 FL compared with grade 3 (Ganti et al. 2006), others have not (Shustik et al. 2011; Chau et al. 2003). While grade 3B disease is often considered to be akin to DLBCL and treated as such, the literature is not consistent in this regard (Shustik et al. 2011; Chau et al. 2003; Ganti et al. 2006; Wahlin et al. 2012). Finally, some studies show an apparent plateau on the relapse-survival curve with anthracycline-based chemotherapy in grade 3 FL (Ganti et al. 2006; Wahlin et al. 2012) while others do not (Shustik et al. 2011; Chau et al. 2003). Thus, many questions remain whether the current grading system of FL can be used for prognostic purposes or to guide therapy.

Numerous other pathological factors have been investigated in FL including chromosomal alterations, overexpression of distinct genes as assessed by immunohistochemistry, genetics of the host, the microenvironment, transformation to high-grade disease, etc. (Relander et al. 2010). Currently, these factors are still poorly understood. How they should impact current management has not been elucidated. Validated prognostic indices, such as the FLIPI, combined with an assessment of disease presentation and clinical course by the oncologist remain the primary factors that guide therapy.

4.3 Positron Emission Tomography

The majority of patients with FL present with advanced disease. Advanced FL is generally considered an indolent

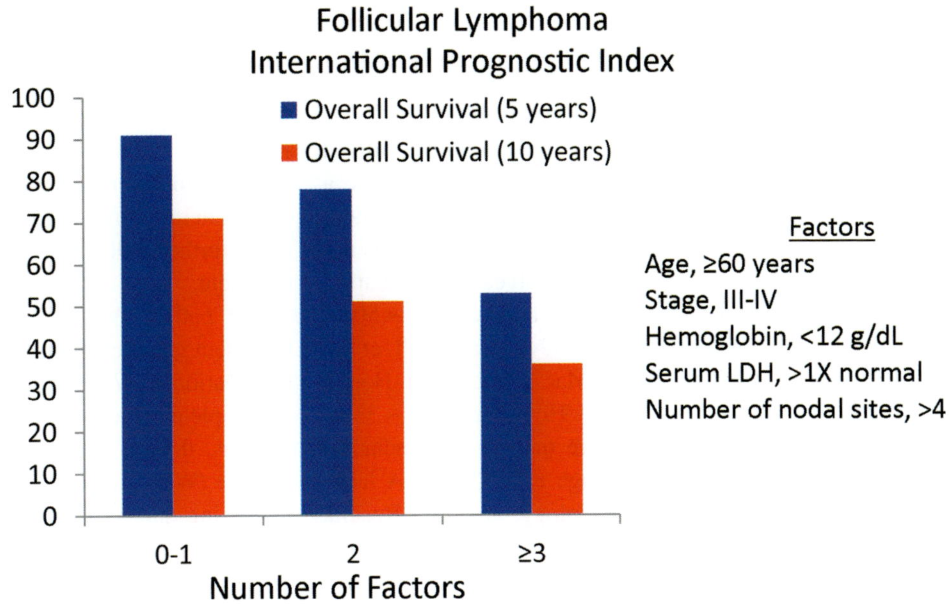

Fig. 4 The Follicular Lymphoma International Prognostic Index (FLIPI). The primary endpoint was overall survival (Blood 2004; 104;1258)

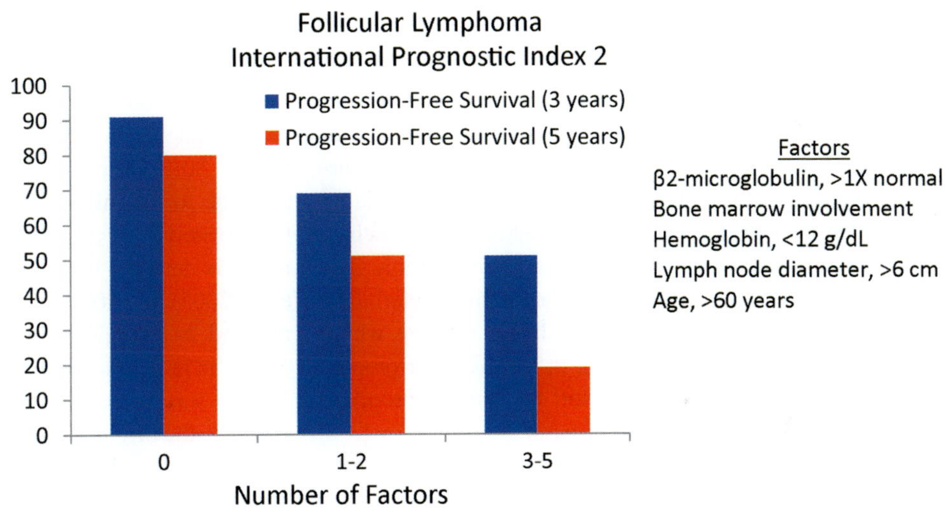

Fig. 5 The Follicular Lymphoma International Prognostic Index 2 (FLIPI2). The primary endpoint was progression-free survival (JCO 2009; 27:4555)

disease, with a long disease course, but not curable with conventional chemotherapy. Patients with a low disease burden and who are asymptomatic do not require immediate treatment. For those requiring treatment, the most appropriate approach is combination chemotherapy with rituximab. Response to chemoimmunotherapy by PET imaging has been shown to be prognostic. In a prospective European study, patients with previously untreated, high-tumor burden FL received 6 cycles of R-CHOP and underwent interim and end of treatment PET imaging (Dupuis et al. 2012). Interim and post-treatment PET responses were closely correlated. Based on post-treatment PET imaging, 2-year progression-free survival was 87 % for PET positive patients vs. 51 % for PET negative patients, respectively ($p = 0.005$). There was also a difference in 2-year survival (100 vs 88 %, $p = 0.13$). Similar findings were observed in a subset of the PRIMA (Primary Rituximab and Maintenance) trial participants where post-treatment PET was predictive of progression-free and overall survival (Trotman et al. 2011).

4.4 Treatment-Specific Factors

Similar to DLBCL, the single most significant advance in the treatment of FL is the contribution of rituximab. Multiple randomized studies have shown that rituximab, added to a variety of different chemotherapy regimens, decreases the risk of progression and improves overall survival (Marcus et al. 2008; Hiddemann et al. 2005; Herold et al. 2007). Maintenance rituximab use, after a course of immunochemotherapy, further decreases the risk of relapse, but its effect on survival has not been conclusively demonstrated (van Oers et al. 2010; Salles et al. 2011). Thus, for patients with symptomatic or large burden advanced FL requiring treatment, a combination chemotherapy regimen combined with rituximab, with or without maintenance rituximab, is currently considered standard of care.

Only ~20 % of patients with FL present with localized disease. As opposed to advanced FL, there seems to be a potential for cure in this subgroup. The optimal treatment for patients with stage I, or localized stage II disease, is not clear. Most guidelines recommend involved-field radiation therapy. Long-term disease control is achieved in ~50 % of patients with low-doses (24–30 Gy) (Campbell et al. 2010; Guadagnolo et al. 2006; Mac Manus and Hoppe 1996; Vaughan Hudson et al. 1994). However, only ~33 % of patients with stage I disease are treated with radiation therapy (Friedberg et al. 2009; Pugh et al. 2010). A large study using Surveillance, Epidemiology, and End Results (SEER) data demonstrated superior survival in patients who received radiation therapy (62 vs. 48 % at 10 years, $p < 0.001$) (Pugh et al. 2010). However, results from the National LymphoCare Study have challenged the paradigm that radiation alone is optimal in stage I FL (Friedberg et al. 2012). With short follow-up, combined approaches using chemotherapy, immunotherapy, and radiation therapy were associated with a lower risk of relapse compared with radiation therapy alone with no difference in overall survival. The rarity of this stage of disease has precluded large phase III studies evaluating differing treatment approaches. With the understanding that neither chemotherapy nor immunotherapy is curative in FL, the minimal morbidity and cost of low-dose involved-field radiation therapy, which provides long-term disease control in a significant proportion of patients, suggests this is still the most appropriate treatment strategy for localized disease.

5 Non-Hodgkin Lymphomas: Other

5.1 Marginal Zone Lymphoma

Marginal zone lymphomas consist of three distinct entities-nodal marginal zone lymphoma, splenic marginal zone lymphoma, and extranodal marginal zone lymphoma of mucosa-associated lymphoid tissue (MALT). The latter is most common and most extensively studied. MALT typically presents with localized disease most commonly involving the stomach, orbital adnexa, salivary glands, thyroid, or skin.

With the exception of *Helicobacter pylori* (*H. pylori*) positive gastric MALT lymphoma, first-line treatment for localized MALT lymphoma is typically radiation therapy. Complete response rates approach 100 % with doses ~25–30 Gy (Goda et al. 2010). The primary prognostic factor is disease site. MALT arising in paired organs (e.g., orbit or salivary gland) appears to have a higher risk of relapse compared with that arising in a single organ (e.g., stomach or thyroid) (Goda et al. 2010; Tsang et al. 2003). Relapse after radiation therapy for cutaneous marginal zone lymphoma is also rather frequent (Senff et al. 2007b). However, many relapses are localized, often in the contralateral paired organ, and after appropriate treatment, often further radiation therapy alone, long-term survival is excellent.

For patients with gastric MALT lymphoma, antibiotic treatment is indicated in the presence of *H. pylori* infection. Eradication of *H. pylori* is near universal after antibiotics. A complete response is achieved in approximately 80 % of patients, though this may take up to 2 years or longer to achieve (Wundisch et al. 2005). As long as the lymphoma is regressing on serial endoscopy, a watch and wait policy is appropriate. Predictive factors associated with a lower chance of achieving a complete response include deep gastric wall invasion (Nakamura et al. 2001; Sackmann et al. 1997; Ruskone-Fourmestraux et al. 2001), nodal involvement (Ono et al. 2010; Ruskone-Fourmestraux et al. 2001), and the translocation t(11;18) (Wundisch et al. 2005; Levy et al. 2005).

Of patients achieving a complete response, approximately 30 % of patients will relapse. The risk of relapse appears to be higher for those patients harboring the translocation t(11;18) and when ongoing B-cell monoclonality is detected by polymerase chain reaction (Wundisch et al. 2005). For patients who are *H. pylori* negative, do not respond to or relapse after antibiotics, the treatment of choice is radiation therapy. Long-term progression-free and overall survival exceeds 90 % (Goda et al. 2010). Interestingly, the original B-cell clone is also detected frequently after radiation therapy for gastric MALT lymphoma but without an associated risk of relapse (Noy et al. 2005).

5.2 Mantle Cell Lymphoma

Mantle cell lymphoma is a rare subtype of NHL. The majority of patients present with advanced disease. It is an aggressive lymphoma, typically arising in older adults, and not considered curable with conventional chemotherapy. The International Prognostic Index, utilized extensively for DLBCL, was not satisfactory in mantle cell lymphoma, which prompted development of a prognostic index specifically for this subtype of NHL.

The German Low Grade Lymphoma Study Group and the European Mantle Cell Lymphoma Network combined data to identify prognostic factors, apply the IPI and FLIPI, and design a specific model for mantle cell lymphoma. Using data from 455 patients with advanced disease entered on three consecutive randomized trials between 1996 and

2004, four independent adverse prognostic factors were identified (Hoster et al. 2008). These included increasing age, compromised performance status, elevated LDH, and elevated white blood cell count. Using a complex formula, a mantle cell lymphoma international prognostic index (MIPI) can be calculated with partitioning of patients into three risk groups. A simplified prognostic index (sMIPI) was also developed. Most studies have shown that the MIPI retains prognostic significance when applied to patients treated with modern rituximab-containing regimens with autologous stem cell transplantation (Budde et al. 2011; Geisler et al. 2010).

A small proportion of patients present with localized mantle cell lymphoma. The optimal treatment for this population is unclear. Based on general principles of lymphoma management, the inclusion of consolidation radiation therapy into the treatment program seems justified. Indeed, retrospective studies have shown favorable outcomes when radiation therapy is employed (Bernard et al. 2013; Leitch et al. 2003).

Finally, mantle cell lymphoma is a heterogeneous disease. Although most cases display aggressive behavior, there is a subset of patients with indolent disease. These patients occasionally present with slowly growing tumors that are amenable to low-dose radiation therapy. Mantle cell lymphoma can be exquisitely radiosensitive, and doses of ~ 10 Gy or even less often provide excellent palliation.

5.3 Systemic Anaplastic Large Cell Lymphoma

Systemic anaplastic large cell lymphoma (ALCL) is a relatively rare subtype of NHL that occurs in both children and adults. ALCL is a CD30 + T-cell neoplasm that often expresses the protein anaplastic lymphoma kinase (ALK), a protein that is not expressed normally in humans except occasionally in the brain. The most common chromosomal abnormality that leads to ALK expression is t(2;5) (p23; q35), though several others have been reported. The World Health Organization currently distinguishes ALK-positive ALCL as a distinct entity and ALK-negative ALCL as a provisional entity. ALK positive cases occur more commonly in the first three decades of life with ALK negative cases occurring predominantly in older adults.

Several studies have shown that survival is significantly better with ALK-positive ALCL (Sibon et al. 2012; Falini et al. 1999; Gascoyne et al. 1999; Savage et al. 2008). The International Peripheral T-cell Lymphoma Project demonstrated 5-year failure-free survival of 60 % for ALK-positive ALCL and 36 % for ALK-negative ALCL ($p = 0.15$). A difference in 5-year overall survival was also observed (70 vs 49 %, $p = 0.16$). There remains some uncertainty whether ALK expression is independently prognostic or simply correlates with other favorable factors (e.g., young age). A recent report from the Groupe D'Etude des Lymphomas de l'Adulte demonstrated only an elevated β2-microglobulin and older age as independent prognostic factors, but not ALK status (Sibon et al. 2012). ALK was also not independently prognostic in the study by Suzuki et al. (2000) However, other reports have demonstrated independent prognostic significance of ALK (Falini et al. 1999; Gascoyne et al. 1999).

5.4 Primary Central Nervous System Lymphoma

Primary central nervous system lymphoma (PCNSL) is a rare subtype of DLBCL that arises in the brain, spinal cord, and/or eyes. Whole brain radiation therapy (WBRT) was historically the treatment of choice with ~ 80 % of patients achieving a complete response. Unfortunately, relapses are common after WBRT alone with a median survival of ~ 12–18 months (Shibamoto et al. 2005). High-dose methotrexate regimens, with or without WBRT, have become the treatment of choice with an improvement in median survival to ~ 50–60 months in many studies (Abrey et al. 2000; Pels et al. 2003).

The contribution of WBRT after high-dose methotrexate regimens is controversial. In older patients (>60 years), conventional doses of radiation therapy (45 Gy) have been associated with unacceptably high rates of severe neurotoxicity, including dementia (Omuro et al. 2005), and should be avoided. Although conventional WBRT may decrease the risk of relapse, it is often counterbalanced by increased toxicity (Abrey et al. 2000). In the setting of a complete response with high-dose methotrexate, lower doses of WBRT may decrease the risk of relapse but avoid the toxicity of full-dose treatment (Shah et al. 2007). However, longer follow-up will be required to confirm these initial findings.

Though a number of prognostic factors have been identified in PCNSL (Corry et al. 1998; Bessell et al. 2004; Ferreri et al. 2003), the most important factors appear to be age and performance status. The Memorial Sloan-Kettering Cancer Center Prognostic Model, using recursive partitioning and external validation, identified three subgroups with distinct survival outcomes: class 1 (<50 years), class 2 ($\geq$50 years, Karnofsky performance score [KPS] $\geq$ 70), and class 3 ($\geq$50 years, KPS < 70) (Abrey et al. 2006). Median survival was 8.5, 3.2, and 1.1 years in classes 1–3, respectively.

5.5 Cutaneous Lymphomas

The cutaneous lymphomas present interesting diagnostic and therapeutic challenges given that they are relatively rare with an incidence of less than 5 per 1,000,000 individuals and present in a variety of different ways. Cutaneous lymphomas present with either a B-cell or T-cell phenotype. Mycosis fungoides (MF) is the most common of all of the cutaneous lymphomas. It is of the T-cell variety and typically presents clinically as patches and plaques on the skin but can involve lymph nodes and visceral organs. Another T-cell lymphoma that commonly involves the skin is anaplastic large cell lymphoma. This must be distinguished from the benign skin disorder lymphomatoid papulosis, another CD30 + lymphoproliferative disorder. Compared to its nodal counterpart discussed above, the cutaneous variant generally does not express the anaplastic lymphoma kinase (ALK). The B-cell lymphomas generally present differently than MF, and tend to be more isolated and often more nodular in appearance. The three most common types are: primary cutaneous diffuse large B-cell lymphoma, leg type, primary cutaneous marginal zone B-cell lymphoma, and primary cutaneous follicle center lymphoma (Senff et al. 2008; Girardi et al. 2004; Smith et al. 2004).

Mycosis fungoides is considered an indolent lymphoma and patients generally receive a variety of treatments during the course of their disease, including RT. With the exception of early, localized disease, treatment is not generally considered curative. Studies have evaluated numerous prognostic factors for different endpoints (overall survival, disease-specific survival, etc.). In terms of overall survival, the most consistent adverse prognostic factors include increasing age, higher T stage, presence of extracutaneous disease, elevated LDH and peripheral blood involvement (Kim et al. 1995, 2003; Diamandidou et al. 1999; Agar et al. 2010; Talpur et al. 2012). Folliculotropic histology (Agar et al. 2010) and large cell transformation also portends poor survival (Diamandidou et al. 1998). Primary cutaneous anaplastic large cell lymphoma, the other common T-cell cutaneous lymphoma, is much less common than MF and generally has a more favorable prognosis. Advancing age appears to be the most significant adverse prognostic factor (Liu et al. 2003; Woo et al. 2009). Progression to extracutaneous disease is also a likely adverse factor (Woo et al. 2009).

The prognosis of primary cutaneous marginal zone B-cell lymphoma and primary cutaneous follicle center lymphoma is excellent. For the majority with localized disease, RT alone produces complete response rates of nearly 100 % with excellent long-term survival (Senff et al. 2007b). Patients with marginal zone lymphoma may be at higher risk of relapse compared with follicle center lymphoma, though most recurrences are confined to the skin and typically amenable to a second course of RT (Senff et al. 2007b). On the other hand, primary cutaneous large B-cell lymphoma, leg type is associated with a much worse prognosis and a combined modality approach, consisting of chemotherapy and radiation therapy, is often employed (Senff et al. 2007a, b; Zinzani et al. 2006).

6 Toxicity

Long-term toxicity from RT is dependent on many variables. These include the type of lymphoma, radiation dose, normal structures within the radiation field, other treatments received (surgery and chemotherapy), age of the patient, and other medical co-morbidities. Unfortunately, many oncologists view risks of long-term toxicity from radiation therapy from a simplistic dichotomous viewpoint- either radiation was administered or it was not. This perception has contributed to the decline in the utilization of radiation therapy for many types of lymphomas. A more comprehensive assessment is necessary to weigh risks and benefits of treatment and to fully inform patients and other providers.

As lymphoma is a systemic disease that can affect any organ, it would be challenging to comprehensively address normal tissue toxicity. The two most troublesome complications after lymphoma treatment, particularly for HL, are secondary malignancies and cardiovascular disease. The most common complication is likely hypothyroidism. These will receive further discussion.

6.1 Secondary Malignancies

6.1.1 Hodgkin Versus Non-Hodgkin Lymphoma

Current survivors of HL are at increased risk of developing secondary malignancies. This is particularly true for patients treated in decades past with historical regimens such as subtotal nodal irradiation and chemotherapy regimens incorporating high doses of alkylating agents. In large registries of patients treated over many decades, second cancer risk has consistently been elevated over expected rates. Using data from 32,591 HL patients from 16 North American and European cancer registries, treated between 1935–1994, the observed-to-expected ratio was 2.3 (95 % CI 2.2–2.4). A similar study of 10,472 survivors from North America between 1940–1987 demonstrated an observed/expected ratio of 2.7 (95 % CI 2.5–4.2) (Boivin et al. 1995). Finally, a standardized incidence ratio of 2.9 (95 % CI 2.6–3.2) was noted in a cohort of 5519 British patients treated between 1963–1993 (Swerdlow et al. 2000). It should be remembered that during these time periods definitive subtotal nodal irradiation was standard and many patients also received alkylating agents.

The risk of developing a secondary malignancy after treatment for NHL has not been as extensively studied compared with HL and is therefore less understood. In an early study from Duke Cancer Institute, among 686 patients with non-Hodgkin lymphoma the risk of developing a solid tumor was similar to the general population. The risk of leukemia was elevated, though the incorporation of radiation therapy did not increase risk (Lavey et al. 1990).

However, subsequent studies using larger databases have demonstrated an elevated risk of developing a secondary malignancy in NHL survivors compared to age-matched controls. In a British cohort study, patients treated for NHL were at 30 % higher risk of developing a secondary cancer compared with the general population (RR 1.3, 95 % CI, 1.1–1.6) (Mudie et al. 2006). Similarly, studies from the United States using the SEER database have demonstrated a 14–18 % increased risk (Travis et al. 1991; Tward et al. 2006). Pooling data from 109,451 patients with NHL from 13 cancer registries demonstrated a 47 % increased risk of developing a second cancer (SIR 1.47, 95 % CI 1.43–1.51) (Brennan et al. 2005). Thus, though rates are elevated, they appear to be less so compared with survivors of HL.

6.1.2 Radiation Dose and Fields

In the setting of a combined modality treatment program for HL, randomized trials have demonstrated that radiation fields encompassing the originally involved lymph node regions, as opposed to more extensive fields encompassing prophylactic areas, is adequate (Bonadonna et al. 2004; Engert et al. 2003; Zittoun et al. 1985). Even more conformal radiation fields, treating only the original extent of nodal disease with an appropriate margin, are currently being explored (Campbell et al. 2008; Eich et al. 2008; Girinsky et al. 2008). This is referred to as involved-site and involved-node radiation therapy, with the latter including only the originally involved lymph nodes with margin. For early-stage DLBCL and FL, the optimal field size has never been tested in a randomized trial though involved-field or involved-site radiotherapy has been used most frequently. In these two diseases, studies from British Columbia have not shown a higher risk of disease recurrence with involved-site radiotherapy compared with involved-field RT (Campbell et al. 2010, 2012).

A decrease in the field size has been associated with a corresponding decrease in radiation dose, for HL, DLBCL, and FL. For early-stage, favorable HL, 20 Gy of radiation therapy was shown to be adequate in GHSG HD10 (Engert et al. 2010). A randomized study by the British National Lymphoma Investigation showed that 24 Gy was sufficient for FL and 30 Gy is as effective as higher doses for DLBCL (Lowry et al. 2011).

Over the last few decades the dose and field size of RT have both decreased in concert, making it somewhat difficult to parse out the contribution of each to the risk of secondary malignancies. In studies in which low doses are administered to involved-fields, the risk of developing a second cancer is dramatically less compared with definitive RT (Koontz et al. 2006; Salloum et al. 1996). In women survivors, RT fields avoiding the axilla are associated with a lower risk of secondary breast cancer (De Bruin et al. 2009). Randomized studies comparing involved-field RT with more extensive fields have shown trends toward a lower risk of second cancer induction, though longer follow-up is required (Engert et al. 2003; Sasse et al. 2012).

6.1.3 Age

For women treated for mediastinal HL, the risk of developing a secondary breast cancer is dependent on multiple factors. The radiation dose and field size are important, as discussed above, but so is the age of the patient. Using historical radiation techniques, studies have shown that the relative risk of developing breast cancer is ~3–5 fold higher compared with age-matched controls (Hancock et al. 1993a; Wolden et al. 2000; Wahner-Roedler et al. 2003) with a latency period of 15–20 years (Yahalom et al. 1992; Gervais-Fagnou et al. 1999; Hancock et al. 1993a; Wahner-Roedler et al. 2003). Increasing age of a female is associated with a lower risk of treatment, until a woman is approximately 30–35 years old when the risk is no longer appreciably increased compared with age-matched controls (De Bruin et al. 2009; Ferme et al. 2007; Hancock et al. 1993a; Wahner-Roedler et al. 2003). There is undoubtedly always an increased risk, even in older patients, but it is probably very small, especially with low doses of radiation therapy avoiding the axilla.

6.2 Cardiovascular Disease

Cardiovascular disease is the second most prevalent serious late effect, behind secondary malignancies, in current HL survivors (Ng et al. 2002). Survivors of NHL also appear to be at greater risk of developing cardiovascular disease, though less thoroughly studied compared with HL patients (Moser et al. 2006). Cardiovascular disease in HL survivors occurs earlier in life and at a higher rate than age-matched controls. The disorders that have been observed include coronary artery disease leading to myocardial infarction, valvular disease, pericardial disease, conduction abnormalities, and cardiomyopathies. In the modern era, when the entire heart is not treated to doses above 20 Gy, the risk of pericarditis is quite low.

Identification of specific risk factors for the development of cardiovascular disease after radiation therapy for lymphoma has been challenging. Radiation-induced cardiac disease is undoubtedly influenced by both the dose of radiation and the field. In terms of dose, many studies have shown that lower radiation doses are associated with a lower risk of cardiac disease (Hull et al. 2003; Hancock et al. 1993b; Kupeli et al. 2010). In a recent study of 1,132 HL survivors treated before age 18, the 25-year actuarial risk of cardiac disease was 21 % after receiving a mediastinal dose of 36 Gy compared with 3 % when 20 Gy was utilized ($p < 0.001$) (Schellong et al. 2010). As for radiation fields, a study from Stanford demonstrated a significantly lower risk of cardiac disease other than acute myocardial infarction when subcarinal and left ventricular blocking was utilized (Hancock et al. 1993b). The location of the coronary arteries often precludes adequate shielding when subcarinal disease is present. In the modern era of conformal fields, avoidance of the valves and coronary arteries is possible in many patients. Geographic avoidance is the best way to decrease the risk of complications.

Other factors also seem to contribute to risk. Anthracyclines, and possibly other chemotherapeutics (Swerdlow et al. 2007), appear to compound the risk of radiation therapy, particularly for congestive heart failure and valvular disorders (Aleman et al. 2007; Myrehaug et al. 2008). Further, patients with known cardiac risk factors (e.g. diabetes, hypertension, hyperlipidemia, smoking) appear to be at much higher risk of developing cardiac complications compared with patients with no cardiac risk factors (Hull et al. 2003; Glanzmann et al. 1998). Thus, mediastinal radiation therapy can be considered a cardiac risk factor, which when compounded by diabetes or other cardiac comorbidities, begins to increase the risk of an adverse event. The effect of age on risk is unclear. While the relative risk appears to increase with age, the absolute excess risk is greatest in older subgroups as cardiac disease is a disease of older adults (Aleman et al. 2007; Swerdlow et al. 2007; Hancock et al. 1993b).

6.3 Hypothyroidism

Thyroid disorders are common when the thyroid gland is within the radiation field. In a large series of patients with HL from Stanford, mostly treated with relatively high doses of radiation therapy (>40 Gy), the actuarial risk of developing thyroid diseases 20 years after treatment was 52 %, and this continued to rise with further follow-up (Hancock et al. 1991). Hypothyroidism was by far the most common finding. Many patients will initially develop subclinical hypothyroidism, defined as elevation of thyroid-stimulating hormone (TSH) with normal thyroxine (T4) levels without any symptoms of hypothyroidism. Whether thyroid replacement should be initiated in such patients is controversial. At a minimum, close follow-up of such patients is necessary.

The primary risk factor for developing hypothyroidism is increasing radiation dose (Bhatia et al. 1996; Constine et al. 1984; Hancock et al. 1991). Female gender, addition of chemotherapy, and age seem to contribute little, if any, to the risk. Chemotherapy alone does not appear to be a significant risk factor for hypothyroidism.

References

Abrey LE, Yahalom J, DeAngelis LM (2000) Treatment for primary CNS lymphoma: the next step. J Clin Oncol 18(17):3144–3150

Abrey LE, Ben-Porat L, Panageas KS, Yahalom J, Berkey B, Curran W, Schultz C, Leibel S, Nelson D, Mehta M, DeAngelis LM (2006) Primary central nervous system lymphoma: the Memorial Sloan-Kettering Cancer Center prognostic model. J Clin Oncol 24(36):5711–5715. doi:10.1200/JCO.2006.08.2941 JCO.2006.08.2941 [pii]

Agar NS, Wedgeworth E, Crichton S, Mitchell TJ, Cox M, Ferreira S, Robson A, Calonje E, Stefanato CM, Wain EM, Wilkins B, Fields PA, Dean A, Webb K, Scarisbrick J, Morris S, Whittaker SJ (2010) Survival outcomes and prognostic factors in mycosis fungoides/Sezary syndrome: validation of the revised International Society for Cutaneous Lymphomas/European Organisation for Research and Treatment of Cancer staging proposal. J Clin Oncol 28(31):4730–4739. doi:10.1200/JCO.2009.27.7665 JCO.2009.27.7665 [pii]

Aleman BM, Raemaekers JM, Tirelli U, Bortolus R, van 't Veer MB, Lybeert ML, Keuning JJ, Carde P, Girinsky T, van der Maazen RW, Tomsic R, Vovk M, van Hoof A, Demeestere G, Lugtenburg PJ, Thomas J, Schroyens W, De Boeck K, Baars JW, Kluin-Nelemans JC, Carrie C, Aoudjhane M, Bron D, Eghbali H, Smit WG, Meerwaldt JH, Hagenbeek A, Pinna A, Henry-Amar M (2003) Involved-field radiotherapy for advanced Hodgkin's lymphoma. N Engl J Med 348(24):2396–2406

Aleman BM, van den Belt-Dusebout AW, De Bruin ML, van 't Veer MB, Baaijens MH, de Boer JP, Hart AA, Klokman WJ, Kuenen MA, Ouwens GM, Bartelink H, van Leeuwen FE (2007) Late cardiotoxicity after treatment for Hodgkin lymphoma. Blood 109(5):1878–1886. doi:10.1182/blood-2006-07-034405 blood-2006-07-034405 [pii]

Alizadeh AA, Eisen MB, Davis RE, Ma C, Lossos IS, Rosenwald A, Boldrick JC, Sabet H, Tran T, Yu X, Powell JI, Yang L, Marti GE, Moore T, Hudson J Jr, Lu L, Lewis DB, Tibshirani R, Sherlock G, Chan WC, Greiner TC, Weisenburger DD, Armitage JO, Warnke R, Levy R, Wilson W, Grever MR, Byrd JC, Botstein D, Brown PO, Staudt LM (2000) Distinct types of diffuse large B-cell lymphoma identified by gene expression profiling. Nature 403(6769):503–511. doi:10.1038/35000501

Aviles A, Delgado S (1998) A prospective clinical trial comparing chemotherapy, radiotherapy and combined therapy in the treatment of early stage Hodgkin's disease with bulky disease. Clin Lab Haematol 20(2):95–99

Aviles A, Delgado S, Nambo MJ, Alatriste S, Diaz-Maqueo JC (1994) Adjuvant radiotherapy to sites of previous bulky disease in patients stage IV diffuse large cell lymphoma. Int J Radiat Oncol Biol Phys 30(4):799–803

Aviles A, Fernandezb R, Perez F, Nambo MJ, Neri N, Talavera A, Castaneda C, Gonzalez M, Cleto S (2004) Adjuvant radiotherapy in stage IV diffuse large cell lymphoma improves outcome. Leuk Lymphoma 45(7):1385–1389

Barnes JA, LaCasce AS, Zukotynski K, Israel D, Feng Y, Neuberg D, Toomey CE, Hochberg EP, Canellos GP, Abramson JS (2011) End-of-treatment but not interim PET scan predicts outcome in nonbulky limited-stage Hodgkin's lymphoma. Ann Oncol 22(4):910–915. doi:10.1093/annonc/mdq549 mdq549 [pii]

Barrans S, Crouch S, Smith A, Turner K, Owen R, Patmore R, Roman E, Jack A (2010) Rearrangement of MYC is associated with poor prognosis in patients with diffuse large B-cell lymphoma treated in the era of rituximab. J Clin Oncol 28(20):3360–3365. doi: 10.1200/JCO.2009.26.3947 JCO.2009.26.3947 [pii]

Bernard M, Tsang RW, Le LW, Hodgson DC, Sun A, Wells W, Kukreti V, Kuruvilla J, Crump M, Gospodarowicz MK (2013) Limited-stage mantle cell lymphoma: treatment outcomes at the Princess Margaret Hospital. Leuk Lymphoma 54(2):261–267. doi: 10.3109/10428194.2012.711828

Bessell EM, Graus F, Lopez-Guillermo A, Lewis SA, Villa S, Verger E, Petit J (2004) Primary non-Hodgkin's lymphoma of the CNS treated with CHOD/BVAM or BVAM chemotherapy before radiotherapy: long-term survival and prognostic factors. Int J Radiat Oncol Biol Phys 59(2):501–508. doi:10.1016/j.ijrobp.2003.11.001 S0360301603022855 [pii]

Bhatia S, Ramsay NK, Bantle JP, Mertens A, Robison LL (1996) Thyroid Abnormalities after therapy for Hodgkin's disease in childhood. Oncologist 1(1 & 2):62–67

Boivin JF, Hutchison GB, Zauber AG, Bernstein L, Davis FG, Michel RP, Zanke B, Tan CT, Fuller LM, Mauch P et al (1995) Incidence of second cancers in patients treated for Hodgkin's disease. J Natl Cancer Inst 87(10):732–741

Bonadonna G, Bonfante V, Viviani S, Di Russo A, Villani F, Valagussa P (2004) ABVD plus subtotal nodal versus involved-field radiotherapy in early-stage Hodgkin's disease: long-term results. J Clin Oncol 22(14):2835–2841

Bonnet C, Fillet G, Mounier N, Ganem G, Molina TJ, Thieblemont C, Ferme C, Quesnel B, Martin C, Gisselbrecht C, Tilly H, Reyes F (2007) CHOP alone compared with CHOP plus radiotherapy for localized aggressive lymphoma in elderly patients: a study by the Groupe d'Etude des Lymphomes de l'Adulte. J Clin Oncol 25(7):787–792. doi:10.1200/JCO.2006.07.0722 JCO.2006.07.0722 [pii]

Borchmann P, Haverkamp H, Diehl V, Cerny T, Markova J, Ho AD, Eich HT, Mueller-Hermelink HK, Kanz L, Greil R, Rank A, Paulus U, Smardova L, Huber C, Dorken B, Nerl C, Krause SW, Mueller RP, Fuchs M, Engert A (2011) Eight cycles of escalated-dose BEACOPP compared with four cycles of escalated-dose BEACOPP followed by four cycles of baseline-dose BEACOPP with or without radiotherapy in patients with advanced-stage hodgkin's lymphoma: final analysis of the HD12 trial of the German Hodgkin Study Group. J Clin Oncol 29(32):4234–4242. doi:10.1200/JCO.2010.33.9549 JCO.2010.33.9549 [pii]

Brennan P, Scelo G, Hemminki K, Mellemkjaer L, Tracey E, Andersen A, Brewster DH, Pukkala E, McBride ML, Kliewer EV, Tonita JM, Seow A, Pompe-Kirn V, Martos C, Jonasson JG, Colin D, Boffetta P (2005) Second primary cancers among 109 000 cases of non-Hodgkin's lymphoma. Br J Cancer 93(1):159–166. doi:10.1038/sj.bjc.6602654 6602654 [pii]

Budde LE, Guthrie KA, Till BG, Press OW, Chauncey TR, Pagel JM, Petersdorf SH, Bensinger WI, Holmberg LA, Shustov AR, Green DJ, Maloney DG, Gopal AK (2011) Mantle cell lymphoma international prognostic index but not pretransplantation induction regimen predicts survival for patients with mantle-cell lymphoma receiving high-dose therapy and autologous stem-cell transplantation. J Clin Oncol 29(22):3023–3029. doi:10.1200/JCO.2010.33.7055 JCO.2010.33.7055 [pii]

Campbell BA, Voss N, Pickles T, Morris J, Gascoyne RD, Savage KJ, Connors JM (2008) Involved-nodal radiation therapy as a component of combination therapy for limited-stage Hodgkin's lymphoma: a question of field size. J Clin Oncol 26(32):5170–5174. doi:10.1200/JCO.2007.15.1001 JCO.2007.15.1001 [pii]

Campbell BA, Voss N, Woods R, Gascoyne RD, Morris J, Pickles T, Connors JM, Savage KJ (2010) Long-term outcomes for patients with limited stage follicular lymphoma: involved regional radiotherapy versus involved node radiotherapy. Cancer 116(16):3797–3806. doi:10.1002/cncr.25117

Campbell BA, Connors JM, Gascoyne RD, Morris WJ, Pickles T, Sehn LH (2012) Limited-stage diffuse large B-cell lymphoma treated with abbreviated systemic therapy and consolidation radiotherapy: involved-field versus involved-node radiotherapy. Cancer 118(17):4156–4165. doi:10.1002/cncr.26687

Cashen AF, Dehdashti F, Luo J, Homb A, Siegel BA, Bartlett NL (2011) 18F-FDG PET/CT for early response assessment in diffuse large B-cell lymphoma: poor predictive value of international harmonization project interpretation. J Nucl Med 52(3):386–392. doi:10.2967/jnumed.110.082586 jnumed.110.082586 [pii]

Chau I, Jones R, Cunningham D, Wotherspoon A, Maisey N, Norman AR, Jain P, Bishop L, Horwich A, Catovsky D (2003) Outcome of follicular lymphoma grade 3: is anthracycline necessary as front-line therapy? Br J Cancer 89(1):36–42. doi: 10.1038/sj.bjc.6601006 6601006 [pii]

Chen RC, Chin MS, Ng AK, Feng Y, Neuberg D, Silver B, Pinkus GS, Stevenson MA, Mauch PM (2010) Early-stage, lymphocyte-predominant Hodgkin's lymphoma: patient outcomes from a large, single-institution series with long follow-up. J Clin Oncol 28(1):136–141. doi:10.1200/JCO.2009.24.0945 JCO.2009.24.0945 [pii]

Choi WW, Weisenburger DD, Greiner TC, Piris MA, Banham AH, Delabie J, Braziel RM, Geng H, Iqbal J, Lenz G, Vose JM, Hans CP, Fu K, Smith LM, Li M, Liu Z, Gascoyne RD, Rosenwald A, Ott G, Rimsza LM, Campo E, Jaffe ES, Jaye DL, Staudt LM, Chan WC (2009) A new immunostain algorithm classifies diffuse large B-cell lymphoma into molecular subtypes with high accuracy. Clin Cancer Res 15(17):5494–5502. doi: 10.1158/1078-0432.CCR-09-0113 1078-0432.CCR-09-0113 [pii]

Constine LS, Donaldson SS, McDougall IR, Cox RS, Link MP, Kaplan HS (1984) Thyroid dysfunction after radiotherapy in children with Hodgkin's disease. Cancer 53(4):878–883

Corry J, Smith JG, Wirth A, Quong G, Liew KH (1998) Primary central nervous system lymphoma: age and performance status are more important than treatment modality. Int J Radiat Oncol Biol Phys 41(3):615–620 S0360-3016(97)00571-3 [pii]

De Bruin ML, Sparidans J, van't Veer MB, Noordijk EM, Louwman MW, Zijlstra JM, van den Berg H, Russell NS, Broeks A, Baaijens MH, Aleman BM, van Leeuwen FE (2009) Breast cancer risk in female survivors of Hodgkin's lymphoma: lower risk after smaller radiation volumes. J Clin Oncol 27(26):4239–4246. doi:10.1200/JCO.2008.19.9174 JCO.2008.19.9174 [pii]

Diamandidou E, Colome-Grimmer M, Fayad L, Duvic M, Kurzrock R (1998) Transformation of mycosis fungoides/Sezary syndrome: clinical characteristics and prognosis. Blood 92(4):1150–1159

Diamandidou E, Colome M, Fayad L, Duvic M, Kurzrock R (1999) Prognostic factor analysis in mycosis fungoides/Sezary syndrome. J Am Acad Dermatol 40(6 Pt 1):914–924 S0190-9622(99)70079-4 [pii]

Diehl V, Sextro M, Franklin J, Hansmann ML, Harris N, Jaffe E, Poppema S, Harris M, Franssila K, van Krieken J, Marafioti T, Anagnostopoulos I, Stein H (1999) Clinical presentation, course, and prognostic factors in lymphocyte-predominant Hodgkin's disease and lymphocyte-rich classical Hodgkin's disease: report from the European Task Force on Lymphoma Project on Lymphocyte-Predominant Hodgkin's Disease. J Clin Oncol 17(3):776–783

Dorth JA, Chino JP, Prosnitz LR, Diehl LF, Beaven AW, Coleman RE, Kelsey CR (2011) The impact of radiation therapy in patients with diffuse large B-cell lymphoma with positive post-chemotherapy FDG-PET or gallium-67 scans. Ann Oncol 22(2):405–410. doi: 10.1093/annonc/mdq389 mdq389 [pii]

Dorth JA, Prosnitz LR, Broadwater G, Diehl LF, Beaven AW, Coleman RE, Kelsey CR (2012) Impact of consolidation radiation therapy in stage III-IV diffuse large B-cell lymphoma with negative post-chemotherapy radiologic imaging. Int J Radiat Oncol Biol Phys 84(3):762–767. doi:10.1016/j.ijrobp.2011.12.067 S0360-3016(11)03771-0 [pii]

Dupuis J, Berriolo-Riedinger A, Julian A, Brice P, Tychyj-Pinel C, Tilly H, Mounier N, Gallamini A, Feugier P, Soubeyran P, Colombat P, Laurent G, Berenger N, Casasnovas RO, Vera P, Paone G, Xerri L, Salles G, Haioun C, Meignan M (2012) Impact of [18F]Fluorodeoxyglucose positron emission tomography response evaluation in patients with high-tumor burden follicular lymphoma treated with immunochemotherapy: a prospective study from the Groupe d'Etudes des Lymphomes de l'Adulte and GOELAMS. J Clin Oncol 30(35):4317–4322. doi:10.1200/JCO.2012.43.0934 JCO.2012.43.0934 [pii]

Eich HT, Muller RP, Engenhart-Cabillic R, Lukas P, Schmidberger H, Staar S, Willich N (2008) Involved-node radiotherapy in early-stage Hodgkin's lymphoma. Definition and guidelines of the German Hodgkin Study Group (GHSG). Strahlenther Onkol 184(8):406–410

Eich HT, Diehl V, Gorgen H, Pabst T, Markova J, Debus J, Ho A, Dorken B, Rank A, Grosu AL, Wiegel T, Karstens JH, Greil R, Willich N, Schmidberger H, Dohner H, Borchmann P, Muller-Hermelink HK, Muller RP, Engert A (2010) Intensified chemotherapy and dose-reduced involved-field radiotherapy in patients with early unfavorable Hodgkin's lymphoma: final analysis of the German Hodgkin Study Group HD11 trial. J Clin Oncol 28(27):4199–4206. doi:10.1200/JCO.2010.29.8018 JCO.2010.29.8018 [pii]

Engert A (2012) Radiotherapy in early-stage Hodgkin lymphoma. The ASCO Post, 15 June 2012

Engert A, Schiller P, Josting A, Herrmann R, Koch P, Sieber M, Boissevain F, De Wit M, Mezger J, Duhmke E, Willich N, Muller RP, Schmidt BF, Renner H, Muller-Hermelink HK, Pfistner B, Wolf J, Hasenclever D, Loffler M, Diehl V (2003) Involved-field radiotherapy is equally effective and less toxic compared with extended-field radiotherapy after four cycles of chemotherapy in patients with early-stage unfavorable Hodgkin's lymphoma: results of the HD8 trial of the German Hodgkin's Lymphoma Study Group. J Clin Oncol 21(19):3601–3608

Engert A, Diehl V, Franklin J, Lohri A, Dorken B, Ludwig WD, Koch P, Hanel M, Pfreundschuh M, Wilhelm M, Trumper L, Aulitzky WE, Bentz M, Rummel M, Sezer O, Muller-Hermelink HK, Hasenclever D, Loffler M (2009) Escalated-dose BEACOPP in the treatment of patients with advanced-stage Hodgkin's lymphoma: 10 years of follow-up of the GHSG HD9 study. J Clin Oncol 27(27):4548–4554. doi:10.1200/JCO.2008.19.8820 JCO.2008.19.8820 [pii]

Engert A, Plutschow A, Eich HT, Lohri A, Dorken B, Borchmann P, Berger B, Greil R, Willborn KC, Wilhelm M, Debus J, Eble MJ, Sokler M, Ho A, Rank A, Ganser A, Trumper L, Bokemeyer C, Kirchner H, Schubert J, Kral Z, Fuchs M, Muller-Hermelink HK, Muller RP, Diehl V (2010) Reduced treatment intensity in patients with early-stage Hodgkin's lymphoma. N Engl J Med 363(7):640–652. doi:10.1056/NEJMoa1000067

Engert A, Haverkamp H, Kobe C, Markova J, Renner C, Ho A, Zijlstra J, Kral Z, Fuchs M, Hallek M, Kanz L, Dohner H, Dorken B, Engel N, Topp M, Klutmann S, Amthauer H, Bockisch A, Kluge R, Kratochwil C, Schober O, Greil R, Andreesen R, Kneba M, Pfreundschuh M, Stein H, Eich HT, Muller RP, Dietlein M, Borchmann P, Diehl V (2012) Reduced-intensity chemotherapy and PET-guided radiotherapy in patients with advanced stage Hodgkin's lymphoma (HD15 trial): a randomised, open-label, phase 3 non-inferiority trial. Lancet 379(9828):1791–1799. doi:10.1016/S0140-6736(11)61940-5 S0140-6736(11)61940-5 [pii]

Fabian CJ, Mansfield CM, Dahlberg S, Jones SE, Miller TP, Van Slyck E, Grozea PN, Morrison FS, Coltman CA Jr, Fisher RI (1994) Low-dose involved field radiation after chemotherapy in advanced Hodgkin disease. A Southwest Oncology Group randomized study. Ann Intern Med 120(11):903–912

Falini B, Pileri S, Zinzani PL, Carbone A, Zagonel V, Wolf-Peeters C, Verhoef G, Menestrina F, Todeschini G, Paulli M, Lazzarino M, Giardini R, Aiello A, Foss HD, Araujo I, Fizzotti M, Pelicci PG, Flenghi L, Martelli MF, Santucci A (1999) ALK + lymphoma: clinico-pathological findings and outcome. Blood 93(8):2697–2706

Federico M, Bellei M, Marcheselli L, Luminari S, Lopez-Guillermo A, Vitolo U, Pro B, Pileri S, Pulsoni A, Soubeyran P, Cortelazzo S, Martinelli G, Martelli M, Rigacci L, Arcaini L, Di Raimondo F, Merli F, Sabattini E, McLaughlin P, Solal-Celigny P (2009) Follicular lymphoma international prognostic index 2: a new prognostic index for follicular lymphoma developed by the international follicular lymphoma prognostic factor project. J Clin Oncol 27(27):4555–4562. doi:10.1200/JCO.2008.21.3991 JCO.2008.21.3991 [pii]

Ferme C, Eghbali H, Meerwaldt JH, Rieux C, Bosq J, Berger F, Girinsky T, Brice P, van't Veer MB, Walewski JA, Lederlin P, Tirelli U, Carde P, Van den Neste E, Gyan E, Monconduit M, Divine M, Raemaekers JM, Salles G, Noordijk EM, Creemers GJ, Gabarre J, Hagenbeek A, Reman O, Blanc M, Thomas J, Vie B, Kluin-Nelemans JC, Viseu F, Baars JW, Poortmans P, Lugtenburg PJ, Carrie C, Jaubert J, Henry-Amar M (2007) Chemotherapy plus involved-field radiation in early-stage Hodgkin's disease. N Engl J Med 357(19):1916–1927. doi:10.1056/NEJMoa064601 357/19/1916 [pii]

Ferreri AJ, Dell'Oro S, Reni M, Ceresoli GL, Cozzarini C, Ponzoni M, Villa E (2000) Consolidation radiotherapy to bulky or semibulky lesions in the management of stage III-IV diffuse large B-cell lymphomas. Oncology 58(3):219–226 ocl58219 [pii]

Ferreri AJ, Blay JY, Reni M, Pasini F, Spina M, Ambrosetti A, Calderoni A, Rossi A, Vavassori V, Conconi A, Devizzi L, Berger F, Ponzoni M, Borisch B, Tinguely M, Cerati M, Milani M, Orvieto E, Sanchez J, Chevreau C, Dell'Oro S, Zucca E, Cavalli F (2003) Prognostic scoring system for primary CNS lymphomas: the International Extranodal Lymphoma Study Group experience. J Clin Oncol 21(2):266–272

Feugier P, Van Hoof A, Sebban C, Solal-Celigny P, Bouabdallah R, Ferme C, Christian B, Lepage E, Tilly H, Morschhauser F, Gaulard P, Salles G, Bosly A, Gisselbrecht C, Reyes F, Coiffier B (2005) Long-term results of the R-CHOP study in the treatment of elderly patients with diffuse large B-cell lymphoma: a study by the Groupe d'Etude des Lymphomes de l'Adulte. J Clin Oncol 23(18):4117–4126. doi:10.1200/JCO.2005.09.131 JCO.2005.09.131 [pii]

Franklin JG, Paus MD, Pluetschow A, Specht L (2005) Chemotherapy, radiotherapy and combined modality for Hodgkin's disease, with emphasis on second cancer risk. Cochrane Database Syst Rev (4):CD003187. doi:10.1002/14651858.CD003187.pub2

Friedberg JW (2012) Double-hit diffuse large B-cell lymphoma. J Clin Oncol 30(28):3439–3443. doi:10.1200/JCO.2012.43.5800 JCO.2012.43.5800 [pii]

Friedberg JW, Taylor MD, Cerhan JR, Flowers CR, Dillon H, Farber CM, Rogers ES, Hainsworth JD, Wong EK, Vose JM, Zelenetz AD, Link BK (2009) Follicular lymphoma in the United States: first report of the national LymphoCare study. J Clin Oncol 27(8):1202–1208. doi:10.1200/JCO.2008.18.1495 JCO.2008.18.1495 [pii]

Friedberg JW, Byrtek M, Link BK, Flowers C, Taylor M, Hainsworth J, Cerhan JR, Zelenetz AD, Hirata J, Miller TP (2012) Effectiveness of first-line management strategies for stage I follicular lymphoma: analysis of the National LymphoCare Study. J Clin

Oncol 30(27):3368–3375. doi:10.1200/JCO.2011.40.6546 JCO.2011.40.6546 [pii]
Gallamini A, Hutchings M, Rigacci L, Specht L, Merli F, Hansen M, Patti C, Loft A, Di Raimondo F, D'Amore F, Biggi A, Vitolo U, Stelitano C, Sancetta R, Trentin L, Luminari S, Iannitto E, Viviani S, Pierri I, Levis A (2007) Early interim 2-[18F]fluoro-2-deoxy-D-glucose positron emission tomography is prognostically superior to international prognostic score in advanced-stage Hodgkin's lymphoma: a report from a joint Italian-Danish study. J Clin Oncol 25(24):3746–3752. doi:10.1200/JCO.2007.11.6525 JCO.2007.11.6525 [pii]
Ganti AK, Weisenburger DD, Smith LM, Hans CP, Bociek RG, Bierman PJ, Vose JM, Armitage JO (2006) Patients with grade 3 follicular lymphoma have prolonged relapse-free survival following anthracycline-based chemotherapy: the Nebraska Lymphoma Study Group Experience. Ann Oncol 17(6):920–927. doi: 10.1093/annonc/mdl039 mdl039 [pii]
Gascoyne RD, Aoun P, Wu D, Chhanabhai M, Skinnider BF, Greiner TC, Morris SW, Connors JM, Vose JM, Viswanatha DS, Coldman A, Weisenburger DD (1999) Prognostic significance of anaplastic lymphoma kinase (ALK) protein expression in adults with anaplastic large cell lymphoma. Blood 93(11):3913–3921
Geisler CH, Kolstad A, Laurell A, Raty R, Jerkeman M, Eriksson M, Nordstrom M, Kimby E, Boesen AM, Nilsson-Ehle H, Kuittinen O, Lauritzsen GF, Ralfkiaer E, Ehinger M, Sundstrom C, Delabie J, Karjalainen-Lindsberg ML, Brown P, Elonen E (2010) The Mantle Cell Lymphoma International Prognostic Index (MIPI) is superior to the International Prognostic Index (IPI) in predicting survival following intensive first-line immunochemotherapy and autologous stem cell transplantation (ASCT). Blood 115(8):1530–1533. doi: 10.1182/blood-2009-08-236570 blood-2009-08-236570 [pii]
Gervais-Fagnou DD, Girouard C, Laperriere N, Pintillie M, Goss PE (1999) Breast cancer in women following supradiaphragmatic irradiation for Hodgkin's disease. Oncology 57(3):224–231 12035 [pii] 12035
Girardi M, Heald PW, Wilson LD (2004) The pathogenesis of mycosis fungoides. N Engl J Med 350(19):1978–1988. doi:10.1056/NEJMra032810 350/19/1978 [pii]
Girinsky T, Specht L, Ghalibafian M, Edeline V, Bonniaud G, Van Der Maazen R, Aleman B, Paumier A, Meijnders P, Lievens Y, Noordijk E, Poortmans P (2008) The conundrum of Hodgkin lymphoma nodes: to be or not to be included in the involved node radiation fields. The EORTC-GELA lymphoma group guidelines. Radiother Oncol 88(2):202–210. doi:10.1016/j.radonc.2008.05.012 S0167-8140(08)00241-7 [pii]
Glanzmann C, Kaufmann P, Jenni R, Hess OM, Huguenin P (1998) Cardiac risk after mediastinal irradiation for Hodgkin's disease. Radiother Oncol 46(1):51–62 S0167814097001254 [pii]
Goda JS, Gospodarowicz M, Pintilie M, Wells W, Hodgson DC, Sun A, Crump M, Tsang RW (2010) Long-term outcome in localized extranodal mucosa-associated lymphoid tissue lymphomas treated with radiotherapy. Cancer 116(16):3815–3824. doi: 10.1002/cncr.25226
Guadagnolo BA, Li S, Neuberg D, Ng A, Hua L, Silver B, Stevenson MA, Mauch P (2006) Long-term outcome and mortality trends in early-stage, Grade 1–2 follicular lymphoma treated with radiation therapy. Int J Radiat Oncol Biol Phys 64(3):928–934. doi: 10.1016/j.ijrobp.2005.08.010 S0360-3016(05)02375-8 [pii]
Habermann TM, Weller EA, Morrison VA, Gascoyne RD, Cassileth PA, Cohn JB, Dakhil SR, Woda B, Fisher RI, Peterson BA, Horning SJ (2006) Rituximab-CHOP versus CHOP alone or with maintenance rituximab in older patients with diffuse large B-cell lymphoma. J Clin Oncol 24(19):3121–3127. doi:10.1200/JCO.2005.05.1003 JCO.2005.05.1003 [pii]
Haioun C, Itti E, Rahmouni A, Brice P, Rain JD, Belhadj K, Gaulard P, Garderet L, Lepage E, Reyes F, Meignan M (2005) [18F]fluoro-2-deoxy-D-glucose positron emission tomography (FDG-PET) in aggressive lymphoma: an early prognostic tool for predicting patient outcome. Blood 106(4):1376–1381. doi:10.1182/blood-2005-01-0272 2005-01-0272 [pii]
Halasz LM, Jacene HA, Catalano PJ, Van den Abbeele AD, Lacasce A, Mauch PM, Ng AK (2012) Combined modality treatment for PET-positive non-Hodgkin lymphoma: favorable outcomes of combined modality treatment for patients with non-Hodgkin lymphoma and positive interim or postchemotherapy FDG-PET. Int J Radiat Oncol Biol Phys 83(5):e647–e654. doi:10.1016/j.ijrobp.2012.01.060 S0360-3016(12)00133-2 [pii]
Hancock SL, Cox RS, McDougall IR (1991) Thyroid diseases after treatment of Hodgkin's disease. N Engl J Med 325(9):599–605. doi:10.1056/NEJM199108293250902
Hancock SL, Tucker MA, Hoppe RT (1993a) Breast cancer after treatment of Hodgkin's disease. J Natl Cancer Inst 85(1):25–31
Hancock SL, Tucker MA, Hoppe RT (1993b) Factors affecting late mortality from heart disease after treatment of Hodgkin's disease. JAMA 270(16):1949–1955
Hans CP, Weisenburger DD, Greiner TC, Gascoyne RD, Delabie J, Ott G, Muller-Hermelink HK, Campo E, Braziel RM, Jaffe ES, Pan Z, Farinha P, Smith LM, Falini B, Banham AH, Rosenwald A, Staudt LM, Connors JM, Armitage JO, Chan WC (2004) Confirmation of the molecular classification of diffuse large B-cell lymphoma by immunohistochemistry using a tissue microarray. Blood 103(1):275–282. doi:10.1182/blood-2003-05-1545 2003-05-1545 [pii]
Herold M, Haas A, Srock S, Neser S, Al-Ali KH, Neubauer A, Dolken G, Naumann R, Knauf W, Freund M, Rohrberg R, Hoffken K, Franke A, Ittel T, Kettner E, Haak U, Mey U, Klinkenstein C, Assmann M, von Grunhagen U (2007) Rituximab added to first-line mitoxantrone, chlorambucil, and prednisolone chemotherapy followed by interferon maintenance prolongs survival in patients with advanced follicular lymphoma: an East German Study Group Hematology and Oncology Study. J Clin Oncol 25(15):1986–1992. doi:10.1200/JCO.2006.06.4618 JCO.2006.06.4618 [pii]
Hiddemann W, Kneba M, Dreyling M, Schmitz N, Lengfelder E, Schmits R, Reiser M, Metzner B, Harder H, Hegewisch-Becker S, Fischer T, Kropff M, Reis HE, Freund M, Wormann B, Fuchs R, Planker M, Schimke J, Eimermacher H, Trumper L, Aldaoud A, Parwaresch R, Unterhalt M (2005) Frontline therapy with rituximab added to the combination of cyclophosphamide, doxorubicin, vincristine, and prednisone (CHOP) significantly improves the outcome for patients with advanced-stage follicular lymphoma compared with therapy with CHOP alone: results of a prospective randomized study of the German Low-Grade Lymphoma Study Group. Blood 106(12):3725–3732
Horning SJ, Weller E, Kim K, Earle JD, O'Connell MJ, Habermann TM, Glick JH (2004) Chemotherapy with or without radiotherapy in limited-stage diffuse aggressive non-Hodgkin's lymphoma: Eastern Cooperative Oncology Group study 1484. J Clin Oncol 22(15):3032–3038. doi:10.1200/JCO.2004.06.088 JCO.2004.06.088 [pii]
Hoster E, Dreyling M, Klapper W, Gisselbrecht C, van Hoof A, Kluin-Nelemans HC, Pfreundschuh M, Reiser M, Metzner B, Einsele H, Peter N, Jung W, Wormann B, Ludwig WD, Duhrsen U, Eimermacher H, Wandt H, Hasford J, Hiddemann W, Unterhalt M (2008) A new prognostic index (MIPI) for patients with advanced-stage mantle cell lymphoma. Blood 111(2):558–565. doi: 10.1182/blood-2007-06-095331 blood-2007-06-095331 [pii]
Hull MC, Morris CG, Pepine CJ, Mendenhall NP (2003) Valvular dysfunction and carotid, subclavian, and coronary artery disease in

survivors of hodgkin lymphoma treated with radiation therapy. JAMA 290(21):2831–2837

Hutchings M, Loft A, Hansen M, Pedersen LM, Buhl T, Jurlander J, Buus S, Keiding S, D'Amore F, Boesen AM, Berthelsen AK, Specht L (2006) FDG-PET after two cycles of chemotherapy predicts treatment failure and progression-free survival in Hodgkin lymphoma. Blood 107(1):52–59

Juweid ME, Wiseman GA, Vose JM, Ritchie JM, Menda Y, Wooldridge JE, Mottaghy FM, Rohren EM, Blumstein NM, Stolpen A, Link BK, Reske SN, Graham MM, Cheson BD (2005) Response assessment of aggressive non-Hodgkin's lymphoma by integrated International Workshop Criteria and fluorine-18-fluorodeoxyglucose positron emission tomography. J Clin Oncol 23(21):4652–4661. doi:10.1200/JCO.2005.01.891 JCO.2005.01.891 [pii]

Juweid ME, Stroobants S, Hoekstra OS, Mottaghy FM, Dietlein M, Guermazi A, Wiseman GA, Kostakoglu L, Scheidhauer K, Buck A, Naumann R, Spaepen K, Hicks RJ, Weber WA, Reske SN, Schwaiger M, Schwartz LH, Zijlstra JM, Siegel BA, Cheson BD (2007) Use of positron emission tomography for response assessment of lymphoma: consensus of the Imaging Subcommittee of International Harmonization Project in Lymphoma. J Clin Oncol 25(5):571–578. doi:10.1200/JCO.2006.08.2305 JCO.2006.08.2305 [pii]

Kim YH, Bishop K, Varghese A, Hoppe RT (1995) Prognostic factors in erythrodermic mycosis fungoides and the Sezary syndrome. Arch Dermatol 131(9):1003–1008

Kim YH, Liu HL, Mraz-Gernhard S, Varghese A, Hoppe RT (2003) Long-term outcome of 525 patients with mycosis fungoides and Sezary syndrome: clinical prognostic factors and risk for disease progression. Arch Dermatol 139(7):857–866. doi:10.1001/archderm.139.7.857 139/7/857 [pii]

Klapper W, Stoecklein H, Zeynalova S, Ott G, Kosari F, Rosenwald A, Loeffler M, Trumper L, Pfreundschuh M, Siebert R (2008) Structural aberrations affecting the MYC locus indicate a poor prognosis independent of clinical risk factors in diffuse large B-cell lymphomas treated within randomized trials of the German High-Grade Non-Hodgkin's Lymphoma Study Group (DSHNHL). Leukemia 22(12):2226–2229. doi:10.1038/leu.2008.230 leu2008230 [pii]

Koontz BF, Kirkpatrick JP, Clough RW, Prosnitz RG, Gockerman JP, Moore JO, Prosnitz LR (2006) Combined-modality therapy versus radiotherapy alone for treatment of early-stage Hodgkin's disease: cure balanced against complications. J Clin Oncol 24(4):605–611

Kupeli S, Hazirolan T, Varan A, Akata D, Alehan D, Hayran M, Besim A, Buyukpamukcu M (2010) Evaluation of coronary artery disease by computed tomography angiography in patients treated for childhood Hodgkin's lymphoma. J Clin Oncol 28(6):1025–1030. doi:10.1200/JCO.2009.25.2627 JCO.2009.25.2627 [pii]

Laskar S, Gupta T, Vimal S, Muckaden MA, Saikia TK, Pai SK, Naresh KN, Dinshaw KA (2004) Consolidation radiation after complete remission in Hodgkin's disease following six cycles of doxorubicin, bleomycin, vinblastine, and dacarbazine chemotherapy: is there a need? J Clin Oncol 22(1):62–68

Lavey RS, Eby NL, Prosnitz LR (1990) Impact on second malignancy risk of the combined use of radiation and chemotherapy for lymphomas. Cancer 66(1):80–88

Leitch HA, Gascoyne RD, Chhanabhai M, Voss NJ, Klasa R, Connors JM (2003) Limited-stage mantle-cell lymphoma. Ann Oncol 14(10):1555–1561

Lenz G, Wright G, Dave SS, Xiao W, Powell J, Zhao H, Xu W, Tan B, Goldschmidt N, Iqbal J, Vose J, Bast M, Fu K, Weisenburger DD, Greiner TC, Armitage JO, Kyle A, May L, Gascoyne RD, Connors JM, Troen G, Holte H, Kvaloy S, Dierickx D, Verhoef G, Delabie J, Smeland EB, Jares P, Martinez A, Lopez-Guillermo A, Montserrat E, Campo E, Braziel RM, Miller TP, Rimsza LM, Cook JR, Pohlman B, Sweetenham J, Tubbs RR, Fisher RI, Hartmann E, Rosenwald A, Ott G, Muller-Hermelink HK, Wrench D, Lister TA, Jaffe ES, Wilson WH, Chan WC, Staudt LM (2008) Stromal gene signatures in large-B-cell lymphomas. N Engl J Med 359(22):2313–2323. doi:10.1056/NEJMoa0802885 359/22/2313 [pii]

Levy M, Copie-Bergman C, Gameiro C, Chaumette MT, Delfau-Larue MH, Haioun C, Charachon A, Hemery F, Gaulard P, Leroy K, Delchier JC (2005) Prognostic value of translocation t(11;18) in tumoral response of low-grade gastric lymphoma of mucosa-associated lymphoid tissue type to oral chemotherapy. J Clin Oncol 23(22):5061–5066

Liu HL, Hoppe RT, Kohler S, Harvell JD, Reddy S, Kim YH (2003) CD30 + cutaneous lymphoproliferative disorders: the Stanford experience in lymphomatoid papulosis and primary cutaneous anaplastic large cell lymphoma. J Am Acad Dermatol 49(6):1049–1058. doi:10.1016/S0190 S0190962203024848 [pii]

Lowry L, Smith P, Qian W, Falk S, Benstead K, Illidge T, Linch D, Robinson M, Jack A, Hoskin P (2011) Reduced dose radiotherapy for local control in non-Hodgkin lymphoma: a randomised phase III trial. Radiother Oncol 100(1):86–92. doi:10.1016/j.radonc.2011.05.013 S0167-8140(11)00205-2 [pii]

Mac Manus MP, Hoppe RT (1996) Is radiotherapy curative for stage I and II low-grade follicular lymphoma? Results of a long-term follow-up study of patients treated at Stanford University. J Clin Oncol 14(4):1282–1290

Marcus R, Imrie K, Solal-Celigny P, Catalano JV, Dmoszynska A, Raposo JC, Offner FC, Gomez-Codina J, Belch A, Cunningham D, Wassner-Fritsch E, Stein G (2008) Phase III study of R-CVP compared with cyclophosphamide, vincristine, and prednisone alone in patients with previously untreated advanced follicular lymphoma. J Clin Oncol 26(28):4579–4586. doi:10.1200/JCO.2007.13.5376 JCO.2007.13.5376 [pii]

Martinelli G, Gigli F, Calabrese L, Ferrucci PF, Zucca E, Crosta C, Pruneri G, Preda L, Piperno G, Gospodarowicz M, Cavalli F, Moreno Gomez H (2009) Early stage gastric diffuse large B-cell lymphomas: results of a randomized trial comparing chemotherapy alone versus chemotherapy + involved field radiotherapy (IELSG 4) [corrected]. Leuk Lymphoma 50(6):925–931. doi:10.1080/10428190902912478 911751509 [pii]

Meyer PN, Fu K, Greiner TC, Smith LM, Delabie J, Gascoyne RD, Ott G, Rosenwald A, Braziel RM, Campo E, Vose JM, Lenz G, Staudt LM, Chan WC, Weisenburger DD (2011) Immunohistochemical methods for predicting cell of origin and survival in patients with diffuse large B-cell lymphoma treated with rituximab. J Clin Oncol 29(2):200–207. doi:10.1200/JCO.2010.30.0368 JCO.2010.30.0368 [pii]

Meyer RM, Gospodarowicz MK, Connors JM, Pearcey RG, Wells WA, Winter JN, Horning SJ, Dar AR, Shustik C, Stewart DA, Crump M, Djurfeldt MS, Chen BE, Shepherd LE (2012) ABVD alone versus radiation-based therapy in limited-stage Hodgkin's lymphoma. N Engl J Med 366(5):399–408. doi:10.1056/NEJMoa1111961

Mikhaeel NG, Timothy AR, O'Doherty MJ, Hain S, Maisey MN (2000) 18-FDG-PET as a prognostic indicator in the treatment of aggressive Non-Hodgkin's Lymphoma-comparison with CT. Leuk Lymphoma 39(5–6):543–553 I308J001131 [pii]

Miller TP, Dahlberg S, Cassady JR, Adelstein DJ, Spier CM, Grogan TM, LeBlanc M, Carlin S, Chase E, Fisher RI (1998) Chemotherapy alone compared with chemotherapy plus radiotherapy for localized intermediate- and high-grade non-Hodgkin's lymphoma. N Engl J Med 339(1):21–26

Moser EC, Noordijk EM, van Leeuwen FE, le Cessie S, Baars JW, Thomas J, Carde P, Meerwaldt JH, van Glabbeke M, Kluin-

Nelemans HC (2006) Long-term risk of cardiovascular disease after treatment for aggressive non-Hodgkin lymphoma. Blood 107(7):2912–2919. doi:10.1182/blood-2005-08-3392 2005-08-3392 [pii]

Mudie NY, Swerdlow AJ, Higgins CD, Smith P, Qiao Z, Hancock BW, Hoskin PJ, Linch DC (2006) Risk of second malignancy after non-Hodgkin's lymphoma: a British Cohort Study. J Clin Oncol 24(10):1568–1574. doi:10.1200/JCO.2005.04.2200 JCO.2005.04.2200 [pii]

Muris JJ, Meijer CJ, Vos W, van Krieken JH, Jiwa NM, Ossenkoppele GJ, Oudejans JJ (2006) Immunohistochemical profiling based on Bcl-2, CD10 and MUM1 expression improves risk stratification in patients with primary nodal diffuse large B-cell lymphoma. J Pathol 208(5):714–723. doi:10.1002/path.1924

Myrehaug S, Pintilie M, Tsang R, Mackenzie R, Crump M, Chen Z, Sun A, Hodgson DC (2008) Cardiac morbidity following modern treatment for Hodgkin lymphoma: supra-additive cardiotoxicity of doxorubicin and radiation therapy. Leuk Lymphoma 49(8):1486–1493. doi:10.1080/10428190802140873 793642260 [pii]

Nachman JB, Sposto R, Herzog P, Gilchrist GS, Wolden SL, Thomson J, Kadin ME, Pattengale P, Davis PC, Hutchinson RJ, White K (2002) Randomized comparison of low-dose involved-field radiotherapy and no radiotherapy for children with Hodgkin's disease who achieve a complete response to chemotherapy. J Clin Oncol 20(18):3765–3771

Nakamura S, Matsumoto T, Suekane H, Takeshita M, Hizawa K, Kawasaki M, Yao T, Tsuneyoshi M, Iida M, Fujishima M (2001) Predictive value of endoscopic ultrasonography for regression of gastric low grade and high grade MALT lymphomas after eradication of *Helicobacter pylori*. Gut 48(4):454–460

Natkunam Y, Farinha P, Hsi ED, Hans CP, Tibshirani R, Sehn LH, Connors JM, Gratzinger D, Rosado M, Zhao S, Pohlman B, Wongchaowart N, Bast M, Avigdor A, Schiby G, Nagler A, Byrne GE, Levy R, Gascoyne RD, Lossos IS (2008) LMO2 protein expression predicts survival in patients with diffuse large B-cell lymphoma treated with anthracycline-based chemotherapy with and without rituximab. J Clin Oncol 26(3):447–454. doi:10.1200/JCO.2007.13.0690 JCO.2007.13.0690 [pii]

Ng AK, Bernardo MP, Weller E, Backstrand KH, Silver B, Marcus KC, Tarbell NJ, Friedberg J, Canellos GP, Mauch PM (2002) Long-term survival and competing causes of death in patients with early-stage Hodgkin's disease treated at age 50 or younger. J Clin Oncol 20(8):2101–2108

Niitsu N, Okamoto M, Miura I, Hirano M (2009) Clinical features and prognosis of de novo diffuse large B-cell lymphoma with t(14;18) and 8q24/c-MYC translocations. Leukemia 23(4):777–783. doi:10.1038/leu.2008.344 leu2008344 [pii]

Nogova L, Reineke T, Eich HT, Josting A, Muller-Hermelink HK, Wingbermuhle K, Brillant C, Gossmann A, Oertel J, Bollen MV, Muller RP, Diehl V, Engert A (2005) Extended field radiotherapy, combined modality treatment or involved field radiotherapy for patients with stage IA lymphocyte-predominant Hodgkin's lymphoma: a retrospective analysis from the German Hodgkin Study Group (GHSG). Ann Oncol 16(10):1683–1687. doi:10.1093/annonc/mdi323 mdi323 [pii]

Nogova L, Reineke T, Brillant C, Sieniawski M, Rudiger T, Josting A, Bredenfeld H, Skripnitchenko R, Muller RP, Muller-Hermelink HK, Diehl V, Engert A (2008) Lymphocyte-predominant and classical Hodgkin's lymphoma: a comprehensive analysis from the German Hodgkin Study Group. J Clin Oncol 26(3):434–439. doi:10.1200/JCO.2007.11.8869 JCO.2007.11.8869 [pii]

Nooka AK, Nabhan C, Zhou X, Taylor MD, Byrtek M, Miller TP, Friedberg JW, Zelenetz AD, Link BK, Cerhan JR, Dillon H, Sinha R, Shenoy PJ, Levy D, Dawson K, Hirata JH, Flowers CR (2012) Examination of the follicular lymphoma international prognostic index (FLIPI) in the National LymphoCare study (NLCS): a prospective US patient cohort treated predominantly in community practices. Ann Oncol. doi:10.1093/annonc/mds429 mds429 [pii]

Noordijk EM, Thomas J, Ferme C, van 't Veer MB, Brice P, Divine M, Morschhauser F, Carde P, Eghbali H, Henry-Amar M (2005) First results of the EORTC-GELA H9 randomized trials: the H9-F trial (comparing 3 radiation dose levels) and H9-U trial (comparing 3 chemotherapy schemes) in patients with favorable or unfavorable early stage Hodgkin's lymphoma (HL). Proc ASCO 23(June 1 Supplement):6505

Noy A, Yahalom J, Zaretsky L, Brett I, Zelenetz AD (2005) Gastric mucosa-associated lymphoid tissue lymphoma detected by clonotypic polymerase chain reaction despite continuous pathologic remission induced by involved-field radiotherapy. J Clin Oncol 23(16):3768–3772. doi:10.1200/JCO.2005.10.018 23/16/3768 [pii]

Nyman H, Jerkeman M, Karjalainen-Lindsberg ML, Banham AH, Leppa S (2009) Prognostic impact of activated B-cell focused classification in diffuse large B-cell lymphoma patients treated with R-CHOP. Mod Pathol 22(8):1094–1101. doi:10.1038/modpathol.2009.73 modpathol200973 [pii]

Omuro AM, Ben-Porat LS, Panageas KS, Kim AK, Correa DD, Yahalom J, Deangelis LM, Abrey LE (2005) Delayed neurotoxicity in primary central nervous system lymphoma. Arch Neurol 62(10):1595–1600. doi:10.1001/archneur.62.10.1595 62/10/1595 [pii]

Ono S, Kato M, Takagi K, Kodaira J, Kubota K, Matsuno Y, Komatsu Y, Asaka M (2010) Long-term treatment of localized gastric marginal zone B-cell mucosa associated lymphoid tissue lymphoma including incidence of metachronous gastric cancer. J Gastroenterol Hepatol 25(4):804–809. doi:10.1111/j.1440-1746.2009.06204.x JGH6204 [pii]

Pavlovsky S, Maschio M, Santarelli MT, Muriel FS, Corrado C, Garcia I, Schwartz L, Montero C, Sanahuja FL, Magnasco O et al (1988) Randomized trial of chemotherapy versus chemotherapy plus radiotherapy for stage I-II Hodgkin's disease. J Natl Cancer Inst 80(18):1466–1473

Pels H, Schmidt-Wolf IG, Glasmacher A, Schulz H, Engert A, Diehl V, Zellner A, Schackert G, Reichmann H, Kroschinsky F, Vogt-Schaden M, Egerer G, Bode U, Schaller C, Deckert M, Fimmers R, Helmstaedter C, Atasoy A, Klockgether T, Schlegel U (2003) Primary central nervous system lymphoma: results of a pilot and phase II study of systemic and intraventricular chemotherapy with deferred radiotherapy. J Clin Oncol 21(24):4489–4495. doi:10.1200/JCO.2003.04.056 JCO.2003.04.056 [pii]

Pfreundschuh M, Trumper L, Osterborg A, Pettengell R, Trneny M, Imrie K, Ma D, Gill D, Walewski J, Zinzani PL, Stahel R, Kvaloy S, Shpilberg O, Jaeger U, Hansen M, Lehtinen T, Lopez-Guillermo A, Corrado C, Scheliga A, Milpied N, Mendila M, Rashford M, Kuhnt E, Loeffler M (2006) CHOP-like chemotherapy plus rituximab versus CHOP-like chemotherapy alone in young patients with good-prognosis diffuse large-B-cell lymphoma: a randomised controlled trial by the MabThera International Trial (MInT) Group. Lancet Oncol 7(5):379–391

Phan J, Mazloom A, Jeffrey Medeiros L, Zreik TG, Wogan C, Shihadeh F, Rodriguez MA, Fayad L, Fowler N, Reed V, Horace P, Dabaja BS (2010) Benefit of consolidative radiation therapy in patients with diffuse large B-cell lymphoma treated with R-CHOP chemotherapy. J Clin Oncol 28(27):4170–4176. doi:10.1200/JCO.2009.27.3441 JCO.2009.27.3441 [pii]

Picardi M, De Renzo A, Pane F, Nicolai E, Pacelli R, Salvatore M, Rotoli B (2007) Randomized comparison of consolidation radiation versus observation in bulky Hodgkin's lymphoma with post-chemotherapy negative positron emission tomography scans. Leuk Lymphoma 48(9):1721–1727. doi:10.1080/10428190701559140 781796832 [pii]

Pregno P, Chiappella A, Bello M, Botto B, Ferrero S, Franceschetti S, Giunta F, Ladetto M, Limerutti G, Menga M, Nicolosi M, Priolo G, Puccini B, Rigacci L, Salvi F, Vaggelli L, Passera R, Bisi G, Vitolo U (2012) Interim 18-FDG-PET/CT failed to predict the outcome in diffuse large B-cell lymphoma patients treated at the diagnosis with rituximab-CHOP. Blood 119(9):2066–2073. doi:10.1182/blood-2011-06-359943 blood-2011-06-359943 [pii]

Pugh TJ, Ballonoff A, Newman F, Rabinovitch R (2010) Improved survival in patients with early stage low-grade follicular lymphoma treated with radiation: a surveillance, epidemiology, and end results database analysis. Cancer 116(16):3843–3851. doi:10.1002/cncr.25149

Relander T, Johnson NA, Farinha P, Connors JM, Sehn LH, Gascoyne RD (2010) Prognostic factors in follicular lymphoma. J Clin Oncol 28(17):2902–2913. doi:10.1200/JCO.2009.26.1693 JCO.2009.26.1693 [pii]

Rosenwald A, Wright G, Chan WC, Connors JM, Campo E, Fisher RI, Gascoyne RD, Muller-Hermelink HK, Smeland EB, Giltnane JM, Hurt EM, Zhao H, Averett L, Yang L, Wilson WH, Jaffe ES, Simon R, Klausner RD, Powell J, Duffey PL, Longo DL, Greiner TC, Weisenburger DD, Sanger WG, Dave BJ, Lynch JC, Vose J, Armitage JO, Montserrat E, Lopez-Guillermo A, GroganTM, Miller TP, LeBlanc M, Ott G, Kvaloy S, Delabie J, Holte H, Krajci P, Stokke T, Staudt LM (2002) The use of molecular profiling to predict survival after chemotherapy for diffuse large-B-cell lymphoma. N Engl J Med 346(25):1937–1947

Ruskone-Fourmestraux A, Lavergne A, Aegerter PH, Megraud F, Palazzo L, de Mascarel A, Molina T, Rambaud JL (2001) Predictive factors for regression of gastric MALT lymphoma after anti-Helicobacter pylori treatment. Gut 48(3):297–303

Sackmann M, Morgner A, Rudolph B, Neubauer A, Thiede C, Schulz H, Kraemer W, Boersch G, Rohde P, Seifert E, Stolte M, Bayerdoerffer E (1997) Regression of gastric MALT lymphoma after eradication of Helicobacter pylori is predicted by endosonographic staging. MALT Lymphoma Study Group. Gastroenterology 113(4):1087–1090 S0016508597004599 [pii]

Safar V, Dupuis J, Itti E, Jardin F, Fruchart C, Bardet S, Vera P, Copie-Bergman C, Rahmouni A, Tilly H, Meignan M, Haioun C (2012) Interim [18F]fluorodeoxyglucose positron emission tomography scan in diffuse large B-cell lymphoma treated with anthracycline-based chemotherapy plus rituximab. J Clin Oncol 30(2):184–190. doi:10.1200/JCO.2011.38.2648 JCO.2011.38.2648 [pii]

Salles G, Seymour JF, Offner F, Lopez-Guillermo A, Belada D, Xerri L, Feugier P, Bouabdallah R, Catalano JV, Brice P, Caballero D, Haioun C, Pedersen LM, Delmer A, Simpson D, Leppa S, Soubeyran P, Hagenbeek A, Casasnovas O, Intragumtornchai T, Ferme C, da Silva MG, Sebban C, Lister A, Estell JA, Milone G, Sonet A, Mendila M, Coiffier B, Tilly H (2011) Rituximab maintenance for 2 years in patients with high tumour burden follicular lymphoma responding to rituximab plus chemotherapy (PRIMA): a phase 3, randomised controlled trial. Lancet 377(9759):42–51. doi:10.1016/S0140-6736(10)62175-7 S0140-6736(10)62175-7 [pii]

Salloum E, Doria R, Schubert W, Zelterman D, Holford T, Roberts KB, Farber LR, Kiehl RK, Cardinale J, Cooper DL (1996) Second solid tumors in patients with Hodgkin's disease cured after radiation or chemotherapy plus adjuvant low-dose radiation. J Clin Oncol 14(9):2435–2443

Sasse S, Klimm B, Gorgen H, Fuchs M, Heyden-Honerkamp A, Lohri A, Koch O, Wilhelm M, Trenn G, Finke J, Muller RP, Diehl V, Eich HT, Borchmann P, Engert A (2012) Comparing long-term toxicity and efficacy of combined modality treatment including extended- or involved-field radiotherapy in early-stage Hodgkin's lymphoma. Ann Oncol. doi:10.1093/annonc/mds110 mds110 [pii]

Savage KJ, Harris NL, Vose JM, Ullrich F, Jaffe ES, Connors JM, Rimsza L, Pileri SA, Chhanabhai M, Gascoyne RD, Armitage JO, Weisenburger DD (2008) ALK- anaplastic large-cell lymphoma is clinically and immunophenotypically different from both ALK + ALCL and peripheral T-cell lymphoma, not otherwise specified: report from the International Peripheral T-Cell Lymphoma Project. Blood 111(12):5496–5504. doi:10.1182/blood-2008-01-134270 blood-2008-01-134270 [pii]

Savage KJ, Johnson NA, Ben-Neriah S, Connors JM, Sehn LH, Farinha P, Horsman DE, Gascoyne RD (2009) MYC gene rearrangements are associated with a poor prognosis in diffuse large B-cell lymphoma patients treated with R-CHOP chemotherapy. Blood 114(17):3533–3537. doi:10.1182/blood-2009-05-220095 blood-2009-05-220095 [pii]

Savage KJ, Skinnider B, Al-Mansour M, Sehn LH, Gascoyne RD, Connors JM (2011) Treating limited-stage nodular lymphocyte predominant Hodgkin lymphoma similarly to classical Hodgkin lymphoma with ABVD may improve outcome. Blood 118(17):4585–4590. doi:10.1182/blood-2011-07-365932 blood-2011-07-365932 [pii]

Schellong G, Riepenhausen M, Bruch C, Kotthoff S, Vogt J, Bolling T, Dieckmann K, Potter R, Heinecke A, Bramswig J, Dorffel W (2010) Late valvular and other cardiac diseases after different doses of mediastinal radiotherapy for Hodgkin disease in children and adolescents: report from the longitudinal GPOH follow-up project of the German-Austrian DAL-HD studies. Pediatr Blood Cancer 55(6):1145–1152. doi:10.1002/pbc.22664

Schlembach PJ, Wilder RB, Tucker SL, Ha CS, Rodriguez MA, Hess MA, Cabanillas FF, Cox JD (2000) Impact of involved field radiotherapy after CHOP-based chemotherapy on stage III-IV, intermediate grade and large-cell immunoblastic lymphomas. Int J Radiat Oncol Biol Phys 48(4):1107–1110 S0360-3016(00)00760-4 [pii]

Senff NJ, Hoefnagel JJ, Jansen PM, Vermeer MH, van Baarlen J, Blokx WA, Canninga-van Dijk MR, Geerts ML, Hebeda KM, Kluin PM, Lam KH, Meijer CJ, Willemze R (2007a) Reclassification of 300 primary cutaneous B-Cell lymphomas according to the new WHO-EORTC classification for cutaneous lymphomas: comparison with previous classifications and identification of prognostic markers. J Clin Oncol 25(12):1581–1587. doi:10.1200/JCO.2006.09.6396 JCO.2006.09.6396 [pii]

Senff NJ, Hoefnagel JJ, Neelis KJ, Vermeer MH, Noordijk EM, Willemze R (2007b) Results of radiotherapy in 153 primary cutaneous B-Cell lymphomas classified according to the WHO-EORTC classification. Arch Dermatol 143(12):1520–1526. doi:10.1001/archderm.143.12.1520 143/12/1520 [pii]

Senff NJ, Noordijk EM, Kim YH, Bagot M, Berti E, Cerroni L, Dummer R, Duvic M, Hoppe RT, Pimpinelli N, Rosen ST, Vermeer MH, Whittaker S, Willemze R (2008) European Organization for Research and Treatment of Cancer and International Society for Cutaneous Lymphoma consensus recommendations for the management of cutaneous B-cell lymphomas. Blood 112(5):1600–1609. doi:10.1182/blood-2008-04-152850 blood-2008-04-152850 [pii]

Shah GD, Yahalom J, Correa DD, Lai RK, Raizer JJ, Schiff D, LaRocca R, Grant B, DeAngelis LM, Abrey LE (2007) Combined immunochemotherapy with reduced whole-brain radiotherapy for newly diagnosed primary CNS lymphoma. J Clin Oncol 25(30):4730–4735. doi:10.1200/JCO.2007.12.5062 25/30/4730 [pii]

Shibamoto Y, Ogino H, Hasegawa M, Suzuki K, Nishio M, Fujii T, Kato E, Ishihara S, Sougawa M, Kenjo M, Kawamura T, Hayabuchi N (2005) Results of radiation monotherapy for primary central nervous system lymphoma in the 1990s. Int J Radiat Oncol

Biol Phys 62(3):809–813. doi:10.1016/j.ijrobp.2004.12.043 S0360-3016(04)03166-9 [pii]

Shustik J, Quinn M, Connors JM, Gascoyne RD, Skinnider B, Sehn LH (2011) Follicular non-Hodgkin lymphoma grades 3A and 3B have a similar outcome and appear incurable with anthracycline-based therapy. Ann Oncol 22(5):1164–1169 10.1093/annonc/mdq574mdq574 [pii]

Sibon D, Fournier M, Briere J, Lamant L, Haioun C, Coiffier B, Bologna S, Morel P, Gabarre J, Hermine O, Sonet A, Gisselbrecht C, Delsol G, Gaulard P, Tilly H (2012) Long-term outcome of adults with systemic anaplastic large-cell lymphoma treated within the Groupe d'Etude des Lymphomes de l'Adulte Trials. J Clin Oncol 30(32):3939–3946. doi:10.1200/JCO.2012.42.2345 JCO.2012.42.2345 [pii]

Smith BD, Glusac EJ, McNiff JM, Smith GL, Heald PW, Cooper DL, Wilson LD (2004) Primary cutaneous B-cell lymphoma treated with radiotherapy: a comparison of the European Organization for Research and Treatment of Cancer and the WHO classification systems. J Clin Oncol 22(4):634–639. doi:10.1200/JCO.2004.08.044 JCO.2004.08.044 [pii]

Solal-Celigny P, Roy P, Colombat P, White J, Armitage JO, Arranz-Saez R, Au WY, Bellei M, Brice P, Caballero D, Coiffier B, Conde-Garcia E, Doyen C, Federico M, Fisher RI, Garcia-Conde JF, Guglielmi C, Hagenbeek A, Haioun C, LeBlanc M, Lister AT, Lopez-Guillermo A, McLaughlin P, Milpied N, Morel P, Mounier N, Proctor SJ, Rohatiner A, Smith P, Soubeyran P, Tilly H, Vitolo U, Zinzani PL, Zucca E, Montserrat E (2004) Follicular lymphoma international prognostic index. Blood 104(5):1258–1265

Spaepen K, Stroobants S, Dupont P, Van Steenweghen S, Thomas J, Vandenberghe P, Vanuytsel L, Bormans G, Balzarini J, De Wolf-Peeters C, Mortelmans L, Verhoef G (2001) Prognostic value of positron emission tomography (PET) with fluorine-18 fluorodeoxyglucose ([18F]FDG) after first-line chemotherapy in non-Hodgkin's lymphoma: is [18F]FDG-PET a valid alternative to conventional diagnostic methods? J Clin Oncol 19(2):414–419

Straus DJ, Portlock CS, Qin J, Myers J, Zelenetz AD, Moskowitz C, Noy A, Goy A, Yahalom J (2004) Results of a prospective randomized clinical trial of doxorubicin, bleomycin, vinblastine, and dacarbazine (ABVD) followed by radiation therapy (RT) versus ABVD alone for stages I, II, and IIIA nonbulky Hodgkin disease. Blood 104(12):3483–3489

Suzuki R, Kagami Y, Takeuchi K, Kami M, Okamoto M, Ichinohasama R, Mori N, Kojima M, Yoshino T, Yamabe H, Shiota M, Mori S, Ogura M, Hamajima N, Seto M, Suchi T, Morishima Y, Nakamura S (2000) Prognostic significance of CD56 expression for ALK-positive and ALK-negative anaplastic large-cell lymphoma of T/null cell phenotype. Blood 96(9):2993–3000

Swerdlow AJ, Barber JA, Hudson GV, Cunningham D, Gupta RK, Hancock BW, Horwich A, Lister TA, Linch DC (2000) Risk of second malignancy after Hodgkin's disease in a collaborative British cohort: the relation to age at treatment. J Clin Oncol 18(3):498–509

Swerdlow AJ, Higgins CD, Smith P, Cunningham D, Hancock BW, Horwich A, Hoskin PJ, Lister A, Radford JA, Rohatiner AZ, Linch DC (2007) Myocardial infarction mortality risk after treatment for Hodgkin disease: a collaborative British cohort study. J Natl Cancer Inst 99(3):206–214. doi:10.1093/jnci/djk029 99/3/206 [pii]

Talpur R, Singh L, Daulat S, Liu P, Seyfer S, Trynosky T, Wei W (2009) Duvic M (2012) Long-term outcomes of 1,263 patients with mycosis fungoides and Sezary syndrome from 1982 to. Clin Cancer Res 18(18):5051–5060. doi:10.1158/1078-0432.CCR-12-0604 1078-0432.CCR-12-0604 [pii]

The International Non-Hodgkin's Lymphoma Prognostic Factors Project (1993) A predictive model for aggressive non-Hodgkin's lymphoma. N Engl J Med 329(14):987–994

Travis LB, Curtis RE, Boice JD Jr, Hankey BF, Fraumeni JF Jr (1991) Second cancers following non-Hodgkin's lymphoma. Cancer 67(7):2002–2009

Trotman J, Fournier M, Lamy T, Seymour JF, Sonet A, Janikova A, Shpilberg O, Gyan E, Tilly H, Estell J, Forsyth C, Decaudin D, Fabiani B, Gabarre J, Salles B, Van Den Neste E, Canioni D, Garin E, Fulham M, Vander Borght T, Salles G (2011) Positron emission tomography-computed tomography (PET-CT) after induction therapy is highly predictive of patient outcome in follicular lymphoma: analysis of PET-CT in a subset of PRIMA trial participants. J Clin Oncol 29(23):3194–3200. doi:10.1200/JCO.2011.35.0736 JCO.2011.35.0736 [pii]

Tsang RW, Gospodarowicz MK, Pintilie M, Wells W, Hodgson DC, Sun A, Crump M, Patterson BJ (2003) Localized mucosa-associated lymphoid tissue lymphoma treated with radiation therapy has excellent clinical outcome. J Clin Oncol 21(22):4157–4164

Tward JD, Wendland MM, Shrieve DC, Szabo A, Gaffney DK (2006) The risk of secondary malignancies over 30 years after the treatment of non-Hodgkin lymphoma. Cancer 107(1):108–115. doi:10.1002/cncr.21971

van Oers MH, Van Glabbeke M, Giurgea L, Klasa R, Marcus RE, Wolf M, Kimby E, van t Veer M, Vranovsky A, Holte H, Hagenbeek A (2010) Rituximab maintenance treatment of relapsed/resistant follicular non-Hodgkin's lymphoma: long-term outcome of the EORTC 20981 phase III randomized intergroup study. J Clin Oncol 28(17):2853–2858. doi:10.1200/JCO.2009.26.5827 JCO.2009.26.5827 [pii]

Vaughan Hudson B, Vaughan Hudson G, MacLennan KA, Anderson L, Linch DC (1994) Clinical stage 1 non-Hodgkin's lymphoma: long-term follow-up of patients treated by the British National Lymphoma Investigation with radiotherapy alone as initial therapy. Br J Cancer 69(6):1088–1093

von Tresckow B, Plutschow A, Fuchs M, Klimm B, Markova J, Lohri A, Kral Z, Greil R, Topp MS, Meissner J, Zijlstra JM, Soekler M, Stein H, Eich HT, Mueller RP, Diehl V, Borchmann P, Engert A (2012) Dose-intensification in early unfavorable Hodgkin's lymphoma: final analysis of the German Hodgkin study group HD14 trial. J Clin Oncol 30(9):907–913. doi:10.1200/JCO.2011.38.5807 JCO.2011.38.5807 [pii]

Wahlin BE, Yri OE, Kimby E, Holte H, Delabie J, Smeland EB, Sundstrom C, Christensson B, Sander B (2012) Clinical significance of the WHO grades of follicular lymphoma in a population-based cohort of 505 patients with long follow-up times. Br J Haematol 156(2):225–233. doi:10.1111/j.1365-2141.2011.08942.x

Wahner-Roedler DL, Nelson DF, Croghan IT, Achenbach SJ, Crowson CS, Hartmann LC, O'Fallon WM (2003) Risk of breast cancer and breast cancer characteristics in women treated with supradiaphragmatic radiation for Hodgkin lymphoma: Mayo clinic experience. Mayo Clin Proc 78(6):708–715. doi:10.4065/78.6.708 S0025-6196(11)62460-9 [pii]

Weihrauch MR, Re D, Scheidhauer K, Ansen S, Dietlein M, Bischoff S, Bohlen H, Wolf J, Schicha H, Diehl V, Tesch H (2001) Thoracic positron emission tomography using 18F-fluorodeoxyglucose for the evaluation of residual mediastinal Hodgkin disease. Blood 98(10):2930–2934

Wolden SL, Hancock SL, Carlson RW, Goffinet DR, Jeffrey SS, Hoppe RT (2000) Management of breast cancer after Hodgkin's disease. J Clin Oncol 18(4):765–772

Woo DK, Jones CR, Vanoli-Storz MN, Kohler S, Reddy S, Advani R, Hoppe RT, Kim YH (2009) Prognostic factors in primary cutaneous anaplastic large cell lymphoma: characterization of clinical subset with worse outcome. Arch Dermatol 145(6):667–674 10.1001/archdermatol.2009.74145/6/667 [pii]

Wundisch T, Thiede C, Morgner A, Dempfle A, Gunther A, Liu H, Ye H, Du MQ, Kim TD, Bayerdorffer E, Stolte M, Neubauer A (2005) Long-term follow-up of gastric MALT lymphoma after Helicobacter pylori eradication. J Clin Oncol 23(31):8018–8024. doi:10.1200/JCO.2005.02.3903 JCO.2005.02.3903 [pii]

Yahalom J, Petrek JA, Biddinger PW, Kessler S, Dershaw DD, McCormick B, Osborne MP, Kinne DA, Rosen PP (1992) Breast cancer in patients irradiated for Hodgkin's disease: a clinical and pathologic analysis of 45 events in 37 patients. J Clin Oncol 10(11):1674–1681

Yang DH, Min JJ, Song HC, Jeong YY, Chung WK, Bae SY, Ahn JS, Kim YK, Bom HS, Chung IJ, Kim HJ, Lee JJ (2011) Prognostic significance of interim (1)(8)F-FDG PET/CT after three or four cycles of R-CHOP chemotherapy in the treatment of diffuse large B-cell lymphoma. Eur J Cancer 47(9):1312–1318. doi:10.1016/j.ejca.2010.12.027 S0959-8049(11)00038-4 [pii]

Ziepert M, Hasenclever D, Kuhnt E, Glass B, Schmitz N, Pfreundschuh M, Loeffler M (2010) Standard International prognostic index remains a valid predictor of outcome for patients with aggressive CD20 + B-cell lymphoma in the rituximab era. J Clin Oncol 28(14):2373–2380. doi:10.1200/JCO.2009.26.2493

Zinzani PL, Quaglino P, Pimpinelli N, Berti E, Baliva G, Rupoli S, Martelli M, Alaibac M, Borroni G, Chimenti S, Alterini R, Alinari L, Fierro MT, Cappello N, Pileri A, Soligo D, Paulli M, Pileri S, Santucci M, Bernengo MG (2006) Prognostic factors in primary cutaneous B-cell lymphoma: the Italian Study Group for Cutaneous Lymphomas. J Clin Oncol 24(9):1376–1382. doi:10.1200/JCO.2005.03.6285 JCO.2005.03.6285 [pii]

Zinzani PL, Gandolfi L, Broccoli A, Argnani L, Fanti S, Pellegrini C, Stefoni V, Derenzini E, Quirini F, Baccarani M (2011) Midtreatment 18F-fluorodeoxyglucose positron-emission tomography in aggressive non-Hodgkin lymphoma. Cancer 117(5):1010–1018. doi:10.1002/cncr.25579

Zinzani PL, Rigacci L, Stefoni V, Broccoli A, Puccini B, Castagnoli A, Vaggelli L, Zanoni L, Argnani L, Baccarani M, Fanti S (2012) Early interim 18F-FDG PET in Hodgkin's lymphoma: evaluation on 304 patients. Eur J Nucl Med Mol Imaging 39(1):4–12. doi:10.1007/s00259-011-1916-8

Zittoun R, Audebert A, Hoerni B, Bernadou A, Krulik M, Rojouan J, Eghbali H, Merle-Beral H, Parlier Y, Diebold J et al (1985) Extended versus involved fields irradiation combined with MOPP chemotherapy in early clinical stages of Hodgkin's disease. J Clin Oncol 3(2):207–214

Brain Metastases

Paul W. Sperduto and Laurie E. Gaspar

...tract

...ı metastases are a common problem historically ...ated with poor outcomes, however the past sense ...ıpeutic nihilism is no longer appropriate because ... understand prognosis and the factors determin- ...osis vary widely by diagnosis. Fifty years of ...ials have demonstrated a gradual shift in the ... of death from neurologic to non-neurologic (50 % ...eurologic in the early trials to less than 20 % in recent trials). This shift correlates with improvements in local control rates in the radiosurgery era. One-year local control with WBRT alone, SRS alone, and WBRT plus SRS is approximately 50 %, 70–80 %, and 80–90 %, respectively. Evidence-based guidelines and randomized trials are reviewed and elucidate the general principles of management, aiding the clinician regarding choice of treatment (surgery, stereotactic radiosurgery (SRS) and whole brain radiation therapy). Notably, 15 randomized trials of chemotherapy or radiosensitizers have failed to improve survival. On-going trials address quality-of-life and cognitive outcomes (i.e., the extent to which cognitive decline is due to tumor progression versus treatment-related toxicity). Better control of extra-cranial tumor will be necessary in order to improve overall survival for most patients

1 Introduction

In 2012, over 1.6 million people were diagnosed with cancer in the United States (American Cancer Society 2012). Approximately 15 % of these patients (240,000) will develop brain metastases (Zimm et al. 1981; Wen et al. 2001). The incidence of brain metastases is more than 10 times that of primary malignant brain tumors. If untreated, the median survival is about 10 weeks. (Horton et al. 1971) Thus, brain metastases are a common and serious problem

P. W. Sperduto (✉)
Minneapolis Radiation Oncology, University of Minnesota, Gamma Knife Center, Minneapolis, MN, USA
e-mail: Psperduto@mropa.com

L. E. Gaspar
University of Colorado, Denver, CO, USA

C. Nieder and L. E. Gaspar (eds.), *Decision Tools for Radiation Oncology*, Medical Radiology. Radiation Oncology,
DOI: 10.1007/174_2013_856, © Springer-Verlag Berlin Heidelberg 2013
Published Online: 15 June 2013

Table 1 Incidence of brain metastases by primary tumor type and median interval from primary diagnosis to brain metastases

Primary site	Percentage of all brain metastases	Median interval (mo) Dx to brain metastases
Lung cancer	51	2–9
Non-small cell	44	
Small cell lung cancer	7	
Breast cancer	15	24–40
Melanoma	11	15–41
Renal cell carcinoma	7	12–27
Gastrointestinal cancers	5	22–33
Other	11	

in oncology. In the past, survival was uniformly poor and a fatalistic futility dominated management recommendations. With advances in systemic therapy and technology such as stereotactic radiosurgery, this nihilism has been replaced with the ability to tailor therapy to appropriate subgroups, based on expected survival. It is now understood that the prognosis for patients with brain metastases varies widely and a one-size-fits-all treatment paradigm is no longer appropriate. Prognosis and the factors that determine prognosis vary by diagnosis (Sperduto et al. 2012a, b; Suki 2004). These diagnosis-specific prognostic factors include a variety of clinical factors and genetic mutations. It is incumbent upon the physician to understand the prognosis in order to assist the patient and his/her family in making appropriate choices regarding treatment and end-of-life care.

Table 1 shows the primary tumor most commonly associated with the development of brain metastases (Sperduto et al. 2012b). Lung cancer accounts for the highest number of cases of brain metastases but patients with melanoma have the highest incidence of developing brain metastases. Melanoma represents only 4 % of all cancers but 11 % of melanoma patients will develop brain metastases (Suki 2004; Ribalta and Fuller 2004).

2 Prognosis

2.1 Natural Course and Cause of Death

If brain metastases are not treated, the median survival is expected to be approximately 10 weeks (Horton et al. 1971). With steroids and whole brain radiation, the median survival is 4–6 months (Patchell et al. 1990; Noordjik et al. 1994; Mintz et al. 1996; Andrews et al. 2004). Clinical trials over the past 50 years have demonstrated a gradual shift in the cause of death from neurologic to non-neurologic. The early RTOG trials (Borgelt et al. 1980; Kurtz et al. 1981) showed approximately 50 % of patients died of neurologic causes whereas the most recent trials show less than 20 % of patients with brain metastases die from neurologic causes (Sperduto et al. 2013). This reflects not only the improvements in treatment for brain metastases as well as the refractory nature of systemic disease.

2.2 Prognostic Indices

As recently as 1997, a radiation oncology textbook recommended the following rudimentary functional scale be used to assess prognosis in patients with brain metastases: Level I—fully functional, able to work; Level II—fully functional, not able to work; Level III—stays in bed, needs help half the time, and; Level IV—requires help all the time (Kagan 1997). The original work on more formal prognostic indices for patients with brain metastases dates back to 1997, when Gaspar et al. published a seminal manuscript on a prognostic index for patients with brain metastases, the Radiation Therapy Oncology Group's Recursive Partitioning Analysis (RTOG-RPA) (Fig. 1) (Gaspar et al. 1997). The RTOG-RPA was based on age, Karnofsky performance status (KPS), whether the primary tumor was controlled, whether extracranial metastases were present or absent. The median survival for patients with RPA class I, II and III were 7.1, 4.2 and 2.3 months, respectively. The index was validated and quickly adopted for purposes of stratification in clinical trials (Gaspar et al. 2000). (Weaknesses of the RTOG-RPA are that it is not diagnosis-specific and the determination of both primary tumor control and the presence of extracranial metastases can vary widely based on the type, technique and timing of restaging studies. Other previously published indices (Score Index for Radiosurgery (SIR) and the Basic Score for Brain Metastases (BSBM)) share the same weaknesses (Weltman et al. 2000; Lorenzoni et al. 2004) (Tables 2, 3). The SIR was found to be more predictive of survival in radiosurgery patients than the RPA. The median survival for patients who scored from 1–3, 4–7, and 8–10 was 2.91, 7 and 31.38 months, respectively ($p = 0.0001$) Similarly, the BSBM was more predictive of survival following radiosurgery than the RPA but was proposed as a simpler method than SIR. The median survival for patients who scored 3, 2, 1 or 0 was more than 32, 13.1, 3.3, and 1.9 months, respectively ($p < 0.0001$).

The graded prognostic assessment (GPA) is a newer prognostic index for patients with brain metastases (Sperduto et al. 2008). This prognostic index was originally developed from a database of 1,960 patients accrued to four Radiation Therapy Oncology Group (RTOG) protocols for patients with brain metastases treated with whole brain radiation therapy (WBRT) (Sause et al. 1993; Murray et al.

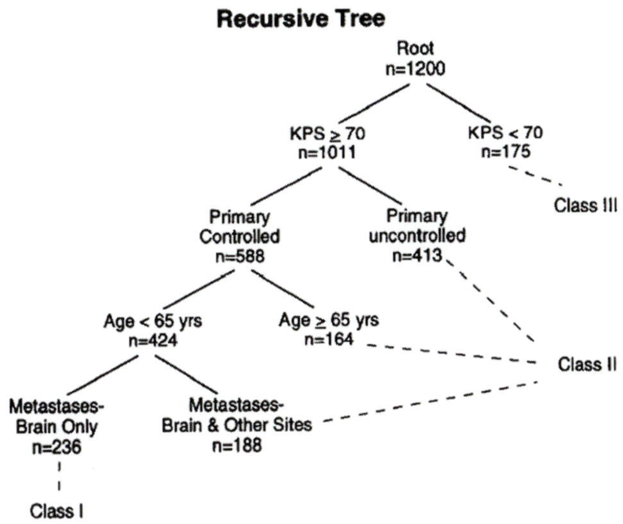

Fig. 1 Recursive partitioning analysis (RPA)

Table 2 Score index for radiosurgery (SIR)

	0	1	2
Age (years)	≥60	51–59	≤50
Karnofsky performance status	<50	60–70	>70
Systemic disease status	PD	PR-SD	CR-NED
Largest lesion volume (cc)	>13	5–13	<5
Number lesions	>3	2	1

PD Progressive disease, *PR* Partial remission, *SD* Stable disease, *CR* Complete clinical remission, *NED* No evidence of disease

Table 3 Basic score for brain metastases (BS-BM)

	0	1
KPS	50–70	80–100
Control of primary tumor	No	Yes
Extracranial metastases	Yes	No

1997; Komarnicky et al. 1991; Phillips et al. 1994). The diagnosis-specific prognostic indices was then refined based on a second, independent multi-institutional retrospective analysis of 4,259 other patients with brain metastases from breast carcinoma, small cell and non-small cell lung carcinoma, gastrointestinal cancers, melanoma and renal cell carcinoma treated with WBRT and/or SRS (Sperduto et al. 2010). The breast cancer-specific GPA index was then further refined using additional variables, including HER2 and ER/PR status (Sperduto et al. 2012b). In that study, two statistical methodologies, multivariate Cox regression (MCR) and recursive partitioning analysis (RPA), were used to identify and weight the prognostic factors that were significant for each diagnosis. The prognostic factors significant for survival vary by diagnosis and each are weighted in proportion to their regression coefficients. All of the diagnosis-specific GPA scales are set on a 4.0 scale in which a GPA of 4.0 represents the best prognosis and 0.0, the worst. A user-friendly worksheet to calculate a patient's GPA is shown in Table 4 (Sperduto et al. 2012a). The median survival by diagnosis and GPA is shown in Table 5.

The GPA has been independently validated by multiple centers (Likacheva et al. 2012; Guo et al. 2012; Viana et al. 2012; Nieder and Mehta 2009; Nieder et al. 2008, 2009a, b, 2012; Villa et al. 2011) and is now being used to stratify patients in multiple on-going clinical trials of the RTOG.

3 Treatment Options, Outcomes and Toxicity

3.1 General Principles

Recently published evidence-based guidelines reflect the many options and nuances of managing this patient population (Linskey et al. 2010; Tsao et al. 2012; Mehta et al. 2005; Kalkanis et al. 2010). A common problem faced by clinicians when attempting to interpret guidelines is that the term "in selected patients" has become so ubiquitous in guidelines and review articles that it renders them edentulous. This creates a heuristic imbroglio of clinical science, defeating the purpose of the guidelines and suggesting almost any treatment option is acceptable. Only randomized trials provide Level I evidence and are summarized in Table 6. Notably 11 randomized trials of chemotherapy and four randomized trials of radiosensitizers have failed to a survival benefit. (Sperduto 2013, French, Robinet, DeAngelis 1989a, Postmus, Ushio, Antonadou, Mornex, Knisely, Neuhaus, Lee, Aiken, Suh, Mehta, Eyre).

3.2 Local Control of Brain Metastases

Reports on 1-year local control rates for brain metastases treated with WBRT alone, WBRT plus SRS and SRS alone vary widely, even among randomized trials. The 1-year local control rate for WBRT alone ranges from 0 to 71 % (Patchell et al. 1990; Andrews et al. 2004; Kondziolka et al. 1999). 1 year local control with WBRT plus SRS was 80–90 % in two randomized trials (Andrews et al. 2004; Aoyama et al. 2006). The 1-year local control rate for SRS alone is 73 % (Aoyama et al. 2006).

4 Toxicity

4.1 Radiation Necrosis

Radiation necrosis is extremely rare after WBRT alone but not uncommon after SRS. The toxicity associated with

Table 4 Diagnosis-specific prognostic factors and graded prognostic assessment (GPA) worksheet to estimate survival for newly diagnosed brain metastases

		GPA scoring criteria					Patient
Non-small cell and small cell lung cancer	Prognostic factor	0	0.5	1.0			Score
	Age	>60	50–60	<50			—
	KPS	<70	70–80	90–100			—
	ECM	Present	–	Absent			—
	#BM	>3	2–3	1			—
				Sum total			—
MST (mo) by GPA: 0–1.0 = 3.0, 1.5–2.0 = 5.5, 2.5–3.0 = 9.4, 3.5–4.0 = 14.8							
Melanoma	Prognostic factor	0		1.0		2.0	Score
	KPS	<70		70–80		90–100	—
	#BM	>3		2–3		1	—
						Sum total	—
MST (mo) by GPA: 0–1.0 = 3.4, 1.5–2.0 = 4.7, 2.5–3.0 = 8.8, 3.5–4.0 = 13.2							
Breast cancer	Prognostic factor	0	0.5	1.0	1.5	2.0	Score
	KPS	≤50	60	70–80	90–100	N/a	—
	Subtype	Basal	N/a	LumA	HER2	LumB	—
	Age	≥60	<60	N/a	N/a	N/a	—
						Sum total	—
Subtype:	Basal = Triple negative (ER/PR/HER2-neg)						
	LumA = Luminal A (ER/PR-pos, HER2-neg)						
	LumB = Luminal B (Triple Positive, ER/PR/HER2-pos)						
	HER2 = HER2-pos, ER/PR-neg						
MST (mo) by GPA: 0–1.0 = 3.4, 1.5–2.0 = 7.7, 2.5–3.0 = 15.1, 3.5–4.0 = 25.3							
Renal cell carcinoma	Prognostic factor	0		1.0		2.0	Score
	KPS	<70		70–80		90-100	—
	#BM	>3		2–3		1	—
						Sum total	—
MST (mo) by GPA: 0–1.0 = 3.3, 1.5–2.0 = 7.3, 2.5–3.0 = 11.3, 3.5–4.0 = 14.8							
GI cancers	Prognostic Factor	0	1	2	3	4	Score
	KPS	<70	70	80	90	100	—
MST (mo) by GPA: 0–1.0 = 3.1, 2.0 = 4.4, 3.0 = 6.9, 4.0 = 13.5							

GPA Graded prognostic assessment, *KPS* Karnofsky performance score, *ECM* Extra-cranial metastases, *#BM* Number of brain metastases, *ER* Estrogen receptor, *PR* Progesterone receptor, *HER2* Human epidermal growth factor receptor 2

Table 5 Median survival time (MST) by graded prognostic assessment (GPA) score

Diagnosis	Overall MST (months)	MST (months) by diagnosis-specific GPA			
		GPA 0–1	GPA 1.5–2	GPA 2.5–3	GPA 3.5–4
NSCLC	7.0	3.0	5.5	9.4	14.8
SCLC	4.9	2.8	4.9	7.7	17.1
Melanoma	6.7	3.4	4.7	8.8	13.2
Renal cell	9.6	3.3	7.3	11.3	14.8
GI	5.4	3.1	4.4	6.9	13.5
Breast	13.8	3.4	7.7	15.1	25.3
Total	7.2	3.1	5.4	9.6	16.7

NSCLC Non small cell lung cancer, *SCLC* Small cell lung cancer, *GI* Gastrointestinal

Table 6 Selected randomized trials in patients with brain metastases and summary conclusions

Topic	Author	Year	N	Conclusion
A. WBRT versus WBRT + S in patients with solitary operable brain metastases	Patchell (NEJM)	1990	48	Surgery improves survival from 15 to 40 weeks ($p < 0.01$)
	Noordjik (IJROP)	1994	63	Surgery improves survival from 6 to 10 months ($p < 0.04$)
	Mintz (Cancer)	1996	84	Surgery did not improve survival
B. S versus S + WBRT in patients with solitary operable brain metastasis	Patchell (JAMA)	1998	95	WBRT decreases recurrence rate in brain from 70 to 18 % ($p < 0.001$), not powered to assess survival
	Kocher (JCO)	2011	359	Schema was S or SRS ± WBRT in pts with 1–3 metastases. WBRT reduced recurrence rate in brain and neurologic death but did not improve duration of functional independence. The study was not powered to assess survival
C. WBRT versus WBRT + SRS in patients with 1–3 brain metastases	Andrews (Lancet)	2004	333	WBRT + SRS improves survival for patients with one metastasis from 4.9 to 6.5 months ($p < 0.04$) and improves local control, response rate, performance status and steroid dependence in patients with 1–3 metastases. Unplanned subset analysis shows improved survival in NSCLC from 3.9 to 5.9 months ($p = 0.05$)
D. SRS versus SRS + WBRT in patients with 1-4 brain metastases	Aoyama (JAMA)	2006	132	WBRT + SRS improves recurrence rate in brain from 76 to 47 % ($p < 0.001$) but did not improve survival. WBRT provided neurological and neurocognitive function protection, not decline. Study was not powered to assess survival
E. WBRT + SRS versus WBRT + SRS + chemo	11 trials (Sperduto et al. 2013; French et al. 1952; Robinet et al. 2001; DeAngelis et al.1989a; Postmus et al. 2000; Ushio et al. 1991; Antonadou et al. 2002; Mornex et al. 2003; Knisely et al. 2008; Neuhaus et al. 2009; Lee et al. 2008)			No survival benefit with addition of chemotheraphy
F. WBRT versus WBRT + radiosensitizer	Four trials (Aiken et al. 1984; Suh et al. 2006; Mehta et al. 2003, 2005; Eyre et al. 1984)			No survival benefit with addition of radiosensitizers

stereotactic radiosurgery was well-defined by RTOG 9005, a dose escalation study (Shaw et al. 1996, 2000). The maximum tolerated dose (MTD) was found to vary with tumor size as follows: for tumors <2.0 cm, 2.1–3.0 cm and 3.1–4.0 cm, the MTD was 24, 18 and 15 Gy. The risk of radiation necrosis following SRS is dependent on both radiation dose and volume (Flickinger 1989). It may not develop until 6–36 months after SRS.

Differentiating radiation necrosis from tumor recurrence radiographically can be difficult. Advanced imaging techniques such as MR perfusion scan may be of benefit in distinguishing tumor recurrence from radiation necrosis (Hoefnagels et al. 2009; Mitsuya et al. 2010). Dequesada et al. (2008) studied a novel parameter, the "Lesion Quotient" (LQ), defined as "the ratio of maximal cross-sectional area of a definable nodule on T2-weighted imaging to the corresponding maximal cross-sectional area of T1-contrast enhancement," and found a LQ of <0.3, between 0.3 and 0.6, and >0.6 correlated well with radiation necrosis, mixed findings of necrosis and tumor, and tumor progression/recurrence, respectively. Others have studied a ratio known as a "T1/T2 mismatch," defined as "lack of a clear and defined lesion margin on T2-weighted images compared to the margin of contrast uptake on T1-weighted images," and found mismatches correlated with radiation necrosis (Kano et al. 2010).

Sneed reported a retrospective analysis of 436 patients with 2,057 brain metastases in which they used surgical pathology, serial MRI and perfusion MRI to determine the risk factors for radiation necrosis after radiosurgery for brain metastases (Sneed et al. 2012). The appearance of necrosis was noted to be variable and frequently indistinguishable from tumor progression at single points in time. Review of serial imaging was key, along with surgical pathology when available. The risk of necrosis at 1 year after SRS varies significantly by primary tumor type, diameter of brain metastasis and prior radiation. Specifically, the risk of necrosis was 3–6 % for breast, 6–9 % for melanoma, 10–16 % for lung, and 15–23 % for kidney. The risk was 0, 2–4, 8–14, 17–24, 22–32 and 25–30 % for tumors of maximum diameter of ≤0.5, 0.6–1.0, 1.1–1.5, 1.6–2.0, 2.1–3.0 and >3 cm, respectively. Regarding the technique of, the risk of necrosis was 6–9 % for SRS alone, 7–15 % after prior WBRT, 12–17 % with concurrent WBRT and 35–43 % for repeat SRS after prior SRS.

4.2 Neurocognitive Dysfunction

Patients with brain metastases often have neurocognitive deficits prior to radiation therapy. Certainly, cognitive impairment is a common presenting symptom of patients with brain metastases resulting directly from the tumor burden in the brain. One trial demonstrated significant baseline neurocognitive abnormalities prior to treatment in 90.5 % of patients presenting with brain metastases (Mehta et al. 2003). Neurocognitive reassessment of patients in this trial following WBRT showed further decline in neurocognitive function strongly correlated with progressive disease in the brain (Meyers et al. 2004). Furthermore, many patients had received prior chemotherapy for their primary tumor, a well-documented cause of cognitive impairment. (Tannock et al. 2004).

Patchell found that giving WBRT after surgery actually improved neurologic outcomes compared to those who did not receive WBRT after surgery (Patchell et al. 1998). Regine demonstrated an increased rate of symptomatic recurrences and neurologic deficits when the tumor recurred (Regine et al. 2002). These findings are consistent with those of Aoyama et al. (2006). These studies raise concern that progression of brain metastases, seen commonly after local treatments such as surgery or SRS, is a much greater cause of neurocognitive dysfunction than WBRT.

Nonetheless, there is evidence that WBRT can cause neurocognitive decline. In an older study, DeAngelis found an association between dose per fraction and the risk of neurocognitive dysfunction at 1 year or longer (DeAngelis et al. 1989a, b). No dementia was found in the patients who received ≤300 cGy per fraction. Total WBRT dose is also likely related to the risk of cognitive decline (Le Pechoux et al. 2011). One randomized trial of SRS versus SRS plus WBRT was closed early after 58 patients were accrued because interim analysis suggested a high probability that patients in the SRS plus WBRT arm were significantly more likely to show a decline in learning and memory function at four months compared to those in the SRS alone arm (Chang et al. 2009). Because of concerns about the neurocognitive effects of WBRT, the RTOG recently completed a placebo-controlled, double-blind randomized trial of WBRT with and without memantine has previously been shown to be of benefit in vascular and Alzheimer's dementia (Brown et al. 2012). Even though no statistically significant difference was seen in delayed recall, patients treated with had better cognitive function over time. Memantine delayed time to cognitive decline and reduced the rate of decline in recognition memory, executive function and processing speed in patients receiving WBRT. An ongoing clinical trial of SRS versus SRS plus WBRT (NCCTG 0574/RTOG 0671) will further elucidate quality-of-life and cognitive outcomes for patients with brain metastases.

5 Conclusions and Future Directions

5.1 Conclusions

Take-home lessons from the aforementioned literature include the following.

- There is marked heterogeneity in outcomes for patients with brain metastases and these outcomes vary not only by diagnosis but also by diagnosis-specific prognostic factors.
- If the patient has a single brain metastasis with symptomatic mass effect in an operable location, surgery is appropriate. For operable patients with good performance status (e.g., KPS ≥ 70), limited extracranial disease, and a resectable brain metastasis, complete resection of the single brain metastasis improves the probability of extended survival. The addition of postoperative whole brain radiotherapy improves local and overall brain control.
- There have been no high quality randomized trials that have assessed whether selected patients with a small single brain metastasis, in surgically accessible sites, should undergo radiosurgery or resection. Adding WBRT did not improve overall survival or functional independence.
- For good prognosis patients with single brain metastases (less than 4 cm in size, in patients with good performance status and controlled extracranial disease), the use of radiosurgery added to WBRT improves survival, treated brain lesion control, and overall brain control as compared with WBRT alone.
- In good prognosis patients with multiple brain metastases (all less than 4 cm in size and up to 4 brain metastases in number), radiosurgery boost when added to WBRT improves treated brain lesion and overall brain control as compared with WBRT alone. As there is no survival advantage with radiosurgery added to WBRT in patients

with multiple brain metastases, WBRT alone may be considered.

- For selected patients with poor life expectancy (less than 3 months), the use of whole brain radiotherapy may or may not significantly improve symptoms from brain metastases. Comfort measures only, or short course (20 Gy in 5 daily fractions) whole brain radiotherapy, are reasonable options.
- Performance status is a key prognostic factor for all patients with brain metastases.
- Serial imaging and awareness of the risk factors for radiation necrosis are key to interpretation of follow-up brain MRIs in patients previously treated with radiation for brain metastases.
- Treating with SRS alone (omitting WBRT) is associated with an increased risk of recurrence elsewhere in the brain which is associated with neurocognitive decline. However, treating with SRS alone (omitting WBRT) does not negatively affect survival.
- Neurocognitive decline is more closely correlated with progressive tumor than with whole brain radiation therapy.

5.2 Future Directions

One of the first and most important lessons taught to radiation oncology residents is that for each patient, the physician must determine if the intent of treatment is curative or palliative. Historically and in almost all cases still today, if the patient has biopsy-proven or persuasive radiographic evidence of metastases, the patient was considered incurable and the entire focus turns to palliative care and quality of life. There is even some provocative literature to suggest cure with brain metastases is possible in oligometastatic disease (Weichselbaum and Hellman 2011). More recently, there is evidence of an abscopal effect consistent with radiation-induced immune enhancement (Postow et al. 2012; Stamell et al. 2013). The future directions of care for patients with brain metastases will ride the wave of personalized oncology care with improving systemic therapies based on the specific genetic mutations of the patient's tumor, immunotherapies (which may include radiation-induced immune enhancement—the abscopal effect) in conjunction with highly localized radiation, such as SRS or stereotactic body radiation therapy (SBRT). These developments should result in increased local control and survival, decreased toxicity, and improved quality of life.

References

Aiken R, Leavengood JM, Kim JH et al (1984) Metronidazole in the treatment of metastatic brain tumors: results of a controlled clinical trial. J Neurooncol 2:105–111

American Cancer Society (2012) Cancer facts and figures 2012. American Cancer Society, Atlanta

Andrews DW, Scott CB, Sperduto PW et al (2004) Whole brain radiation therapy with and without stereotactic radiosurgery boost for patients with one to three brain metastases: phase III results of the RTOG 9508 randomised trial. Lancet 363:1665–1672

Antonadou D, Paraskevaidis M, Saris G et al (2002) Phase II randomized trial of temozolomide and concurrent radiotherapy in patients with brain metastases. J Clin Oncol 20:3644–3650

Aoyama H, Shirato H, Tago M et al (2006) Stereotatic radiosurgery plus whole brain radiation therpay vs. stereotactic radiosurgery alone for treatment of brain metastases: a randomized controlled trial. JAMA 295:2483–2491

Borgelt B, Delber R, Kramer S et al (1980) The palliation of brain metastases: final results of the first two studies by the radiation therapy oncology group. Int J Radiat Oncol Biol Phys 6:1–9

Brown PD, Shook S, Laack NN et al (2012) Memantine for the prevention of cognitive dysfunction in patients receiving whole-brain radiation therapy (WBRT): first report of RTOG 0614, a placebo-controlled, double-blind randomized trial. Int J Radiat Oncol Biol Phys 84(supp):pS1

Chang EL, Wefel JS, Hess KR et al (2009) Neurocognition in patients with brain metastases treated with radiosurgery or radiosurgery plus whole-brain irradiation: a randomised controlled trial. Lancet Oncology 10(11):1037–1044

DeAngelis LM, Currie VE, Kim JH et al (1989a) The combined use of radiation therapy and lonidamide in the treatment of brain metastases. J Neurooncol 7:241–247

DeAngelis LM, Mandell LR, Thaler HT (1989b) The role of postoperative radiotherapy after resection of single brain metastasis. Neurosurgery 24:798–805

Dequesada IM, Quisling RG, Yachnis A et al (2008) Can standard magnetic resonance imaging reliably distinguish recurrent tumor from radiation necrosis after radiosurgery for brain metastasis? A radiographic-pathologic study. Neurosurgery 63(5):898–903.

Eyre HJ, Ohlsen JD, Frank J et al (1984) Randomized trial of radiotherapy versus radiotherapy plus metronidazole for the treatment of metastatic cancer to brain. J Neurooncol 2:325–330

Flickinger JC (1989) An integrated logistic formula for prediction of complications from radiosurgery. Int J Radiat Oncol Biol Phys 17:879–885

French JD, West PM, Von Amerongen FK et al (1952) Effects of intracarotid adminsitration of nitrogen mustard on normal brain and brain tumors. J Neurosurg 9:378–389

Gaspar L, Scott C, Murray K et al (2000) Validation of the RTOG recursive partitioning analysis (RPA) classification for brain metastases. Int J Radiat Oncol Biol Phys 47:1001–1006

Gaspar L, Scott C, Rotman M et al (1997) Recursive partitioning analysis (RPA) of prognostic factors in three radiation therapy oncology group (RTOG) brain metastases trials. Int J Radiat Oncol Biol Phys 37:745–751

Guo S, Reddy CA, Chao ST et al (2012) Impact of non-small cell lung cancer histology on survival predicted from the graded prognostic assessment for patients with brain metastases. Lung Cancer 77:389–393

Hoefnagels FW, Lagerwaard FJ, Sanchez E, Haasbeek CJ, Knol DL, Slotman BJ, Vandertop WP (2009) Radiological progression of cerebral metastases after radiosurgery: assessment of perfusion MRI for differentiating between necrosis and recurrence. J Neurol 256(6):878–887. doi:10.1007/s00415-009-5034-5, Epub Mar 10, 2009

Horton J, Baxter DH, Olson KB (1971) The management of metastases to the brain by irradiation and corticosteroids. Am J Roentgenol 111:334–336

Kagan AB (1997) Palliation of brain and spinal cord metastases. In: Perez CA, Brady LW (eds) Principles and practice of radiation oncolgoy, 3rd edn. JB Lippincott, Philadelphia, pp 2187–2197

Kalkanis SN, Kondziolka D, Gaspar L et al (2010) The role of surgical resection in the management of newly diagnosed brain metastases: a systematic review and evidence-based clinical practice guideline. J Neurooncol 96:33–43

Kano H, Kondziolka D, Lobato-Polo J, Zorro O, Flickinger JC, Lunsford LD (2010) T1/T2 matching to differentiate tumor growth from radiation effects after stereotactic radiosurgery. Neurosurgery 66(3):486–491 (discussion 491–492). doi: 10.1227/01.NEU.0000360391.35749.A5

Knisely JPS, Berkey B, Chakravarti A et al (2008) A phase III study of conventional radiation therapy plus thalidomide versus conventional radiation therapy for multiple brain metastases (RTOG 0118). Int J Radiat Oncol Biol Phys 71:79–86

Kocher M, Soffieti R, Abacioglu U et al (2011) Adjuvant whole-brain radiotherapy versus observation after radiosurgery or surgical resection of one to three cerebral metastases: results of the EORTC 22952–26001 study. J Clin Oncol 29:134–141

Komarnicky LT, Phillips TL, Martz K et al (1991) A randomized phase III protocol for the evaluation of misonidazole combined with radiation in the treatment of patients with brain metastases (RTOG 79–16). Int J Radiat Oncol Biol Phys 20:53–58

Kondziolka D, Patel A, Lunsford LD et al (1999) Stereotactic radiosurgery plus whole brain radiotherapy versus radiotherapy alone for patients with multiple brain metastases. Int J Radiat Oncol Biol Phys 45:427–434

Kurtz JM, Gelber R, Brady LW et al (1981) The palliation of brain metastases in a favorable patient population: a randomized clinical trial by the radiation therapy oncology group. Int J Radiat Oncol Biol Phys 7:891–895

Le Péchoux C, Laplanche A, Faivre-Finn C, Ciuleanu T, Wanders R, Lerouge D, Keus R, Hatton M, Videtic GM, Senan S, Wolfson A, Jones R, Arriagada R, Quoix E, Dunant A, Prophylactic Cranial Irradiation (PCI) Collaborative Group (2011) Clinical neurological outcome and quality of life among patients with limited small-cell cancer treated with two different doses of prophylactic cranial irradiation in the intergroup phase III trial (PCI99-01, EORTC 22003-08004, RTOG 0212 and IFCT 99-01). Ann Oncol 22(5):1154–1163. doi: 10.1093/annonc/mdq576. Epub Dec 7, 2010

Lee DH, Han J-Y, Kim HT et al (2008) Primary chemotherapy for newly diagnosed NSCLC with synchronous brain metastases compared with WBRT administered first. Result of a randomized pilot study. Cancer 113:143–149

Likacheva A, Pinnix CC, Parikh N et al (2012) Validation of recursive partitioning analysis and diagnosis-specific graded prognostic assessment in patients treated initially with radiosurgery alone. J Neurosurg 117(supp):38–44

Linskey ME, Andrews DW, Asher AL et al (2010) The role of stereotactic radiosurgery in the management of with newly diagnosed brain metastases: a systematic review and evidence-based clinical practice guideline. J Neurooncol 96:45–68

Lorenzoni J, Devriendt D, Massager N et al (2004) Radiosurgery for treatment of brain metastases: estimation of patient eligibility using three stratification systems. Int J Radiat Oncol Biol Phys 60:218–224

Mehta MP, Rodrigus P, Terhaard CHJ et al (2003) Survival and neurologic outcomes in a randomized trial of motexafin gadolinium and whole-brain radiation therapy in brain metastases. J Clin Oncol 21:2529–2536

Mehta MP, Tsao MN, Whelan TJ et al (2005) The American Society for Therapeutic Radiology and Oncology (ASTRO) evidence-based review of the role of radiosurgery for brain metastases. Int J Radiat Oncol Biol Phys 63:37–46

Meyers CA, Smith JA, Bezjak A et al (2004) Neurocognitive function and progression in patients with brain metastases treated with whole-brain radiation and motexafin gadolinium: results of a randomized phse III trial. J Clin Oncol 22:157–165

Mintz AH, Kestle J, Rathbone MP et al (1996) A randomized trial to assess the efficacy of surgery in addition to radiotherapy in patients with single brain metastasis. Cancer 78:1470–1476

Mitsuya K, Nakasu Y, Horiguchi S, Harada H, Nishimura T, Bando E, Okawa H, Furukawa Y, Hirai T, Endo M (2010) Perfusion weighted magnetic resonance imaging to distinguish the recurrence of metastatic brain tumors from radiation necrosis after stereotactic radiosurgery. J Neurooncol 99(1):81–88. doi:10.1007/s11060-009-0106-z, Epub Jan 8, 2010

Mornex F, Thomas L, Mohr P et al (2003) Randomized phase III trial of fotemustine versus fotemustine plus whole brain irradiation in cerebral metastases of melanoma (article in French). Cancer Radiother 7:1–8

Murray KJ, Scott C, Greenberg HM et al (1997) A randomized phase III study of accelerated hyperfractionation versus standard fractionation in patients with brain metastases: a report of the Radiation Therapy Oncology Group (RTOG 9104). Int J Radiat Oncol Biol Phys 39:571–574

Neuhaus T, Ko Y, Muller RP et al (2009) A phase III trial of topotecan and whole brain radiation therapy for patients with CNS-metastases due to lung cancer. Br J Cancer 100:291–297

Nieder C, Andratschke NH, Geinitz H et al (2012) Diagnosis-specific graded prognostic assessment score is valid in patients with brain metastases treated in routine clinical practice in two European countries. Med Sci Monit 18:CR450–CR455

Nieder C, Geinitz H, Molls M (2008) Validation of the graded prognostic assessment index for surgically treated patients with brain metastases. Anticancer Res 28:3015–3017

Nieder C, Mehta MP (2009) Prognostic indices for brain metastases—usefulness and challenges. Radiat Oncol 4:10

Nieder C, Bremnes RM, Andratschke NH (2009a) Prognostic scores in patients with brain metastases from non-small cell lung cancer. J Thor Oncol 11:1337–1341

Nieder C, Marienhagen K, Geinitz H et al (2009b) Validation of the graded prognostic assessment index for patients with brain metastases. Acta Oncol 48:457–459

Noordjik EM, Vecht CJ, Haaxma-Reiche H et al (1994) The choice of treatment of single brain metastasis should be based on extracranial tumor activity and age. Int J Radiat Oncol Biol Phys 29:711–717

Patchell RA, Tibbs PA, Walsh JW et al (1990) A randomized trial of surgery in the treatment of single metastasis to the brain. N Engl J Med 322:494–500

Patchell RA, Tibbs PA, Regine WF et al (1998) Postoperative radiotherapy in the treatment of single metastasis to the brain. JAMA 280:1485–1489

Phillips TL, Scott CB, Leibel S et al (1994) Results of a randomized comparison of radiotherapy and bromodeoxyuridine to radiotherapy alone for brain metastases: Report of RTOG trial 89–05. Int J Radiat Oncol Biol Phys 30:215

Postmus PE, Haaxma-Reiche H, Smit EF et al (2000) Treatment of brain metastases of small-cell lung cancer: comparing teniposide and teniposide with whole brain radiotherapy- a phase III study of the European Organization for the Research and Treatment of Lung Cancer Cooperative Group. J Clin Oncol 18:3400–3408

Postow MA, Callahan MK, Barker CA et al (2012) Immunologic correlates of the abscopal effect in a patient with melanoma. N Engl J Med 366:925–931

Regine WF, Huhn JL, Patchell RA et al (2002) Risk of symptomatic brain tumor recurrence and neurologic deficit after radiosurgery

alone in patients with newly diagnosed brain metastases: results and implications. Int J Radiat Oncol Biol Phys 52:333–338
Ribalta T, Fuller GN (2004) Brain metastases: histopathological evaluation and diagnostic pitfalls. In: Sawaya R (ed) Intracranial metastases: current management strategies. Blackwell Publishing, Malden, pp 55–70
Robinet G, Thomas P, Breton JL et al (2001) Results of a phase III study of early versus delayed whole brain radiotherapy with concurrent cisplatin and vinorelbine combination in inoperable brain metastasis of non-small cell lung cancer: Groupe Français de Pneumo-Cancérologie (GFPC) Protocol 95–1. Ann Oncol 12:59–67
Sause WT, Scott C, Kirsch R et al (1993) Phase I/II trial of accelerated fractionation in brain metastases, RTOG 85–28. Int J Radiat Oncol Biol Phys 26:653–657
Shaw E, Scott C, Souhami L et al (1996) Radiosurgery for the treatment of previously irradiated recurrent primary brain tumors and brain metastasis: initial report of Radiation Therapy Oncology Group protocol (90–05). Int J Radiat Oncol Biol Phys 34:647–654
Shaw E, Scott C, Souhami L et al (2000) Single dose radiosurgical treatment of recurrent previously irradiated primary brain tumors and brain metastases: final report of RTOG protocol 90–05. Int J Radiat Oncol Biol Phys 47:291–298
Sneed PK, Mendez J, Fogh SE et al (2012) Risk factors for radiation necrosis after radiosurgery for brain metastases. Int J Radiat Oncol Biol Phys 84(supp):pS118
Sperduto PW, Berkey B, Gaspar LE et al (2008) A new prognostic index and comparison to three other indices for patients with brain metastases: an analysis of 1960 patients in the RTOG database. Int J Radiat Oncol Biol Phys 70:510–514
Sperduto PW, Chao ST, Sneed P et al (2010) Diagnosis-specific prognostic factors, indices and treatment outcomes for patients with newly diagnosed brain metastases: a multi-institutional analysis of 4,259 patients. Int J Radiat Oncol Biol Phys 77:655–661
Sperduto PW, Kased N, Roberge D et al (2012a) Summary report on the graded prognostic assessment (GPA): an accurate and facile diagnosis-specific tool to estimate survival, guide treatment and stratify clinical trials for patients with brain metastases. J Clin Onc 30:419–425
Sperduto PW, Kased N, Roberge D et al (2012b) The graded prognostic assessment (GPA): a new diagnosis-specific prognostic index for women with breast cancer and brain metastases. Int J Radiat Oncol Biol Phys 82(5):2111–2117
Sperduto PW, Wang M, Robins HI et al (2013) RTOG 0320: a phase III trial of whole brain radiation therapy (WBRT) and stereotactic radiosurgery (SRS) alone versus WBRT & SRS with temozolomide (TMZ) or erlotinib for non-small cell lung cancer and 1–3 brain metastases. Int J Radiat Oncol Biol Phys 85:1312–1318
Stamell EF, Wolchok JD, Gnjatic S et al (2013) The abscopal effect associated with a systemic anti-melanoma immune response. Int J Radiat Oncol Biol Phys 85:293–295
Suh JH, Stea B, Nabid A et al (2006) Phase III study of efaproxiral as an adjunct to whole-brain radiation therapy for brain metastases. J Clin Oncol 24:106–114
Suki D (2004) The epidemiology of brain metastasis. In: Sawaya R (ed) Intracranial metastases: current management strategies. Blackwell Publishing, Malden, pp 20–34
Tannock IF, Ahles TA, Ganz PA et al (2004) Cognitive impairment associated with chemotherapy for cancer: report of a workshop. J Clin Oncol 22:2233–2239
Tsao MN, Rades D, Wirth A et al (2012) Radiotherapeutic and surgical management for newly diagnosed brain metastasis(es): an American society for radiation oncology evidence-based guideline. Pract Radiat Oncol 2:210–225
Ushio Y, Arita N, Hayakawa T et al (1991) Chemotherapy of brain metastases from lung carcinoma: a controlled randomized study. Neurosurg 28:201–205
Viana GA, da Silva LG, Stefano EJ (2012) Prognostic indexes for brain metastases: which is the most powerful. Int J Radiat Oncol Biol Phys 83:e325–e330
Villa S, Weber DC, Moretones C et al (2011) Validation of the new graded prognostic assessment scale for brain metastases: a multicenter prospective study. Radiat Oncol 6:23
Weltman E, Salvajoli JV, Brandt RA et al (2000) Radiosurgery for brain metastases: a score for predicting prognosis. Int J Radiat Oncol Biol Phys 46:1155–1161
Wen PY, Black PM, Loeffler JS (2001) Metastatic brain cancer. In: DeVita V, Hellman S, Rosenberg SA (eds) Cancer: principles and practice of oncology, 6th edn. Williams and Wilkins, Philadelphia, pp 2655–2670
Weichselbaum RR, Hellman S (2011) Oligometastases revisited. Nat Rev Clin Oncol 8(6):378–382
Zimm S, Wampler GL, Stablein D et al (1981) Intracerebral metastases in solid-tumor patients: natural history and results of treatment. Cancer 48:384–394

Bone Metastases

Marko Popovic, Michael Poon, Erin Wong, Danielle Rodin, Kenneth Li, Florence Mok, and Edward Chow

Contents

Abstract

Bone is one of the most common sites of metastasis. This chapter addresses three notable issues for bone metastases patients receiving radiotherapy: prognosis, complications affecting this patient population and predictive factors for various toxicities. Overall survival estimates for bone metastases patients have improved considerably over the past 50 years and vary with respect to primary tumour location. Numerous general and tumour-specific predictors influence survival in this patient population; when combined, these covariates have been used to develop relevant predictive models for survival. Toxicities in bone metastases patients are generally mild, and risk is determined by radiation site and dose. One noteworthy toxicity that has garnered significant research in recent years is radiotherapy-induced nausea and vomiting, for which risk factors include the anatomic site being irradiated, a greater radiotherapy field size, a female gender and anxiety. Complications that may affect bone metastases patients are spinal cord compression, impending or pathologic fractures, neuropathic pain and recurrence of bone metastasis. In closing, this chapter contains essential information that should be considered in the delivery of treatment; ultimately, however, treatment choice should be tailored to the individual patient and should be based on a variety of clinical and sociodemographic factors.

M. Popovic · M. Poon · E. Wong · D. Rodin · E. Chow (✉)
Rapid Response Radiotherapy Program, Department of Radiation Oncology, University of Toronto, Odette Cancer Centre, Sunnybrook Health Sciences Centre, Toronto, ON M4N 3M5, Canada
e-mail: Edward.Chow@sunnybrook.ca

K. Li
Department of Clinical Oncology, Queen Elizabeth Hospital, Hong Kong SAR, China

F. Mok
Department of Clinical Oncology, Prince of Wales Hospital, Hong Kong SAR, China

1 Introduction

Bone is one of the most common sites of metastasis. It has been shown that radiation is effective in pain relief in around 60 % of patients (Chow et al. 2012), and is also effective in preventing and treating skeletal related events (Harada et al. 2010). In this chapter, relevant issues to patients with bone metastases receiving radiotherapy, such

C. Nieder and L. E. Gaspar (eds.), *Decision Tools for Radiation Oncology*, Medical Radiology. Radiation Oncology,
DOI: 10.1007/174_2013_836, © Springer-Verlag Berlin Heidelberg 2013
Published Online: 30 June 2013

as prognosis and predictive factors of toxicities will be discussed. Complications that affect this patient population, such as spinal cord compression, impending or pathologic fracture, and neuropathic bone pain will also be addressed.

2 Prognosis

In the last 50 years, prognosis for patients with bone metastases has improved considerably. Harrington noted that the mean survival for bone metastases patients referred for orthopaedic fixation increased from seven to 19 months from 1960 to 1980 (Harrington 1988).

2.1 Survival by Primary Tumour Type

Median survival for patients with bone metastases varies widely with respect to primary tumour location. Prostate and breast patients have a median survival of 29.3 and 22.6 months, respectively, while renal-cell and lung patients have a markedly shorter expected survival of 11.8 and 3.6 months, respectively (Harrington 1988). Regardless of primary tumour location, for patients with bone-only metastases, expected median survival is 52 months (Perez et al. 1990; Yamashita et al. 1991, 1992).

Patients with primary breast and prostate cancers account for the majority of bone metastases patients as a result of high prevalence and lengthy duration of these diseases (Plunkett and Rubens 2005). Although bone metastases can occur in patients with any primary cancer, three primary sites are especially favoured: the breast, prostate and lung.

2.1.1 Breast Cancer

Breast cancer carries a high metastatic affinity for the skeletal system; the majority of patients with advanced breast cancer have bone metastases by the time of death (Galasko 1986). Overall, it has been cited that the median survival from diagnosis of bone metastases from breast cancer is approximately 20 months (Plunkett and Rubens 2005). At first relapse, breast cancer patients with bone metastases have significantly better survival than patients with visceral metastases (median survival: 24 months versus 12 months, respectively) (Solomayer et al. 2000). Similar results are obtained with regard to overall survival (71 months for bone metastases versus 48 months for visceral metastases) (Solomayer et al. 2000).

Patients with advanced breast cancer and with bone-only metastases have favourable prognosis. Coleman et al. reported a median survival of 24 months in patients with skeleton-only metastases and only 3 months for patients who had a relapse in the liver (Coleman and Rubens 1987). Similar findings are found in more recent studies, as patients with solely osseous metastases have a better prognosis than patients with visceral-only metastases (Solomayer et al. 2000).

2.1.2 Prostate Cancer

Bone metastasis is frequent in cancers of the prostate—approximately 10 % of prostate patients present with bone metastases, and almost all patients who die from the disease are found to have bony metastases at autopsy (Landis et al. 1999). As with breast cancer, median survival from diagnosis of bone metastases from prostate cancer is expected at 20 months (Plunkett and Rubens 2005).

A bone scan index (BSI) quantifies the extent of metastatic skeletal involvement by tumour type (Sabbatini et al. 1999). In patients with androgen-independent prostate cancer, patients with low, intermediate or extensive skeletal involvement have median survivals of 18.3, 15.8 and 8.1 months, respectively (Sabbatini et al. 1999).

2.1.3 Lung Cancer

Approximately 30–40 % of patients with lung cancer have developed metastatic disease to the bone (Coleman 2001); with the introduction of more sensitive screening technologies, this value is expected to increase (Iordanidou et al. 2006; Shaham et al. 2006). With the advancement of new therapeutic methods, survival for lung cancer patients with bone metastases has dramatically increased; in 2003, a study cited that median survival for this patient population was 6 months (Rosen et al. 2003), while in 2006 it doubled to 12 months (Sandler et al. 2006).

2.2 Factors Affecting Prognosis

Both general and tumour-specific factors which influence prognosis in bone metastases patients receiving radiotherapy have been identified. A summary of these determinants is presented in the following section.

In prostate cancer patients, prognostic predictors include performance status, tumour grade, haemoglobin concentration, serum lactate dehydrogenase levels and prostate-specific antigen levels (Robson and Dawson 1996; Eisenberger et al. 1994; Matzkin et al. 1993). In the same population, it has also been found that patients with low serum levels of C-terminal telopeptide of type I procollagen, C-terminal telopeptide of type I collagen (ICTP) and alkaline phosphatase had significantly better survival when compared to patients with high levels of these markers (Akimoto et al. 1999; Izumi et al. 2012). Further, elevated levels in the following biomarkers have also been proven to significantly reduce overall survival in prostate cancer patients: type I procollagen N-terminal propeptide (Brasso et al. 2006), parathyroid hormone (Berruti et al. 2012), osteoprotegerin, bone sialoprotein, cross-linked N-telopeptides of type I collagen (NTX) and tartrate-resistant acid phosphatase isoenzyme 5b (Jung et al. 2004). Extent of skeletal metastatic involvement has, according to bone scintigraphy, shown a significant correlation to survival in this patient group (Crawford et al. 1989). Bone scintigraphy has also revealed a relationship between the number of metastatic lesions and survival (Soloway et al. 1988). In devising these two correlations, the studies by Crawford et al. and Soloway et al. (Crawford et al. 1989; Soloway et al. 1988) managed to differentiate between patients at the extremes of their respective scales. However neither managed to successfully discriminate between more moderate cases.

A recent clinical trial of 132 patients with pathologically confirmed bone metastases from lung cancer analyzed 11 potential covariates for their prognostic significance in this population after radiotherapy (Komatsu et al. 2012). Upon univariate analysis, surgery as a treatment for primary lung cancer (vs. other treatments), solitary bone metastasis (vs. multiple), no visceral organ metastasis (vs. 1 and ≥ 2), no symptoms or numbness (vs. numbness vs. paresis), no pain (vs. mild or severe pain), Eastern Cooperative Oncology Group (ECOG) performance status <2 (vs. ≥ 2), biological effective radiation dose of ≥ 40 Gy (vs. <40 Gy), adenocarcinoma histology (versus others), and the use of epidermal growth factor receptor (EGFR)-targeted agents significantly correlated to improved survival in this patient population. Further multivariate analysis revealed that a solitary bone metastasis ($p = 0.038$), performance status <2 ($p = 0.006$), biological effective radiation dose ≥ 40 Gy ($p = 0.003$), adenocarcinoma histology ($p = 0.014$), and the use of EGFR-targeted agents ($p < 0.001$) significantly correlated with improved survival. In the same year, Bae et al. examined 220 patients with non-small cell lung cancer presenting with bone metastases to determine prognostic predictors of overall survival at diagnosis (Bae et al. 2012). It was found that patients with squamous cell carcinoma (vs. non-squamous cell carcinoma) and patients with a single bone metastasis had a 1.8-times higher risk of shorter survival ($p = 0.016$) and 2.4-times longer survival ($p = 0.008$), respectively. A biomarker study (Brown et al. 2005) discovered that, when compared to non-small cell lung cancer patients with low urinary levels of NTX, patients with high NTX levels had a more than threefold increased risk of death (RR = 3.03, $p < 0.001$), as well as a 5-month reduction in median survival (8.2 months versus 3.2 months, respectively). Additionally, patients with high bone-specific alkaline phosphatase (BALP) levels (≥ 146 IU/L) also had significantly increased risk of death when compared to patients with low BALP levels (<146 IU/L) (RR = 1.53; $p = 0.003$).

Coleman et al. analyzed 367 women with breast cancer to assess the impact of certain patient characteristics on the development and prognosis of bone metastases (Coleman et al. 1998). On multivariate analysis, they found 5 factors that had great prognostic importance in their population: histological grade ($p < 0.0001$), oestrogen receptor status ($p < 0.0001$), bone disease at initial presentation ($p < 0.0001$), disease-free interval ($p = 0.002$) and age ($p = 0.006$). Biomarker analysis by Brown et al. (Brown et al. 2012) revealed that serum lactate dehydrogenase was a significant prognostic predictor of survival, along with Functional Assessment of Cancer Therapy-General (FACT-G) score of less than 65 ($p < 0.05$ vs. FACT-G ≥ 75), ECOG performance status of ≥ 1 versus 0 (RR 1.74, $p < 0.01$) and prior chemotherapy (RR 1.97, $p < 0.01$ vs. no prior chemotherapy). It was also determined that, for breast cancer patients with bone metastases, elevated baseline serum N-telopeptide (663 days vs. 941 days; $p < 0.001$) (Ali et al. 2004), elevated serum ICTP ($p = 0.02$) (Lipton et al. 2011), and expression of receptor activator for nuclear factor kappa B (Zhang et al. 2012) significantly shortened survival. Interestingly, in the breast cancer setting, >30 ng/mL of vitamin D at diagnosis significantly ameliorated overall survival ($p = 0.0101$) (Hatse et al. 2012). As well, in this patient population it has been shown that the maximum standardized uptake value on positron emission tomography/computed tomography images was strongly associated with overall survival in both univariate ($n = 141$, hazard ratio: 3.13, $p < 0.001$) and multivariate analyses (hazard ratio: 3.19, $p = 0.002$) (Morris et al. 2012).

In a literature review, Popovic et al. aimed to determine prognostic factors in patients with spinal metastases (Popovic et al. 2012). It was found that primary cancer site, extent of metastases, as well as general condition and performance score were most consistently identified as prognostic predictors in spinal metastases patients; age, neurological deficit and previous treatments were also candidates for predicting survival.

2.3 Development of Predictive Models for Survival

Based on prognostic factors, Chow et al. aimed to develop a model for prediction of survival in advanced cancer patients (Chow et al. 2002). Using a prospective database from an outpatient palliative radiotherapy clinic, the work analyzed 16 potential covariates in 395 patients to determine their predictive value of survival in this patient population. Of these patients, 70 % were diagnosed with bone metastases, while a total of 113 of 395 patients (28.6 %) had bone-only metastases. Compared to the cohort with other forms of metastatic involvement, the bone metastases-only cohort survived notably longer (median survival: 29 vs. 16 weeks;

$p < 0.0001$). Upon univariate analysis, 12 of the 16 studied factors entered the initial regression model by satisfying the selection criterion of log-rank $p \leq 0.01$ (Table 1). The 12 included covariates were primary cancer site, site of metastases (bone-only vs. others), weight loss ($\geq$10 % over the last 6 months vs. <10 %), Karnofsky Performance Status (KPS) (>50 vs. $\leq$ 50), time from first cancer diagnosis to first consultation at the outpatient clinic (>12 months vs. $\leq$12 months), and the Edmonton Symptom Assessment System (ESAS) scores of fatigue, nausea, depression, drowsiness, appetite, sense of well-being and shortness of breath. Upon multivariate analysis, six covariates were retained: primary cancer site, site of metastases, KPS, and the ESAS scores of fatigue, appetite and shortness of breath (Table 2). With these six factors, they devised two models with different scoring summations. In the first, each predictor was assigned a partial score, and summation of all six partial scores led to a survival prediction score; the second method involved identifying the number of risk factors, of a possible six, that the patient had. To evaluate the performance of the models, a C index was used, which quantified the probability that, for a randomly chosen pair of patients, the patient having the better outcome was the one having the better-predicted outcome. For the C index, a value of 0.5 indicated no predictive discrimination while a value of 1.0 indicated perfect separation of patients with different outcomes. Overall, the models had C index values that were consistently >0.7 at 3, 6 and 12 months. When actual survival was compared to predicted survival, a R^2 value of 0.31 was calculated.

After the establishment of the initial models, the same team worked on performing temporal validation of the models by testing them on patients attending the same clinic in a different year (Chow et al. 2009). This work utilized a third form of test called the D index to assess the performance of the models. The D index quantified the discrimination of the models based on their abilities to separate the risk of death among groups of patients; for this statistical test, the larger the D statistic, the greater the degree of separation. The models had C index values ranging from 0.65 to 0.68, which represented reasonable concordance, and D index values of 0.99 to 1.41, representing good separation of prognostic groups. However, generalized R^2 values remained poor (range: 0.27–0.31), indicating that the models accounted for less than one-third of the variability in survival.

Chow and colleagues aimed to simplify their original prognostication models (Chow et al. 2008). They cited difficulty in extracting ESAS scores as the reason why they believed a simpler model made up of only three readily available factors—primary cancer site (breast, prostate, lung and others), site of metastases (bone vs. others) and KPS—deserved consideration. As with their previous models, they utilized two scoring approaches: the partial score method and the number of risk factors method. In order to validate these new models, they conducted both temporal and external validation by comparing cohorts from different years and at different institutions. In evaluation of the performance of these predictive models, C index values ranged from 0.63 to 0.66 and D index values ranged from 0.81 to 1.09, indicating reasonable separation of the three prognostic groups formed by the models. In addition, it was noted that the models were not hindered by over-optimism. In contrast to the previous R^2 values for the initial ($R^2 = 0.31$) and temporal validation ($R^2 = 0.27$) cohorts of the six-factor models, the R^2 values for the three-variable models were lower across the initial, temporal and external validation sets ($R^2 = 0.23$, 0.24, 0.15, respectively). The reduction in the generalized R^2 values indicated that the three ESAS variables that were omitted did contribute statistical significance to the six-factor model. However, these statistics should be considered with reservation, as R^2 values are generally not reported in predictive models, and when they are reported, values are generally low despite successful validation (Toscani and Brunelli 2005).

Although some factors were not included in the models by Chow et al., in general, survival of metastatic cancer patients is dependent on performance status (Chow et al. 2002), symptoms comprising part of the "terminal cancer syndrome" (Reuben et al. 1988), and other patient symptoms which include asthenia, anorexia, cachexia, weight loss, dysphagia, xerostomia, delirium and cognitive impairment (Llobera et al. 2000; Maltoni et al. 2005). Additionally, some studies state that nonclinical factors, such as social support (Schoenbach et al. 1986) and religion (Phillips and Smith 1990; Jarvis and Northcott 1987) also influence survival in this patient population, although others have concluded that psychosocial factors are not associated with survival in palliative advanced cancer patients (Chow et al. 2008; Chow et al. 2002).

3 Risk Factors for Toxicities

3.1 Radiotherapy-Induced Nausea and Vomiting

The earliest studies reported the incidence of vomiting as 60 % in those receiving fractionated radiotherapy to the whole abdomen (Priestman and Priestman 1984) and 80 % when single fractions were given (Danjoux et al. 1979; Priestman et al. 1990). Dennis et al. (2011a) summarize the risk factors for radiotherapy-induced nausea and vomiting (RINV) (Table 3). These predictors include a younger age, female gender, low alcohol consumption, and previous experience of emesis (Feyer et al. 1998). In addition, radiation to the upper abdomen is well recognized as one of the most emetogenic sites for radiation (Coates et al. 1983).

Table 1 Univariate survival analysis of 16 prognostic factors as reported by Chow et al. (2002)

	Covariates	Subgroups	Number of patients	Missing values (%)	Survival at 6 months (%)	Median survival (weeks)	Log-rank *p value*[a]
1	Age at 1st visit	≤68 years	207	0	47	21	0.18
		>68 years	188		39	19	
2	Primary cancer site	Lung	143	0	34	16	<0.0001
		Breast	80		65	52	
		Prostate	56		60	39	
		Others	116		31	14	
3	Site of metastases	Bone only	113	0	55	29	<0.0001
		Others	282		38	16	
4	Weight loss (≥10 % over last 6 months)	Yes	132		30	14	<0.0001
		No	263		49	26	
5	KPS	>50	278	0	52	27	<0.0001
		≤50	117		20	8	
6	Time from 1st diagnosis of cancer to 1st consultation	>12 months	202	0.5	51	26	<0.0001
		≤12 months	191		33	15	
7	Analgesic consumption within last 24 h of 1st consultation	None	102	0	53	30	0.25
		Non-opioids	44		36	19	
		Weak-opioids	54		50	26	
		Strong-opioids	195		37	17	
8	Pain	0	87	6	45	20	0.1
		1–3	126		49	25	
		4–7	111		34	16	
		8–10	49		47	21	
9	Fatigue	0	26	9	64	63	<0.0001
		1–3	87		60	35	
		4–7	165		39	19	
		8–10	83		32	13	
10	Nausea	0	200	7	4S	24	0.0004
		1–3	111		44	19	
		4–7	41		37	19	
		8–10	16		6	10	
11	Depression	0	92	13	49	24	0.004
		1–3	149		49	25	
		4–7	32		41	20	
		8–10	19		16	S	
12	Anxiety	0	72	13	50	24	0.5
		1–3	143		46	19	
		4–7	95		41	19	
		8–10	33		40	16	

(continued)

Table 1 (continued)

	Covariates	Subgroups	Number of patients	Missing values (%)	Survival at 6 months (%)	Median survival (weeks)	Log-rank *p value*[a]
13	Drowsiness	0	71	9	64	36	<0.0001
		1–3	137		50	24	
		4–7	112		33	17	
		8–10	39		18	8	
14	Appetite	0	73	7	54	33	<0.000 1
		1–3	102		50	24	
		4–7	128		45	I8	
		8–10	63		19	11	
15	Sense of well-being	0	16	15	69	56	<0.0001
		1–3	130		52	27	
		4–7	151		39	18	
		8–10	40		29	14	
16	Shortness of breath	0	131	7	58	34	<0.0001
		1–3	126		39	18	
		4–7	74		30	14	
		8–10	36		36	14	

[a] Replace the missing value of a covariate with the median of that covariate
KPS Karnofsky performance score Reprinted from Chow et al. (2002) with permission from Elsevier

In an Italian Group for Antiemetic Research in Radiotherapy (IGARR) observational trial, the irradiated site being the upper abdomen and field size (>400 cm^2) were statistically significant therapy-related risk factors for radiation-induced emesis, while concomitant chemotherapy and previous vomiting induced by chemotherapy were the only significant patient-related risk factors (Feyer et al. 1998). Although not statistically significant, a relatively high incidence of RINV was also found in patients receiving radiotherapy to the thorax (31 %), head and neck region (30.5 %), brain (35 %), and pelvis (24.1 %). These findings were concurrent with an earlier IGARR observational trial (The Italian Group for Antiemetic Research in Radiotherapy 1999). The reported incidence of RINV, by irradiated site, was 71.4 % for upper abdomen patients, 48.4 % for thorax patients, 40.4 % for head and neck patients, 40.4 % for brain patients, and 39 % for pelvis patients. Enblom et al. reported a high incidence of nausea in patients receiving radiotherapy to the abdominal or pelvic regions (63 %) and the brain or head and neck regions (48 %) (Enblom et al. 2009).

Due to the unexpected higher incidence of RINV in patients receiving head and neck and brain radiation (Enblom et al. 2009; Maranzano et al. 2010), reclassification of both head and neck and brain radiation from minimal to low emetogenic risk group status was adopted by the Multinational Association of Supportive Care in Cancer (MASCC) and the European Society of Clinical Oncology (ESMO) in their updated 2009 antiemetic guidelines (Feyer et al. 2011), as well as in the 2011 updated antiemetic recommendations from the American Society of Clinical Oncology (ASCO) (Basch et al. 2011).

3.2 Other Toxicities

Additional toxicities are summarized in two systematic analyses published by Chow et al. (2012, 2007), who reported that risk of toxicities is determined by radiation site and dose. In general, they found that toxicities were mild and patients who received single fraction or multiple fractions treatment experienced similar acute toxicities. In contradiction, three trials have reported more acute toxicities in patients receiving multiple fractions (Hartsell et al. 2005; Kaasa et al. 2006; Foro et al. 2008). Acute toxicities reported from various studies are summarized in Table 4.

4 Complications Affecting Patients with Bone Metastases

4.1 Spinal Cord Compression

Spinal cord compression occurs when an extradural tumour compresses on the dural sac which surrounds the spinal cord or cauda equina. Approximately 5–10 % of patients with

Table 2 Multivariate analysis of six prognostic factors included in predictive survival models by Chow et al. (2002)

	p value	Hazard ratio (95 % CI)
Primary cancer site	<0.0001	
Breast		1.00
Prostate		1.94 (1.25–3.01)
Lung		2.10 (1.48–2.96)
Others		2.49 (1.75–3.50)
Site of metastases	<0.0001	
Bone metastases only		1.00
Others		2.07 (1.54–2.78)
KPS	<0.0001	
>50		1.00
≤50		2.10 (1.64–2.69)
ESAS fatigue score	0.005	
0		1.00
1–3		1.26 (0.71–2.21)
4–7		1.66 (0.96–2.86)
8–10		1.84 (1.02–3.32)
ESAS appetite score	0.009	
0		1.00
1–3		1.00 (0.69–1.43)
4–7		1.00 (0.71–1.42)
8–10		1.78 (1.15–2.68)
ESAS shortness of breath score	0.04	
0		1.00
1–3		1.30 (0.97–1.74)
4–7		1.67 (1.18–2.35)
8–10		1.33 (0.85–2.08)

Reprinted from Chow et al. (2002) with permission from Elsevier

Table 3 Risk factors for the development of radiotherapy-induced nausea and vomiting

Anatomic site being irradiated[a]
Concurrent chemotherapy[a]
Previous chemotherapy-induced nausea and vomiting[a]
Radiotherapy field size greater than 400 cm^2[a]
Age less than 55 years
Female
Anxiety
Daily alcohol consumption less than 100 g
High dose per radiotherapy fraction
High total cumulative radiotherapy dose

[a] Indicates statistically significant risk factor based on the Italian Group for Antiemetic Research in Radiotherapy (IGARR) observational trial (The Italian Group for Antiemetic Research in Radiotherapy 1999)

bone metastases develop spinal cord compression (Rades and Abrahm 2010; Sejpal et al. 2007). This complication is considered an oncologic emergency, because if left alone, it can lead to devastating consequences such as paralysis, significant pain, sensory loss and incontinence (Kwok et al. 2005; Loblaw et al. 2005). The incidence of spinal cord compression is related to the primary tumour type, most commonly occurring in patients with breast, prostate, and lung cancers (Sejpal et al. 2007). Radiation is a common treatment for patients with spinal cord compression since it can be used alone or after surgical interventions (Rades and Abrahm 2010). In patients suffering from spinal cord compression, radiation or surgery is usually combined with corticosteroids (Rades and Abrahm 2010; Sejpal et al. 2007). Shiue et al. noted that using radiation therapy for spinal cord compression shows significant improvements in multiple areas; pain reduction occurred in 57–73 % of patients, motor function improvement occurred in 26–42 %

Table 4 Summary of acute toxicities reported by the literature

Reference	Nausea and vomiting	Lethargy/tiredness	Diarrhoea	Skin reaction	Additional	Overall
Price et al. (1986)						No statistically significant difference between arms in acute morbidity
Cole (1989)	Single: 77 %; only beyond first week in 23 %; multiple: 33 %; persisted beyond first week; effects did not correlate with site of radiation	No statistically significant difference between arms; increased with larger field size	Single: 30 %; multiple: 22 %; mild; no temporal relationship to radiation	Single: 30 %; multiple: 22 %; no statistically significant difference between arms; one severe reaction; one reaction to aminoglutethimide		
Kagei et al. (1990)	Single: 14 %; multiple: 23 %		Single: 21 %; multiple: 15 %		Transient pain augment: 8 % multiple; transient haemoptysis: 7 % single	
Gaze et al. (1997)	Single: G0 60 %; G1 18 %; G2 10 %; G3 11 %; G4 1 %; multiple: G0 65 %; G1 8 %; G2 11 %; G3 15 %	Single: G0 29 %; G1 35 %; G2 24 %; G3 10 %; G4 3 %; multiple: G0 25 %; G1 30 %; G2 29 %; G3 14 %; G4 2 %; same degree of tiredness				No statistically significant difference between arms in acute adverse effects
Foro et al. (1998)				Total: G1 12 %; no statistically significant difference between arms		
Nielson et al. (1998)	Very modest; no statistically significant difference between arms	Very modest; no statistically significant difference between arms		Very modest; no statistically significant difference between arms		
Bone Pain Trial Working Party (1999)	Single: 56 % nausea; 30 % vomiting; multiple: 65 % nausea; 32 % vomiting; no statistically significant difference between arms					
Steenland et al. (1999)	No statistically significant difference between arms	No statistically significant difference between arms		No statistically significant difference between arms	Single: 1 case of radiation enteritis (post re-treatment); multiple: 1 case of small bowel ileus	

(continued)

Table 4 (continued)

Reference	Nausea and vomiting	Lethargy/tiredness	Diarrhoea	Skin reaction	Additional	Overall
Ozsaran et al. (2001)					G1 or G2 acute toxicity (mainly GI) in 16.1 % of patients	No G3 or G4 toxicity; no significant difference in frequency or severity between treatment groups ($p = 0.382$)
Sarkar et al. (2002)	Single: 29 % nausea; 3 % vomiting; multiple: 35 % nausea; 4 % vomiting; mild nausea; moderate vomiting		Single: 10 %; multiple: 7 %; mild cases	Single: 23 %; multiple: 21 %; mild erythema		
Altundag et al. (2002)	Mild nausea and vomiting					No other early or late complications
Hartsell et al. (2005)	(gastrointestinal toxicity); single: G1 7 %; G2 5 %; G3 1 %; multiple: G1 11 %; G2 7 %; G3 1 %			Single: G1 3 %; multiple: G1 8 %; G2 4 %	Lung, central nervous system, haematological, and other toxicities	More acute toxicities (G2-4) in multiple (17 %) arm than single (10 %; $P = 0.02$)
Roos et al. (2005)	G3 1 % (upper gastrointestinal toxicity)				G3 lung 1 %; pain flare worse in single than multiple	Toxicities were generally absent or mild
Kaasa et al. (2006)	Fewer patients with nausea in first 4 weeks in single arm	No statistically significant differences in fatigue	Fewer patients with diarrhoea in first 4 weeks in single arm			
El-Shenshawy et al. (2006)	Single: G0 62 %; G1 12 %; G2 12 %; G3 12 %; G4 2 %; multiple: G0 66 %; G1 14 %; G2 10 %; G3 10 %; G4 2 %; Not statistically significant ($p = 0.496$)	Single: G0 30 %; G1 36 %; G2 22 %; G3 10 %; G4 2 %; multiple: G0 26 %; G1 32 %; G2 26 %; G3 14 %; G4 0 %; Not statistically significant ($p = 0.286$)			During the 18 month follow-up period, no late adverse effects were noted	No difference in acute toxicities between the two groups
Hamouda et al. (2007)	Very modest	Very modest			No late adverse effect noted	
Foro et al. (2008)	(Gastrointestinal toxicity): Single: G1 2 %; multiple: G1 2 %			Single: G1 8 %; G2 2 %; multiple: G1 10 %; G2 5 %		Acute toxicity greater in multiple arm without significant differences
Amouzegar-Hashemi et al. (2008)	Mild gastrointestinal disturbances: nausea. Single: 3 patients; multiple: 5 patients					

G0 Grade 0; *G1* Grade 1; *G2* Grade 2; *G3* Grade 3; *G4* Grade 4 of patients, and mobility was regained in 26–35 % of treated patients (Shiue et al. 2010).

4.1.1 Prognosis

For most patients with metastatic spinal cord compression, prognosis is at most 6 months; however, there are some patients who may live for a few years (Maranzano et al. 2005; Rades et al. 2006). Prognostic factors for patients with spinal cord compression are an important consideration as they affect the optimal dosage and fractionation of radiation treatment. For example, single radiation fraction therapies are recommended for patients with poor prognosis (i.e. ≤6 months) whereas more protracted radiotherapy can be considered for patients with longer expected prognosis (i.e. >6 months) (Holt et al. 2012). Rades et al. determined several prognostic factors for patients with spinal cord compression, irrespective of primary cancer: ECOG performance status, type of primary tumour time between diagnosis of primary to diagnosis of metastases, presence of visceral metastases during radiation, degree of motor function before radiation, and length of time from the onset of motor deficit to radiation (Rades et al. 2006, 2008). They used these prognostic factors to develop a scoring system to help physicians determine the appropriate radiation amount and fractionation schedule for different patients (Rades et al. 2008). A 2010 study determined that a later onset of motor deficit is additionally related to better functional outcome and survival (Shiue et al. 2010). Abrahm et al. reported that pre-treatment ambulatory status was the most important predictor of survival in spinal cord compression patients (Abrahm et al. 2008).

4.2 Impending or Pathologic Fractures

Pathologic or impending fractures can occur in patients with bone metastases. They are frequently associated with breast, lung, prostate, kidney, and thyroid primary cancers (Coleman 1997). Impending or pathologic fractures are considered a complication because they can cause hospitalization, significant pain and urgent need for surgery in unfavourable circumstances (Jawad and Scully 2010).

4.2.1 Prognosis

The occurrence of pathologic fracture or the suggestion of an impending fracture has become more frequent as palliation of cancer has improved. Thus far, it has been found that prognosis of patients with pathologic fracture is affected by the number of other, non-osseous metastases and the primary tumour type. Ruggieri et al. noted that the occurrence of fracture negatively affects prognosis and quality of life of cancer patients (Ruggieri et al. 2010). They also suggested that a pathologic fracture within the upper extremities is associated with better prognosis than a pathologic fracture in the lower extremities (Ruggieri et al. 2010). In a large analysis of 619 patients with metastatic involvement to the spine or to the extremities, the presence of complete pathologic fracture was shown to hinder prognosis ($p = 0.03$) (Wedin 2001).

4.3 Neuropathic Pain from Bone Metastases

Neuropathic pain can be defined by certain characteristics. First, it is pain that does not correlate to an area of disease or damage and can be explained by impingement or damage to neural structure. Second, neuropathic pain is usually described as a burning or prickling sensation or a shooting or stabbing-like sensation. Third, the pain is usually associated with abnormal autonomic, sensory, or motor functions (Grond et al. 1999).

Neuropathic pain has been previously described as being difficult to palliate and can be resistant to opioids (Kerba et al. 2010). For neuropathic pain to be due to bone metastases, the metastases would have to be close by so that it can aggravate or compress the nerve involved, either mechanically or chemically (Kerba et al. 2010; Dennis et al. 2011b). A survey conducted by Kerba et al. to assess the prevalence of neuropathic pain in cancer patients found that approximately 17 % of patients experienced neuropathic pain (Kerba et al. 2010). Neuropathic pain is considered a complication of bone metastases due to its negative impact on quality of life and functional ability of patients (Urch and Dickenson 2008).

4.3.1 Treatment

Common treatments for neuropathic pain include antidepressants, corticosteroids, opioids, and radiation (Grond et al. 1999; Roos et al. 2005). Previous literature has revealed that approximately 60 % of patients treated with radiation to bone experience pain relief due to the treatment; however, there lacks distinction between neuropathic bone pain and non-neuropathic bone pain. There is currently a paucity of evidence on the efficacy and recommended dosage of radiotherapy for exclusively bone metastases-induced neuropathic pain, as well as on specific prognostic factors in this patient population. There has been only one study on the efficacy of different dose fractionation schedules for the palliation of neuropathic pain caused by bone metastases (Roos et al. 2005). Roos et al. found that a dose fractionation schedule of 8 Gy in one fraction cannot be conclusively determined to be just as effective as 20 Gy in five fractions; however, a conclusion that 8 Gy in one fraction performed worse than 20 Gy in five fractions could not be drawn as well (Roos et al. 2005). As such, the efficacy of single treatment versus protracted treatment for palliation of neuropathic pain caused by bone metastases still seems to be inconclusive. It is suggested that a single fraction of 8 Gy should be considered for patients with shorter prognosis and decreased performance status (Chow et al. 2012; Lo et al. 2010).

4.4 Recurrence of Bone Metastasis

The predictive risk factors for recurrence of bone metastasis correspond to the risks for initial bone metastasis. Factors associated with higher rates of metastatic recurrence include higher numbers of involved lymph nodes, larger tumour size, and estrogen receptor expression in breast cancer patients. Bisphosphonates can offer an effective adjuvant therapy to reduce recurrence of bone metastases in breast cancer patients. Further research is needed to identify additional predictive factors for recurrence of bone metastases, both in general and site-specific cases.

5 Closing Remarks

Radiotherapy for bone metastases patients is a seemingly simple science but consists of a sophisticated art. This chapter contains important information that should be considered in the delivery of treatment tailored to the individual patient that is based on a variety of clinical and socio-demographic factors.

References

Abrahm JL, Banffy MB, Harris MB (2008) Spinal cord compression in patients with advanced metastatic cancer. J Am Med Assoc 299(8):937–946

Akimoto S et al (1999) Inability of bone turnover marker as a strong prognostic indicator in prostate cancer patients with bone metastasis: comparison with the extent of disease (EOD) grade. Prostate 38:28–34

Ali SM, Demers LM, Leitzel K, Harvey HA, Clemens D, Mallinak N et al (2004) Baseline serum NTx levels are prognostic in metastatic breast cancer patients with bone-only metastasis. Ann Oncol 15(3):455–459

Altundag MB, Ucer AR, Calikoglu T, Guran Z (2002) Single (500 cGy, 800 cGy) and multifraction (300 X 10 cGy) radiotherapy schedules in the treatment of painful bone metastases. Turk J Hematol Oncol 12:16–21

Amouzegar-Hashemi F, Behrouzi H, Kazemian A et al (2008) Single versus multiple fractions of palliative radiotherapy for bone metastases: a randomized clinical trial in Iranian patients. Curr Oncol 15:151

Bae HM, Lee SH, Kim TM, Kim DW, Yang SC, Wu HG, Kim YW, Heo DS (2012) Prognostic factors for non-small cell lung cancer with bone metastasis at the time of diagnosis. Lung Cancer 77(3):572–577

Basch E, Prestrud AA, Hesketh PJ et al (2011) Antiemetics: American Society of Clinical Oncology clinical practice guideline update. J Clin Oncol 29(31):4189–4198

Berruti A, Cook R, Saad F, Buttigliero C, Lipton A, Tampellini M et al (2012) Prognostic role of serum parathyroid hormone levels in advanced prostate cancer patients undergoing zoledronic acid administration. Oncologist 17(5):645–652

Bone Pain Trial Working Party (1999) 8 Gy single fraction radiotherapy for the treatment of metastatic skeletal pain: randomized comparison with multi-fraction schedule over 12 months of patient follow-up. Radiother Oncol 52(2):111–121

Brasso K, Christensen IJ, Johansen JS, Teisner B, Garnero P, Price PA et al (2006) Prognostic value of PINP, bone alkaline phosphatase, CTX-I, and YKL-40 in patients with metastatic prostate carcinoma. Prostate 66(5):503–513

Brown JE, Cook RJ, Major P et al (2005) Bone turnover markers as predictors of skeletal complications in prostate cancer, lung cancer, and other solid tumors. J Natl Cancer Inst 97:59–69

Brown JE, Cook RJ, Lipton A, Coleman RE (2012) Serum lactate dehydrogenase is prognostic for survival in patients with bone metastases from breast cancer: a retrospective analysis in bisphosphonate-treated patients. Clin Cancer Res 18(22):6348–6355

Chow E, Fung KW, Panzarella T, Bezjak A, Danjoux C, Tannock I (2002) A predictive model for survival in metastatic cancer patients attending an outpatient palliative radiotherapy clinic. Int J Radiat Oncol Biol Phys 53(5):1291–1302

Chow E, Harris K, Fan G, Tsao M, Sze WM (2007) Palliative radiotherapy trials for bone metastases: a systematic review. J Clin Oncol 25(11):1423–1436

Chow E, Abdolell M, Panzarella T, Harris K, Bezjak A, Warde P, Tannock I (2008) Predictive model for survival in patients with advanced cancer. J Clin Oncol 26(36):5863–5869

Chow E, Abdolell M, Panzarella T, Harris K, Bezjak A, Warde P, Tannock I (2009) Validation of a predictive model for survival in metastatic cancer patients attending an outpatient palliative radiotherapy clinic. Int J Radiat Oncol Biol Phys 73(1):280–287

Chow E, Zeng L, Salvo N, Dennis K, Tsao M, Lutz S (2012) Update on the systemic review of palliative radiotherapy trials for bone metastases. Clin Oncol (R Coll Radiol) 24(2):112–124

Coates A, Abraham SK, Kaye SB (1983) On the receiving end: patient perception of the side effects of cancer chemotherapy. Eur J Cancer Clin Oncol 19:203

Cole D (1989) A randomized trial of a single treatment versus conventional fractionation in the palliative radiotherapy of painful bone metastases. Clin Oncol 1:59–62

Coleman RE (1997) Skeletal complications of malignancy. Cancer 80(8 Suppl):1588–1594

Coleman RE (2001) Metastatic bone disease: clinical features, pathophysiology and treatment strategies. Cancer Treat Rev 27:165–176

Coleman R, Rubens R (1987) The clinical course of bone metastases in breast cancer. Br J Cancer 77:336–340

Coleman RE, Smith P, Rubens RD (1998) Clinical course and prognostic factors following bone recurrence from breast cancer. Br J Cancer 77(2):336–340

Crawford E, Eisenberger M, McLeod K (1989) A controlled trial of leuprolide with and without flutamide in prostatic carcinoma. N Engl J Med 321:419–424

Danjoux CE, Rider WD, Fitzpatrick PJ (1979) The acute radiation syndrome. A memorial to William Michael Court-Brown. Clin Radiol 30:581–584

Dennis K, Maranzano E, De Angelis C et al (2011a) Radiotherapy-induced nausea and vomiting. Exp Rev Pharmacoecon Outcomes Res 11:685–692

Dennis K, Chow E, Roos D, DeAngelis C, Hartsell W, van der Linden Y, Hoskin P (2011b) Should bone metastases causing neuropathic pain be treated with single-dose radiotherapy? Clin Oncol 23(7):482–484
Eisenberger M, Crawford E, Wolf M (1994) Prognostic factors in stage D2 prostate cancer: important implications for future trials. Semin Oncol 21:613–619
El-Shenshawy H, Kandeel A, El-Essawy S (2006) The effect of a single fraction compared to multiple fractions radiotherapy on painful bone metastases with evaluation of computed tomography bone density in osteolytic bone metastases. Bull Alex Fac Med 42:439
Enblom A, Bergius AB, Steineck G, Hammar M, Borjeson S (2009) One third of patients with radiotherapy-induced nausea consider their antiemetic treatment insufficient. Support Care Cancer 17(1):23–32
Feyer PC, Stewart AL, Titlbach OJ (1998) Aetiology and prevention of emesis induced by radiotherapy. Support Care Cancer 6(3):253–260
Feyer PC, Maranzano E, Molassiotis A, Roila F, Clark-Snow RA, Jordan K (2011) Radiotherapy-induced nausea and vomiting (RINV): MASCC/ESMO guideline for antiemetics in radiotherapy: update 2009. Support Care Cancer 19(Suppl. 1):S5–S14
Foro P, Algara M, Reig A et al (1998) Randomized prospective trial comparing three schedules of palliative radiotherapy. Preliminary results. Oncologia 21:55–60
Foro P, Fontanals AV, Galceran JC et al (2008) Randomized clinical trial with two palliative radiotherapy regimens in painful bone metastases: 30 Gy in 10 fractions compared with 8 Gy in single fraction. Radiother Oncol 89:150–155
Galasko CSB (1986) Skeletal metastases. Butterworths, London
Gaze MN, Kelly CG, Kerr GR et al (1997) Pain relief and quality of life following radiotherapy for bone metastases: a randomized trial of two fractionation schedules. Radiother Oncol 45:109–116
Grond S, Radbruch L, Meuser T, Sabatowski R, Loick G, Lehmann KA (1999) Assessment and treatment of neuropathic cancer pain following WHO guidelines. Pain 79(1):15–20
Hamouda WE, Roshdy W, Teema M (2007) Single versus conventional fractionated radiotherapy in the palliation of painful bone metastases. Gulf J Oncol 1:35–41
Harada H, Katagiri H, Kamata M, Yoshioka Y, Asakura H, Hashimoto T, Furutani K, Takahashi M, Sakahara H, Nishimura T (2010) Radiological response and clinical outcome in patients with femoral bone metastases after radiotherapy. J Radiat Res 51(2):131–136
Harrington KD (1988) Prophylactic management of impending fractures. In: Harrington KD (ed) Orthopaedic management of metastatic bone disease. CV Mosby, St. Louis
Hartsell W et al (2005) Randomized trial of short versus long-course radiotherapy for palliation of painful bone metastases. J Natl Cancer Inst 97:798–804
Hatse S, Lambrechts D, Verstuyf A, Smeets A, Brouwers B, Vandorpe T et al (2012) Vitamin D status at breast cancer diagnosis: correlation with tumor characteristics, disease outcome, and genetic determinants of vitamin D insufficiency. Carcinogenesis 33(7):1319–1326
Holt T, Hoskin P, Maranzano E, Sahgal A, Schild SE, Ryu S, Loblaw A (2012) Malignant epidural spinal cord compression: the role of external beam radiotherapy. Curr Opin Support Palliat Care 6(1):103–108
Iordanidou L, Trivizaki E, Saranti S et al (2006) Is there a role of whole body bone scan in early stages of non small cell lung cancer patients. J Buon 11:491–497
Izumi K, Mizokami A, Itai S, Shima T, Shigehara K, Miwa S et al (2012) Increases in bone turnover marker levels at an early phase after starting zoledronic acid predicts skeletal-related events in patients with prostate cancer with bone metastasis. BJU Int 109(3):394–400
Jarvis GK, Northcott HC (1987) Religion and differences in morbidity and mortality. Soc Sci Med 25:813–824
Jawad MU, Scully SP (2010) In brief: classifications in brief: Mirels' classification: metastatic disease in long bones and impending pathologic fracture. Clin Orthop Relat Res 468(10):2825–2827
Jung K, Lein M, Stephan C, Von Hosslin K, Semjonow A, Sinha P et al (2004) Comparison of 10 serum bone turnover markers in prostate carcinoma patients with bone metastatic spread: diagnostic and prognostic implications. Int J Cancer 111(5):783–791
Kaasa S, Brenne E, Lund J et al (2006) Prospective randomized multicentre trial on single fraction radiotherapy (8 Gy X 1) versus multiple fractions (3 Gy X 10) in the treatment of painful bone metastases: Phase III randomized trial. Radiother Oncol 79:278–284
Kagei K, Suzuki K, Shirato H et al (1990) A randomized trial of single and multifraction radiation therapy for bone metastasis: a preliminary report. Gan No Rinsho 36:2553–2558
Kerba M, Wu JS, Duan Q, Hagen NA, Bennett MI (2010) Neuropathic pain features in patients with bone metastases referred for palliative radiotherapy. J Clin Oncol 28(33):4892–4897
Komatsu T, Kunieda E, Oizumi Y, Tamai Y, Akiba T (2012) An analysis of the survival rate after radiotherapy in lung cancer patients with bone metastasis: is there an optimal subgroup to be treated with high-dose radiation therapy? Neoplasma 59(6):650–657
Kwok Y, Regine WF, Patchell RA (2005) Radiation therapy alone for spinal cord compression: time to improve upon a relatively ineffective status quo. J Clin Oncol 23(15):3308–3310
Landis S et al (1999) Cancer statistics. CA Cancer J Clin 49:8–29
Lipton A, Chapman JA, Demers L, Shepherd LE, Han L, Wilson CF et al (2011) Elevated bone turnover predicts for bone metastasis in postmenopausal breast cancer: results of NCIC CTG MA. 14. J Clin Oncol 29(27):3605–3610
Llobera J, Esteva M, Rifa J et al (2000) Terminal cancer: duration and prediction of survival time. Eur J Cancer 36:2036–2043
Lo SS, Holden L, Lutz ST, Liu RK, Chow E (2010) Should all patients with uncomplicated bone metastases be treated with a single 8-gy fraction? Exp Rev Pharmacoecon Outcomes Res 10(2):95–98
Loblaw DA, Perry J, Chambers A, Laperriere NJ (2005) Systematic review of the diagnosis and management of malignant extradural spinal cord compression: the cancer care Ontario practice guidelines initiative's neuro-oncology disease site group. J Clin Oncol 23(9):2028–2037
Maltoni M, Caraceni A, Brunelli C et al (2005) Prognostic factors in advanced cancer patients: evidence-based clinical recommendations—a study by the steering committee of the European Association for Palliative Care. J Clin Oncol 23:6340–6348
Maranzano E, Bellavita R, Rossi R, DeAngelis V, Frattegiani A, Bagnoli R et al (2005) Short-course versus split-course radiotherapy in metastatic spinal cord compression: results of a phase III, randomized, multicenter trial. J Clin Oncol 23(15):3358–3365
Maranzano E, De Angelis V, Pergolizzi S et al (2010) A prospective observational trial on emesis in radiotherapy: analysis of 1020 patients recruited in 45 Italian radiation oncology centres. Radiother Oncol 94(1):36–41
Matzkin H, Perito P, Soloway M (1993) Prognostic factors in metastatic prostate cancer. Cancer 72(suppl 12):3788–3792
Morris PG, Ulaner GA, Eaton A et al (2012) Standardized uptake value by position emission tomography/computed tomography as a prognostic variable in metastatic breast cancer. Cancer 118(22):5454–5462
Nielson O et al (1998) Randomized trial of single dose versus fractionated palliative radiotherapy of bone metastases. Radiother Oncol 47:233–240

Ozsaran Z, Yalman D, Anacek Y et al (2001) Palliative radiotherapy in bone metastases: results of a randomized trial comparing three fractionation schedules. J Buon 6:43–48

Perez JE, Machiavelli M, Leone BA, Romero A, Rabinovich MG, Vallejo CT, Bianco A, Rodriguez R, Cuevas MA, Alvarez LA (1990) Bone-only versus visceral-only metastatic pattern in breast cancer: analysis of 150 patients. Am J Clin Oncol 13:294–298

Phillips DP, Smith DG (1990) Postponement of death until symbolically meaningful occasions. J Am Med Assoc 263:1947–1951

Plunkett TA, Rubens RD (2005) Clinical features and prognosis of bone metastases. In: Jasmin C, Coleman RE, Coia LR, Capanna R, Saillant G (eds) Textbook of bone metastases. Wiley, Chichester

Popovic M et al (2012) Comparing prognostic factors in patients with spinal metastases: a literature review. Exp Rev Pharmacoecon Outcomes Res 12(3):345–356

Price P, Hoskin PJ, Easton D et al (1986) Prospective randomized trial of single and multifraction radiotherapy schedules in the treatment of painful bony metastases. Radiother Oncol 6:247–255

Priestman TJ, Priestman SG (1984) An initial evaluation of Nabilone in the control of radiotherapy-induced nausea and vomiting. Clin Radiol 35(4):265–266

Priestman TJ, Roberts JT, Lucraft H et al (1990) Results of a randomized, double-blind comparative study of ondansetron and metoclopramide in the prevention of nausea and vomiting following high-dose upper abdominal irradiation. Clin Oncol 2(2):71–75

Rades D, Abrahm JL (2010) The role of radiotherapy for metastatic epidural spinal cord compression. Nat Rev Clin Oncol 7(10):590–598

Rades D, Fehlauer F, Schulte R, Veninga T, Stalpers LJ, Basic H et al (2006) Prognostic factors for local control and survival after radiotherapy of metastatic spinal cord compression. J Clin Oncol 24(21):3388–3393

Rades D, Rudat V, Veninga T, Stalpers LJ, Basic H, Karstens JH et al (2008) A score predicting post treatment ambulatory status in patients irradiated for metastatic spinal cord compression. Int J Radiat Oncol Biol Phys 72(3):905–908

Reuben DB, Mor V, Hiris J (1988) Clinical symptoms and length of survival in patients with terminal cancer. Arch Intern Med 148:1586–1591

Robson M, Dawson N (1996) How is androgen-dependent metastatic prostate cancer best treated? Hemat Oncol Clin North Am 10:727–747

Roos D et al (2005) Randomized trial of 8 Gy in 1 versus 20 Gy in 5 fractions of radiotherapy for neuropathic pain due to bone metastases (Trans-Tasman Radiation Oncology Group, TROG 96.05). Radiother Oncol 75:54–63

Rosen LS, Gordon D, Tchekmedyian S et al (2003) Zoledronic acid versus placebo in the treatment of skeletal metastases in patients with lung cancer and other solid tumors: a phase III, double-blind, randomized trial—the Zoledronic Acid Lung Cancer and Other Solid Tumors Study Group. J Clin Oncol 21:3150–3157

Ruggieri P, Mavrogenis AF, Casadei R, Errani C, Angelini A, Calabro T (2010) Protocol of surgical treatment of long bone pathologic fractures. Injury 41(11):1161–1167

Sabbatini P et al (1999) Prognostic significance of extent of disease in bone in patients with androgen-independent prostate cancer. J Clin Oncol 17:948–957

Sandler A, Gray R, Perry MC et al (2006) Paclitaxel-carboplatin alone or with bevacizumab for non-small-cell lung cancer. N Engl J Med 355:2542–2550

Sarkar SK, Sarkar S, Pahari B et al (2002) Multiple and single fraction palliative radiotherapy in bone secondaries: a prospective study. Ind J Radiol Imag 12:281–284

Schoenbach VJ, Kaplan BH, Fredman L et al (1986) Social ties and mortality in Evans County, Georgia. Am J Epidemiol 123:577–591

Sejpal SV, Bhate A, Small W (2007) Palliative radiation therapy in the management of brain metastases, spinal cord compression, and bone metastases. Semin Intervent Radiol 24(4):363–374

Shaham D, Breuer R, Copel L et al (2006) Computed tomography screening for lung cancer: applicability of an international protocol in a single-institution environment. Clin Lung Cancer 7:262–267

Shiue K, Sahgal A, Chow E, Lutz ST, Chang EL, Mayr NA et al (2010) Management of metastatic spinal cord compression. Expert Rev Anticancer Ther 10(5):697–708

Solomayer EF, Diel IJ, Meyberg GC, Gollan Ch, Bastert G (2000) Metastatic breast cancer: clinical course, prognosis and therapy related to the first site of metastases. Breast Cancer Res Treat 59:271–278

Soloway M, Hardeman S, Hickey D (1988) Stratification of patients with metastatic prostate cancer based on extent of disease on initial bone scan. Cancer 61:195–202

Steenland E et al (1999) The effect of a single fraction compared to multiple fractions on painful bone metastases: a global analysis of the Dutch Bone Metastasis Study. Radiother Oncol 52:101–109

The Italian Group for Antiemetic Research in Radiotherapy (1999) Radiation-induced emesis: a prospective observational multicenter Italian trial. Int J Radiat Oncol Biol Phys 44(3):619–625

Toscani F, Brunelli C (2005) Predicting survival in terminal cancer patients: clinical observation or quality-of-life evaluation? Palliat Med 19:220–227

Urch CE, Dickenson AH (2008) Neuropathic pain in cancer. Eur J Cancer 44(8):1091–1096

Wedin R (2001) Surgical treatment for pathologic fractures. Acta Orthop Scand 72(Suppl 302):1–29

Yamashita K, Ueda T, Komatsubara Y, Koyama H, Inaji H, Yonenobu K, Ono K (1991) Breast cancer with bone-only metastases: visceral metastases-free rate in relation to anatomic distribution of bone metastases. Cancer 68:634–637

Yamashita K, Ueda T, Komatsubara Y, Koyama H, Inaji H, Ono K, Yonenobu K (1992) A classification of bone metastases from breast cancer. In: Uchida A, Ono K (eds) Recent advances in musculoskeletal oncology. Springer, Berlin

Zhang L, Teng Y, Zhang Y et al (2012) Receptor activator for nuclear factor κ B expression predicts poor prognosis in breast cancer patients with bone metastasis but not in patients with visceral metastasis. J Clin Pathol 65:36–40

Index

C. Nieder and L. E. Gaspar (eds.), *Decision Tools for Radiation Oncology*, Medical Radiology. Radiation Oncology,
DOI: 10.1007/978-3-642-37102-8, © Springer-Verlag Berlin Heidelberg 2014

Printing and Binding: Stürtz GmbH, Würzburg